# THE
## DICTIONARY OF
# SODIUM,
# FATS, AND
# CHOLESTEROL
## Second Edition

# THE DICTIONARY OF
# SODIUM, FATS, AND CHOLESTEROL

## Second Edition

## BY BARBARA KRAUS

A PERIGEE BOOK

In memory of Mary V. Reilly

Perigee Books
are published by
The Putnam Publishing Group
200 Madison Avenue
New York, NY 10016

Library of Congress Cataloging-in-Publication Data

Kraus, Barbara.
  The dictionary of sodium, fats, and cholesterol / by Barbara
Kraus.—2nd ed.
    p.   cm.
  "A Perigee book."
  Includes bibliographical references.
    1. Food—Sodium content—Tables.   2. Food—Cholesterol content—
Tables.   3. Food—Fat content—Tables.   I. Title.
TX553.S65K7425   1990                89-35280 CIP
641.1′021—dc20
ISBN 0-399-51572-0

Printed in the United States of America
    2   3   4   5   6   7   8   9   10

This book is printed on acid-free paper.

# CONTENTS

# INTRODUCTION

This dictionary lists the total fat, saturated and unsaturated fatty acids, cholesterol, and sodium content of several thousand food items. These nutrients have been receiving increasing attention by nutritionists and the medical profession because of their possible relationship to atherosclerosis (coronary heart disease). Of course, diet is not the only factor to be considered in heart disease. Other considerations are heredity, obesity, high blood pressure, blood cholesterol, blood lipids, cigarette smoking, lack of exercise, stress, and certain ailments such as diabetes.

Patients with coronary disease and high blood pressure are often placed on diets in which one or more of these nutrients is controlled. Since physicians now believe that the conditions leading to early heart attacks are the result of a lifetime of habits that predispose individuals to such attacks, they recommend that certain changes in dietary patterns be made also in early childhood.

## Total Fat

The caloric intake from fat is often as much as 45 to 50 percent of the American diet. In the past 25 years, the consumption of fats and oils alone has increased, on the average, about 20 percent. In the same period, Americans have consumed over 18 percent more meat, which is also high in fat content. It is now frequently recommended that only about one-third of the calories be from fat, and of this amount, about two-thirds should be from polyunsaturated and monounsaturated fatty acids, amounting to approximately 10 to 15 percent of the diet.

Some fat in the diet is essential. It is used in the body to supply energy, yielding about nine calories per gram, more than twice as much as either protein or carbohydrate (the other energy-yielding nutrients in foods), which each supply about four calories per gram. Fat is also important in supplying essential fatty acids (those that cannot be synthesized by the body) and in the supply and utilization of fat soluble vitamins A, D, E, and K. Fat adds flavor and satiety value to otherwise bulky and bland diets.

## Fatty Acids

Fats are composed of "saturated" and "unsaturated" fatty acids. In scientific terms, they are saturated if the carbon atoms contain all the hydrogen they can hold. If there is one double bond where hydrogen can be added, the fat is monounsaturated; if there are two or more, the fat is polyunsaturated. In layman's terms: if the fat is solid at room temperature it is saturated, if liquid, it is unsaturated. This is a very rough rule of thumb and there are exceptions to it. Most foods contain both kinds of fat in varying proportions. Oils from plant foods and fish contain the most abundant amounts of polyunsaturated fats. Coconut oil is an exception. It is high in saturated fatty acids and is solid at room temperature.

Meats, cheeses, eggs, and most animal products are high in saturated fatty acids. The listings in this book showing the values for unsaturated fatty acids include both mono and polyunsaturated fats. At this time, the available information for many foods is not adequate to give a breakdown between these two forms. New federal requirements for labeling commercial products will result in more complete information in the future, and later editions of this book will incorporate such values.

Since the values for saturated and unsaturated fats are rounded to the nearest whole number they may add up to more or less than the figure given for total fat. In many cases, the values for unsaturated fat were derived by the subtraction of the saturated from the total fats. In a very few cases, manufacturers reported analyzed saturated and unsaturated fats which did not add up to the total fat shown, because the undetermined fatty acids were, in their opinion, not present in significant amounts.

# Cholesterol

Cholesterol is one of the complex compounds known as sterols. It is an essential nutrient in normal metabolic processes and is synthesized in the body. It is also present in many foods of animal origin that we consume. Plant foods do not contain cholesterol in any significant amounts. Foods such as chocolate, cocoa, olive oil, coconut butter, and peanut butter are devoid of it since they are plant products.

Animal products are generally high in cholesterol. Organ and glandular meats such as brains, kidney, liver, sweetbreads, and heart are especially high in cholesterol. Egg yolk contains high concentrations of cholesterol, but it is absent in the white.

Cholesterol occurs in both the lean portions and the fatty portions of meat; the removal of fatty tissue if replaced by an equal amount of lean does not reduce the cholesterol intake. This is unlike the effect on the amount of fatty acids and must be taken into account in planning low cholesterol diets.

# Sodium

Sodium is an essential element in the growth of animals. It occurs naturally in many foods but the principle source in diets is sodium chloride or ordinary table salt. Salt is used in the processing of many foods in freezing, canning, and other manufacturing methods. It is also added in the home in cooking and at the table.

For some people, the use of salt is excessive and low-sodium diets are prescribed by physicians. Low-sodium diets are used in the treatment of diseases such as cardiac failure, edema formation, and high blood pressure.

# Summary

Always keep in mind that in making any drastic changes in dietary habits the advice and guidance of a competent physician should be sought. It is an essential of good health that the diet contain all the nutrients required by the individual and in adequate amounts. Reductions or increases in one or more of the essential nutrients may bring about adverse effects.

The tables given here are intended to provide basic information to help plan a varied and attractive diet within broad guidelines that are nutritionally adequate when one or more of the nutrients must be controlled.

## ARRANGEMENT OF THIS BOOK

Foods are listed alphabetically by brand name or by the name of the food. The singular form is used for the entries, that is, blackberry instead of blackberries. Most items are listed individually although a few are grouped (see p. 11). For example, all candies are listed together so that if you are looking for *Mars* bar, you look first under Candy, then under *M* in alphabetical order. But, if you are looking for a breakfast food such as Oatmeal, you will find it under *O* in the main alphabet. Many cross references are included to assist you in finding items known by different names.

Under the main headings, it was often not possible nor even desirable to follow an alphabetical arrangement. For basic foods, such as apricots, the first entries are for the fresh product weighed with seeds as it is purchased in the store, then the fruit in small portions as they may be eaten or measured. These entries are followed by the processed products, canned (although it may actually be a bottle or a jar), dehydrated, dried, and frozen items. This basic plan, with adaptations where necessary, was followed for fruits, vegetables, and meats.

In almost all entries, where data were available, the U.S. Department of Agriculture figures are shown first. The Department values represent averages from several manufacturers and are shown for comparison with the values from individual companies or for use where particular brands are not available.

All brand-name products have been italicized and company names appear in parentheses.

## Portions Used

The portion column is a most important one to read and note. Common household measures are used wherever possible. For some items, the amounts given are those commonly purchased in the store, such as one pound of meat, or a 15-ounce package of cake mix. These quantities can be divided into the number of servings used in the home and the nutritive values in each portion can then be readily determined. Any ingredients added in preparing such products must also be taken into account.

The smaller portions given are for foods as served or measured in moderate amounts, such as one-half cup of reconstituted juice, or four ounces of meat. Be sure to adjust the amount of the nutrients to the actual portions you use. For example, if you serve one cup of juice instead of one-half cup, multiply the amount of the nutrients shown for the smaller amount by two.

The size of portions you use is extremely important in controlling the intake of any nutrient. The amount of a nutrient is directly related to the weight of the food served. The weight of a volumetric measure, such as a cup or a pint may vary considerably depending on many factors; four ounces by weight may be very different from one-half cup or four fluid ounces. Ounces in the tables are always ounces by weight unless specified as fluid ounces, fractions of a cup, or other volumetric measure. Foods that are fluffy in texture such as flaked coconut and bean sprouts vary greatly in weight per cup, depending on how tightly they are packed. Such foods as canned green beans also vary when measured with and without liquid; for instance, canned beans with liquid weigh 4.2 ounces for one-half cup, but drained beans weigh 2.5 ounces for the same half cup. Check the weights of your serving portions regularly. Bear in mind that you can reduce or increase the intake of any nutrient by changing the serving size.

It was impossible to convert all the portions to a uniform basis. Some sources were able to report data only in terms of weights with no information on cup or other volumetric measures. We have shown small portions in quantities that might reasonably be expected to be served or measured in the home or institution.

You will find in the portion column the phrases "weighed with bone," and "weighed with skin and seeds." These descriptions apply to the products as you purchase them in the markets, but the nutritive values as shown are for the amount of edible food after you discard the bone, skin, seed, or other inedible part. The weight given in the "measure" or "quantity" column is to the nearest gram or fraction of an ounce.

Data on the composition of foods are constantly changing for many reasons. Better sampling and analytical methods, improvements in marketing procedures, and changes in formulas of mixed products may alter values for all of the nutrients. Weights of packaged foods are frequently changed. It is essential to read label information in order to be knowledgeable about these matters and to make intelligent use of food tables.

## Other Nutrients

These tables are not intended as a dietary guide. Any drastic change from a normal mixed diet should be undertaken only under the guidance of a qualified physician. Do not forget that other nutrients—protein, carbohydrate, minerals, and vitamins— are extremely important in diet planning. From a nutritional viewpoint, perhaps the best advice that can be given is to eat a varied diet with all classes of food represented. Meat, fish, chicken, fats and oils, milk, vegetables, fruits, and grain products are all important sources of essential nutrients and some foods from each of these classes should be included in the diet every day.

If your doctor has recommended the control of one or more of the nutrients shown in these tables, you can choose foods from this book under the doctor's guidance that will fit his specifications and will provide a varied selection of products that are acceptable. Control of certain nutrients such as cholesterol or sodium does not condemn you to a monotonous diet. There is a rich and varied assortment of foods in our markets that will meet any medical requirements. Choose wisely and eat well.

## Sources of Data

Values in this dictionary are based on publications issued by the U.S. Department of Agriculture and on data submitted by manufacturers and processors. The U.S.

Department of Agriculture issues basic tables on food composition for use in the United States. The commercial products from U.S.D.A. publications represent average values obtained on products of more than one company. The figures designated as "home recipe" are based on recipes on file with the Department of Agriculture. Data on commercial products listed by brand name in this publication are based on values supplied by manufacturers and processors for their own individual products. Supermarket brand names, such as the A & P's *Ann Page,* or private labels could not be included in this book inasmuch as they are not usually analyzed under these trade names. Every care has been taken to interpret the data and the descriptions supplied by the companies as fully and as accurately as possible. Many values have been recalculated to different portions from those submitted, in order to bring about greater uniformity among similar items.

Analysis of foods to provide information on nutritive values are extremely expensive to conduct. Many small companies cannot afford to have their products analyzed and were unable to provide data or were able to provide only a portion of the data requested. Other companies have simply never gotten around to having the analyses done. New requirements for labeling nutritive values for products may provide information on additional items in the future. Wherever data were unavailable blank spaces were left which may be filled in by the reader at a later time.

## Foods Listed by Groups

Foods in the following classes are reported together rather than as individual items in the main alphabet: baby food, bread, cake, cake icing, cake icing mix, cake mix, candy, cheese, cookies, cookie mix, crackers, gravy, pie, pudding & pie filling, salad dressing, sauce, soft drink, and soup.

BARBARA KRAUS

# ABBREVIATIONS AND SYMBOLS

(USDA) = United States Department
of Agriculture
* = prepared as packaging directs [1]
< = less than
> = more than
& = and
″ = inch
+ = values do not include amount
of sodium found in the local
water used in packaging
canned = bottles or jars as well as cans
dia. = diameter
DNA = data not available
fl. = fluid
liq. = liquid

lb. = pound
med. = medium
oz. = ounce
pkg. = package
pt. = pint
qt. = quart
sq. = square
T. = tablespoon
Tr. = trace
tsp. = teaspoon
wt. = weight
mg. = milligram
gr. = gram

Italics or name in parentheses = registered trademark, ®.
Where zero in parenthesis appears in the tabular column it means that (0) zero is imputed by author wherever there is a reasonable assumption that that nutrient is not present.

# EQUIVALENTS

| By Weight | By Volume |
|---|---|
| 1 pound = 16 ounces | 1 quart = 4 cups |
| 1 ounce = 28.35 grams | 1 cup = 8 fluid ounces |
| 3.52 ounces = 100 grams | 1 cup = ½ pint |
| 1 milligram = .001 gram | 1 cup = 16 tablespoons |
| | 2 tablespoons = 1 fluid ounce |
| | 1 tablespoon = 3 teaspoons |
| | 1 pound butter = 4 sticks or 2 cups |

[1]If the package directions call for whole or skim milk, the data given here are for whole milk, unless otherwise stated.

# THE DICTIONARY OF
# SODIUM, FATS, AND CHOLESTEROL

## Second Edition

| Food and Description | Measure or Quantity | Sodium (mg.) | Total | —Fats in grams—<br>Satu-<br>rated | Unsatu-<br>rated | Choles-<br>terol<br>(mg.) |
|---|---|---|---|---|---|---|

# A

**ABALONE** (USDA):
| | | | | | | |
|---|---|---|---|---|---|---|
| Raw, meat only | 4 oz. | | .6 | | | |
| Canned | 4 oz. | | .3 | | | |

**AC'CENT**
| | | | | | | |
|---|---|---|---|---|---|---|
| | ¼ tsp. (1 gram) | 129 | 0.0 | | | 0 |

**ACEROLA,** fresh (USDA):
| | | | | | | |
|---|---|---|---|---|---|---|
| Fruit | ½ lb. (weighed with seeds) | 15 | .6 | | | 0 |
| Juice | ½ cup (4.3 oz.) | 4 | .4 | | | 0 |

**ALBACORE,** raw, meat only
| | | | | | | |
|---|---|---|---|---|---|---|
| (USDA) | 4 oz. | 45 | 8.6 | 3. | 5. | |

**ALCOHOLIC BEVERAGES**
(See individual listings)

**ALEWIFE** (USDA):
| | | | | | | |
|---|---|---|---|---|---|---|
| Raw, meat only | 4 oz. | | 5.6 | | | |
| Canned, solids & liq. | 4 oz. | | 9.1 | | | |

**ALLSPICE** (Spice Islands):
| | | | | | | |
|---|---|---|---|---|---|---|
| Ground | 1 tsp. | 2 | | | | (0) |
| Whole | 1 tsp. | 1 | | | | (0) |

**ALMOND:**
In shell:
| | | | | | | |
|---|---|---|---|---|---|---|
| (USDA) | 4 oz. (weighed in shell) | 2 | 31.4 | 2. | 29. | 0 |
| (USDA) | 1 cup (2.8 oz.) | 2 | 21.7 | 2. | 20. | 0 |
| Shelled: | | | | | | |
| Plain, unsalted: | | | | | | |
| Whole (USDA) | 1 oz. | 1 | 15.4 | 1. | 14. | 0 |
| Whole (USDA) | 1 cup (5 oz.) | 6 | 77.0 | 6. | 71. | 0 |
| Whole (USDA) | 13-15 almonds (.6 oz.) | <1 | 9.5 | <1. | 9. | 0 |
| Chopped (USDA) | 1 cup (4.5 oz.) | 5 | 68.8 | 5. | 64. | 0 |
| (Blue Diamond) | 1 cup (5.6 oz.) | 6 | 83.8 | 10. | 74. | (0) |
| Blanched: | | | | | | |
| Salted (USDA) | 1 cup (5.5 oz.) | 311 | 90.6 | 8. | 83. | 0 |

(USDA): United States Department of Agriculture
*Prepared as Package Directs

17

| Food and Description | Measure or Quantity | Sodium (mg.) | Total | Fats in grams — Satu- rated | Unsatu- rated | Choles- terol (mg.) |
|---|---|---|---|---|---|---|
| Slivered (Blue Diamond) | 1 cup (5.6 oz.) | 6 | 86.2 | 10. | 76. | (0) |
| Chocolate-covered (See **CANDY**) | | | | | | |
| Flavored (Blue Diamond) barbecue, cheese, French-fried, onion-garlic or smokehouse-style | 1 oz. | 56 | | | | (0) |
| Roasted, salted: | | | | | | |
| (USDA) | 1 oz. | 56 | 16.4 | 1. | 15. | 0 |
| (USDA) | 1 cup (5.5 oz.) | 311 | 90.6 | 8. | 83. | 0 |
| (Fisher): | | | | | | |
| Dry roasted, smoked | 1 oz. | 220 | 14 | | | 0 |
| Honey roasted | 1 oz. | 75 | 14 | | | 0 |
| (Flavor-House) dry | 1 oz. | 56 | 16.4 | | | 0 |
| (Planters): | | | | | | |
| Dry roasted | 1 oz. | 200 | 15 | | | 0 |
| Smoked | 1 oz. | 170 | 15 | | | 0 |
| (Tom's) oil roasted | 1 oz. | 120 | 16 | | | 0 |
| **ALMOND MEAL,** partially defatted (USDA) | 1 oz. | 2 | 5.2 | Tr. | 5. | 0 |
| **ALPHABITS,** oat cereal (Post) | 1 cup (1 oz.) | 150 | 1.1 | | | 0 |
| **AMARANTH,** raw (USDA): | | | | | | |
| Untrimmed | 1 lb. (weighed untrimmed) | | 1.4 | | | 0 |
| Trimmed | 4 oz. | | .6 | | | 0 |
| **AMBROSIA,** chilled, bottled (Kraft) | 4 oz. | 115 | 2.4 | | | (0) |
| **A.M.,** fruit juice drink (Mott's) | ½ cup | | .1 | | | (0) |
| **ANCHOVY PASTE,** canned (Crosse & Blackwell) | 1 T. (.5 oz.) | 1,540 | .5 | | | |
| **ANCHOVY, PICKLED,** canned: (USDA) with or without added oil, not heavily salted | 1 oz. | | 2.9 | | | |

(USDA): United States Department of Agriculture
*Prepared as Package Directs

| Food and Description | Measure or Quantity | Sodium (mg.) | Total | Satu-rated | Unsatu-rated | Choles-terol (mg.) |
|---|---|---|---|---|---|---|
| | | | — Fats in grams — | | | |
| (Granadaisa) pickled | 1 oz. | 1,587 | 2.5 | | | |

**ANGEL FOOD CAKE,** (See **CAKE**, Angel Food)

**ANGEL FOOD CAKE MIX** (See **CAKE MIX,** Angel Food)

| | | | | | | |
|---|---|---|---|---|---|---|
| **ANISE SEED** (Spice Islands) | 1 tsp. | < 1 | | | | (0) |

**APPLE,** any variety:
Fresh (USDA):

| | | | | | | |
|---|---|---|---|---|---|---|
| Eaten with skin | 1 lb. (weighed with skin & core) | 4 | 2.5 | | | 0 |
| Eaten with skin | 1 med., 2½″ dia. (about 3 per lb.) | 1 | .8 | | | 0 |
| Eaten without skin | 1 lb. (weighed with skin & core) | 4 | 1.2 | | | 0 |
| Eaten without skin | 1 med., 2½″ dia. (about 3 per lb.) | 1 | .4 | | | 0 |
| Pared, diced | 1 cup (3.8 oz.) | 1 | .3 | | | 0 |
| Pared, quartered | 1 cup (4.3 oz.) | 1 | .4 | | | 0 |

Canned (See also **APPLESAUCE**):

| | | | | | | |
|---|---|---|---|---|---|---|
| (Comstock) rings | 1.1-oz. piece | 8 | .5 | | | |
| (Del Monte) uncooked, evaporated | 2 oz. | 57 | 1.0 | | | 0 |

(White House):

| | | | | | | |
|---|---|---|---|---|---|---|
| Rings, spiced | .5-oz. ring | 5 | 0.0 | | | 0 |
| Sliced | ½ cup (4 oz.) | 10 | 0.0 | | | 0 |

Dehydrated:

| | | | | | | |
|---|---|---|---|---|---|---|
| Uncooked (USDA) | 1 oz. | 2 | .6 | | | 0 |
| Cooked, sweetened (USDA) | ½ cup (4.2 oz.) | 1 | .4 | | | 0 |

Dried:

| | | | | | | |
|---|---|---|---|---|---|---|
| Uncooked (USDA) | 1 cup (3 oz.) | 4 | 1.4 | | | 0 |
| Uncooked (Del Monte) | 1 cup (3 oz.) | 75 | 1.6 | | | 0 |
| Cooked, unsweetened (USDA) | ½ cup (4.3 oz.) | 1 | .6 | | | 0 |
| Cooked, sweetened (USDA) | ½ cup (4.9 oz.) | 1 | .6 | | | 0 |

(USDA): United States Department of Agriculture
*Prepared as Package Directs

| Food and Description | Measure or Quantity | Sodium (mg.) | Fats in grams — Total | Satu- rated | Unsatu- rated | Choles- terol (mg.) |
|---|---|---|---|---|---|---|
| Frozen, sweetened, slices, not thawed (USDA) | 4 oz. | 16 | .1 | | | 0 |
| **APPLE BROWN BETTY,** home recipe (USDA)[1] | 1 cup (8.1 oz.) | 352 | 8.0 | 2. | 6. | |
| **APPLE BUTTER:** | | | | | | |
| (USDA) | ½ cup (5 oz.) | 3 | 1.1 | | | 0 |
| (USDA) | 1 T. (.6 oz.) | <1 | .1 | | | 0 |
| (Bama) | 1 T. (.6 oz.) | 1 | <.1 | | | (0) |
| (Smucker's) spiced | 1 T. (.6 oz.) | 4 | .1 | | | (0) |
| **APPLE-CHERRY BERRY DRINK,** canned | | | | | | |
| (Lincoln) | 6 fl. oz. | 30 | 0 | | | 0 |
| **APPLE CIDER** (USDA) | ½ cup (4.4 oz.) | 1 | Tr. | | | 0 |
| **APPLE-CRANBERRY JUICE DRINK:** | | | | | | |
| Canned: | | | | | | |
| (Hi-C) | 6 fl. oz. | 23 | Tr. | | | |
| (Mott's): | | | | | | |
| Aseptic carton | 8.45-fl.-oz. cont. | 24 | 0.0 | | | |
| Can | 9.5-fl.-oz. can | 27 | 0.0 | | | |
| Glass jar | 6-fl.-oz. serving | 24 | 0.0 | | | |
| *Mix (Hi-C) | 6 fl. oz. | 11 | Tr. | | | |
| **APPLE DRINK:** | | | | | | |
| Canned: | | | | | | |
| (USDA) | ½ cup (4.4 oz.) | 1 | Tr. | | | 0 |
| (Johanna Farms) | ½ cup | 1 | 0.0 | | | 0 |
| (Mott's) sweet | ½ cup | Tr. | 0 | | | 0 |
| (Tree Top) | 6 fl. oz. | 10 | 0 | | | 0 |
| *Mix (Country Time) | 8 fl. oz. | 94 | 0 | | | 0 |
| **APPLE DUMPLING,** frozen | | | | | | |
| (Pepperidge Farm) | 1 dumpling (3.3 oz.) | 206 | 16.4 | | | |
| **APPLE, ESCALLOPED:** | | | | | | |
| Canned (White House) | ½ cup (4.5 oz.) | 60 | 1 | | | |
| Frozen (Stouffer's) | 4-oz. serving | 50 | 3 | | | |

(USDA): United States Department of Agriculture
*Prepared as Package Directs
[1]Principal sources of fat: butter, bread crumbs.

| Food and Description | Measure or Quantity | Sodium (mg.) | — Fats in grams — | | | Choles- terol (mg.) |
|---|---|---|---|---|---|---|
| | | | Total | Satu- rated | Unsatu- rated | |

**APPLE-GRAPE JUICE,** canned:
| | | | | | | |
|---|---|---|---|---|---|---|
| (Mott's) | 6 fl. oz. | 17 | 0.0 | | | |
| (Red Cheek) | 6 fl. oz. | 9 | 0.0 | | | |

***APPLE JACKS,*** cereal
| | | | | | | |
|---|---|---|---|---|---|---|
| (Kellogg's) | 1 cup (1 oz.) | 68 | .2 | | | (0) |

**APPLE JELLY:**
Regular:
| | | | | | | |
|---|---|---|---|---|---|---|
| (Bama) | 1 T. | 7 | 0.0 | | | 0 |
| (Home Brands) | 1 T. | 7 | 0.0 | | | 0 |

Dietetic:
| | | | | | | |
|---|---|---|---|---|---|---|
| (Diet Delight) | 1 T. | 25 | 0.0 | | | 0 |
| (Estee) | 1 T. | <3 | 0.0 | | | 0 |
| (Featherweight) | 1 T. | 40-50 | 0.0 | | | 0 |
| (Louis Sherry) | 1 T. | <3 | 0.0 | | | 0 |

**APPLE JUICE:**
Canned:
| | | | | | | |
|---|---|---|---|---|---|---|
| (USDA) | ½ cup (4.3 oz.) | 1 | Tr. | | | 0 |
| (Borden's) *Sippin' Pak* | 8.45-fl.-oz. cont. | 25 | 0.0 | | | (0) |
| (Johanna Farms): | | | | | | |
| Florida citrus | 10 fl. oz. | 5 | Tr. | | | (0) |
| *Tree-Ripe* | 8.45-fl.-oz. cont. | 2 | Tr. | | | (0) |
| (Minute Maid) | 6 fl. oz. | 2 | Tr. | | | (0) |
| (Mott's) | 6 fl. oz. | 13 | 0.0 | | | (0) |
| (Ocean Spray) | 6 fl. oz. | 14 | 0.0 | | | (0) |
| (Red Cheek): | | | | | | |
| Natural | 6 fl. oz. | 16 | 0.0 | | | (0) |
| 100% pure | 6 fl. oz. | 7 | 0.0 | | | (0) |
| (Thank You Brand): | | | | | | |
| Regular | 6 fl. oz. | 37 | 0.0 | | | (0) |
| With vitamin C | 6 fl. oz. | 28 | 0.0 | | | (0) |
| (Tree Top) regular | 6 fl. oz. | 10 | 0.0 | | | (0) |
| (White House) | 6 fl. oz. | 5 | 0.0 | | | (0) |
| Chilled (Minute Maid) | 6 fl. oz. | 2 | Tr. | | | (0) |
| *Frozen: | | | | | | |
| (Minute Maid) | 6 fl. oz. | 2 | Tr. | | | (0) |
| (Tree Top) regular | 6 fl. oz. | 10 | 0.0 | | | (0) |

**APPLE PIE** (See **PIE,** Apple)

(USDA): United States Department of Agriculture
*Prepared as Package Directs

| Food and Description | Measure or Quantity | Sodium (mg.) | Fats in grams — Total | Satu- rated | Unsatu- rated | Choles- terol (mg.) |
|---|---|---|---|---|---|---|
| **APPLE PIE FILLING** (See **PIE FILLING,** Apple) | | | | | | |
| **APPLE RAISIN CRISP,** cereal | | | | | | |
| (Kellogg's) | 1 cup (1 oz.) | 200 | 0.0 | | | |
| **APPLESAUCE,** canned: | | | | | | |
| Sweetened: | | | | | | |
| (USDA) | ½ cup (4.5 oz.) | 3 | .1 | | | 0 |
| (Comstock) | ½ cup (4.4 oz.) | 90 | 0.0 | | | (0) |
| (Del Monte) | ½ cup (4 oz.) | <5 | 0.0 | | | (0) |
| (Hunt's) *Snack-Pak* | 4.25-oz. container | 0 | 0.0 | | | (0) |
| (Mott's): | | | | | | |
| Jarred: | | | | | | |
| Regular or cinnamon | 6 oz. | <1 | 0.0 | | | (0) |
| Chunky | 6 oz. | 11 | 0.0 | | | (0) |
| Single-serve cups: | | | | | | |
| Regular or cinnamon | 4-oz. container | <1 | 0.0 | | | (0) |
| Cherry | 3.75-oz. container | 8 | 0.0 | | | (0) |
| Peach | 4-oz. container | 7 | 0.0 | | | (0) |
| Pineapple | 3.75-oz. container | 2 | 0.0 | | | (0) |
| Strawberry | 3.75-oz. container | 10 | 0.0 | | | (0) |
| (Thank You Brand) | ½ cup (4.5 oz.) | 26 | 0.0 | | | (0) |
| (Tree Top) any type | ½ cup | Tr. | 0.0 | | | (0) |
| (White House) | ½ cup (5 oz.) | 5 | 0.0 | | | (0) |
| Unsweetened, dietetic or low calorie: | | | | | | |
| (USDA) | ½ cup (4.3 oz.) | 2 | .2 | | | 0 |
| (Del Monte) *Lite* | ½ cup (4 oz.) | <10 | 0.0 | | | (0) |
| (Diet Delight) | ½ cup (4.3 oz.) | 5 | 0.0 | | | (0) |
| (Mott's): | | | | | | |
| Jarred | 6 oz. | 3 | 0.0 | | | (0) |
| Single-serve cup | 4-oz. container | 2 | 0.0 | | | (0) |
| (Thank You Brand) | ½ cup (4.3 oz.) | 12 | 0.0 | | | (0) |
| (White House) regular or with apple juice added | ½ cup | 5 | 0.0 | | | (0) |
| **APPLE STRUDEL,** frozen | | | | | | |
| (Pepperidge Farm) | 3-oz. serving | 220 | 11.0 | | | |
| **APPLE TURNOVER,** frozen (See **TURNOVER,** Apple) | | | | | | |

(USDA): United States Department of Agriculture
*Prepared as Package Directs

| Food and Description | Measure or Quantity | Sodium (mg.) | Fats in grams — Total | Satu- rated | Unsatu- rated | Choles- terol (mg.) |
|---|---|---|---|---|---|---|
| **APRICOT:** | | | | | | |
| Fresh (USDA): | | | | | | |
| Whole | 1 lb. (weighed with pits) | 4 | .9 | | | 0 |
| Whole | 3 apricots (about 12 per lb.) | 1 | .2 | | | 0 |
| Halves | 1 cup (5.5 oz.) | 2 | .3 | | | 0 |
| Canned, regular pack, solids & liq.: | | | | | | |
| Juice pack (USDA) | 4 oz. | 1 | .2 | | | 0 |
| Light syrup (USDA) | 4 oz. | 1 | .1 | | | 0 |
| Heavy syrup: | | | | | | |
| Halves & syrup (USDA) | ½ cup (4.4 oz.) | 1 | .1 | | | 0 |
| Halves & syrup (USDA) | 4 med. halves with 2 T. syrup (4.3 oz.) | 1 | .1 | | | 0 |
| (Del Monte) | ½ cup (4.4 oz.) | < 1 | 0.0 | | | 0 |
| Extra heavy syrup (USDA) | 4 oz. | 1 | .1 | | | 0 |
| Canned, unsweetened or low calorie: | | | | | | |
| Water pack, halves & liq. (USDA) | 4 oz. | 1 | .1 | | | 0 |
| Water pack, halves & liq. (USDA) | ½ cup (4.3 oz.) | 1 | .1 | | | 0 |
| (Diet Delight) | ½ cup (4.4 oz.) | 5 | <.1 | | | (0) |
| (Featherweight) juice or water pack | ½ cup | <10 | 0.0 | | | (0) |
| (Libby's) lite | ½ cup (4.4 oz.) | 10 | 0.0 | | | (0) |
| (S&W) *Nutradiet,* blue or white label | ½ cup | 2 | 0.0 | | | (0) |
| Dehydrated (USDA): | | | | | | |
| Uncooked | 4 oz. | 37 | 1.1 | | | 0 |
| Cooked, sugar added, solids & liq. | 4 oz. | 9 | .2 | | | 0 |
| Dried: | | | | | | |
| Uncooked: | | | | | | |
| (USDA) | 1 lb. | 118 | 2.3 | | | 0 |
| (USDA) | 14 large halves (½ cup or 2.8 oz.) | 21 | .4 | | | 0 |

(USDA): United States Department of Agriculture
*Prepared as Package Directs

APRICOT (Continued)

| Food and Description | Measure or Quantity | Sodium (mg.) | Fats in grams — Total | Satu- rated | Unsatu- rated | Choles- terol (mg.) |
|---|---|---|---|---|---|---|
| (USDA) | 10 small halves (¼ cup or 1.3 oz.) | 10 | .2 | | | 0 |
| (USDA) | ½ cup (2.3 oz.) | 17 | .3 | | | 0 |
| (Del Monte) | ½ cup (2.3 oz.) | <10 | 0.0 | | | 0 |
| Cooked (USDA): | | | | | | |
| Sweetened | ½ cup with liq. (12-13 halves, 5.7 oz.) | 11 | .2 | | | 0 |
| Unsweetened | ½ cup with liq. (4.3 oz.) | 10 | .2 | | | 0 |
| Frozen, sweetened, not thawed (USDA) | 4 oz. | 5 | .1 | | | 0 |
| **APRICOT, CANDIED** (USDA) | 1 oz. | | <.1 | | | 0 |
| **APRICOT LIQUEUR** (Leroux) 60 proof | 1 fl. oz. | <1 | (0.0) | | | (0) |
| **APRICOT NECTAR,** canned, sweetened: | | | | | | |
| (USDA) | ½ cup (4.2 oz.) | Tr. | .1 | | | 0 |
| (Del Monte) | ½ cup (4.3 oz.) | <10 | 0.0 | | | 0 |
| (Libby's) | 6-fl.-oz. can | 5 | 0.0 | | | (0) |
| **APRICOT & PINEAPPLE NECTAR** (S&W) *Nutradiet,* unsweetened | 4 oz. (by wt.) | 2 | 0.0 | | | (0) |
| **APRICOT & PINEAPPLE PRESERVE:** | | | | | | |
| Sweetened (Bama) | 1 T. (.7 oz.) | 2 | <.1 | | | (0) |
| Dietetic or low calorie: | | | | | | |
| (Diet Delight) | 1 T. (.6 oz.) | 4 | 0.0 | | | (0) |
| (S&W) *Nutradiet,* red label | 1 T. (.5 oz.) | | 0.0 | | | (0) |
| (Tillie Lewis) | 1 T. (.5 oz.) | | Tr. | | | 0 |
| **APRICOT PRESERVE:** | | | | | | |
| Sweetened (Home Brand) | 1 T. | 7 | 0.0 | | | (0) |
| Dietetic or low calorie: | | | | | | |
| (Estee) | 1 T. (.6 oz.) | <3 | 0.0 | | | (0) |

(USDA): United States Department of Agriculture
*Prepared as Package Directs

| Food and Description | Measure or Quantity | Sodium (mg.) | Fats in grams — Total | Satu- rated | Unsatu- rated | Choles- terol (mg.) |
|---|---|---|---|---|---|---|
| (Featherweight) | 1 T. | 40–50 | 0.0 | | | (0) |
| (Louis Sherry) | 1 T. (.6 oz.) | <3 | 0.0 | | | (0) |

**APRICOT, STRAINED,** canned
| | | | | | | |
|---|---|---|---|---|---|---|
| (Larsen) no salt added | ½ cup (4.3 oz.) | 12 | 0.0 | | | (0) |

***ARBY'S:***
| | | | | | | |
|---|---|---|---|---|---|---|
| Bac'n Cheddar Deluxe | 7.85-oz. serving | 1,385 | 34.0 | | | 78 |
| Beef'n Cheddar | 6-oz. serving | 1,520 | 21.0 | | | 51 |
| Chicken breast sandwich | 7¼-oz. serving | 1,340 | 27.0 | | | 57 |
| Croissant: | | | | | | |
| Bacon & egg | 4½-oz. serving | 550 | 25.0 | | | 440 |
| Butter | 2-oz. serving | 725 | 10.0 | | | 50 |
| Chicken salad | 5-oz. serving | 725 | 36.0 | | | 111 |
| Ham & swiss | 4-oz. serving | 995 | 15.0 | | | 70 |
| Mushroom & swiss | 4-oz. serving | 630 | 18.0 | | | 60 |
| Sausage & egg | 5¾-oz. serving | 745 | 35.0 | | | 645 |
| French fries | 2½-oz. serving | 30 | 8.0 | | | 6 |
| Ham & cheese, hot | 1 serving | 1,655 | 13.0 | | | 50 |
| Potato cake | 3-oz. serving | 425 | 14.0 | | | 13 |
| Potato, super stuffed: | | | | | | |
| Broccoli & cheddar | 12-oz. serving | 475 | 22.0 | | | 24 |
| Deluxe | 11.1-oz. serving | 475 | 38.0 | | | 72 |
| Mushroom & cheese | 10½-oz. serving | 635 | 22.0 | | | 21 |
| Plain | 11-oz. serving | 12 | .5 | | | 0 |
| Taco | 15-oz. serving | 1,065 | 27.0 | | | 145 |
| Roast beef: | | | | | | |
| Regular | 5.2-oz. serving | 590 | 15.0 | | | 39 |
| Junior | 3-oz. serving | 345 | 8.0 | | | 20 |
| King | 6.7-oz. serving | 765 | 19.0 | | | 49 |
| Super | 8.3-oz. serving | 800 | 22.0 | | | 40 |
| Shake: | | | | | | |
| Chocolate | 10.6-oz. serving | 300 | 11.0 | | | 32 |
| Jamocha | 10.8-oz. serving | 280 | 10.0 | | | 31 |
| Vanilla | 8.8-oz. serving | 245 | 10.0 | | | 30 |
| Turkey, deluxe, sandwich | 7-oz. serving | 850 | 17.0 | | | 39 |

**ARTICHOKE,** Globe or French
(See also **JERUSALEM ARTICHOKE**):
| | | | | | | |
|---|---|---|---|---|---|---|
| Raw, whole (USDA) | 1 lb. (weighed untrimmed) | 78 | .4 | | | 0 |

(USDA): United States Department of Agriculture
*Prepared as Package Directs

25

| Food and Description | Measure or Quantity | Sodium (mg.) | Fats in grams — Total | Satu-rated | Unsatu-rated | Choles-terol (mg.) |
|---|---|---|---|---|---|---|
| Boiled without salt, drained (USDA) | 4 oz. | 34 | .2 | | | 0 |
| Frozen, hearts (Birds Eye) | 5-6 hearts (3 oz.) | 40 | .4 | | | 0 |
| **ASPARAGUS:** | | | | | | |
| Raw, whole spears (USDA) | 1 lb. (weighed untrimmed) | 5 | .5 | | | 0 |
| Boiled without salt, whole spears (USDA) | 4 spears (1/2" dia. at base, 2.1 oz.) | < 1 | .1 | | | 0 |
| Boiled without salt, 1 1/2"-2" pieces, drained | 1 cup (5.1 oz.) | 1 | .3 | | | 0 |
| Canned, regular pack: | | | | | | |
| Green: | | | | | | |
| (USDA): | | | | | | |
| Spears & liq. | 4 oz. | 268 | .3 | | | 0 |
| Spears & liq. | 1 cup (8.6 oz.) | 576 | .7 | | | 0 |
| Spears only | 1 cup (7.6 oz.) | 507 | .9 | | | 0 |
| Spears only | 6 med. spears (3.4 oz.) | 227 | .4 | | | 0 |
| Liq. only | 2 T. (1.1 oz.) | 71 | Tr. | | | 0 |
| Cut spears & liq. (Green Giant) | 1/2 of 10 1/2-oz. can | 492 | .1 | | | (0) |
| Spears & liq. (Green Giant) | 1/3 of 15-oz. can | 468 | .1 | | | (0) |
| (Del Monte) spears & tips, solids & liq. | 1/2 cup (4 oz.) | 355 | Tr. | | | (0) |
| (Green Giant) solids & liq.: | | | | | | |
| Cuts | 1/2 of 8-oz. can | 450 | 0.0 | | | (0) |
| Spears | 1/2 cup (4 oz.) | 353 | Tr. | | | (0) |
| Spears & liq., *LeSueur* | 1/4 of 1-lb. 3-oz. can | 446 | .1 | | | (0) |
| Solids & liq. (Stokely-Van Camp's) | 1/2 cup (3.9 oz.) | | .4 | | | (0) |
| Drained solids (Del Monte) | 1 cup (7.8 oz.) | 417 | .8 | | | 0 |
| White (USDA): | | | | | | |
| Spears & liq. | 4 oz. | 268 | .3 | | | 0 |
| Spears & liq. | 1 cup (8.4 oz.) | 564 | .7 | | | 0 |
| Spears only | 1 cup (7.6 oz.) | 507 | 1.1 | | | 0 |

(USDA): United States Department of Agriculture
*Prepared as Package Directs

| Food and Description | Measure or Quantity | Sodium (mg.) | Total | Satu-rated | Unsatu-rated | Choles-terol (mg.) |
|---|---|---|---|---|---|---|
| Spears only | 6 med. spears (3.4 oz.) | 227 | .5 | | | 0 |
| Liq. only | 2 T. (1.1 oz.) | 71 | Tr. | | | 0 |
| Canned, dietetic pack: | | | | | | |
| Green: | | | | | | |
| (USDA): | | | | | | |
| Spears & liq. | 4 oz. | 3 | .2 | | | 0 |
| Liquid only | 4 oz. | 3 | Tr. | | | 0 |
| (Diet Delight) solids & liq. | ½ cup (4.2 oz.) | 5 | 0.0 | | | (0) |
| (S&W) *Nutradiet*, spears, green label, solids & liq. | ½ cup | <10 | 0.0 | | | (0) |
| White (USDA): | | | | | | |
| Spears & liq. | 4 oz. | 5 | .2 | | | 0 |
| Drained solids | 4 oz. | 5 | .2 | | | 0 |
| Drained liq. | 4 oz. | 5 | Tr. | | | 0 |
| Frozen: | | | | | | |
| (USDA): | | | | | | |
| Cuts & tips, not thawed | 4 oz. | 2 | .2 | | | 0 |
| Cuts & tips, boiled without salt, drained | 4 oz. | 1 | .2 | | | 0 |
| Cuts & tips, boiled without salt, drained | ½ cup (3.2 oz.) | <1 | .2 | | | 0 |
| Spears, not thawed | 4 oz. | 2 | .2 | | | 0 |
| Spears, boiled without salt, drained | 4 oz. | 1 | .2 | | | 0 |
| (Birds Eye): | | | | | | |
| Cuts | ⅓ of 10-oz. pkg. | 5 | 0.0 | | | 0 |
| Spears | ⅓ of 10-oz. pkg. | 0 | 0.0 | | | 0 |
| (Green Giant) cut spears in butter sauce | ½ cup | 725 | 4 | | | |
| (McKenzie) spears | 3⅓ oz. | 19 | 0.0 | | | |

**AUNT JEMIMA SYRUP** (See **SYRUP,** Pancake or Waffle)

**AVOCADO,** peeled, pitted (USDA): All commercial varieties:

| | | | | | | |
|---|---|---|---|---|---|---|
| Whole | 1 lb. (weighed with seed & skin) | 14 | 55.8 | 11. | 45. | 0 |
| Diced | ½ cup (2.6 oz.) | 3 | 12.1 | 2 | 10. | 0 |
| Mashed | ½ cup (4.1 oz.) | 5 | 19.0 | 3. | 16. | 0 |

(USDA): United States Department of Agriculture
*Prepared as Package Directs

27

| Food and Description | Measure or Quantity | Sodium (mg.) | Fats in grams Total | Saturated | Unsaturated | Cholesterol (mg.) |
|---|---|---|---|---|---|---|
| California varieties, mainly Fuerte: | | | | | | |
| Whole | ½ avocado (3⅛" dia.) | 4 | 18.4 | 3. | 15. | 0 |
| ½" cubes | ½ cup (2.7 oz.) | 3 | 12.9 | 2. | 11. | 0 |
| Florida varieties: | | | | | | |
| Whole | ½ avocado (3⅝" dia.) | 6 | 16.7 | 3. | 14. | 0 |
| ½" cubes | ½ cup (2.7 oz.) | 3 | 8.4 | 2. | 7. | 0 |
| *AWAKE (Birds Eye) | ½ cup (4.4 oz.) | 14 | .3 | | | 0 |

# B

**BABY FOOD:**

| Food and Description | Measure or Quantity | Sodium (mg.) | Fats in grams Total | | | |
|---|---|---|---|---|---|---|
| Apple: | | | | | | |
| & apricot, junior (Beech-Nut) | 7¾ oz. | <1 | Tr. | | | |
| & apricot, strained (Beech-Nut) | 4¾ oz. | <1 | Tr. | | | |
| Apple Betty (Beech-Nut): | | | | | | |
| Junior | 7¾ oz. | 1 | Tr. | | | |
| Strained | 4¾ oz. | <1 | Tr. | | | |
| Apple-cherry juice: | | | | | | |
| Strained (Beech-Nut) | 4⅕ fl. oz. (4.4 oz.) | 6 | Tr. | | | |
| Strained (Gerber) | 4⅕ fl. oz. (4.6 oz.) | Tr. | .1 | | | |
| Apple-grape juice: | | | | | | |
| Strained (Beech-Nut) | 4⅕ fl. oz. (4.4 oz.) | 6 | Tr. | | | |
| Strained (Gerber) | 4.2 fl. oz. | 2 | .1 | | | |
| Apple juice: | | | | | | |
| Strained (Beech-Nut) | 4⅕ fl. oz. (4.4 oz.) | 6 | Tr. | | | |
| Strained (Gerber) | 4⅕ fl. oz. (4.6 oz.) | 2 | .2 | | | |
| Applesauce: | | | | | | |
| Junior (Beech-Nut) | 7¾ oz. | 5 | Tr. | | | |
| Junior (Gerber) | 7⅘ oz. | 2 | .5 | | | |
| Strained (Beech-Nut) | 4¾ oz. | <1 | Tr. | | | |
| Strained (Gerber) | 4⁷⁄₁₀ oz. | 3 | .3 | | | |
| & apricots, junior (Gerber) | 7½ oz. | 6 | Tr. | | | |

(USDA): United States Department of Agriculture
*Prepared as Package Directs

| Food and Description | Measure or Quantity | Sodium (mg.) | —Fats in grams— | | | Cholesterol (mg.) |
|---|---|---|---|---|---|---|
| | | | Total | Saturated | Unsaturated | |
| & apricots, strained (Gerber) | 4½ oz. | 3 | Tr. | | | |
| & cherries, junior (Beech-Nut) | 7¾ oz. | 5 | Tr. | | | |
| & cherries, strained (Beech-Nut) | 4¾ oz. | 3 | Tr. | | | |
| & pineapple, strained (Gerber) | 4½ oz. | 3 | Tr. | | | |
| & raspberries, junior (Beech-Nut) | 7¾ oz. | 5 | Tr. | | | |
| & raspberries, strained (Beech-Nut) | 4¾ oz. | 3 | Tr. | | | |
| Apricot with tapioca: | | | | | | |
| Junior (Beech-Nut) | 7¾ oz. | 15 | Tr. | | | |
| Junior (Gerber) | 7¾ oz. | 22 | Tr. | | | |
| Strained (Gerber) | 4¾ oz. | 8 | Tr. | | | |
| Banana: | | | | | | |
| & pineapple with tapioca: | | | | | | |
| Junior (Gerber) | 7½ oz. | 8 | .3 | | | |
| Strained (Gerber) | 4½ oz. | 6 | Tr. | | | |
| Dessert, junior (Beech-Nut) | 7½ oz. | 10 | Tr. | | | |
| With tapioca: | | | | | | |
| Strained (Beech-Nut) | 4¾ oz. | 6 | .3 | | | |
| Strained (Gerber) | 4½ oz. | 22 | Tr. | | | |
| Bean, green: | | | | | | |
| Junior (Beech-Nut) | 7¼ oz. | 5 | .2 | | | |
| Strained (Beech-Nut) | 4½ oz. | 3 | .3 | | | |
| Strained (Gerber) | 4½ oz. | 4 | .1 | | | |
| Creamed with bacon, junior (Gerber) | 7½ oz. | 19 | Tr. | | | |
| With potatoes & ham, casserole, toddler (Gerber) | 6¼ oz. | 538 | 5.0 | | | |
| Beef: | | | | | | |
| Junior (Gerber) | 3½ oz. | 52 | 4.0 | | | |
| Strained (Gerber) | 3½ oz. | 52 | 4.1 | | | |
| Beef & beef broth (Beech-Nut): | | | | | | |
| Junior | 7½ oz. | 162 | 13.2 | | | |
| Strained | 4½ oz. | 88 | 9.1 | | | |
| Beef & beef heart, strained (Gerber) | 3½ oz. | 58 | 4.2 | | | |
| Beef dinner: | | | | | | |
| & noodles, junior (Beech-Nut) | 7½ oz. | 54 | 4.3 | | | |

(USDA): United States Department of Agriculture
*Prepared as Package Directs

| Food and Description | Measure or Quantity | Sodium (mg.) | —Fats in grams— | | | Cholesterol (mg.) |
|---|---|---|---|---|---|---|
| | | | Total | Saturated | Unsaturated | |
| & noodles, junior (Gerber) | 7½ oz. | 36 | 4.0 | | | |
| & noodles, strained | | | | | | |
| (Beech-Nut) | 4½ oz. | 32 | 2.7 | | | |
| With vegetables: | | | | | | |
| Junior (Gerber) | 4½ oz. | 36 | 6.5 | | | |
| Strained (Gerber) | 4½ oz. | 31 | 6.5 | | | |
| Strained (Heinz) | 4¾ oz. | 126 | 5.4 | | | |
| Beef lasagna, toddler (Gerber) | 6¼ oz. | 685 | 1.9 | | | |
| Beef liver, strained (Gerber) | 3½ oz. | 47 | 3.4 | | | |
| Beef stew, toddler (Gerber) | 6 oz. | 593 | 2.4 | | | |
| Beet, strained (Gerber) | 4½ oz. | 119 | .1 | | | |
| Carrot: | | | | | | |
| Junior (Gerber) | 7½ oz. | 111 | .4 | | | |
| Strained (Beech-Nut) | 4½ oz. | 88 | .1 | | | |
| Strained (Gerber) | 4½ oz. | 47 | Tr. | | | |
| Cereal, dry: | | | | | | |
| Barley (Gerber) | 4 T. | 4 | .3 | | | |
| Hi-protein (Beech-Nut) | 1 oz. | <40 | .5 | | | |
| Mixed (Beech-Nut) | 1 oz. | <40 | 1.4 | | | |
| Mixed (Gerber) | 4 T. | 4 | .7 | | | |
| Mixed, honey (Beech-Nut) | 1 oz. | 29 | 1.4 | | | |
| Mixed, with banana (Gerber) | 4 T. | 13 | 1.2 | | | |
| Oatmeal (Beech-Nut) | 1 oz. | <40 | 1.8 | | | |
| Oatmeal (Gerber) | 4 T. | 8 | 1.1 | | | |
| Oatmeal, honey (Beech-Nut) | 1 oz. | 34 | 1.8 | | | |
| Rice (Beech-Nut) | 1 oz. | <40 | 1.1 | | | |
| Rice (Gerber) | 4 T. | 4 | .8 | | | |
| Cereal, or mixed cereal: | | | | | | |
| With applesauce & banana: | | | | | | |
| Junior (Gerber) | 7½ oz. | 8 | 1.3 | | | |
| Strained (Gerber) | 4½ oz. | 3 | .9 | | | |
| With egg yolks & bacon: | | | | | | |
| Junior (Beech-Nut) | 7½ oz. | 168 | 10.8 | | | |
| Junior (Gerber) | 7½ oz. | 4 | 1.5 | | | |
| Strained (Gerber) | 4½ oz. | 3 | 1.1 | | | |
| Cherry vanilla pudding (Gerber): | | | | | | |
| Junior | 7½ oz. | 17 | 1.9 | | | |
| Strained | 4½ oz. | 9 | 1.3 | | | |
| Chicken: | | | | | | |
| Junior (Beech-Nut) | 3½ oz. | 39 | 8.5 | | | |

(USDA): United States Department of Agriculture
*Prepared as Package Directs

| Food and Description | Measure or Quantity | Sodium (mg.) | — Fats in grams — | | | Cholesterol (mg.) |
|---|---|---|---|---|---|---|
| | | | Total | Saturated | Unsaturated | |
| Strained (Gerber) | 3½ oz. | 39 | 8.9 | | | |
| Chicken dinner: | | | | | | |
| Noodle: | | | | | | |
| Junior (Beech-Nut) | 7½ oz. | 44 | .6 | | | |
| Junior (Gerber) | 7½ oz. | 28 | 3.2 | | | |
| Strained (Beech-Nut) | 4½ oz. | 26 | .9 | | | |
| Strained (Gerber) | 4½ oz. | 20 | 2.2 | | | |
| With vegetables: | | | | | | |
| Junior (Gerber) | 4½ oz. | 33 | 7.4 | | | |
| Strained (Gerber) | 4½ oz. | 33 | 6.8 | | | |
| Chicken soup, cream of, strained (Gerber) | 4½ oz. | 29 | 2.5 | | | |
| Chicken stew, toddler (Gerber) | 6 oz. | 651 | 6.8 | | | |
| Chicken sticks, junior (Gerber) | 2½ oz. | 323 | 8.4 | | | |
| Cookie, animal-shaped (Gerber) | 1 cookie (6 grams) | 13 | 1.0 | | | |
| Corn, creamed: | | | | | | |
| Junior (Gerber) | 7½ oz. | 34 | .5 | | | |
| Strained (Beech-Nut) | 4½ oz. | 20 | .3 | | | |
| Strained (Gerber) | 4½ oz. | 11 | .3 | | | |
| Custard: | | | | | | |
| Junior (Beech-Nut) | 7¾ oz. | 54 | 1.3 | | | |
| Chocolate, strained (Gerber) | 4½ oz. | 30 | 2.1 | | | |
| Vanilla, strained (Gerber) | 4½ oz. | 31 | 1.6 | | | |
| Egg yolk: | | | | | | |
| Strained (Beech-Nut) | 3⅓ oz. | 57 | 16.0 | | | |
| Strained (Gerber) | 3⅓ oz. | 45 | 16.7 | | | |
| Fruit dessert: | | | | | | |
| Junior (Beech-Nut) | 7¾ oz. | 46 | Tr. | | | |
| Strained (Heinz) | 4½ oz. | 13 | .1 | | | |
| Tropical, junior (Beech-Nut) | 7¾ oz. | 35 | Tr. | | | |
| With tapioca, strained (Beech-Nut) | 4½ oz. | 26 | Tr. | | | |
| Fruit juice: | | | | | | |
| Mixed, strained (Beech-Nut) | 4⅕ fl. oz. (4.4 oz.) | 6 | Tr. | | | |
| Mixed, strained (Gerber) | 4⅕ fl. oz. (4.6 oz.) | 2 | Tr. | | | |

(USDA): United States Department of Agriculture
*Prepared as Package Directs

| Food and Description | Measure or Quantity | Sodium (mg.) | Fats in grams — Total | Saturated | Unsaturated | Cholesterol (mg.) |
|---|---|---|---|---|---|---|
| **Ham:** | | | | | | |
| Junior (Gerber) | 3½ oz. | 39 | 5.8 | | | |
| Strained (Beech-Nut) | 3½ oz. | 40 | 5.8 | | | |
| **Ham dinner:** | | | | | | |
| Junior (Gerber) | 3½ oz. | 39 | 6.9 | | | |
| Strained (Beech-Nut) | 4½ oz. | 76 | 8.8 | | | |
| With vegetables: | | | | | | |
| Junior (Gerber) | 4½ oz. | 24 | 3.6 | | | |
| Strained (Gerber) | 4½ oz. | 22 | 3.6 | | | |
| **Lamb:** | | | | | | |
| Junior (Gerber) | 3½ oz. | 53 | 4.1 | | | |
| Strained (Gerber) | 3½ oz. | 51 | 4.0 | | | |
| **Lamb & lamb broth (Beech-Nut):** | | | | | | |
| Junior | 7½ oz. | 172 | 15.9 | | | |
| Strained | 3½ oz. | 97 | 9.5 | | | |
| **Macaroni:** | | | | | | |
| With tomato & beef: | | | | | | |
| Junior (Gerber) | 7½ oz. | 34 | Tr. | | | |
| Strained (Gerber) | 4½ oz. | 18 | Tr. | | | |
| Meat sticks, junior (Gerber) | 2½ oz. | 326 | 9.3 | | | |
| **Orange-apple juice, strained:** | | | | | | |
| (Beech-Nut) | 4⅕ fl. oz. (4.4 oz.) | 3 | Tr. | | | |
| (Gerber) | 4⅕ fl. oz. (4.6 oz.) | 5 | Tr. | | | |
| **Orange-apricot juice, strained** | | | | | | |
| (Gerber) | 4⅕ fl. oz. (4.6 oz.) | 7 | Tr. | | | |
| **Orange-banana juice, strained** | | | | | | |
| (Beech-Nut) | 4⅕ fl. oz. (4.4 oz.) | 3 | Tr. | | | |
| **Orange juice, strained:** | | | | | | |
| (Beech-Nut) | 4⅕ fl. oz. (4.4 oz.) | 3 | Tr. | | | |
| (Gerber) | 4⅕ fl. oz. (4.6 oz.) | 4 | Tr. | | | |
| **Orange-pineapple dessert, strained (Beech-Nut)** | 4¾ oz. | 28 | Tr. | | | |
| **Orange-pineapple juice, strained:** | | | | | | |
| (Beech-Nut) | 4⅕ fl. oz. (4.4 oz.) | 3 | .4 | | | |

(USDA): United States Department of Agriculture
*Prepared as Package Directs

| Food and Description | Measure or Quantity | Sodium (mg.) | Fats in grams Total | Satu- rated | Unsatu- rated | Choles- terol (mg.) |
|---|---|---|---|---|---|---|
| (Gerber) | 4 1/5 fl. oz. (4.6 oz.) | 1 | .2 | | | |
| Orange pudding, strained | | | | | | |
| (Gerber) | 4 3/4 oz. | 28 | 1.2 | | | |
| Pea: | | | | | | |
| Strained (Beech-Nut) | 4 1/2 oz. | 3 | .5 | | | |
| Strained (Gerber) | 4 1/2 oz. | 11 | .4 | | | |
| Peach: | | | | | | |
| Junior (Beech-Nut) | 7 3/4 oz. | 15 | Tr. | | | |
| Junior (Gerber) | 7 1/2 oz. | 6 | .7 | | | |
| Strained (Beech-Nut) | 4 3/4 oz. | 9 | Tr. | | | |
| Strained (Gerber) | 4 7/10 oz. | 4 | .4 | | | |
| Peach cobbler (Gerber): | | | | | | |
| Junior | 7 3/4 oz. | 20 | .3 | | | |
| Strained | 4 7/10 oz. | 9 | .4 | | | |
| Peach Melba (Beech-Nut): | | | | | | |
| Junior | 7 3/4 oz. | 20 | Tr. | | | |
| Strained | 4 3/4 oz. | 12 | Tr. | | | |
| Pear: | | | | | | |
| Junior (Beech-Nut) | 7 1/2 oz. | 5 | Tr. | | | |
| Junior (Gerber) | 7 1/2 oz. | 6 | .4 | | | |
| Strained (Beech-Nut) | 4 1/2 oz. | 3 | Tr. | | | |
| Strained (Gerber) | 4 1/2 oz. | 4 | .3 | | | |
| Pear & pineapple: | | | | | | |
| Junior (Beech-Nut) | 7 1/2 oz. | 10 | Tr. | | | |
| Junior (Gerber) | 7 1/2 oz. | 4 | .6 | | | |
| Strained (Beech-Nut) | 4 1/2 oz. | 6 | Tr. | | | |
| Strained (Gerber) | 4 1/2 oz. | 3 | Tr. | | | |
| Pineapple dessert, strained | | | | | | |
| (Beech-Nut) | 4 3/4 oz. | 12 | Tr. | | | |
| Plum with tapioca: | | | | | | |
| Junior (Gerber) | 7 3/4 oz. | 12 | .4 | | | |
| Strained (Gerber) | 4 3/4 oz. | 5 | .2 | | | |
| Pork, strained (Gerber) | 3 1/2 oz. | 38 | 6.0 | | | |
| Pretzel (Gerber) | 1 piece (5 grams) | 15 | .1 | | | |
| Prune-orange juice, strained | | | | | | |
| (Beech-Nut) | 4 1/2 oz. | 6 | Tr. | | | |
| Prune with tapioca: | | | | | | |
| Junior (Beech-Nut) | 7 3/4 oz. | 10 | .2 | | | |
| Junior (Gerber) | 7 3/4 oz. | 20 | .5 | | | |
| Strained (Beech-Nut) | 4 3/4 oz. | 6 | .1 | | | |

(USDA): United States Department of Agriculture
*Prepared as Package Directs

| Food and Description | Measure or Quantity | Sodium (mg.) | — Fats in grams — | | | Cholesterol (mg.) |
|---|---|---|---|---|---|---|
| | | | Total | Saturated | Unsaturated | |
| Strained (Gerber) | 4¾ oz. | 13 | .4 | | | |
| *Similac:* | | | | | | |
| Advance | 1 fl. oz. (1 oz.) | 12 | .5 | | | <1 |
| Isomil | 1 fl. oz. (1 oz.) | 9 | 1.0 | | | 0 |
| *Powder | 1 fl. oz. (1 oz.) | 11 | 1.0 | | | Tr. |
| Ready-to-feed | 1 fl. oz. (1 oz.) | 9 | 1.0 | | | Tr. |
| Spaghetti & meat balls, toddler (Gerber) | 6½ oz. | 629 | 1.8 | | | |
| Spaghetti, tomato sauce & beef: | | | | | | |
| Junior (Beech-Nut) | 7½ oz. | 74 | 4.0 | | | |
| Junior (Gerber) | 7½ oz. | 58 | 2.5 | | | |
| Spinach, creamed, strained (Gerber) | 4½ oz. | 49 | 1.7 | | | |
| Squash: | | | | | | |
| Junior (Beech-Nut) | 7½ oz. | 5 | .4 | | | |
| Junior (Gerber) | 7½ oz. | 4 | .5 | | | |
| Strained (Beech-Nut) | 4½ oz. | 3 | .4 | | | |
| Strained (Gerber) | 4½ oz. | 5 | .3 | | | |
| Sweet potato: | | | | | | |
| Junior (Beech-Nut) | 7¾ oz. | 111 | Tr. | | | |
| Junior (Gerber) | 7¾ oz. | 51 | Tr. | | | |
| Strained (Gerber) | 4¾ oz. | 24 | .3 | | | |
| Turkey: | | | | | | |
| Junior (Gerber) | 3½ oz. | 50 | 7.7 | | | |
| Strained (Gerber) | 3½ oz. | 56 | 7.8 | | | |
| Turkey dinner: | | | | | | |
| With rice: | | | | | | |
| Junior (Beech-Nut) | 7½ oz. | 55 | .8 | | | |
| Strained (Beech-Nut) | 4½ oz. | 33 | .8 | | | |
| With rice & vegetables, junior (Beech-Nut) | 7½ oz. | 36 | 4.3 | | | |
| With vegetables: | | | | | | |
| Junior (Gerber) | 4½ oz. | 40 | 7.3 | | | |
| Strained (Gerber) | 4½ oz. | 37 | 6.0 | | | |
| Tutti frutti dessert (Heinz): | | | | | | |
| Junior | 7¾ oz. | 79 | .5 | | | |
| Strained | 4½ oz. | 69 | .5 | | | |
| Veal: | | | | | | |
| Junior (Gerber) | 3½ oz. | 55 | 4.2 | | | |
| Strained (Gerber) | 3½ oz. | 52 | 4.0 | | | |
| Veal dinner: | | | | | | |

(USDA): United States Department of Agriculture
*Prepared as Package Directs

34

| Food and Description | Measure or Quantity | Sodium (mg.) | — Fats in grams — | | | Choles-terol (mg.) |
|---|---|---|---|---|---|---|
| | | | Total | Satu-rated | Unsatu-rated | |
| Junior (Beech-Nut) | 4½ oz. | 145 | 8.2 | | | |
| Strained (Beech-Nut) | 4½ oz. | 177 | 6.9 | | | |
| With vegetables: | | | | | | |
| Junior (Gerber) | 4½ oz. | 31 | 2.0 | | | |
| Strained (Gerber) | 4½ oz. | 27 | 1.8 | | | |
| Vegetables: | | | | | | |
| Garden, strained (Beech-Nut) | 4½ oz. | 50 | Tr. | | | |
| Garden, strained (Gerber) | 4½ oz. | 28 | .3 | | | |
| Mixed, junior (Gerber) | 7½ oz. | 77 | .4 | | | |
| Mixed, strained (Gerber) | 4½ oz. | 27 | .1 | | | |
| Vegetables & bacon: | | | | | | |
| Junior (Gerber) | 7½ oz. | 121 | 7.7 | | | |
| Strained (Beech-Nut) | 4½ oz. | 141 | 4.4 | | | |
| Strained (Gerber) | 4½ oz. | 79 | 4.7 | | | |
| Vegetables & beef: | | | | | | |
| Junior (Beech-Nut) | 7½ oz. | 55 | 4.0 | | | |
| Junior (Gerber) | 7½ oz. | 26 | 3.6 | | | |
| Strained (Beech-Nut) | 4½ oz. | 33 | 4.1 | | | |
| Strained (Gerber) | 4½ oz. | 17 | 2.9 | | | |
| Vegetables & chicken (Gerber): | | | | | | |
| Junior | 7½ oz. | 21 | 2.8 | | | |
| Strained | 4½ oz. | 14 | 1.7 | | | |
| Vegetables & ham: | | | | | | |
| Junior (Gerber) | 7½ oz. | 30 | 3.8 | | | |
| Strained (Beech-Nut) | 4½ oz. | 33 | 2.0 | | | |
| Vegetables & lamb: | | | | | | |
| Junior (Gerber) | 7½ oz. | 26 | 5.0 | | | |
| Strained (Gerber) | 4½ oz. | 15 | 2.8 | | | |
| Vegetables & liver: | | | | | | |
| Junior (Gerber) | 7½ oz. | 28 | .8 | | | |
| Strained (Gerber) | 4½ oz. | 19 | .5 | | | |
| Vegetables & turkey: | | | | | | |
| Junior (Gerber) | 7½ oz. | 32 | 2.3 | | | |
| Strained (Gerber) | 4½ oz. | 20 | 1.9 | | | |
| Toddler, casserole (Gerber) | 6¼ oz. | 577 | 6.2 | | | |
| | | | | | | |
| **BACON,** cured: | | | | | | |
| Raw (USDA): | | | | | | |
| Sliced | 1 lb. | 3,084 | 314.3 | 101. | | 213.0 |
| Sliced | 1 oz. | 193 | 19.6 | 6. | | 13.0 |
| Slab | 1 lb. (weighed with rind) | 2,900 | 295.5 | 95. | | 200.0 |

(USDA): United States Department of Agriculture
*Prepared as Package Directs

35

| Food and Description | Measure or Quantity | Sodium (mg.) | —Fats in grams— | | | Choles-terol (mg.) |
|---|---|---|---|---|---|---|
| | | | Total | Satu-rated | Unsatu-rated | |
| Broiled or fried, crisp, drained: | | | | | | |
| (USDA) thin slice | 1 slice (5 grams) | 51 | 2.6 | <1. | 2. | |
| (USDA) medium slice | 1 slice (8 grams) | 77 | 3.9 | 1. | 3. | |
| (USDA) thick slice | 1 slice (.4 oz.) | 123 | 6.2 | 2. | 4. | |
| (Hormel): | | | | | | |
| Black Label | 1 slice | 149 | 2.5 | | | |
| Range Brand | 1 slice | 186 | 4.5 | | | |
| (Oscar Mayer): | | | | | | |
| Regular | 6-gram slice | 118 | 3.1 | 1.2 | 1.9 | 5 |
| Center cut | 4.5-gram slice | 96 | 2.0 | .9 | 1.4 | 5 |
| Lower salt | 6.1-gram slice | 85 | 2.7 | | | 5 |
| Thick slice | 11-gram slice | 208 | 5.7 | 2.2 | 3.5 | 10 |
| Canned (USDA) | 3 oz. | | 60.8 | 20. | 41. | |

**BACON BITS:**
| Real: | | | | | | |
|---|---|---|---|---|---|---|
| Bac*Os (General Mills) | 1 tsp. | 77 | .7 | | | |
| (Oscar Mayer) | 1 tsp. (.1 oz.) | 56 | .3 | .1 | .2 | 2 |
| Imitation: | | | | | | |
| (Durkee) | 1 tsp. | 229 | .4 | | | |
| (Estee) | 1 tsp. | 30 | | | | |
| Crumbles (French's) | 1 tsp. | 55 | Tr. | | | |

**BACON, CANADIAN:**
| Unheated: | | | | | | |
|---|---|---|---|---|---|---|
| (USDA) | 1 oz. | 538 | 4.1 | 1. | 3. | |
| (Eckrich) | 1-oz. slice | 460 | 1.0 | | | |
| (Hormel): | | | | | | |
| Regular | 1 oz. | 315 | 2.0 | | | |
| Light & Lean | 1 slice | | .5 | | | |
| (Oscar Mayer) | 1-oz. slice | 389 | 1.4 | | | 12 |
| Broiled or fried, drained | | | | | | |
| (USDA) | 1 oz. | 724 | 5.0 | 2. | 3. | |

**BACON, SIMULATED, COOKED:**
| (Oscar Mayer) Lean 'N Tasty: | | | | | | |
|---|---|---|---|---|---|---|
| Beef | 12-gram strip | 190 | 3.8 | 1.5 | 2.2 | 13 |
| Pork | 13-gram strip | 215 | 4.7 | 1.8 | 2.9 | 14 |
| (Swift) Sizzlean, pork | .4-oz. strip | 159 | 4.2 | | | |

**BACO NOIR BURGUNDY**

(USDA): United States Department of Agriculture
*Prepared as Package Directs

| Food and Description | Measure or Quantity | Sodium (mg.) | Fats in grams Total | Satu-rated | Unsatu-rated | Choles-terol (mg.) |
|---|---|---|---|---|---|---|
| (Great Western) 12.5% alcohol | 3 fl. oz. | 36 | 0.0 | | | 0 |
| **BAGEL:** | | | | | | |
| (USDA): | | | | | | |
| Egg | 3″ dia. (1.9 oz.) | | 2.0 | | | |
| Water | 3″ dia. (1.9 oz.) | | 2.0 | | | |
| (Lender's): | | | | | | |
| Plain | 2-oz. piece | 350 | | | | |
| *Bagelettes* | .9-oz. piece | Tr. | | | | |
| Onion | 1 bagel | 290 | | | | |
| Raisin & honey or wheat & raisin with honey | 2.5-oz. bagel | 310 | | | | |
| **BAKING POWDER:** | | | | | | |
| Regular: | | | | | | |
| Phosphate (USDA) | 1 tsp. (5 grams) | 386 | Tr. | | | 0 |
| SAS (USDA) | 1 tsp. (4 grams) | 405 | Tr. | | | 0 |
| Tartrate (USDA) | 1 tsp. (4 grams) | 270 | Tr. | | | 0 |
| (Calumet) SAS | 1 tsp. (4 grams) | 396 | Tr. | | | 0 |
| (Davis) | 1 tsp. (4 grams) | 326 | 0.0 | | | 0 |
| Low sodium, commercial: | | | | | | |
| (USDA) | 1 tsp. (4 grams) | <1 | Tr. | | | 0 |
| (Featherweight) | 1 tsp. | 2 | 0.0 | | | 0 |
| **BAMBOO SHOOT:** | | | | | | |
| Raw (USDA): | | | | | | |
| Untrimmed | ½ lb. (weighed untrimmed) | | .2 | | | 0 |
| Trimmed | 4 oz. | | .3 | | | 0 |
| Canned, drained solids: | | | | | | |
| (Chun King) | 8½-oz. can | 0 | .7 | | | 0 |
| (La Choy) | ¼ cup | 0 | <1.0 | | | 0 |
| **BANANA** (USDA): | | | | | | |
| Common: | | | | | | |
| Fresh: | | | | | | |
| Whole | 1 lb. (weighed with skin) | 3 | .6 | | | 0 |
| Small size | 4.9-oz. banana (7¾″ × 1¹¹⁄₃₂″) | 1 | .2 | | | 0 |
| Medium size | 6.2-oz. banana (8¾″ × 1¹³⁄₃₂″) | 1 | .2 | | | 0 |

(USDA): United States Department of Agriculture
*Prepared as Package Directs

BANANA (Continued)

| Food and Description | Measure or Quantity | Sodium (mg.) | Total | Fats in grams — Satu-rated | Unsatu-rated | Choles-terol (mg.) |
|---|---|---|---|---|---|---|
| Large size | 7-oz. banana (9¾" × 1⁷⁄₁₆") | 1 | 3 | | | 0 |
| Chunks | 1 cup (5 oz.) | 1 | .3 | | | 0 |
| Mashed | 1 cup (2 med., 7.8 oz.) | 2 | .4 | | | 0 |
| Sliced | 1 cup (1¼ med., 5.1 oz.) | 1 | .3 | | | 0 |
| Dehydrated: | | | | | | |
| Flakes | ½ cup (1.8 oz.) | 2 | .4 | | | 0 |
| Powder | 1 oz. | 1 | .2 | | | 0 |
| Red, fresh, whole | 1 lb. (weighed with skin) | 3 | .6 | | | 0 |
| Red, fresh, peeled | 4 oz. | 1 | .2 | | | 0 |

**BANANA, BAKING** (See **PLANTAIN**)

**BANANA NECTAR,** canned
(Libby's)     6 fl. oz.    5    0.

**BANANA PIE,** cream or custard
(See **PIE,** Banana)

**BANANA PUDDING & PIE FILLING** (See **PUDDING OR PIE FILLING**)

**BARBADOS CHERRY**
(See **ACEROLA**)

**BARBECUE SAUCE** (See **SAUCE,** Barbecue)

**BARBECUE SEASONING**
(French's)    1 tsp. (2 grams)    70    Tr.

**BARLEY,** pearled, dry:
Light:
(USDA)    ¼ cup (1.8 oz.)    2    .5    0

(USDA): United States Department of Agriculture
*Prepared as Package Directs

| Food and Description | Measure or Quantity | Sodium (mg.) | —Fats in grams— | | | Choles- terol (mg.) |
|---|---|---|---|---|---|---|
| | | | Total | Satu- rated | Unsatu- rated | |
| (Quaker Scotch) | ¼ cup (1.7 oz.) | 5 | .5 | | | (0) |
| Pot or Scotch (USDA) | 2 oz. | | .6 | | | 0 |
| **BARRACUDA,** raw, meat only | | | | | | |
| (USDA) | 4 oz. | | 2.9 | | | |
| **BASS** (USDA): | | | | | | |
| Black sea: | | | | | | |
| Raw, whole | 1 lb. (weighed whole) | 120 | 2.1 | | | |
| Baked, home recipe[1] | 4 oz. | | 17.9 | | | |
| Smallmouth & largemouth, raw: | | | | | | |
| Whole | 1 lb. (weighed whole) | | 3.7 | | | |
| Meat only | 4 oz. | | 2.9 | | | |
| Striped: | | | | | | |
| Raw, whole | 1 lb. (weighed whole) | | 5.3 | | | |
| Raw, meat only | 4 oz. | | 3.1 | | | |
| Oven-fried[2] | 4 oz. | | 9.6 | | | |
| White, raw, whole | 1 lb. (weighed whole) | | 4.1 | | | |
| White, raw, meat only | 4 oz. | | 2.6 | | | |
| **BASIL** (Spice Islands) | 1 tsp. | Tr. | | | | (0) |
| **BAY LEAF** (Spice Islands) | 1 med. leaf | Tr. | | | | (0) |
| **BEAN, BAKED,** canned: | | | | | | |
| (USDA): | | | | | | |
| With pork & molasses sauce[3] | 1 cup (9 oz.) | 969 | 12.0 | 5. | 7. | |
| With pork & tomato sauce[3] | 1 cup (9 oz.) | 1,181 | 6.6 | 3. | 4. | |
| With tomato sauce | 1 cup (9 oz.) | 862 | 1.3 | | | 0 |
| (Allen) *Wagon Master,* with pork | ½ cup (4 oz.) | 600 | 2.0 | | | |
| (B&M) Brick Oven: | | | | | | |
| Barbecue | ⅞ cup (8 oz.) | 960 | 6.0 | | | |
| Honey | ⅞ cup (8 oz.) | 940 | 2.0 | | | |

(USDA): United States Department of Agriculture
*Prepared as Package Directs
[1]Prepared with bacon, butter, onion, celery & bread cubes.
[2]Prepared with milk, bread crumbs, butter & salt.
[3]Principal source of fat: pork.

39

| Food and Description | Measure or Quantity | Sodium (mg.) | Total | —Fats in grams— Satu- rated | Unsatu- rated | Choles- terol (mg.) |
|---|---|---|---|---|---|---|
| Pea bean, small, in pork & molasses sauce | 7/8 cup (8 oz.) | 750 | 7.0 | | | |
| Red kidney in brown sugar sauce | 7/8 cup (8 oz.) | 640 | 7.0 | | | |
| In tomato sauce | 7/8 cup (8 oz.) | 1,010 | 3.0 | | | |
| Vegetarian | 7/8 cup (8 oz.) | 750 | 7.0 | | | |
| Yellow eye bean in brown sugar sauce | 7/8 cup (8 oz.) | 770 | 7.0 | | | |
| (Campbell's): | | | | | | |
| Home style | 8 oz. | 1,130 | 4.0 | | | |
| Old fashioned, in molasses & brown sugar sauce | 8 oz. | 1,060 | 3.0 | | | |
| & pork in tomato sauce | 8 oz. | 820 | 3.0 | | | |
| (Friend's): | | | | | | |
| Pea bean | 1 cup (9 oz.) | 1,270 | 5.0 | | | |
| Red kidney bean | 1 cup (9 oz.) | 1,320 | 4.0 | | | |
| Yellow eye bean | 1 cup (9 oz.) | 1,470 | 6.0 | | | |
| (Furman's) & pork in tomato sauce | 8 oz. | 718 | 1.7 | | | |
| (Hormel) Short Orders: | | | | | | |
| With bacon | 7 1/2 oz. | 813 | 12.0 | | | |
| With ham | 7 1/2 oz. | 1,182 | 18.0 | | | |
| (Hunt's) & pork [1] | 8 oz. | 800 | 2.0 | | | |
| (Van Camp's): | | | | | | |
| & pork | 8 oz. | 1,005 | 1.9 | | | |
| Vegetarian | 8 oz. | 959 | .6 | | | |
| **BEAN, BAYO,** dry (USDA) | 4 oz. | 28 | 1.7 | | | 0 |
| ***BEAN 'N BEEF*** (Campbell's) | 1 cup | 1211 | 6.1 | | | |
| **BEAN, BLACK,** dry (USDA) | 4 oz. | 28 | 1.7 | | | 0 |
| **BEAN, BROWN,** dry (USDA) | 4 oz. | 28 | 1.7 | | | 0 |
| **BEAN, CALICO,** dry (USDA) | 4 oz. | 11 | 1.4 | | | 0 |
| **BEAN, CHILI,** canned (Hunt's) | 1/2 cup (3.5 oz.) | 430 | < 1.0 | | | |
| **BEAN & FRANKFURTER,** canned: | | | | | | |
| (USDA) | 1 cup (9 oz.) | 1,374 | 18.1 | | | |

(USDA): United States Department of Agriculture
*Prepared as Package Directs
[1]Principal source of fat: bacon.

| Food and Description | Measure or Quantity | Sodium (mg.) | — Fats in grams — | | | Cholesterol (mg.) |
|---|---|---|---|---|---|---|
| | | | Total | Saturated | Unsaturated | |

| Food and Description | Measure or Quantity | Sodium (mg.) | Total | Cholesterol (mg.) |
|---|---|---|---|---|
| (Campbell's) in tomato & molasses sauce | 7⁷/₈-oz. serving | 1,140 | 14.0 | |
| (Hormel) *Short Orders* | 7¹/₂-oz. can | 1,342 | 14.0 | |
| **BEAN & FRANKFURTER DINNER,** frozen: | | | | |
| (Banquet) *American Favorites* | 10¹/₄ oz. | 1,377 | 19.0 | |
| (Morton) | 10³/₄-oz. dinner | 1,000 | 14.6 | |
| (Swanson) | 12¹/₂-oz. dinner | 1,100 | 20.0 | |
| **BEAN, GARBANZO,** canned, solids & liq.: | | | | |
| Regular (Old El Paso) | ¹/₂ cup | 247 | 1.3 | |
| Dietetic (S&W) *Nutradiet,* green label, low sodium | ¹/₂ cup | < 10 | 1.0 | |
| **BEAN, GREAT NORTHERN** (See **BEAN, WHITE**) | | | | |
| **BEAN, GREEN OR SNAP:** | | | | |
| Fresh (USDA): | | | | |
| Whole | 1 lb. (weighed untrimmed) | 28 | .8 | 0 |
| 1¹/₂" to 2" pieces | ¹/₂ cup (1.8 oz.) | 4 | .1 | 0 |
| French-style | ¹/₂ cup (1.4 oz.) | 3 | < .1 | 0 |
| Boiled without salt, drained, whole (USDA) | ¹/₂ cup (2.2 oz.) | 2 | .1 | 0 |
| Boiled without salt, drained, 1¹/₂" to 2" pieces (USDA) | ¹/₂ cup (2.4 oz.) | 3 | .1 | 0 |
| Canned, regular pack: (USDA): | | | | |
| Solids & liq. | ¹/₂ cup (4.2 oz.) | 283 | .1 | 0 |
| Drained solids, whole | 4 oz. | 268 | .2 | 0 |
| Drained solids, cut | ¹/₂ cup (2.5 oz.) | 165 | .1 | 0 |
| Drained liq. | 4 oz. | 268 | .1 | 0 |
| (Allen) solids & liq.: | | | | |
| Regular, any style | ¹/₂ cup (4 oz.) | 350 | 0.0 | |
| Cut, with dry, shelled beans | ¹/₂ cup (4 oz.) | 230 | 0.0 | |
| (Comstock) solids & liq. | ¹/₂ cup (4.2 oz.) | 400 | 0.0 | |
| (Del Monte) any style, solids & liq. | ¹/₂ cup (4 oz.) | 355 | Tr. | |

(USDA): United States Department of Agriculture
*Prepared as Package Directs

| Food and Description | Measure or Quantity | Sodium (mg.) | — Fats in grams — | | | Choles- terol (mg.) |
|---|---|---|---|---|---|---|
| | | | Total | Satu- rated | Unsatu- rated | |
| (Green Giant) any style, solids & liq. | ½ cup (4.2 oz.) | 270 | .1 | | | |
| (Larsen) *Freshlike*, solids & liq. | ½ cup | 340 | 0.0 | | | |
| (Sunshine) solids & liq. | ½ cup (4.2 oz.) | 312 | .1 | | | |
| Canned, dietetic pack: | | | | | | |
| (USDA): | | | | | | |
| Solids & liq. | 4 oz. | 2 | .1 | | | 0 |
| Drained solids | 4 oz. | 2 | .1 | | | 0 |
| Drained liq. | 4 oz. | 2 | .1 | | | 0 |
| (Allen) no added salt, solids & liq. | ½ cup (4 oz.) | 10 | 0.0 | | | |
| (Del Monte) no added salt, solids & liq. | ½ cup (4 oz.) | < 10 | 0.0 | | | |
| (Diet Delight) solids & liq. | ½ cup (4.2 oz.) | 5 | 0.0 | | | |
| (Featherweight) solids & liq. | ½ cup (4 oz.) | < 10 | 0.0 | | | |
| (Larsen) *Fresh-Lite*, water pack, solids & liq. | ½ cup (4.2 oz.) | 6 | 0.0 | | | |
| (S&W) *Nutradiet*, green label, solids & liq. | ½ cup | < 10 | 0.0 | | | |
| Frozen: | | | | | | |
| (USDA): | | | | | | |
| Cut: | | | | | | |
| Not thawed | 10-oz. pkg. | 3 | .3 | | | 0 |
| Boiled without salt, drained | 4 oz. | 1 | .1 | | | 0 |
| French style: | | | | | | |
| Not thawed | 10-oz. pkg. | 6 | .3 | | | 0 |
| Boiled, drained | ½ cup (2.8 oz.) | 2 | .1 | | | 0 |
| (Birds Eye): | | | | | | |
| Cut | 3 oz. | 3 | .1 | | | 0 |
| French-style | 3 oz. | 2 | .1 | | | 0 |
| Whole, deluxe | 3 oz. | 2 | .2 | | | 0 |
| (Green Giant): | | | | | | |
| Cut or french-style in butter sauce | ½ cup | 355 | 1.0 | | | |
| Cut, *Harvest Fresh* | ½ cup | 175 | 0.0 | | | |
| With mushrooms in cream sauce | ½ cup | 280 | 4.0 | | | |
| Polybag | ½ cup (2.5 oz.) | 5 | 0.0 | | | (0) |
| (Larsen) any style | 3 oz. | 5 | 0.0 | | | (0) |
| (McKenzie) any style | 3 oz. | 17 | 0.0 | | | (0) |
| (Southland) | ⅕ of 16-oz. pkg. | 0 | 0.0 | | | (0) |

(USDA): United States Department of Agriculture
*Prepared as Package Directs

| Food and Description | Measure or Quantity | Sodium (mg.) | Total | —Fats in grams— Satu- rated | Unsatu- rated | Choles- terol (mg.) |
|---|---|---|---|---|---|---|
| **BEAN, GREEN, & MUSHROOM CASSEROLE,** frozen (Stouffer's) | ½ of 9.5-oz. pkg. | 675 | 9.0 | | | |
| **BEAN, GREEN, & POTATO,** canned (Sunshine) solids & liq. | ½ cup (4.5 oz.) | 398 | .1 | | | |
| **BEAN, GREEN, PUREE,** canned (Larsen) no salt added | ½ cup (4.4 oz.) | 6 | .5 | | | |
| **BEAN, ITALIAN** (See **BROADBEAN**) | | | | | | |
| **BEAN, KIDNEY OR RED:** Dry: | | | | | | |
| (USDA) | 4 oz. | 11 | 1.7 | | | 0 |
| (USDA) | ½ cup (3.3 oz.) | 9 | 1.4 | | | 0 |
| Cooked without salt (USDA) | ½ cup (3.3 oz.) | 3 | .5 | | | 0 |
| Canned, solids & liq.: Regular: | | | | | | |
| (USDA) | ½ cup (4.5 oz.) | 4 | .5 | | | 0 |
| (Allen) dark, light, or red | ½ cup (4.1 oz.) | 290 | 1.0 | | | (0) |
| (Comstock) | ½ cup (4.4 oz.) | 410 | 0.0 | | | (0) |
| (Hunt's): | | | | | | |
| Red | ½ cup (3.5 oz.) | 500 | <1.0 | | | (0) |
| Small | 4 oz. | 400 | 0.0 | | | (0) |
| (Van Camp's): Kidney: | | | | | | |
| Dark | 4 oz. | 366 | .2 | | | (0) |
| Light | 4 oz. | 340 | .2 | | | (0) |
| New Orleans style | 4 oz. | 386 | .2 | | | (0) |
| Red | 4 oz. | 465 | .3 | | | (0) |
| Dietetic (S&W) *Nutradiet,* green label, low sodium | ½ cup | <10 | 0.0 | | | (0) |
| **BEAN, LIMA,** young: | | | | | | |
| Raw, whole (USDA) | 1 lb. (weighed in pod) | 4 | .9 | | | 0 |
| Raw, without shell (USDA) | 1 lb. (weighed shelled) | 9 | 2.3 | | | 0 |

(USDA): United States Department of Agriculture
*Prepared as Package Directs

| Food and Description | Measure or Quantity | Sodium (mg.) | — Fats in grams — | | | Cholesterol (mg.) |
|---|---|---|---|---|---|---|
| | | | Total | Saturated | Unsaturated | |
| Boiled without salt, drained (USDA) | ½ cup (3 oz.) | <1 | .4 | | | 0 |
| Canned, regular pack: | | | | | | |
| (USDA): | | | | | | |
| Solids & liq. | ½ cup (4.4 oz.) | 293 | .4 | | | 0 |
| Drained solids | ½ cup (3.1 oz.) | 205 | .3 | | | 0 |
| Drained liquid | 4 oz. | 268 | Tr. | | | 0 |
| (Allen) solids & liq.: | | | | | | |
| Regular | 4 oz. | 370 | <1.0 | | | (0) |
| Baby butter | 4 oz. | | <1.0 | | | (0) |
| Large butter | 4 oz. | 330 | 1.0 | | | (0) |
| (Comstock) solids & liq.: | | | | | | |
| Regular | ½ cup (4.4 oz.) | 400 | 0.0 | | | (0) |
| Butter | ½ cup (4.1 oz.) | 500 | 0.0 | | | (0) |
| (Del Monte) solids & liq. | 4 oz. | 355 | Tr. | | | (0) |
| (Furman's) solids & liq. | ½ cup (3.9 oz.) | 459 | .3 | | | (0) |
| (Larsen) Freshlike, solids & liq. | ½ cup (4 oz.) | 320 | 0.0 | | | (0) |
| Canned, dietetic pack: | | | | | | |
| (USDA) low sodium: | | | | | | |
| Solids & liq. | 4 oz. | 5 | .3 | | | 0 |
| Drained solids | 4 oz. | 5 | .3 | | | 0 |
| (Featherweight) solids & liq. | ½ cup | 25 | 0.0 | | | (0) |
| (Larsen) Fresh-Lite, water packed, solids & liq. | ½ cup (4.4 oz.) | 6 | 0.0 | | | (0) |
| Frozen: | | | | | | |
| Baby butter beans (Birds Eye) | ⅓ of 10-oz. pkg. | 211 | .7 | | | 0 |
| Baby limas: | | | | | | |
| Not thawed (USDA) | 4 oz. | 167 | .2 | | | 0 |
| Boiled, drained (USDA) | ½ cup (3 oz.) | 111 | .2 | | | 0 |
| (Birds Eye) | ½ cup (3.3 oz.) | 116 | .2 | | | 0 |
| (Green Giant) in butter sauce | ⅓ of 10-oz. pkg. | 445 | 2.0 | | | |
| (Larsen) | 3.3-oz. serving | 100 | 1.0 | | | (0) |
| Fordhooks: | | | | | | |
| Not thawed (USDA) | 4 oz. | 146 | .1 | | | 0 |
| Boiled, drained (USDA) | ½ cup (3 oz.) | 85 | <.1 | | | 0 |
| (Birds Eye) | ⅓ of 10-oz. pkg. | 102 | .1 | | | 0 |
| **BEAN, LIMA,** mature: | | | | | | |
| Dry: | | | | | | |
| Baby (USDA) | ½ cup (3.4 oz.) | 4 | 1.5 | | | 0 |

(USDA): United States Department of Agriculture
*Prepared as Package Directs

| Food and Description | Measure or Quantity | Sodium (mg.) | Total | Fats in grams —<br>Satu-rated | Unsatu-rated | Choles-terol (mg.) |
|---|---|---|---|---|---|---|
| Large (USDA) | ½ cup (3.1 oz.) | 4 | 1.4 | | | 0 |
| Boiled without salt, drained (USDA) | ½ cup (3.4 oz.) | 2 | .6 | | | 0 |
| **BEAN, MUNG,** dry (USDA) | ½ cup (3.7 oz.) | 6 | 1.4 | | | 0 |
| **BEAN, NAVY OR PEA** (See **BEAN, WHITE**) | | | | | | |
| **BEAN, PINTO:** | | | | | | |
| Dry (USDA) | 4 oz. | 11 | 1.4 | | | 0 |
| Dry (USDA) | ½ cup (3.4 oz.) | 10 | 1.2 | | | 0 |
| **BEAN, RED** (See **BEAN, KIDNEY** or **BEAN, RED MEXICAN**) | | | | | | |
| **BEAN, RED MEXICAN,** dry (USDA) | 4 oz. | 11 | 1.4 | | | 0 |
| **BEAN, REFRIED,** canned, solids & liq.: | | | | | | |
| (Del Monte): | | | | | | |
| Regular | ½ cup (4.3 oz.) | 530 | 2.0 | | | |
| Spicy | ½ cup (4.3 oz.) | 480 | 2.0 | | | |
| (Gebhardt): | | | | | | |
| Regular | 4 oz. | 490 | 2.0 | | | |
| Jalapeno | 4 oz. | 320 | 2.0 | | | |
| *Little Pancho* (Borden's) & green chili | ½ cup | 330 | 0.0 | | | |
| (Old El Paso): | | | | | | |
| Plain | 4 oz. | 593 | 1.1 | | | |
| With green chili pepper | 4 oz. | 317 | 0.0 | | | |
| With sausage | 4 oz. | 355 | 13.6 | | | |
| (Rosarita): | | | | | | |
| Regular or vegetarian | 4 oz. | 460 | 2.0 | | | |
| With green chilis | 4 oz. | 430 | 2.0 | | | |
| Spicy | 4 oz. | 440 | 2.0 | | | |
| **BEAN SALAD,** canned, solids & liq. (Green Giant) | 4¼ oz. | 540 | .2 | | | |

(USDA): United States Department of Agriculture
\*Prepared as Package Directs

| Food and Description | Measure or Quantity | Sodium (mg.) | Total | —Fats in grams— Satu- rated | Unsatu- rated | Choles- terol (mg.) |
|---|---|---|---|---|---|---|
| **BEANS 'N FIXIN'S,** canned | | | | | | |
| (Hunt's) *Big John's:* | | | | | | |
| Beans | 3 oz. | 370 | < 1.0 | | | |
| Fixin's | 1 oz. | 125 | 2.0 | | | |
| | | | | | | |
| **BEAN SOUP** (See **SOUP,** Bean) | | | | | | |
| | | | | | | |
| **BEAN SPROUT:** | | | | | | |
| Mung: | | | | | | |
| Raw (USDA) | ½ lb. | 12 | .4 | | | 0 |
| Raw (USDA) | ½ cup (1.6 oz.) | 2 | < .1 | | | 0 |
| Boiled without salt, drained | | | | | | |
| (USDA) | ½ cup (2.2 oz.) | 2 | .1 | | | 0 |
| Soy: | | | | | | |
| Raw (USDA) | ½ lb. | | 3.2 | | | 0 |
| Raw (USDA) | ½ cup (1.9 oz.) | | .8 | | | 0 |
| Boiled without salt, drained | | | | | | |
| (USDA) | 4 oz. | | 1.6 | | | 0 |
| Canned, (La Choy) drained | | | | | | |
| solids | ⅔ cup | 18 | < 1.0 | | | (0) |
| | | | | | | |
| **BEAN, WHITE,** dry: | | | | | | |
| Raw: | | | | | | |
| Great Northern (USDA) | ½ cup (3.1 oz.) | 17 | 1.4 | | | 0 |
| Navy or pea (USDA) | ½ cup (3.7 oz.) | 20 | 1.7 | | | 0 |
| All other white (USDA) | 1 oz. | 5 | .5 | | | 0 |
| Cooked without salt: | | | | | | |
| Great Northern (USDA) | ½ cup (3 oz.) | 6 | .5 | | | 0 |
| Navy or pea (USDA) | ½ cup (3.4 oz.) | 7 | .6 | | | 0 |
| All other white (USDA) | 4 oz. | 8 | .7 | | | 0 |
| | | | | | | |
| **BEAN, YELLOW OR WAX:** | | | | | | |
| Raw, whole (USDA) | 1 lb. (weighed untrimmed) | 28 | .8 | | | 0 |
| Boiled without salt, drained | | | | | | |
| (USDA) | 4 oz. | 3 | .2 | | | 0 |
| Boiled without salt, drained 1″ | | | | | | |
| pieces (USDA) | ½ cup (2.9 oz.) | 2 | .2 | | | 0 |
| Canned, regular pack: | | | | | | |
| (USDA): | | | | | | |
| Solids & liq. | ½ cup (4.2 oz.) | 283 | .2 | | | 0 |
| Drained solids | ½ cup (2.2 oz.) | 146 | .2 | | | 0 |

(USDA): United States Department of Agriculture
*Prepared as Package Directs

| Food and Description | Measure or Quantity | Sodium (mg.) | —Fats in grams— | | | Choles-terol (mg.) |
|---|---|---|---|---|---|---|
| | | | Total | Satu-rated | Unsatu-rated | |
| Drained liquid | 4 oz. | 268 | .1 | | | 0 |
| (Comstock) solids & liq. | 1/2 cup (4.2 oz.) | 370 | 0.0 | | | (0) |
| (Del Monte) solids & liq. | 4 oz. | 355 | 0.0 | | | (0) |
| (Larsen) *Freshlike,* cut, solids & liq. | 1/2 cup (4.2 oz.) | 320 | 0.0 | | | (0) |
| Canned, dietetic pack: (USDA): | | | | | | |
| Solids & liq. | 4 oz. | 2 | .1 | | | 0 |
| Drained solids | 4 oz. | 2 | .1 | | | 0 |
| Drained liquid | 4 oz. | 2 | .1 | | | 0 |
| (Featherweight) solids & liq. | 1/2 cup (4 oz.) | < 10 | 0.0 | | | (0) |
| (Larsen) *Fresh-Lite,* water pack, solids & liq. | 1/2 cup (4.2 oz.) | 6 | 0.0 | | | (0) |
| Frozen: | | | | | | |
| Cut, not thawed (USDA) | 4 oz. | 1 | .1 | | | 0 |
| Boiled, drained (USDA) | 4 oz. | 1 | .1 | | | 0 |
| Cut (Larsen) | 3 oz. | 5 | 0.0 | | | (0) |
| **BEAVER,** roasted (USDA) | 4 oz. | | 15.5 | | | |
| **BEECHNUT:** | | | | | | |
| Whole (USDA) | 4 oz. (weighed in shell) | | 34.6 | 3. | 32. | 0 |
| Shelled (USDA) | 1 oz. (weighed shelled) | | 14.2 | 1. | 13. | 0 |

**BEEF.** Values for beef cuts are given below for "lean and fat" and for "lean only." Beef purchased by the consumer at the retail store usually is trimmed to about one-half inch layer of fat. This is the meat described as "lean and fat." If all the fat that can be cut off with a knife is removed, the remainder is the "lean only." These cuts still contain flecks of fat known as "marbling" distributed through the meat. Cooked meats are medium done. Choice grade cuts (USDA):

(USDA): United States Department of Agriculture
*Prepared as Package Directs

| Food and Description | Measure or Quantity | Sodium (mg.) | Total | —Fats in grams— Satu- rated | Unsatu- rated | Choles- terol (mg.) |
|---|---|---|---|---|---|---|
| **Brisket:** | | | | | | |
| Raw, lean & fat | 1 lb. (weighed with bone) | 248 | 112.4 | 54. | 58. | 259 |
| Raw, lean & fat | 1 lb. (weighed without bone) | 295 | 133.8 | 64. | 69. | 308 |
| Raw, lean only | 1 lb. | 295 | 37.2 | 18. | 20. | 295 |
| Braised: | | | | | | |
| Lean & fat | 4 oz. | 68 | 39.5 | 19. | 21. | 107 |
| Lean only | 4 oz. | 68 | 11.9 | 6. | 6. | 103 |
| **Chuck:** | | | | | | |
| Raw, lean & fat | 1 lb. (weighed with bone) | 248 | 75.0 | 36. | 39. | 259 |
| Raw, lean & fat | 1 lb. (weighed without bone) | 295 | 88.9 | 43. | 46. | 308 |
| Raw, lean only | 1 lb. | 295 | 33.6 | 18. | 15. | 295 |
| Braised or pot-roasted: | | | | | | |
| Lean & fat | 4 oz. | 68 | 27.1 | 13. | 14. | 107 |
| Lean only | 4 oz. | 68 | 10.8 | 5. | 6. | 103 |
| **Dried (See BEEF, CHIPPED)** | | | | | | |
| Fat, separable, raw | 1 oz. | | 21.6 | 10. | 11. | 21 |
| Fat, separable, cooked | 1 oz. | | 22.1 | 10. | 12. | |
| Filet Mignon. There is no data available on its composition. For dietary estimates, the data for sirloin steak, lean only, afford the closest approximation. | | | | | | |
| **Flank:** | | | | | | |
| Raw, 100% lean | 1 lb. | 295 | 25.9 | 12. | 13. | 295 |
| Braised, 100% lean | 4 oz. | 68 | 8.3 | 4. | 4. | 103 |
| **Foreshank:** | | | | | | |
| Raw, lean & fat | 1 lb. (weighed with bone) | 156 | 34.8 | 17. | 18. | 163 |
| Simmered: | | | | | | |
| Lean & fat | 4 oz. | 68 | 19.4 | 9. | 10. | 107 |
| Lean only | 4 oz. | 68 | 6.6 | 3. | 3. | 103 |
| **Ground:** | | | | | | |
| Regular: | | | | | | |
| Raw | 1 lb. | 118 | 96.2 | 48. | 48. | 308 |
| Raw | 1 cup (8 oz.) | 104 | 47.9 | 23. | 25. | 154 |
| Broiled | 4 oz. | 53 | 23.0 | 11. | 12. | 107 |

(USDA): United States Department of Agriculture
*Prepared as Package Directs

| Food and Description | Measure or Quantity | Sodium (mg.) | — Fats in grams — | | | Cholesterol (mg.) |
|---|---|---|---|---|---|---|
| | | | Total | Saturated | Unsaturated | |
| **Lean:** | | | | | | |
| Raw | 1 lb. | 236 | 45.4 | 22. | 23. | 295 |
| Raw | 1 cup (8 oz.) | 118 | 22.6 | 11. | 11. | 147 |
| Broiled | 4 oz. | 54 | 12.8 | 6. | 7. | 103 |
| **Heel of round:** | | | | | | |
| Raw, lean & fat | 1 lb. | 295 | 64.4 | 31. | 34. | 308 |
| Raw, lean only | 1 lb. | 295 | 21.3 | 9. | 12. | 295 |
| **Roasted:** | | | | | | |
| Lean & fat | 4 oz. | 68 | 18.3 | 9. | 10. | 107 |
| Lean only | 4 oz. | 68 | 6.5 | 3. | 3. | 103 |
| **Hindshank:** | | | | | | |
| **Raw:** | | | | | | |
| Lean & fat | 1 lb. (weighed with bone) | 136 | 48.9 | 23. | 25. | 142 |
| Lean & fat | 1 lb. (weighed without bone) | 295 | 106.1 | 51. | 55. | 308 |
| Lean only | 1 lb. | 295 | 20.9 | 10. | 11. | 295 |
| **Simmered:** | | | | | | |
| Lean & fat | 4 oz. | 68 | 31.9 | 15. | 17. | 107 |
| Lean only | 4 oz. | 68 | 6.7 | 3. | 4. | 103 |
| **Neck:** | | | | | | |
| Raw, lean & fat | 1 lb. (weighed with bone) | 237 | 57.7 | 28. | 30. | 247 |
| **Pot-roasted:** | | | | | | |
| Lean & fat | 4 oz. | 68 | 22.3 | 11. | 12. | 107 |
| Lean only | 4 oz. | 68 | 8.3 | 4. | 4. | 103 |
| Oxtail, raw | 1 lb. (weighed with bone) | 73 | 7.9 | 4. | 4. | 73 |
| Oxtail, raw | 1 lb. (weighed without bone) | 295 | 31.8 | 15. | 17. | 295 |
| **Plate:** | | | | | | |
| **Raw:** | | | | | | |
| Lean & fat | 1 lb. (weighed with bone) | 263 | 150.6 | 72. | 78. | 275 |
| Lean & fat | 1 lb. (weighed without bone) | 295 | 169.2 | 81. | 88. | 308 |
| Lean only | 1 lb. | 295 | 37.2 | 18. | 20. | 295 |
| **Simmered:** | | | | | | |
| Lean & fat | 4 oz. | 68 | 48.5 | 23. | 25. | 107 |
| Lean only | 4 oz. | 68 | 11.9 | 6. | 6. | 103 |

(USDA): United States Department of Agriculture
*Prepared as Package Directs

| Food and Description | Measure or Quantity | Sodium (mg.) | Total | — Fats in grams — Satu-rated | Unsatu-rated | Choles-terol (mg.) |
|---|---|---|---|---|---|---|
| Rib roast: | | | | | | |
| Raw: | | | | | | |
| Lean & fat | 1 lb. (weighed with bone) | 271 | 156.1 | 75. | 81. | 284 |
| Lean & fat | 1 lb. (weighed without bone) | 295 | 169.6 | 81. | 88. | 308 |
| Lean only | 1 lb. | 295 | 52.6 | 27. | 25. | 295 |
| Roasted: | | | | | | |
| Lean & fat | 4 oz. | 68 | 44.7 | 21. | 23. | 107 |
| Lean only | 4 oz. | 68 | 15.2 | 7. | 8. | 103 |
| Lean only, chopped | 1 cup (4.5 oz.) | 77 | 17.2 | 8. | 9. | 116 |
| Lean only, diced | 1 cup (5 oz.) | 86 | 19.2 | 9. | 10. | 130 |
| Round: | | | | | | |
| Raw: | | | | | | |
| Lean & fat | 1 lb. (weighed with bone) | 286 | 53.9 | 26. | 28. | 299 |
| Lean & fat | 1 lb. (weighed without bone) | 295 | 55.8 | 27. | 29. | 308 |
| Lean only | 1 lb. | 295 | 21.3 | 9. | 12. | 295 |
| Broiled: | | | | | | |
| Lean & fat | 4 oz. | 68 | 17.5 | 8. | 9. | 107 |
| Lean only | 4 oz. | 68 | 6.9 | 3. | 4. | 103 |
| Rump: | | | | | | |
| Raw: | | | | | | |
| Lean & fat | 1 lb. (weighed with bone) | 251 | 97.4 | 47. | 50. | 262 |
| Lean & fat | 1 lb. (weighed without bone) | 295 | 114.8 | 55. | 60. | 308 |
| Lean only | 1 lb. | 295 | 34.0 | 15. | 19. | 295 |
| Roasted: | | | | | | |
| Lean & fat | 4 oz. | 68 | 31.0 | 15. | 16. | 107 |
| Lean only | 4 oz. | 68 | 10.5 | 5. | 5. | 103 |
| Steak, club: | | | | | | |
| Raw: | | | | | | |
| Lean & fat | 1 lb. (weighed with bone) | 229 | 132.1 | 63. | 69. | 259 |
| Lean & fat | 1 lb. (weighed without bone) | 295 | 157.9 | 76. | 82. | 308 |
| Lean only | 1 lb. | 295 | 46.7 | 22. | 25. | 295 |
| Broiled: | | | | | | |
| Lean & fat | 4 oz. | 68 | 46.0 | 22. | 24. | 107 |
| Lean only | 4 oz. | 68 | 14.7 | 7. | 8. | 103 |

(USDA): United States Department of Agriculture
*Prepared as Package Directs

| Food and Description | Measure or Quantity | Sodium (mg.) | —Fats in grams— Total | Saturated | Unsaturated | Cholesterol (mg.) |
|---|---|---|---|---|---|---|
| One 8-oz. steak (weighed without bone before cooking) will give you: | | | | | | |
| Lean & fat | 5.9 oz. | 100 | 67.4 | 32. | 35. | 156 |
| Lean only | 3.4 oz. | 58 | 12.5 | 6. | 7. | 87 |
| Steak, porterhouse: | | | | | | |
| Raw, lean & fat | 1 lb. (weighed with bone) | 268 | 148.8 | 71. | 78. | 281 |
| Broiled: | | | | | | |
| Lean & fat | 4 oz. | 68 | 47.9 | 23. | 25. | 107 |
| Lean only | 4 oz. | 68 | 11.9 | 6. | 6. | 103 |
| One 16-oz. steak (weighed with bone before cooking) will give you: | | | | | | |
| Lean & fat | 10.2 oz. | 173 | 121.5 | 59. | 63. | 271 |
| Lean only | 5.9 oz. | 100 | 17.4 | 8. | 9. | 151 |
| Steak, ribeye, broiled: | | | | | | |
| One 10-oz. steak (weighed without bone before cooking) will give you: | | | | | | |
| Lean & fat | 7.3 oz. | 124 | 81.6 | 39. | 42. | 195 |
| Lean only | 3.8 oz. | 64 | 14.3 | 7. | 7. | 97 |
| Steak, sirloin, double-bone: | | | | | | |
| Raw: | | | | | | |
| Lean & fat | 1 lb. (weighed with bone) | 242 | 108.4 | 52. | 56. | 253 |
| Lean & fat | 1 lb. (weighed without bone) | 295 | 132.0 | 63. | 69. | 308 |
| Lean only | 1 lb. | 295 | 33.6 | 18. | 15. | 295 |
| Broiled: | | | | | | |
| Lean & fat | 4 oz. | 68 | 39.3 | 19. | 20. | 107 |
| Lean only | 4 oz. | 68 | 10.8 | 5. | 6. | 103 |
| One 16-oz. steak (weighed with bone before cooking) will give you: | | | | | | |
| Lean & fat | 8.9 oz. | 151 | 87.4 | 42. | 45. | 237 |
| Lean only | 5.9 oz. | 100 | 15.8 | 8. | 8. | 151 |
| One 12-oz. steak (weighed with bone before cooking) will give you: | | | | | | |
| Lean & fat | 6.6 oz. | 113 | 65.2 | 31. | 34. | 177 |
| Lean only | 4.4 oz. | 74 | 11.8 | 6. | 6. | 113 |

(USDA): United States Department of Agriculture
*Prepared as Package Directs

| Food and Description | Measure or Quantity | Sodium (mg.) | Total | Fats in grams — Satu- rated | Unsatu- rated | Choles- terol (mg.) |
|---|---|---|---|---|---|---|
| Steak, sirloin, hipbone: | | | | | | |
| Raw: | | | | | | |
| Lean & fat | 1 lb. (weighed with bone) | 251 | 149.3 | 72. | 78. | 262 |
| Lean & fat | 1 lb. (weighed without bone) | 295 | 176.0 | 84. | 92. | 308 |
| Lean only | 1 lb. | 295 | 44.9 | 21. | 24. | 295 |
| Broiled: | | | | | | |
| Lean & fat | 4 oz. | 68 | 50.9 | 24. | 26. | 107 |
| Lean only | 4 oz. | 68 | 14.2 | 7. | 7. | 103 |
| Steak, sirloin, wedge & roundbone: | | | | | | |
| Raw: | | | | | | |
| Lean & fat | 1 lb. (weighed with bone) | 274 | 112.3 | 54. | 58. | 287 |
| Lean & fat | 1 lb. (weighed without bone) | 295 | 121.1 | 58. | 63. | 308 |
| Lean only | 1 lb. | 295 | 25.9 | 12. | 14. | 295 |
| Broiled: | | | | | | |
| Lean & fat | 4 oz. | 68 | 36.3 | 17. | 19. | 107 |
| Lean only | 4 oz. | 68 | 8.7 | 4. | 5. | 103 |
| Steak, T-bone: | | | | | | |
| Raw, lean & fat | 1 lb. (weighed with bone) | 263 | 149.1 | 72. | 78. | 275 |
| Broiled: | | | | | | |
| Lean & fat | 4 oz. | 68 | 49.0 | 24. | 26. | 107 |
| Lean only | 4 oz. | 68 | 11.7 | 6. | 6. | 103 |
| One 16-oz. steak (weighed with bone before cooking) will give you: | | | | | | |
| Lean & fat | 9.8 oz. | 167 | 120.1 | 58. | 63. | 261 |
| Lean only | 5.5 oz. | 94 | 16.1 | 8. | 8. | 142 |
| **BEEFARONI**, canned (Chef Boy-Ar-Dee) | ⅕ of 40-oz. can | 1,371 | 6.4 | | | |
| **BEEF BOUILLON/BROTH,** cubes or powder (See also **SOUP,** Beef) | | | | | | |
| (Featherweight) low sodium | 1 tsp. | 10 | 1.0 | | | |
| (Herb-Ox): | | | | | | |
| Cube | 1 cube | 500 | .1 | | | |
| Packet | 1 packet | 1,040 | .1 | | | |

(USDA): United States Department of Agriculture
*Prepared as Package Directs

| Food and Description | Measure or Quantity | Sodium (mg.) | — Fats in grams — | | | Choles- terol (mg.) |
|---|---|---|---|---|---|---|
| | | | Total | Satu- rated | Unsatu- rated | |
| *Lite-Line* (Borden's) instant, low sodium | 1 tsp. | 5 | < 1.0 | | | |
| (Maggi) cube | 1 cube | 743 | 1.0 | | | |
| (Wyler's) | 1 cube or 1 tsp. | 930 | < 1.0 | | | |
| **BEEF, CHIPPED:** | | | | | | |
| Uncooked: | | | | | | |
| (USDA) | 2 oz. (about ⅓ cup) | 2,451 | 3.6 | 2. | 2. | |
| (USDA) | ½ cup (2.9 oz.) | 3,526 | 5.2 | 2. | 3. | |
| (Armour Star) | 1 oz. | | .7 | | | |
| Cooked, creamed, home recipe | | | | | | |
| (USDA)[1] | 1 cup (8.6 oz.) | 1,754 | 25.2 | 15. | 11. | 66 |
| Frozen: | | | | | | |
| (Banquet) creamed | 5-oz bag | | 4.1 | | | |
| (Banquet) *Entree for One,* creamed | 4-oz. serving | 818 | 2.0 | | | 25 |
| (Stouffer's) creamed | 5.5-oz. serving | 900 | 16.0 | | | |
| (Swanson) creamed | 10½-oz. entree | 1,545 | 23.0 | | | |
| **BEEF, CORNED** (See **CORNED BEEF**) | | | | | | |
| **BEEF DINNER,** frozen: | | | | | | |
| (Armour): | | | | | | |
| *Classic Lite,* Steak Diane | 10-oz. pkg. | 770 | 9.0 | | | 90 |
| *Dinner Classics:* | | | | | | |
| Burgundy | 10½-oz. pkg. | 990 | 15.0 | | | 95 |
| Sirloin tips | 11-oz. pkg. | 1,180 | 16.0 | | | 100 |
| (Blue Star) *Dining Lite,* teriyaki with vegetables & rice | 8⅝-oz. pkg. | 980 | 3.0 | | | |
| (Conagra) *Light & Elegant:* | | | | | | |
| Burgundy | 9-oz. entree | 1,240 | 4.0 | | | 55 |
| Julienne | 8½-oz. entree | 990 | 7.0 | | | |
| (Le Menu): | | | | | | |
| Chopped sirloin | 12¼-oz. dinner | 1,080 | 23.0 | | | |
| Sirloin tips | 11½-oz. meal | 840 | 18.0 | | | |
| Yankee pot roast | 11-oz. dinner | 810 | 15.0 | | | |
| (Morton): | | | | | | |
| Regular | 11-oz. dinner | 700 | 5.5 | | | |
| Light, sliced | 11-oz. dinner | 850 | 7.0 | | | |
| (Stouffer's) *Lean Cuisine,* oriental, in sauce with vegetables & rice | 8⅝-oz. pkg. | 1,150 | 8.0 | | | 35 |

(USDA): United States Department of Agriculture
*Prepared as Package Directs
[1]Principal sources of fat: milk, butter & beef.

| Food and Description | Measure or Quantity | Sodium (mg.) | Total | Fats in grams Satu- rated | Unsatu- rated | Choles- terol (mg.) |
|---|---|---|---|---|---|---|
| (Swanson): | | | | | | |
| 4-compartment dinner: | | | | | | |
| Regular | 11½-oz. dinner | 870 | 8.0 | | | |
| Chopped sirloin | 11½-oz. dinner | 930 | 17.0 | | | |
| *Hungry-Man:* | | | | | | |
| Chopped | 17¼-oz. meal | 1,640 | 29.0 | | | |
| Sliced | 16-oz. dinner | 1,150 | 12.0 | | | |
| Sliced | 12¼-oz. entree | 1,040 | 8.0 | | | |
| (Weight Watchers): | | | | | | |
| Beefsteak, chopped | 8 15/16-oz. meal | 980 | 20.0 | | | |
| Oriental | 10-oz. meal | 1,130 | 4.0 | | | |
| | | | | | | |
| **BEEF, DRIED,** packaged | | | | | | |
| (Hormel) sliced | 1 oz. | 822 | 1.0 | | | |
| | | | | | | |
| **BEEF, GROUND,** seasoning | | | | | | |
| mix: | | | | | | |
| *(Durkee): | | | | | | |
| Plain | 1 cup | 799 | 48.5 | | | |
| With onion | 1 cup | 1,099 | 48.0 | | | |
| (French's) With onions | 1⅛-oz. pkg. | 1,760 | 0. | | | |
| | | | | | | |
| **BEEF HASH, ROAST:** | | | | | | |
| Canned (Hormel) *Mary Kitchen* | 7½ oz. | 1,142 | 22.0 | | | |
| Frozen (Stouffer's) | 11½-oz. pkg. | 1,520 | 16.0 | | | |
| | | | | | | |
| **BEEF, PACKAGED:** | | | | | | |
| (Carl Buddig) | 1 oz. | 426 | 1.7 | .9 | .8 | 16 |
| (Hormel) | 1 oz. | 382 | 2.0 | | | |
| | | | | | | |
| **BEEF PEPPER ORIENTAL** | | | | | | |
| (La Choy): | | | | | | |
| Canned | ¾ cup | 1,060 | 2.0 | | | |
| Frozen | 12-oz. dinner | 1,985 | 3.0 | | | |
| | | | | | | |
| **BEEF PIE:** | | | | | | |
| Baked, home recipe (USDA)[1] | 4¼″ pie (8 oz. before baking) | 645 | 32.9 | 9. | 24. | 48 |
| Baked, home recipe (USDA)[1] | ⅓ of 9″ pie (7.4 oz.) | 596 | 30.4 | 8. | 22. | 44 |

(USDA): United States Department of Agriculture
*Prepared as Package Directs
[1]Principal sources of fat: vegetable shortening & beef.

| Food and Description | Measure or Quantity | Sodium (mg.) | — Fats in grams — | | | Choles- terol (mg.) |
|---|---|---|---|---|---|---|
| | | | Total | Satu- rated | Unsatu- rated | |
| **Frozen:** | | | | | | |
| Commercial, unheated (USDA)[1] | 1 pie (7.6 oz.) | 791 | 21.4 | 6. | 15. | 39 |
| (Banquet) | 8-oz. pie | 1,292 | 24.0 | | | |
| (Stouffer's) | 10-oz. pkg. | 1,600 | 36.0 | | | |
| (Swanson): | | | | | | |
| Regular | 8-oz. pie | 900 | 21.0 | | | |
| Chunky | 10-oz. pie | 900 | 28.0 | | | |
| *Hungry-Man:* | | | | | | |
| Regular | 16-oz. pie | 1,750 | 34.0 | | | |
| Steak burger | 16-oz. pie | 1,520 | 41.0 | | | |
| **BEEF, POTTED** (USDA) | 1 oz. | | 5.4 | | | |
| **BEEF SOUP** (See **SOUP,** Beef) | | | | | | |
| **BEEF SOUP MIX** (See **SOUP MIX,** Beef.) | | | | | | |
| **BEEF ROLL** (Hormel) *Lumberjack* | 1 oz. | 304 | 9.0 | | | |
| **BEEF RIBS,** frozen: | | | | | | |
| (Armour) *Dinner Classics,* boneless, with barbecue sauce | 10½-oz. pkg. | 1,180 | 26.0 | | | 95 |
| (Stouffer's) boneless, with vegetable gravy | 11½-oz. pkg. | 1,120 | 50.0 | | | |
| **BEEF SPREAD, ROAST** canned (Underwood) | ½ of 4¾-oz. can | 515 | 10.0 | | | |
| **BEEF STEW:** | | | | | | |
| Home recipe, made with lean beef chuck (USDA)[2] | 1 cup (8.6 oz.) | 91 | 10.5 | 5. | 6. | 64 |
| Canned: | | | | | | |
| Regular: | | | | | | |
| (USDA) | 1 cup (8.6 oz.) | 1,007 | 7.6 | | | 34 |
| *Dinty Moore:* | | | | | | |
| Regular | ½ of 24-oz. can | 980 | 12.0 | | | |
| Regular | ⅕ of 40-oz. can | 971 | 11.0 | | | |
| *Short Orders* | 7½-oz. serving | 939 | 9.0 | | | |

(USDA): United States Department of Agriculture
*Prepared as Package Directs
[1]Principal sources of fat: vegetable shortening & beef.
[2]Principal source of fat: beef.

| Food and Description | Measure or Quantity | Sodium (mg.) | Total | Fats in grams — Satu- rated | Unsatu- rated | Choles- terol (mg.) |
|---|---|---|---|---|---|---|
| (Libby's) | ½ of 24-oz. can | | 6.0 | | | |
| Dietetic: | | | | | | |
| (Estee) | 7½-oz. serving | 110 | 9.0 | | | |
| (Featherweight) | 7½-oz. serving | 96 | 8.0 | | | |
| Frozen: | | | | | | |
| Buffet: | | | | | | |
| (Banquet) *Family Entree* | 2-lb. pkg. | 3,908 | 52.0 | | | |
| (Green Giant) flavor tight pouch | 9-oz. entree | 275 | 3.0 | | | |
| (Stouffer's) | 10-oz. serving | 1,675 | 17.0 | | | |

**BEEF STEW SEASONING MIX:**

| | | | | | | |
|---|---|---|---|---|---|---|
| *(Durkee) | 1 cup | 975 | 24.0 | | | |
| (French's) | 1 pkg. (1⅞ oz.) | 4,620 | Tr. | | | |

**BEEF STOCK BASE** (French's)    1 tsp. (4 grams)    500    Tr.

**BEEF STROGANOFF,** frozen:

| | | | | | | |
|---|---|---|---|---|---|---|
| (Armour) *Dinner Classics* | 11¼-oz. meal | 1,330 | 17.0 | | | 85 |
| (Conagra) *Light & Elegant* | 9-oz. entree | 790 | 6.0 | | | 65 |
| (Green Giant) twin pouch, with noodles | 9-oz. entree | 820 | 16.0 | | | |
| (Le Menu) | 9¼-oz. dinner | 930 | 24.0 | | | |
| (Stouffer's) with parsley noodles | 9¾-oz. pkg. | 1,300 | 19.9 | | | |

**\*BEEF STROGANOFF SEASONING MIX** (Durkee)    1 cup    870    71.2

**BEER,** canned:

Regular:

| | | | | | | |
|---|---|---|---|---|---|---|
| (USDA) 4.5% alcohol | 12 fl. oz. | 25 | 0.0 | | | 0 |
| *Black Label* | 12 fl. oz. | 17 | 0.0 | | | 0 |
| *Blatz* | 12 fl. oz. | 14 | 0.0 | | | 0 |
| *Budweiser,* 4.9% alcohol | 12 fl. oz. | 20-40 | 0.0 | | | 0 |
| *Budweiser,* 3.9% alcohol | 12 fl. oz. | 20-40 | 0.0 | | | 0 |
| *Busch Bavarian,* 3.9% alcohol | 12 fl. oz. | 5-15 | 0.0 | | | 0 |
| *Michelob,* 4.9% alcohol | 12 fl. oz. | 20-40 | 0.0 | | | 0 |
| *Pabst Blue Ribbon* | 12 fl. oz. | 7 | (0.0) | | | (0) |

(USDA): United States Department of Agriculture
\*Prepared as Package Directs

| Food and Description | Measure or Quantity | Sodium (mg.) | —Fats in grams— | | | Cholesterol (mg.) |
|---|---|---|---|---|---|---|
| | | | Total | Saturated | Unsaturated | |
| *Schlitz* | 12 fl. oz. | 24 | (0.0) | | | (0) |
| Low carbohydrate: | | | | | | |
| *Gablinger's,* 4.5% alcohol | 12 fl. oz. | 21 | 0.0 | | | (0) |
| *Meister Brau Light,* 4.6% alcohol | 12 fl. oz. | Tr. | 0.0 | | | (0) |
| **BEER, NEAR,** *Kingsbury* (Heileman) 0.4% alcohol | 12 fl. oz. | 41 | | | | 0 |
| **BEET:** | | | | | | |
| Raw (USDA) | 1 lb. (weighed with skins, part tops) | 133 | .2 | | | 0 |
| Raw (USDA) | 1 lb. (weighed with skins, without tops) | 190 | .3 | | | 0 |
| Raw, diced (USDA) | ½ cup (2.4 oz.) | 40 | <.1 | | | 0 |
| Boiled without salt (USDA): | | | | | | |
| Whole, drained | 2 beets (2″ dia., 3.5 oz.) | 43 | .1 | | | 0 |
| Diced, drained | ½ cup (3 oz.) | 37 | <.1 | | | 0 |
| Sliced, drained | ½ cup (3.6 oz.) | 44 | .1 | | | 0 |
| Canned, regular pack: (USDA): | | | | | | |
| Solids & liq. | ½ cup (4.3 oz.) | 290 | .1 | | | 0 |
| Drained solids, whole | ½ cup (2.8 oz.) | 188 | <.1 | | | 0 |
| Drained solids, diced | ½ cup (2.9 oz.) | 194 | <.1 | | | 0 |
| Drained solids, sliced | ½ cup (3.1 oz.) | 208 | <.1 | | | 0 |
| Drained liq. | 4 oz. | 268 | Tr. | | | 0 |
| (Blue Boy) harvard, solids & liq. | ½ cup (4.2 oz.) | 350 | 0.0 | | | (0) |
| (Comstock) solids & liq.: | | | | | | |
| Regular | ½ cup (4.2 oz.) | 100 | 0.0 | | | (0) |
| Pickled | ½ cup (4.2 oz.) | 500 | 0.0 | | | (0) |
| (Del Monte) solids & liq.: | | | | | | |
| Pickled, sliced | 4 oz. | 375 | 0.0 | | | (0) |
| Sliced or whole | ½ cup (4 oz.) | 290 | 0.0 | | | (0) |
| (Larsen) *Freshlike:* | | | | | | |
| Pickled | ½ cup (4.7 oz.) | 260 | 0.0 | | | (0) |
| Sliced or whole | ½ cup (4.3 oz.) | 650 | 0.0 | | | (0) |
| Canned, dietetic pack: (USDA): | | | | | | |
| Solids & liq. | 4 oz. | 52 | Tr. | | | 0 |

(USDA): United States Department of Agriculture
*Prepared as Package Directs

| Food and Description | Measure or Quantity | Sodium (mg.) | —Fats in grams— | | | Cholesterol (mg.) |
|---|---|---|---|---|---|---|
| | | | Total | Saturated | Unsaturated | |
| Drained solids | 4 oz. | 52 | .1 | | | 0 |
| Drained liq. | 4 oz. | 52 | Tr. | | | 0 |
| (Comstock) solids & liq. | ½ cup (4 oz.) | 100 | 0.0 | | | (0) |
| (Del Monte) sliced, low salt, solids & liq. | ½ cup (4 oz.) | 100 | 0.0 | | | (0) |
| (Featherweight) sliced, solids & liq. | ½ cup (4 oz.) | 55 | 0.0 | | | (0) |
| (Larsen) Fresh-Lite, sliced, solids & liq. | ½ cup (4.3 oz.) | 49 | 0.0 | | | (0) |
| (S&W) Nutradiet, green label, sliced, solids & liq. | ½ cup | 50 | 0.0 | | | (0) |
| **BEET GREENS** (USDA): | | | | | | |
| Raw, whole | 1 lb. (weighed untrimmed) | 330 | .8 | | | 0 |
| Boiled without salt, leaves & stems, drained | ½ cup (2.6 oz.) | 55 | .1 | | | 0 |
| **BERRY, MIXED, DRINK,** canned (Johanna Farms) Ssips | 8.45 fl. oz. | 15 | 0.0 | | | |
| **BEVERAGE** (See individual listings) | | | | | | |
| **BIG H BURGER SAUCE** (Hellmann's) | 1 T. (.5 oz.) | 143 | 7.1 | | | 4 |
| **BIG MAC** (See **MCDONALD'S**) | 1 hamburger (6.5 oz.) | 1,064 | 31.9 | | | |
| **BIG WHEEL** (Hostess) | 1 cake (1.3 oz.) | 132 | 9.1 | | | 7 |
| **BISCUIT:** | | | | | | |
| Baking powder, home recipe (USDA)[1]: | | | | | | |
| Made with regular flour & lard[2] | 1-oz. biscuit (2″ dia.) | 175 | 4.8 | 2. | 3.0 | |

(USDA): United States Department of Agriculture
*Prepared as Package Directs
[1]Made with sodium aluminum sulfate-type baking powder.
[2]Principal source of fat: lard.

58

| Food and Description | Measure or Quantity | Sodium (mg.) | — Fats in grams — | | | Choles-terol (mg.) |
|---|---|---|---|---|---|---|
| | | | Total | Satu-rated | Unsatu-rated | |
| Made with regular flour & vegetable shortening [1] | 1-oz. biscuit (2" dia.) | 175 | 4.8 | 1. | 4. | |
| Made with self-rising flour & lard [2] | 1-oz. biscuit (2" dia.) | 185 | 4.9 | 2. | 3. | |
| Made with self-rising flour & vegetable shortening [1] | 1-oz. biscuit (2" dia.) | 185 | 4.9 | 1. | 4. | |
| Egg (Stella D'oro): | | | | | | |
| Dietetic | 1 piece (.4 oz.) | 1 | 1.0 | | | |
| Regular | 1 piece (.4 oz.) | | 1.0 | | | |
| Roman | 1 piece (1.1 oz.) | | 5.2 | | | |
| Sugared | 1 piece (.5 oz.) | | 1.1 | | | |

**BISCUIT DOUGH:**

| Food and Description | Measure or Quantity | Sodium (mg.) | Total | Satu-rated | Unsatu-rated | Choles-terol (mg.) |
|---|---|---|---|---|---|---|
| Frozen, commercial (USDA) [1] | 1 oz. | 258 | 3.4 | <1. | 2. | |
| Refrigerated: | | | | | | |
| (USDA) commercial | 1 oz. | 258 | 3.4 | <1. | <2. | |
| (Pillsbury): | | | | | | |
| Baking powder: | | | | | | |
| *1869 Brand* | 1 biscuit | 245 | 5.0 | | | |
| *Tender Flake* | 1 biscuit | 170 | 2.5 | | | |
| Buttermilk: | | | | | | |
| Regular | 1 biscuit | 180 | 1.0 | | | |
| *Ballard,* oven ready | 1 biscuit | 180 | 1.0 | | | |
| *1869 Brand* | 1 biscuit | 245 | 5.0 | | | |
| *Heat 'N Eat* | 1 biscuit | 215 | 2.5 | | | |
| *Hungry Jack:* | | | | | | |
| Extra rich | 1 biscuit | 170 | 1.0 | | | |
| Flaky | 1 biscuit | 300 | 4.0 | | | |
| Fluffy | 1 biscuit | 280 | 4.0 | | | |
| *Butter Tastin',* flaky | 1 biscuit | 280 | 4.0 | | | |
| Good'n buttery | 1 biscuit | 365 | 5.0 | | | |

**BISCUIT MIX:**

| Food and Description | Measure or Quantity | Sodium (mg.) | Total | Satu-rated | Unsatu-rated | Choles-terol (mg.) |
|---|---|---|---|---|---|---|
| Dry, with enriched flour (USDA) [1] | 1 oz. | 369 | 3.6 | <1. | | 3 |

(USDA): United States Department of Agriculture
*Prepared as Package Directs
[1] Principal source of fat: vegetable shortening.
[2] Principal source of fat: lard.

| Food and Description | Measure or Quantity | Sodium (mg.) | Total | Fats in grams — Saturated | Unsaturated | Cholesterol (mg.) |
|---|---|---|---|---|---|---|
| *Baked from mix, with added milk (USDA)[1] | 1-oz. biscuit | 276 | 2.6 | < 1. | 2 | |
| *Bisquick* (Betty Crocker) | 1 cup | 1,475 | 17.2 | | | |
| **BITTERS** (Angostura) | | | | | | |
| 45% alcohol | 1 tsp. (5 grams) | Tr. | | | | (0) |
| **BLACKBERRY:** | | | | | | |
| Fresh (includes boysenberry, dewberry, youngberry): | | | | | | |
| With hulls (USDA) | 1 lb. (weighed untrimmed) | 4 | 3.9 | | | 0 |
| Hulled (USDA) | ½ cup (2.6 oz.) | < 1 | .7 | | | 0 |
| Canned, regular, solids & liq. (USDA): | | | | | | |
| Juice pack | 4 oz. | 1 | .9 | | | 0 |
| Light syrup | 4 oz. | 1 | .7 | | | 0 |
| Heavy syrup | ½ cup (4.6 oz.) | 1 | .8 | | | 0 |
| Extra heavy syrup | 4 oz. | 1 | .7 | | | 0 |
| Canned, water pack, solids & liq. (USDA) | ½ cup (4.3 oz.) | 1 | .7 | | | 0 |
| Frozen (USDA): | | | | | | |
| Sweetened, not thawed | 4 oz. | 1 | .3 | | | 0 |
| Unsweetened, not thawed | 4 oz. | 1 | .3 | | | 0 |
| **BLACKBERRY JELLY:** | | | | | | |
| Sweetened: | | | | | | |
| (Home Brand) | 1 T. | 15 | 0.0 | | | (0) |
| (Smucker's) | 1 T. | 4 | Tr. | | | (0) |
| Dietetic: | | | | | | |
| (Diet Delight) | 1 T. (.6 oz.) | 45 | 0.0 | | | (0) |
| (Featherweight) imitation | 1 T. | 40-50 | 0.0 | | | (0) |
| **BLACKBERRY JUICE,** canned, unsweetened (USDA) | ½ cup (4.3 oz.) | 1 | .7 | | | 0 |

(USDA): United States Department of Agriculture
*Prepared as Package Directs
[1]Principal source of fat: vegetable shortening.

| Food and Description | Measure or Quantity | Sodium (mg.) | — Fats in grams — Total | Satu-rated | Unsatu-rated | Choles-terol (mg.) |
|---|---|---|---|---|---|---|
| **BLACKBERRY PRESERVE OR JAM:** | | | | | | |
| Sweetened (Home Brand) | 1 T. (.7 oz.) | 15 | 0.0 | | | (0) |
| Low calorie: | | | | | | |
| Estee | 1 T. (.6 oz.) | Tr. | 0.0 | | | (0) |
| (Featherweight) imitation | 1 T. | 40-50 | 0.0 | | | (0) |
| (Louis Sherry) | 1 T. (.6 oz.) | <3 | 0.0 | | | (0) |
| (S&W) *Nutradiet,* red label | 1 T. (.5 oz.) | | <.1 | | | (0) |
| **BLACK-EYED PEA:** | | | | | | |
| Canned, regular pack, solids & liq.: | | | | | | |
| (Allen) regular | ½ cup (4 oz.) | 370 | 0.0 | | | |
| (Goya) | ½ cup (4 oz.) | 486 | 0.0 | | | |
| (Sunshine) with pork | ½ cup (4 oz.) | 464 | .6 | | | |
| Frozen: | | | | | | |
| (USDA): | | | | | | |
| Not thawed | 10-oz. pkg. | 142 | 1.1 | | | 0 |
| Boiled without salt, drained | ½ cup | 33 | .3 | | | 0 |
| (Birds Eye) | ½ of 10-oz. pkg. | 6 | .6 | | | 0 |
| (Larsen) | 3.3 oz. | 5 | .1 | | | (0) |
| (McKenzie) | 3.3 oz. | 19 | 1.0 | | | (0) |
| (Southland) | ⅕ of 16-oz. pkg. | 5 | 1.0 | | | (0) |
| **BLANCMANGE** (See **VANILLA PUDDING**) | | | | | | |
| **BLINTZ,** frozen: | | | | | | |
| (Empire Kosher Foods): | | | | | | |
| Apple | 2½-oz. piece | 115 | 1.0 | | | 28 |
| Blueberry | 2½-oz. piece | 116 | 1.0 | | | 27 |
| Cherry | 2½-oz. piece | 105 | 1.0 | | | 28 |
| Cheese | 2½-oz. piece | 126 | 1.0 | | | 32 |
| Potato | 2½-oz. piece | 224 | 4.0 | | | 19 |
| (King Kold) cheese | 2½-oz. piece | 250 | 1.9 | | | 8 |

(USDA): United States Department of Agriculture
*Prepared as Package Directs

| Food and Description | Measure or Quantity | Sodium (mg.) | Fats in grams — Total | Satu- rated | Unsatu- rated | Choles- terol (mg.) |
|---|---|---|---|---|---|---|
| **BLOOD PUDDING or SAUSAGE** (USDA) | 1 oz. | | 10.5 | 4. | 7. | |
| **BLOODY MARY MIX** (Holland House) liquid | 1 oz. | 329 | 0.0 | | | (0) |
| **BLUEBERRY:** | | | | | | |
| Fresh, whole (USDA) | 1 lb. (weighed untrimmed) | 4 | 2.1 | | | 0 |
| Fresh, trimmed (USDA) | ½ cup (2.6 oz.) | <1 | .4 | | | 0 |
| Canned, solids & liq. (USDA): | | | | | | |
| Syrup pack, extra heavy | ½ cup (4.4 oz.) | 1 | .2 | | | 0 |
| Water pack | ½ cup (4.3 oz.) | 1 | .2 | | | 0 |
| Frozen (USDA): | | | | | | |
| Sweetened, solids & liq. | ½ cup (4 oz.) | 1 | .3 | | | 0 |
| Unsweetened, solids & liq. | ½ cup (2.9 oz.) | <1 | .4 | | | 0 |
| **BLUEBERRY PIE** (See **PIE,** Blueberry) | | | | | | |
| **BLUEBERRY PIE FILLING** (See **PIE FILLING**) | | | | | | |
| **BLUEBERRY PRESERVE OR JAM:** | | | | | | |
| Sweetened: | | | | | | |
| (Home Brand) | 1 T. | 7 | 0.0 | | | (0) |
| (Smucker's) | 1 T. | 6 | Tr. | | | (0) |
| Dietetic: | | | | | | |
| (Estee) | 1 T. (.6 oz.) | <3 | 0.0 | | | (0) |
| (Louis Sherry) | 1 T. | <3 | 0.0 | | | (0) |
| **BLUEFISH** (USDA): | | | | | | |
| Raw, whole | 1 lb. (weighed whole) | 171 | 7.6 | | | |
| Raw, meat only | 4 oz. | 84 | 3.7 | | | |
| Baked or broiled[1] | 4.4-oz. piece (3½ × 3″ × ½″) | 130 | 6.5 | | | |

(USDA): United States Department of Agriculture
*Prepared as Package Directs
[1]Prepared with butter or margarine.

# BOLOGNA

| Food and Description | Measure or Quantity | Sodium (mg.) | Total | Saturated | Unsaturated | Cholesterol (mg.) |
|---|---|---|---|---|---|---|
| Fried [1] | 5.3-oz. piece (3½″ × 3″ × ½″) | 219 | 14.7 | | | |
| **BOCKWURST** (USDA) | 1 oz. | | 6.7 | 3. | 4. | |
| **BODY BUDDIES,** cereal (General Mills): | | | | | | |
| Brown sugar & honey | 1 cup (1 oz.) | 290 | <1.0 | | | |
| Natural fruit | 1 cup (1 oz.) | 285 | 1.0 | | | |
| **BOLOGNA:** | | | | | | |
| (USDA): | | | | | | |
| All meat | 1 oz. | | 6.5 | | | |
| All meat, very thin slice | ½-oz. slice (3″ × ⅛″) | | 3.0 | | | |
| With cereal | 1 oz. | | 5.8 | | | |
| (Eckrich): | | | | | | |
| Beef: | | | | | | |
| Regular | 1-oz. slice | 280 | 8.0 | | | |
| Smorgas-Pac | ¾-oz. slice | 230 | 6.0 | | | |
| Thick sliced | 1½-oz. slice | 400 | 12.0 | | | |
| Thick sliced | 1.8-oz. slice | 510 | 14.0 | | | |
| Thin sliced | 1 slice | 160 | 4.5 | | | |
| Garlic | 1-oz. slice | 290 | 8.0 | | | |
| German brand: | | | | | | |
| Sliced | 1-oz. slice | 350 | 7.0 | | | |
| Chub | 1-oz. serving | 360 | 7.0 | | | |
| Lunch, chub | 1-oz. serving | 290 | 9.0 | | | |
| Meat: | | | | | | |
| Regular | 1-oz. slice | 290 | 8.0 | | | |
| Smorgas-Pac | ¾-oz. slice | 230 | 6.0 | | | |
| Thick sliced | 1.7-oz. slice | 490 | 14.0 | | | |
| Thin sliced | 1 slice | 160 | 5.0 | | | |
| Ring: | | | | | | |
| Regular | 1 oz. | 280 | 8.0 | | | |
| Pickled | 1 oz. | 290 | 8.0 | | | |
| Sandwich | 1-oz. slice | 310 | 8.0 | | | |
| (Hormel): | | | | | | |
| Beef: | | | | | | |
| Regular | 1 slice | 296 | 8.0 | | | |
| Ring, coarse ground | 1 oz. | 288 | 7.0 | | | |

(USDA): United States Department of Agriculture
*Prepared as Package Directs
[1] Prepared with egg, milk or water, & bread crumbs.

BOLOGNA (Continued)

| Food and Description | Measure or Quantity | Sodium (mg.) | Total | Fats in grams — Saturated | Unsaturated | Cholesterol (mg.) |
|---|---|---|---|---|---|---|
| Coarse ground, ring | 1 oz. | 289 | 7.0 | | | |
| Fine ground, ring | 1 oz. | 298 | 8.0 | | | |
| Meat: | | | | | | |
| Regular | 1 slice | 300 | 8.0 | | | |
| *Light & Lean:* | | | | | | |
| Regular | 1 slice | | 6.0 | | | |
| Thin sliced | 1 slice | | 6.0 | | | |
| (Ohse): | | | | | | |
| Beef | 1 oz. | 310 | 8.0 | | | |
| Chicken, 15% | 1 oz. | 320 | 8.0 | | | |
| Chicken, beef & pork | 1 oz. | 290 | 6.0 | | | |
| (Oscar Mayer): | | | | | | |
| Beef | .5-oz. slice | 165 | 4.3 | | | 8 |
| Beef | 1-oz. slice | 308 | 8.2 | | | 16 |
| Beef Lebanon | .8-oz. slice | 297 | 3.3 | | | 16 |
| Garlic Beef | 1-oz. slice | 294 | 8.3 | | | 16 |
| Meat | .5-oz. slice | 157 | 4.5 | | | 9 |
| Meat | 1-oz. slice | 298 | 8.5 | | | 17 |
| Meat | 2-oz. slice | 516 | 17.0 | | | 34 |

**BOLOGNA & CHEESE:**

| | | | | | | |
|---|---|---|---|---|---|---|
| (Eckrich) | .7-oz. slice | 290 | 8.0 | | | |
| (Oscar Mayer) | .8-oz. slice | 242 | 6.7 | | | 14 |

**BONITO,** raw (USDA):

| | | | | | | |
|---|---|---|---|---|---|---|
| Whole | 1 lb. (weighed whole) | | 19.2 | | | |
| Meat only | 4 oz. | | 8.3 | | | |

**BOO'BERRY,** cereal (General Mills)

| | | | | | | |
|---|---|---|---|---|---|---|
| Mills) | 1 cup (1 oz.) | 210 | 1.0 | | | |

**BORSCHT,** canned:

| | | | | | | |
|---|---|---|---|---|---|---|
| Regular (Mother's) old fashioned | 8 fl. oz. | 907 | .2 | | | |
| Dietetic (Mother's): | | | | | | |
| Artificially sweetened | 8 fl. oz. | 943 | .2 | | | |
| Unsalted | 8 fl. oz. | 51 | .3 | | | |

**BOSTON BROWN BREAD**
  (See **BREAD**)

(USDA): United States Department of Agriculture
*Prepared as Package Directs

64

| Food and Description | Measure or Quantity | Sodium (mg.) | Total | — Fats in grams — Satu- rated | Unsatu- rated | Choles- terol (mg.) |
|---|---|---|---|---|---|---|
| **BOSTON CREAM PIE** (See **PIE,** Boston cream) | | | | | | |
| **BOUILLON CUBE** (See also individual flavors) (USDA) flavor not indicated | 1 cube (approx. 1/2", 4 grams) | 960 | .1 | | | |
| **BOURBON WHISKEY** (See **DISTILLED LIQUOR**) | | | | | | |
| **BOYSENBERRY:** | | | | | | |
| Fresh (See **BLACKBERRY,** fresh) | | | | | | |
| Canned, unsweetened or low calorie | | | | | | |
| Water pack, solids & liq. (USDA) | 4 oz. | 1 | .1 | | | 0 |
| Frozen, not thawed (USDA): | | | | | | |
| Sweetened | 4 oz. | 1 | .3 | | | 0 |
| Unsweetened | 4 oz. | 1 | .3 | | | 0 |
| **BOYSENBERRY PRESERVE OR JAM,** low calorie (S & W) *Nutradiet* | 1 T. (.5 oz.) | | <.1 | | | (0) |
| **BRAINS,** all animals, raw (USDA) | 4 oz. | 142 | 9.8 | | | 2268 |
| **BRAN** (USDA): | | | | | | |
| Crude | 1 oz. | 3 | 1.3 | | | 0 |
| With added sugar & defatted wheat germ | 1 oz. | 139 | .5 | | | 0 |
| With added sugar & malt extract | 1 oz. | 301 | .9 | | | 0 |
| **BRAN BREAKFAST CEREAL:** | | | | | | |
| (Kellogg's): | | | | | | |
| *All-Bran* | 1/3 cup (1 oz.) | 270 | 1.0 | | | (0) |
| *All-Bran Buds* | 1/3 cup (1 oz.) | 150 | 1.0 | | | (0) |
| *Cracklin' Oat Bran* | 1/2 cup (1 oz.) | 190 | 4.0 | | | (0) |
| 40% bran flakes | 3/4 cup (1 oz.) | 220 | 0.0 | | | (0) |

(USDA): United States Department of Agriculture
*Prepared as Package Directs

| Food and Description | Measure or Quantity | Sodium (mg.) | Total | Fats in grams Satu-rated | Unsatu-rated | Choles-terol (mg.) |
|---|---|---|---|---|---|---|
| *Fruitful Bran* | ¾ cup (1 oz.) | 230 | | | | (0) |
| Raisin bran | ¾ cup (1 oz.) | 210 | 1.0 | | | (0) |
| (Loma Linda) | ⅓ cup (1 oz.) | 115 | <1.0 | | | 0 |
| (Nabisco) 100% | ½ cup (1 oz.) | 190 | 2.0 | | | (0) |
| (Post): | | | | | | |
| 40% bran flakes | ⅔ cup (1 oz.) | 260 | .5 | | | 0 |
| With raisins | ½ cup (1 oz.) | 185 | .5 | | | 0 |
| With raisins, *Honey Nut Crunch* | ½ cup (1 oz.) | 150 | .3 | | | 0 |
| (Quaker) Corn bran | ⅔ cup (1 oz.) | 245 | .9 | | | |
| (Ralston Purina): | | | | | | |
| Bran *Chex* | ⅔ cup (1 oz.) | 267 | .8 | | | |
| Honey bran | ⅞ cup (1 oz.) | 157 | .5 | | | |
| Raisin bran | ¾ cup (1.3 oz.) | 286 | .4 | | | |

**BRANDY** (See **DISTILLED LIQUOR**)

**BRAUNSCHWEIGER:**

| | | | | | | |
|---|---|---|---|---|---|---|
| (USDA) | 2 slices (2″ × ¼″, .7 oz.) | | 5.5 | 2. | 4. | |
| (Eckrich) chub | 1 oz. | 400 | 6.0 | | | |
| (Hormel) | 1 oz. | 322 | 7.0 | | | |
| (Oscar Mayer): | | | | | | |
| Chub | 1 oz. | 319 | 8.8 | | | 44 |
| Sliced | 1-oz. slice | 327 | 8.7 | | | 50 |
| Tube, German brand | 1-oz. serving | 341 | 8.4 | | | 46 |

**BRAZIL NUT** (USDA):

| | | | | | | |
|---|---|---|---|---|---|---|
| Whole | 1 lb. (weighed in shell) | 2 | 145.6 | 29. | 117. | 0 |
| Whole | 1 cup (14 nuts, 4.3 oz. with shell) | 1 | 39.2 | 8. | 31. | 0 |
| Shelled | ½ cup (2.5 oz.) | <1 | 46.8 | 9. | 38. | 0 |
| Shelled | 4 nuts (.6 oz.) | <1 | 11.7 | 2. | 9. | 0 |

**BREAD** (listed by type or brand name; toasting does not affect these nutritive values, only weight):

| | | | | | | |
|---|---|---|---|---|---|---|
| Boston brown (USDA) | 1.7-oz. slice (3″ × ¾″) | 120 | .6 | | | |

(USDA): United States Department of Agriculture
*Prepared as Package Directs

| Food and Description | Measure or Quantity | Sodium (mg.) | — Fats in grams — | | | Choles- terol (mg.) |
|---|---|---|---|---|---|---|
| | | | Total | Satu- rated | Unsatu- rated | |
| *Bran'nola* (Arnold) | 1.3-oz. slice | 135 | 1.0 | | | 0 |
| Cinnamon (Pepperidge Farm) | .9-oz. slice | 100 | 2.0 | | | |
| Cornbread (See **CORNBREAD**) | | | | | | |
| Cracked-wheat: | | | | | | |
| (USDA) | .8-oz. slice | 122 | .5 | | | |
| (USDA) 20 slices to 1 lb. | .9-oz. slice | 132 | .6 | | | |
| (Pepperidge Farm) | .9-oz. slice | 145 | 1.0 | | | |
| (Wonder) | 1-oz. slice | 151 | 1.1 | | | Tr. |
| *Daffodil Farm* (Wonder) | .8-oz. slice | 140 | .6 | | | |
| Date nut roll (Dromedary) | ½" slice (1 oz.) | | 2.0 | | | |
| Flatbread, *Ideal:* | | | | | | |
| Bran | 5-gram slice | 47 | Tr. | | | |
| Extra thin | 3-gram slice | 25 | .1 | | | |
| Whole grain | 5-gram slice | 47 | .1 | | | |
| French: | | | | | | |
| (USDA) 20 slices to 1 lb.[1] | .8-oz. slice | 133 | .7 | Tr. | < 1. | |
| (Arnold) *Francisco,* regular or international | ¹⁄₁₆ of loaf (1 oz.) | 110 | 1.0 | | | |
| (Wonder) | 1-oz. slice | 170 | .9 | | | 0 |
| Garlic (Arnold) | 1-oz. slice | 120 | 3.0 | | | |
| *Hi-Fiber* (Monks') | 1-oz. slice | 110 | 1.0 | | | 0 |
| *Hillbilly Old Fashion Bread* | 1-oz. slice | 170 | .9 | | | Tr. |
| *Hollywood:* | | | | | | |
| Dark | 1-oz. slice | 167 | 1.1 | | | Tr. |
| Light | 1-oz. slice | 170 | .9 | | | Tr. |
| Honey bran (Pepperidge Farm) | 1.2-oz. slice | 175 | 1.0 | | | |
| Honey wheatberry: | | | | | | |
| (Arnold) | 1.1-oz. slice | 140 | 2.0 | | | |
| (Pepperidge Farm) | .9-oz. slice | 163 | 1.0 | | | |
| (Pepperidge Farm) | 1.2-oz. slice | 105 | 1.0 | | | |
| Italian: | | | | | | |
| (USDA) 20 slices to 1 lb. | .8-oz. slice | 135 | .2 | | | |
| (Arnold) *Francisco* | 1 slice | 110 | 1.0 | | | |
| Low sodium (Wonder) | 1-oz. slice | 3 | .8 | | | Tr. |
| Multi-grain: | | | | | | |
| (Arnold) *Milk & Honey* | 1-oz. slice | 150 | 1.0 | | | |
| (Pepperidge Farm) very thin sliced | .5-oz. slice | 75 | .5 | | | |
| Natural grain (Arnold) | .8-oz. slice | 110 | 1.0 | | | |

(USDA): United States Department of Agriculture
*Prepared as Package Directs
[1]Principal source of fat: vegetable shortening.

| Food and Description | Measure or Quantity | Sodium (mg.) | Total | Satu-rated | Unsatu-rated | Choles-terol (mg.) |
|---|---|---|---|---|---|---|
| | | | — Fats in grams — | | | |
| Oat (Arnold): | | | | | | |
| *Bran'nola,* country | 1.3-oz. slice | 170 | 1.0 | | | |
| *Milk & Honey* | 1-oz. slice | 150 | 1.0 | | | |
| Oatmeal (Pepperidge Farm) | | | | | | |
| thin | 1 slice | 185 | 1.5 | | | |
| Protein (Thomas') | .7-oz. slice | 94 | .4 | | | 0 |
| Pumpernickel: | | | | | | |
| (USDA) 20 slices to 1 lb. | .8-oz. slice | 131 | .3 | | | |
| (Arnold) Jewish | 1-oz. slice | 200 | 1.0 | | | |
| (Levy's) | 1.1-oz. slice | 200 | 1.0 | | | 0 |
| (Pepperidge Farm) family | 1-oz. slice | 305 | 1.0 | | | |
| (Pepperidge Farm) party | 1 slice (6 grams) | 55 | .2 | | | |
| Raisin: | | | | | | |
| (USDA) 18 slices to 1 lb. [1] | .9-oz. slice | 91 | .7 | Tr. | Tr. | |
| (Arnold): | | | | | | |
| *Sun-Maid* | .8-oz. slice | 85 | 1.0 | | | |
| Tea | .9-oz. slice | 85 | 1.5 | | | < 5 |
| (Monks') cinnamon | 1-oz. slice | 85 | 2.0 | | | 0 |
| (Pepperidge Farm) | | | | | | |
| cinnamon, fresh or frozen | .9-oz. slice | 95 | 1.5 | | | |
| *Roman Meal* | 1-oz. slice | 159 | 1.1 | | | Tr. |
| Rye: | | | | | | |
| Light, 18 slices to 1 lb. | | | | | | |
| (USDA) | .9-oz. slice | 139 | .3 | | | |
| (Arnold): | | | | | | |
| Dill, with seeds | 1.1-oz. slice | 190 | 1.0 | | | 0 |
| Jewish, with or without | | | | | | |
| seeds | 1.1-oz. slice | 170 | 1.0 | | | < 5 |
| Melba thin | .7-oz. slice | 110 | .5 | | | 0 |
| (Levy's) real | 1.1-oz. slice | 170 | 1.0 | | | 0 |
| (Pepperidge Farm): | | | | | | |
| Family, with or without | | | | | | |
| seeds | 1.1-oz. slice | 245 | 1.5 | | | |
| Party, fresh or frozen | .2-oz. slice | 104 | .2 | | | |
| (Wonder) | 1-oz. slice | 170 | .9 | | | Tr. |
| *Sahara* (Thomas'): | | | | | | |
| White: | | | | | | |
| Regular | 2-oz. piece | 300 | 1.0 | | | 0 |
| Mini | 1-oz. piece | 150 | 1.0 | | | 0 |
| Large | 3-oz. piece | 440 | 2.0 | | | 0 |
| Whole wheat: | | | | | | |
| Regular | 2-oz. piece | 320 | 2.0 | | | 0 |
| Mini | 1-oz. piece | 150 | 1.0 | | | 0 |

(USDA): United States Department of Agriculture
*Prepared as Package Directs
[1]Prepared with vegetable shortening & nonfat dry milk.

| Food and Description | Measure or Quantity | Sodium (mg.) | — Fats in grams — | | | Cholesterol (mg.) |
|---|---|---|---|---|---|---|
| | | | Total | Saturated | Unsaturated | |
| Salt-rising (USDA) | .9-oz. slice | 66 | .6 | Tr. | Tr. | |
| 7 Whole Grain (Home Pride) | 1-oz. slice | 135 | 1.1 | | | Tr. |
| Sour dough, DiCarlo | 1-oz. slice | 156 | .6 | | | 0 |
| Sunflower bran (Monks') | 1-oz. slice | 80 | 1.0 | | | 0 |
| Toaster cake (See TOASTER CAKE) | | | | | | |
| Vienna, 20 slices to 1 lb. (USDA) | .8-oz. slice | 133 | .7 | Tr. | Tr. | |
| Wheat: | | | | | | |
| America's Own, cottage (Arnold): | 1-oz. slice | 155 | 1.0 | | | |
| Bran'nola: | | | | | | |
| Dark | 1.3-oz. slice | 170 | 1.0 | | | |
| Hearty | 1.3-oz. slice | 200 | 2.0 | | | |
| Brick Oven: | | | | | | |
| 8-oz. loaf | .8-oz. slice | 100 | 2.0 | | | |
| 1-lb. loaf | .84-oz. slice | 105 | 2.0 | | | |
| 2-lb. loaf | 1.1-oz. slice | 130 | 2.0 | | | |
| Country | 1.3-oz. slice | 150 | 1.0 | | | |
| Less | .8-oz. slice | 120 | 0.0 | | | |
| Milk & Honey | 1-oz. slice | 160 | 1.0 | | | |
| Fresh Horizon | 1-oz. slice | 148 | .6 | | | 0 |
| Home Pride, butter topped (Pepperidge Farm): | 1-oz. slice | 156 | 1.1 | | | Tr. |
| Family | .9-oz. slice | 195 | 1.5 | | | |
| Sandwich | .8-oz. slice | 115 | 1.0 | | | |
| (Wonder) family | 1-oz. slice | 148 | 1.1 | | | Tr. |
| Wheatberry, Home Pride: | | | | | | |
| Regular | 1 oz. | 151 | 1.1 | | | 0 |
| Honey | 1 oz. | 163 | 1.1 | | | Tr. |
| White, enriched or unenriched: | | | | | | |
| Prepared with 1-2% nonfat dry milk (USDA)[1] | .8-oz. slice | 117 | .7 | Tr. | <1. | |
| Prepared with 3-4% nonfat dry milk (USDA)[1] | .8-oz. slice | 117 | .7 | Tr. | <1. | |
| Prepared with 5-6% nonfat dry milk (USDA)[1] | .8-oz. slice | 114 | .9 | Tr. | <1. | |
| America's Own, cottage (Arnold): | 1 oz. | 180 | 1.0 | | | 0 |
| Brick Oven: | | | | | | |
| 8-oz. loaf | .8-oz. slice | 130 | 1.0 | | | |
| 1-lb. loaf | .84-oz. slice | 135 | 1.0 | | | |

(USDA): United States Department of Agriculture
*Prepared as Package Directs
[1]Principal source of fat: vegetable shortening.

BREAD (Continued)

| Food and Description | Measure or Quantity | Sodium (mg.) | — Fats in grams — | | | Cholesterol (mg.) |
|---|---|---|---|---|---|---|
| | | | Total | Saturated | Unsaturated | |
| 2-lb. loaf | 1.1-oz. slice | 160 | 2.0 | | | |
| Country | 1.3-oz. slice | 200 | 2.0 | | | |
| *Less* | .8-oz. slice | 120 | 0.0 | | | |
| *Lite Way* | .8-oz. slice | 130 | 0.0 | | | |
| *Milk & Honey* | 1-oz. slice | 160 | 1.0 | | | |
| Very thin | .5-oz. slice | 85 | 1.0 | | | |
| *Fresh Horizon* | 1 oz. | 142 | .6 | | | 0 |
| *Home Pride* | 1 oz. | 149 | 1.1 | | | Tr. |
| (Monks') | 1 oz. | 95 | 1.0 | | | 0 |
| (Pepperidge Farm): | | | | | | |
| Regular | 1.2-oz. slice | 135 | 1.5 | | | |
| Toasting | 1.1-oz. slice | 230 | 1.0 | | | |
| Very thin slice | .6-oz. slice | 85 | .5 | | | |
| (Wonder): | | | | | | |
| Regular | 1 oz. | 153 | .8 | | | Tr. |
| *Butterworth* | 1 oz. | 170 | 1.1 | | | Tr. |
| Whole-wheat: | | | | | | |
| Made with 2% nonfat dry milk (USDA)[1] | .9-oz. slice | 132 | .8 | Tr. | < 1. | |
| Made with water (USDA)[1] | .8-oz. slice | 122 | .6 | < 1 | Tr. | |
| Made with water (USDA)[1] | .9-oz. slice | 132 | .6 | Tr. | Tr. | |
| (Arnold) stone ground | .8-oz. slice | 100 | 1.0 | | | 0 |
| *Home Pride* | 1 oz. | 142 | 1.1 | | | Tr. |
| (Monks') stone ground | 1 oz. | 110 | 1.0 | | | 0 |
| (Pepperidge Farm) fresh or frozen: | | | | | | |
| Thin sliced | .9-oz. slice | 125 | 1.5 | | | |
| Very thin sliced | .6-oz. slice | 80 | 1.0 | | | |
| (Wonder) 100% | 1 oz. | 121 | 1.1 | | | Tr. |

**BREAD, CANNED:**

| Food and Description | Measure or Quantity | Sodium (mg.) | Total | Saturated | Unsaturated | Cholesterol (mg.) |
|---|---|---|---|---|---|---|
| (B & M) plain or raisin | 1/2″ slice | 220 | Tr. | | | |
| (Friend's) | 1/2″ slice | 220 | Tr. | | | |

**BREAD CRUMBS:**

| Food and Description | Measure or Quantity | Sodium (mg.) | Total | Saturated | Unsaturated | Cholesterol (mg.) |
|---|---|---|---|---|---|---|
| (USDA) Dry, grated | 1 cup (3.5 oz.) | 736 | 4.6 | 1. | 4. | |
| (USDA)[1] Dry, grated | 1 T. (6 grams) | 47 | .3 | Tr. | Tr. | |
| (Contadina): | | | | | | |
| Seasoned | 1 rnd. T. | 249 | .3 | | | Tr. |
| Seasoned | 1/2 cup (2.1 oz.) | 1,491 | 1.8 | | | Tr. |
| (Pepperidge Farm) Premium: | | | | | | |
| Regular | 1 oz. | 255 | 1.0 | | | |

(USDA): United States Department of Agriculture
*Prepared as Package Directs
[1]Principal source of fat: vegetable shortening.

| Food and Description | Measure or Quantity | Sodium (mg.) | — Fats in grams — | | | Choles- terol (mg.) |
|---|---|---|---|---|---|---|
| | | | Total | Satu- rated | Unsatu- rated | |
| Herb seasoned | 1 oz. | 260 | 1.0 | | | |

## BREAD DOUGH:
Frozen:
  (Pepperidge Farm):

| | | | | | | |
|---|---|---|---|---|---|---|
| Rye, country | ¹⁄₁₀ of loaf | 185 | 2.0 | | | |
| Wheat, stone ground | ¹⁄₁₀ of loaf | 127 | 1.5 | | | |
| White | ¹⁄₁₀ of loaf | 165 | 1.5 | | | |

(Rich's):

| | | | | | | |
|---|---|---|---|---|---|---|
| French | ¹⁄₂₀ of loaf | 138 | .6 | | | 0 |
| Italian | ¹⁄₂₀ of loaf | 300 | 1.0 | | | 0 |
| Raisin | ¹⁄₂₀ of loaf | 107 | 1.0 | | | 3 |
| Wheat | .5-oz. serving | 375 | .5 | | | 0 |
| White | .8-oz. serving | 96 | .6 | | | 0 |
| White | .9-oz. serving | 107 | .7 | | | 0 |

Refrigerated (Pillsbury):

| | | | | | | |
|---|---|---|---|---|---|---|
| French | 1″ slice | 110 | <1.0 | | | |
| Wheat or white | 1″ slice | 170 | 2.0 | | | |

## BREADFRUIT, fresh (USDA):

| | | | | | | |
|---|---|---|---|---|---|---|
| Whole | 1 lb. (weighed untrimmed) | 52 | 1.0 | | | 0 |
| Peeled & trimmed | 4 oz. | 17 | .3 | | | 0 |

## *BREAD MIX:
*Home Hearth:*

| | | | | | | |
|---|---|---|---|---|---|---|
| French | ³⁄₈″ slice | 160 | 1.5 | | | |
| Rye | ³⁄₈″ slice | 180 | .5 | | | |
| White | ³⁄₈″ slice | 130 | .5 | | | |

(Pillsbury):

| | | | | | | |
|---|---|---|---|---|---|---|
| Banana | ¹⁄₁₂ of loaf | 200 | 6.0 | | | |
| Blueberry nut | ¹⁄₁₂ of loaf | 150 | 4.0 | | | |
| Cherry nut | ¹⁄₁₂ of loaf | 150 | 5.0 | | | |
| Cranberry | ¹⁄₁₂ of loaf | 160 | 4.0 | | | |
| Date | ¹⁄₁₂ of loaf | 150 | 3.0 | | | |
| Nut | ¹⁄₁₂ of loaf | 190 | 6.0 | | | |

## BREAD STICK (USDA):

| | | | | | | |
|---|---|---|---|---|---|---|
| Salt [1] | 1 piece (3 grams) | 50 | <.1 | Tr. | Tr. | |
| Vienna type | 1 piece (3 grams) | 47 | <.1 | Tr. | Tr. | |

(USDA): United States Department of Agriculture
*Prepared as Package Directs
[1]Principal source of fat: vegetable shortening.

| Food and Description | Measure or Quantity | Sodium (mg.) | Total | Fats in grams — Satu- rated | Unsatu- rated | Choles- terol (mg.) |
|---|---|---|---|---|---|---|
| **\*BREAD STICK DOUGH,** refrigerated (Pillsbury) | 1 piece | 230 | 2.0 | | | |
| | | | | | | |
| **BREAD STUFFING MIX** (See **STUFFING MIX**) | | | | | | |
| | | | | | | |
| **BREAKFAST DRINK,** instant (Pillsbury): | | | | | | |
| Chocolate or chocolate malt | 1 pouch | 185 | 0.0 | | | |
| \*Chocolate or chocolate malt | 8 fl. oz. | 310 | 9.0 | | | |
| Strawberry | 1 pouch | 180 | 0.0 | | | |
| \*Strawberry | 8 fl. oz. | 300 | 9.0 | | | |
| Vanilla | 1 pouch | 210 | 0.0 | | | |
| \*Vanilla | 8 fl. oz. | 330 | 9.0 | | | |
| | | | | | | |
| **BREAKFAST SQUARES** (General Mills) all flavors | 1½-oz. bar | 255 | 8.5 | | | |
| | | | | | | |
| **BROADBEAN:** | | | | | | |
| Immature seed (USDA) | 1 lb. (weighed in pod) | 6 | .6 | | | 0 |
| Immature seed (USDA) | 1 oz. (without pod) | 1 | .1 | | | 0 |
| Mature seed, dry (USDA) | 1 oz. | | .5 | | | 0 |
| Canned, regular pack, drained solids (Del Monte) | ½ cup (2.5 oz.) | 368 | <.1 | | | (0) |
| Frozen, Italian bean (Birds Eye) | ⅓ of 9-oz. pkg. | 36 | .1 | | | 0 |
| Frozen, Italian bean, tomato sauce (Green Giant) | ⅓ of 10-oz. pkg. | 340 | .9 | | | |
| | | | | | | |
| **BROCCOLI:** | | | | | | |
| Raw, whole (USDA) | 1 lb. (weighed untrimmed) | 42 | .8 | | | 0 |
| Raw, large leaves removed (USDA) | 1 lb. (weighed partially trimmed) | 53 | 1.1 | | | 0 |
| Boiled without salt, drained (USDA): | | | | | | |
| Whole stalk | 1 stalk (6.3 oz.) | 18 | .5 | | | 0 |
| ½" pieces | ½ cup (2.8 oz.) | 18 | .2 | | | 0 |

(USDA): United States Department of Agriculture
\*Prepared as Package Directs

| Food and Description | Measure or Quantity | Sodium (mg.) | Fats in grams Total | Satu- rated | Unsatu- rated | Choles- terol (mg.) |
|---|---|---|---|---|---|---|
| Frozen: | | | | | | |
| (USDA): | | | | | | |
| Chopped or cut, not thawed | 10-oz. pkg. | 48 | .8 | | | 0 |
| Chopped or cut, boiled without salt, drained | 1⅜ cups (10-oz. pkg. | 25 | .8 | | | 0 |
| Spears, not thawed | 10-oz. pkg. | 37 | .6 | | | 0 |
| Spears, boiled without salt, drained | ½ cup (3.3 oz.) | 11 | .2 | | | 0 |
| (Birds Eye): | | | | | | |
| With almonds and selected seasonings | ⅓ of 10-oz. pkg. | 216 | 2.8 | | | 0 |
| With cheese sauce | ⅓ of 10-oz. pkg. | 337 | 4.4 | | | 4 |
| Chopped | ⅓ of 10-oz. pkg. | 18 | .3 | | | 0 |
| Cuts or deluxe florets | ⅓ of 10-oz. pkg. | 25 | .2 | | | 0 |
| Spears: | | | | | | |
| Regular | ⅓ of 10-oz. pkg. | 21 | .2 | | | 0 |
| With butter sauce | ⅓ of 10-oz. pkg. | 379 | 3.1 | | | 8 |
| Deluxe | ⅓ of 10-oz. pkg. | 14 | .4 | | | 0 |
| & water chestnuts with selected seasonings | ⅓ of 10-oz. pkg. | 215 | .2 | | | 0 |
| (Green Giant) In cheese sauce: | ½ cup | 425 | .2 | | | |
| Cut: | | | | | | |
| *Harvest Fresh* | ½ cup | 160 | 0.0 | | | (0) |
| Polybag | ½ cup | 10 | 0.0 | | | (0) |
| Spears: | | | | | | |
| In butter sauce | 3.3 oz. | 325 | 1.0 | | | |
| *Harvest Fresh:* | | | | | | |
| Regular | ½ cup | 160 | Tr. | | | |
| Mini | ⅛ of pkg. | 10 | 0.0 | | | |
| In white cheddar sauce | ½ cup | 425 | 2.0 | | | |
| (Larsen) | 3.3 oz. | 30 | 0.0 | | | |
| (McKenzie): | | | | | | |
| Chopped | 3.3 oz. | 23 | 0.0 | | | |
| Spears | 3.3 oz. | 28 | 0.0 | | | |
| (Stouffer's) in cheddar cheese sauce | ½ of 9-oz. pkg. | 970 | 8.0 | | | |

**BROWNIE (See COOKIE)**

(USDA): United States Department of Agriculture
*Prepared as Package Directs

| Food and Description | Measure or Quantity | Sodium (mg.) | —Fats in grams— | | | Choles- terol (mg.) |
|---|---|---|---|---|---|---|
| | | | Total | Satu- rated | Unsatu- rated | |

**BRUNSWICK STEW,** canned
(Hormel) *Short Orders* — 7½-oz. serving — 13.0

**BRUSSELS SPROUT:**

| | | | | | | |
|---|---|---|---|---|---|---|
| Raw (USDA) | 1 lb. | 58 | 1.7 | | | 0 |
| Boiled without salt, 1¼"-1½" dia., drained (USDA) | 1 cup (7-8 sprouts, 5.5 oz.) | 16 | .6 | | | 0 |
| Frozen: | | | | | | |
| (USDA): | | | | | | |
| Not thawed | 10-oz. pkg. | 45 | .6 | | | 0 |
| Boiled without salt, drained (USDA) | 4 oz. | 16 | .2 | | | 0 |
| (Birds Eye): | | | | | | |
| Regular | ⅓ of 10-oz. pkg. | 15 | .3 | | | 0 |
| Baby: | | | | | | |
| Butter sauce | ⅓ of 10-oz. pkg. | 304 | 2.0 | | | 5 |
| With cheese sauce | 3 oz. | 291 | 4.5 | | | 3 |
| Deluxe | 3.3 oz. | 9 | .5 | | | 0 |
| (Green Giant): | | | | | | |
| Butter sauce | ½ cup | 275 | 1.0 | | | |
| Cheese sauce | ½ cup | 475 | 2.0 | | | |
| Polybag | ½ cup | 15 | 0.0 | | | |
| (Larsen) | 3.3 oz. | 20 | 0.0 | | | |
| (McKenzie) | 3.3 oz. | 19 | 0.0 | | | |

**BUCKWHEAT:**

| | | | | | | |
|---|---|---|---|---|---|---|
| Flour (See **FLOUR**) | | | | | | |
| Groats: | | | | | | |
| (Pocono) | 1 oz. | | .7 | | | (0) |
| *Wolff's* (Birkett) | 1 oz. | | .5 | | | 0 |
| Whole-grain (USDA) | 1 oz. | | .7 | | | 0 |

**BUC WHEATS** cereal (General Mills) — 1 cup — 235 — 1.0 — — — (0)

**BUFFALOFISH,** raw (USDA):

| | | | | | | |
|---|---|---|---|---|---|---|
| Whole | 1 lb. (weighed whole) | 76 | 6.1 | | | |
| Meat only | 4 oz. | 59 | 4.8 | | | |

(USDA): United States Department of Agriculture
*Prepared as Package Directs

| Food and Description | Measure or Quantity | Sodium (mg.) | — Fats in grams — | | | Choles- terol (mg.) |
|---|---|---|---|---|---|---|
| | | | Total | Satu- rated | Unsatu- rated | |
| **BULGUR** (from hard red winter wheat) (USDA): | | | | | | |
| Dry | 1 lb. | | 6.8 | | | 0 |
| Canned, seasoned | 1 cup (4.8 oz.) | 621 | 4.5 | | | |
| Canned, unseasoned | 4 oz. | 679 | .8 | | | 0 |
| **BULLHEAD,** raw (USDA): | | | | | | |
| Whole | 1 lb. (weighed whole) | | 1.4 | | | |
| Meat only | 4 oz. | | 1.8 | | | |
| **BULLOCK'S-HEART** (See **CUSTARD APPLE**) | | | | | | |
| **BUN** (See **ROLL**) | | | | | | |
| **BURBOT,** raw (USDA): | | | | | | |
| Whole | 1 lb. (weighed whole) | | .6 | | | |
| Meat only | 4 oz. | | 1.0 | | | |
| *BURGER KING:* | | | | | | |
| Apple pie | | 412 | 12.0 | | | 4 |
| *Breakfast Croissantwich:* | | | | | | |
| Bacon | | 762 | 24.0 | | | 249 |
| Ham | | 987 | 20.0 | | | 262 |
| Sausage | | 1,042 | 41.0 | | | 293 |
| Cheeseburger: | | | | | | |
| Regular | | 439 | 15.0 | | | 48 |
| Double: | | | | | | |
| Plain | | 615 | 27.0 | | | 98 |
| Bacon | | 728 | 31.0 | | | 104 |
| Condiments: | | | | | | |
| Ketchup | | 121 | 0.0 | | | 0 |
| Mustard | | 31 | 0.0 | | | 0 |
| Pickles | | 60 | 0.0 | | | 0 |
| Chicken Specialty Sandwich: | | | | | | |
| Plain | | 1,280 | 20.0 | | | 66 |
| Condiments: | | | | | | |
| Lettuce | | 1 | 0.0 | | | 0 |
| Mayonnaise | | 142 | 20.0 | | | 16 |
| Chicken Tenders | 1 piece | 106 | 1.7 | | | 8 |
| Coffee, regular | | 2 | 0.0 | | | 0 |
| Danish, great | | 288 | 36.0 | | | 6 |

(USDA): United States Department of Agriculture
*Prepared as Package Directs

| Food and Description | Measure or Quantity | Sodium (mg.) | — Fats in grams — | | | Choles- terol (mg.) |
|---|---|---|---|---|---|---|
| | | | Total | Satu- rated | Unsatu- rated | |
| Egg platter, scrambled: | | | | | | |
| Bacon | | 167 | 6.0 | | | 8 |
| Croissant | | 298 | 11.0 | | | 11 |
| Hash browns | | 193 | 11.0 | | | 2 |
| Sausage | | 405 | 22.0 | | | 50 |
| French fries | | 160 | 13.0 | | | 14 |
| French toast sticks | | 498 | 29.0 | | | 74 |
| Hamburger, plain | | 297 | 12.0 | | | |
| Condiments: | | | | | | |
| Ketchup | | 121 | 0.0 | | | 0 |
| Mustard | | 31 | 0.0 | | | 0 |
| Pickles | | 60 | 0.0 | | | 0 |
| Ham & cheese, specialty sandwich, plain | | 1,461 | 13.0 | | | 52 |
| Condiments: | | | | | | |
| Lettuce | | 1 | 0.0 | | | 0 |
| Mayonnaise | | 71 | 10.0 | | | 8 |
| Tomato | | 1 | 0.0 | | | 0 |
| Milk: | | | | | | |
| 2% lowfat | | 122 | 5.0 | | | 18 |
| Whole | | 119 | 9.0 | | | 35 |
| Onion rings | | 665 | 16.0 | | | 0 |
| Orange juice | | 2 | 0.0 | | | 0 |
| Salad dressing: | | | | | | |
| Regular: | | | | | | |
| Bleu cheese | | 309 | 16.0 | | | 22 |
| House | | 269 | 13.0 | | | 11 |
| Thousand island | | 228 | 12.0 | | | 17 |
| Dietetic, Italian | | 426 | 0.0 | | | 0 |
| Shake: | | | | | | |
| Chocolate | | 202 | 12.0 | | | DNA |
| Strawberry | | 213 | 10.0 | | | DNA |
| Vanilla | | 205 | 10.0 | | | DNA |
| Soft drink: | | | | | | |
| Sweetened: | | | | | | |
| Pepsi-Cola | | | 0.0 | | | 0 |
| Seven-Up | | | 0.0 | | | 0 |
| Dietetic, Pepsi-Cola | | | 0.0 | | | 0 |
| Whaler, fish sandwich, plain | | 389 | 13.0 | | | 57 |
| Condiments: | | | | | | |
| Lettuce | | 1 | 0.0 | | | 0 |
| Tartar sauce | | 202 | 14.0 | | | 20 |

(USDA): United States Department of Agriculture
*Prepared as Package Directs

| Food and Description | Measure or Quantity | Sodium (mg.) | —Fats in grams— Total | Satu- rated | Unsatu- rated | Choles- terol (mg.) |
|---|---|---|---|---|---|---|
| *Whopper:* | | | | | | |
| Regular: | | | | | | |
| Plain | | 467 | 21.0 | | | 78 |
| With cheese | | 751 | 28.0 | | | 101 |
| Condiments: | | | | | | |
| Ketchup | | 183 | 0.0 | | | 0 |
| Lettuce | | 2 | 0.0 | | | 0 |
| Mayonnaise | | 107 | 15.0 | | | 12 |
| Onion | | 1 | 0.0 | | | 0 |
| Pickles | | 119 | 0.0 | | | 0 |
| Tomatoes | | 1 | 0.0 | | | 0 |
| Junior: | | | | | | |
| Plain | | 297 | 12.0 | | | 37 |
| With cheese | | 439 | 15.0 | | | 48 |
| Condiments: | | | | | | |
| Ketchup | | 91 | 0.0 | | | 0 |
| Lettuce | | 1 | 0.0 | | | 0 |
| Mayonnaise | | 36 | 5.0 | | | 4 |
| Onions | | 1 | 0.0 | | | 0 |
| Pickles | | 60 | 0.0 | | | 0 |
| Tomatoes | | 1 | 0.0 | | | 0 |
| **BURGUNDY WINE:** | | | | | | |
| (Gold Seal) 12% alcohol | 3 fl. oz. | 3 | 0.0 | | | (0) |
| (Great Western) 12.5% alcohol | 3 fl. oz. | 36 | 0.0 | | | 0 |
| **BURGUNDY WINE, SPARKLING** | | | | | | |
| (Gold Seal) 12% alcohol | 3 fl. oz. | 3 | 0.0 | | | (0) |
| **BURRITO:** | | | | | | |
| *Canned (Del Monte) | 1 burrito | 616 | 10.0 | | | |
| Frozen: | | | | | | |
| (Hormel): | | | | | | |
| Beef | 1 burrito | 780 | 8.0 | | | |
| Cheese | 1 burrito | 792 | 5.0 | | | |
| Cheese & rice | 4-oz. serving | 594 | 4.0 | | | |
| Grande | 5½-oz. serving | 877 | 16.0 | | | |
| Hot chili | 1 burrito | 619 | 8.0 | | | |
| (Swanson) bean & beef, 4-compartment | 15¼-oz. serving | 1,630 | 32.0 | | | |
| (Van de Kamp's): | | | | | | |
| Regular, crispy fried | 6-oz. serving | 823 | 15.0 | | | |

(USDA): United States Department of Agriculture
*Prepared as Package Directs

| Food and Description | Measure or Quantity | Sodium (mg.) | Fats in grams — Total | Satu- rated | Unsatu- rated | Choles- terol (mg.) |
|---|---|---|---|---|---|---|
| Grande, with rice & corn | 16¾-oz. pkg. | 1,210 | 20.0 | | | |
| Sirloin, grande | 11-oz. pkg. | 1,120 | 15.0 | | | |
| **BURRITO FILLING MIX,** | | | | | | |
| canned (Del Monte) | ½ cup (4.3 oz.) | 900 | 1.0 | | | |
| **BUTTER:** | | | | | | |
| Salted: | | | | | | |
| (USDA) | ¼ lb. (1 stick, ½ cup) | 1,119 | 92.0 | 52. | 40. | 284 |
| (USDA) | 1 T. (⅛ stick, .5 oz.) | 138 | 11.3 | 6. | 5. | 35 |
| (USDA) | 1 pat (1″ × 1″ × ⅓″, 5 grams) | 49 | 4.0 | 2. | 2. | 12 |
| (Breakstone's) | 1 T. (.5 oz.) | 95 | 11.0 | | | 29 |
| (Sealtest) | 1 T. (.5 oz.) | 117 | 12.1 | | | |
| Whipped (USDA) | 2.7 oz. (1 stick, ½ cup) | 750 | 61.6 | 35. | 27. | 190 |
| Whipped (USDA) | 1 T. (⅛ stick, 9 grams) | 89 | 7.3 | 4. | 3. | 22 |
| Whipped (USDA) | 1 pat (1¼″ × 1¼″ × ⅓″, 4 grams) | 39 | 3.2 | 2. | 1. | 10 |
| Whipped (Breakstone's) | 1 T. (9 grams) | 64 | 7.4 | | | 19 |
| Whipped (Sealtest) | 1 T. (9 grams) | 74 | 7.6 | | | |
| Unsalted: | | | | | | |
| (USDA) | ¼ lb. (1 stick, ½ cup) | 11 | 92.0 | 52. | 40. | 284 |
| (USDA) | 1 T. (⅛ stick, .5 oz.) | 1 | 11.3 | 6. | 5. | 35 |
| (USDA) | 1 pat (1″ × 1″ × ⅓″, 5 grams) | <1 | 4.0 | 2. | 2. | 12 |
| (Breakstone's) | 1 T. (.5 oz.) | <1 | 11.0 | | | 29 |
| (Sealtest) | 1 T. (.5 oz.) | 1 | 12.1 | | | |
| Whipped (USDA) | ½ cup (1 stick, 2.7 oz.) | 8 | 61.6 | 35. | 27. | 190 |
| Whipped (USDA) | 1 T. (⅛ stick, 9 grams) | <1 | 7.3 | 4. | 3. | 22 |
| Whipped (USDA) | 1 pat (1¼″ × 1¼″ × ⅓″, 4 grams) | <1 | 3.2 | 2. | 1. | 10 |
| Whipped (Breakstone's) | 1 T. (9 grams) | <1 | 7.4 | | | 19 |

(USDA): United States Department of Agriculture
*Prepared as Package Directs

| Food and Description | Measure or Quantity | Sodium (mg.) | — Fats in grams — | | | Choles- terol (mg.) |
|---|---|---|---|---|---|---|
| | | | Total | Satu- rated | Unsatu- rated | |

**BUTTER BEAN (See BEAN, LIMA)**

**BUTTERFISH,** raw (USDA):
Gulf:

| Food and Description | Measure or Quantity | Sodium (mg.) | Total | Satu-rated | Unsatu-rated | Choles-terol (mg.) |
|---|---|---|---|---|---|---|
| Whole | 1 lb. (weighed whole) | | 6.7 | | | |
| Meat only | 4 oz. | | 3.3 | | | |
| Northern: | | | | | | |
| Whole | 1 lb. (weighed whole) | | 23.6 | | | |
| Meat only | 4 oz. | | 11.6 | | | |

**BUTTERMILK (See MILK)**

**BUTTERNUT** (USDA):

| | | | | | | |
|---|---|---|---|---|---|---|
| Whole | 1 lb. (weighed in shell) | | 38.9 | | | 0 |
| Shelled | 4 oz. | | 69.4 | | | 0 |

**BUTTER OIL** or dehydrated

| | | | | | | |
|---|---|---|---|---|---|---|
| butter (USDA) | 1 cup (7.2 oz.) | | 203.0 | 112. | 91. | |

**BUTTERSCOTCH MORSELS**

| | | | | | | |
|---|---|---|---|---|---|---|
| (Nestlé) artificial | 1 oz. | | 15.0 | 7. | | 0 |

**BUTTER SUBSTITUTE,**
*Butter-Buds:*

| | | | | | | |
|---|---|---|---|---|---|---|
| Dry | ⅛ oz. | 170 | 0.0 | | | 0 |
| Liquid | 1 oz. | 170 | 0.0 | | | 0 |
| Sprinkle | 1 tsp. | 66 | 0.0 | | | 0 |

# C

**CABBAGE:**
White (USDA):
Raw:

| | | | | | | |
|---|---|---|---|---|---|---|
| Whole | 1 lb. (weighed untrimmed) | 72 | .7 | | | 0 |
| Coarsely shredded or sliced | 1 cup (2.5 oz.) | 14 | .1 | | | 0 |

(USDA): United States Department of Agriculture
*Prepared as Package Directs

| Food and Description | Measure or Quantity | Sodium (mg.) | — Fats in grams — | | | Choles-terol (mg.) |
|---|---|---|---|---|---|---|
| | | | Total | Satu-rated | Unsatu-rated | |
| Finely shredded or chopped | 1 cup (3.2 oz.) | 18 | .2 | | | 0 |
| Wedge | 3½″ × 4½″ wedge (3.5 oz.) | 20 | .2 | | | 0 |
| Boiled without salt, until tender: | | | | | | |
| Shredded, small amount of water, drained | ½ cup (2.6 oz.) | 10 | .1 | | | 0 |
| Wedges, in large amount of water, drained | ½ cup (3.2 oz.) | 12 | .2 | | | 0 |
| Dehydrated | 1 oz. | 54 | .5 | | | 0 |
| Red, raw (USDA): | | | | | | |
| Whole | 1 lb. (weighed untrimmed) | 93 | .7 | | | 0 |
| Coarsely shredded | 1 cup (2.5 oz.) | 18 | .1 | | | 0 |
| Red, canned (Comstock-Greenwood) | 4 oz. | | Tr. | | | (0) |
| Savoy, raw (USDA): | | | | | | |
| Whole | 1 lb. (weighed untrimmed) | 79 | .7 | | | 0 |
| Coarsely shredded | 1 cup (2.5 oz.) | 15 | .1 | | | 0 |
| **CABBAGE, CHINESE OR CELERY,** raw (USDA): | | | | | | |
| Whole | 1 lb. (weighed untrimmed) | 101 | .4 | | | 0 |
| 1″ pieces, leaves with stalk | ½ cup (1.3 oz.) | 9 | Tr. | | | 0 |
| **CABBAGE, SPOON OR WHITE MUSTARD OR PAKCHOY** (USDA): | | | | | | |
| Raw | 1 lb. (weighed untrimmed) | 112 | .9 | | | 0 |
| Boiled without salt, drained | ½ cup (3 oz.) | 15 | .2 | | | 0 |
| **CABBAGE, STUFFED,** frozen (Green Giant) baked, with beef in tomato sauce | ½ of pkg. | 800 | 12.0 | | | |
| **CAKE** (Some cakes are listed by brand name such as *Yankee Doodles,* etc.): | | | | | | |
| Home Recipe (USDA): | | | | | | |
| Plain: | | | | | | |

(USDA): United States Department of Agriculture
*Prepared as Package Directs

CAKE

| Food and Description | Measure or Quantity | Sodium (mg.) | — Fats in grams — | | | Choles- terol (mg.) |
|---|---|---|---|---|---|---|
| | | | Total | Satu- rated | Unsatu- rated | |
| Without icing: | | | | | | |
| Made with butter[1] | 1/9 of 9" sq. cake (3"×3"×1"—3 oz.) | 258 | 10.9 | 6. | 6. | |
| Made with vegetable shortening[2] | 1/9 of 9" sq. cake (3"×3"×1"—3 oz.) | 258 | 12.0 | 3. | 8. | |
| With boiled white icing: | | | | | | |
| Made with butter[1] | 1/9 of 9" sq. cake (4 oz.) | 299 | 12.0 | 7. | 5. | |
| Made with vegetable shortening[2] | 1/9 of 9" sq. cake (4 oz.) | 299 | 12.0 | 3. | 9. | |
| With chocolate icing: | | | | | | |
| Made with butter[3] | 1/16 of 10" layer cake (3.5 oz.) | 229 | 12.7 | 8. | 6. | |
| Made with vegetable shortening[4] | 1/16 of 10" layer cake (3.5 oz.) | 229 | 12.9 | 4. | 9. | |
| With uncooked white icing: | | | | | | |
| Made with butter[1] | 1/16 of 10" layer cake (3.5 oz.) | 227 | 12.7 | 7. | 6. | |
| Made with vegetable shortening[2] | 1/16 of 10" layer cake (3.5 oz.) | 227 | 11.8 | 3. | 9. | |
| Angel food[5] | 1/12 of 8" cake | 113 | <.1 | | | |
| Caramel: | | | | | | |
| Without icing | 1/9 of 9" sq. cake | 262 | 14.9 | .8 | 7. | |
| With caramel icing | 3 oz. | 214 | 12.6 | | | |
| Chocolate: | | | | | | |
| Without icing: | | | | | | |
| Made with butter[3] | 3 oz. | 250 | 14.6 | 8. | 7. | |
| Made with vegetable shortening[4] | 3 oz. | 250 | 14.6 | 4. | 10. | |
| With chocolate icing, 2-layer | 1/16 of 10" cake (4.2 oz.) | 282 | 19.7 | | | 52 |

(USDA): United States Department of Agriculture
*Prepared as Package Directs
[1]Principal sources of fat: butter, egg & milk.
[2]Principal sources of fat: vegetable shortening, egg & milk.
[3]Principal sources of fat: butter, egg, milk & chocolate.
[4]Principal sources of fat: vegetable shortening, egg, milk & chocolate.
[5]Made with sodium aluminum sulfate-type baking powder.

| Food and Description | Measure or Quantity | Sodium (mg.) | —Fats in grams— | | | Choles-terol (mg.) |
|---|---|---|---|---|---|---|
| | | | Total | Satu-rated | Unsatu-rated | |
| With chocolate icing, 2-layer | 1/16 of 9" cake (2.6 oz.) | 176 | 12.3 | | | 32 |
| With uncooked white icing | 1/16 of 10" cake (4.2 oz.) | 281 | 17.5 | | | |
| Devil's food: | | | | | | |
| Without icing | 3" × 2" ×1½" piece (1.9 oz.) | 162 | 9.5 | | | |
| With chocolate icing, 2-layer | 1/16 of 9" cake (2.6 oz.) | 176 | 12.3 | | | 32 |
| With chocolate icing, 2-layer | 1/16 of 10" cake (4.2 oz.) | 282 | 19.7 | | | 52 |
| With uncooked white icing | 1/16 of 10" cake (4.2 oz.) | 281 | 17.5 | | | |
| Fruit cake: | | | | | | |
| Dark, home recipe[1] | 1-lb. loaf | 717 | 69.4 | | | 206 |
| Dark, home recipe[1] | 1/30 of 8" loaf (.5 oz.) | 24 | 2.3 | | | 7 |
| Dark, home recipe[1] | 2" × 2" × ½" slice (1.1 oz.) | 47 | 4.6 | | | 14 |
| Light, home recipe, made with butter[2] | 1-lb. loaf | 875 | 71.2 | 26. | 45. | |
| Light, home recipe, made with butter[2] | 2" × 2" × ½" slice (1.1 oz.) | 58 | 4.7 | 2. | 3. | |
| Light, home recipe, made with butter[2] | 1/30 of 8" loaf (.5 oz.) | 29 | 2.4 | <1. | 1. | |
| Light, home recipe, made with vegetable shortening[3] | 1-lb. loaf | 875 | 74.8 | 16. | 59. | |
| Light, home recipe, made with vegetable shortening[3] | 2" × 2" × ½" slice (1.1 oz.) | 58 | 5.0 | 1. | 4. | |
| Light, home recipe, made with vegetable shortening[3] | 1/30 of 8" loaf (.5 oz.) | 29 | 2.5 | <1. | 2. | |

(USDA): United States Department of Agriculture
*Prepared as Package Directs
[1]Made with sodium aluminum sulfate type baking powder.
[2]Principal sources of fat: butter, almonds & cream.
[3]Principal sources of fat: vegetable shortening, almonds & cream.

| Food and Description | Measure or Quantity | Sodium (mg.) | — Fats in grams — | | | Choles-terol (mg.) |
|---|---|---|---|---|---|---|
| | | | Total | Satu-rated | Unsatu-rated | |
| **Pound cake:** | | | | | | |
| Home recipe, old fashioned, equal weights flour, sugar, eggs & butter [1] | 1.1-oz. slice (3½″ × 3″ × ½″) | 33 | 7.9 | 4. | 4. | |
| Home recipe, old fashioned, equal weights flour, sugar, eggs & vegetable shortening [2] | 1.1-oz. slice (3½″ × 3″ × ½″) | 33 | 8.8 | 2. | 7. | |
| Home recipe, traditional, made with butter [3] | 1.1-oz. slice (3½″ × 3″ × ½″) | 53 | 4.8 | 2. | 2. | |
| Home recipe, traditional, made with vegetable shortening [4] | 1.1-oz. slice (3½″ × 3″ × ½″ | 53 | 5.6 | 2. | 4. | |
| **White:** | | | | | | |
| Without icing: | | | | | | |
| Made with butter [3] | ⅑ of 9″ sq. cake (3″×3″×1″—3 oz.) | 278 | 13.8 | 8. | 6. | |
| Made with vegetable shortening [4] | ⅑ of 9″ sq. cake (3″×3″×1″—3 oz.) | 278 | 13.8 | 4. | 10. | |
| With coconut icing: | | | | | | |
| Made with butter [3] | ⅟₁₆ of 10″ layer cake (3.5 oz.) | 257 | 13.3 | 7. | 6. | |
| Made with vegetable shortening [4] | ⅟₁₆ of 10″ layer cake (3.5 oz.) | 257 | 13.3 | 4. | 9. | |
| With uncooked white icing: | | | | | | |

(USDA): United States Department of Agriculture
*Prepared as Package Directs
[1] Principal sources of fat: egg & butter.
[2] Principal sources of fat: egg & vegetable shortening.
[3] Principal sources of fat: butter, egg & milk.
[4] Principal sources of fat: vegetable shortening, egg & milk.

| Food and Description | Measure or Quantity | Sodium (mg.) | Fats in grams — Total | Satu- rated | Unsatu- rated | Choles- terol (mg.) |
|---|---|---|---|---|---|---|
| Made with butter[1] | 1/16 of 10″ layer cake (3.5 oz.) | 234 | 12.9 | 7. | 6. | |
| Made with vegetable shortening[2] | 1/16 of 10″ layer cake (3.5 oz.) | 234 | 12.9 | 5. | 9. | |
| **Yellow:** | | | | | | |
| **Without icing:** | | | | | | |
| Made with butter[1] | 1/9 of 9″ sq. cake (3″×3″×1″–3 oz.) | 222 | 10.9 | 6. | 5. | |
| Made with vegetable shortening[2] | 1/9 of 9″ sq. cake (3″×3″×1″–3 oz.) | 222 | 10.9 | 3. | 8. | |
| **With caramel icing:** | | | | | | |
| Made with butter[1] | 1/16 of 10″ layer cake (3.5 oz.) | 226 | 11.7 | 6. | 6. | |
| Made with vegetable shortening[2] | 1/16 of 10″ layer cake (3.5 oz.) | 226 | 11.7 | 3. | 9. | |
| **With chocolate icing, 2-layer:** | | | | | | |
| Made with butter[3] | 1/16 of 9″ cake (2.6 oz.) | 156 | 9.8 | 6. | 4. | |
| Made with vegetable shortening[4] | 1/16 of 9″ cake (2.6 oz.) | 156 | 9.8 | 3. | 7. | 33 |
| **Commercial type:** | | | | | | |
| **Not frozen:** | | | | | | |
| Carrot (Hostess) | 3-oz. cake | 179 | 15.3 | | | 77 |
| Crumb (Hostess) | 1 1/4-oz. cake | 98 | 4.3 | | | 11 |
| **Fruit:** | | | | | | |
| (Holland Honey Cake) unsalted | 1/14 of cake (.9 oz.) | 2 | 0.0 | | | 0 |
| (Hostess) loaf | 1/2 of 5-oz. cake | 262 | 4.3 | | | 3 |
| **Frozen:** | | | | | | |
| Butterscotch pecan (Pepperidge Farm) | 1/10 of 17-oz. cake | 110 | 7.0 | | | |

(USDA): United States Department of Agriculture
*Prepared as Package Directs
[1]Principal sources of fat: butter, egg & milk.
[2]Principal sources of fat: vegetable shortening, egg & milk.
[3]Principal sources of fat: butter, egg, milk & chocolate.
[4]Principal sources of fat: vegetable shortening, egg, milk & chocolate.

| Food and Description | Measure or Quantity | Sodium (mg.) | — Fats in grams — | | | Cholesterol (mg.) |
|---|---|---|---|---|---|---|
| | | | Total | Saturated | Unsaturated | |
| Carrot: | | | | | | |
| (Pepperidge Farm) with cream cheese icing | 1/8 of 11¾-oz. | 150 | 8.0 | | | |
| (Weight Watchers) | 3 oz. | 340 | 6.0 | | | |
| Cheese: | | | | | | |
| (Morton) *Great Little Desserts:* | | | | | | |
| Cherry | 6-oz. cake | 350 | 27.0 | | | 106 |
| Cream | 6-oz. cake | 350 | 32.0 | | | 116 |
| Strawberry | 6-oz. cake | 350 | 27.0 | | | 106 |
| (Weight Watchers): | | | | | | |
| Regular | 3.9-oz. | 220 | 8.0 | | | |
| Black cherry | 3.9 oz. | 190 | 7.0 | | | |
| Strawberry | 3.9 oz. | 220 | 6.0 | | | |
| Chocolate: | | | | | | |
| (Pepperidge Farm): | | | | | | |
| Layer, fudge | 1/10 of 17-oz. cake | 140 | 10.0 | | | |
| Supreme, dutch | 1¾ oz. | 115 | 10.0 | | | |
| (Weight Watchers): | | | | | | |
| Regular | 2½ oz. | 290 | 6.0 | | | |
| German | 2½ oz. | 350 | 8.0 | | | |
| Coconut (Pepperidge Farm) | 1/10 of 17-oz. cake | 120 | 9.0 | | | |
| Devil's food (Pepperidge Farm) layer | 1/10 of 17-oz. cake | 135 | 9.0 | | | |
| Golden (Pepperidge Farm) layer | 1/10 of 17-oz. cake | 115 | 9.0 | | | |
| Grand marnier (Pepperidge Farm) supreme | 1½ oz. | 85 | 18.0 | | | |
| Lemon coconut (Pepperidge Farm) supreme | 1/4 of 12¼-oz. cake | 220 | 13.0 | | | |
| Pineapple cream (Pepperidge Farm) supreme | 1/12 of 24-oz. cake | 130 | 7.0 | | | |

(USDA): United States Department of Agriculture
*Prepared as Package Directs

| Food and Description | Measure or Quantity | Sodium (mg.) | —Fats in grams— | | | Choles- terol (mg.) |
|---|---|---|---|---|---|---|
| | | | Total | Satu- rated | Unsatu- rated | |
| Pound (Pepperidge Farm) | 1/10 of 10¾-oz. cake | 150 | 7.0 | | | |
| Spice (Weight Watchers) | 3 oz. | 350 | 6.0 | | | |
| Strawberry cream (Pepperidge Farm) supreme | 1/12 of 24-oz. cake | 120 | 7.0 | | | |
| Vanilla (Pepperidge Farm) layer | 1/10 of 17-oz. cake | 120 | 8.0 | | | |
| **CAKE ICING:** | | | | | | |
| Butter pecan (Betty Crocker) *Creamy Deluxe* | 1/12 of pkg. | 85 | 7.0 | | | |
| Caramel (USDA) home recipe[1] | 4 oz. | 94 | 7.6 | 4.5 | 3.1 | |
| Caramel pecan (Pillsbury) *Frosting Supreme* | 1/12 of pkg. | 70 | 8.0 | | | |
| Cherry (Betty Crocker) *Creamy Deluxe* | 1/12 of pkg. | 95 | 6.0 | | | |
| Chocolate: | | | | | | |
| (USDA) home recipe[2] | 1 cup (9.7 oz.) | 168 | 38.2 | 22. | 16. | |
| (Betty Crocker) *Creamy Deluxe:* | | | | | | |
| Regular | 1/12 of pkg. | 85 | 8.0 | | | |
| Chip | 1/12 of pkg. | 85 | 7.0 | | | |
| Fudge, dark Dutch | 1/12 of pkg. | 125 | 7.0 | | | |
| Milk | 1/12 of pkg. | 95 | 7.0 | | | |
| Nut | 1/12 of pkg. | 85 | 8.0 | | | |
| Sour cream | 1/12 of pkg. | 110 | 7.0 | | | |
| (Duncan Hines): | | | | | | |
| Regular | 1/12 of pkg. | 84 | 7.0 | | | 7 |
| Fudge, dark Dutch | 1/12 of pkg. | 95 | 7.0 | | | 7 |
| Milk | 1/12 of pkg. | 84 | 7.0 | | | 7 |
| (Pillsbury) *Frosting Supreme:* | | | | | | |
| Chip | 1/12 of pkg. | 70 | 5.0 | | | |
| Fudge | 1/12 of pkg. | 80 | 6.0 | | | |
| Milk | 1/12 of pkg. | 60 | 6.0 | | | |
| Mint | 1/12 of pkg. | 80 | 7.0 | | | |
| Coconut, home recipe (USDA)[3] | 1 cup (5.8 oz.) | 196 | 12.8 | 12. | Tr. | |

(USDA): United States Department of Agriculture
*Prepared as Package Directs
[1]Principal sources of fat: butter & milk.
[2]Principal sources of fat: chocolate, butter & milk.
[3]Principal source of fat: coconut.

| Food and Description | Measure or Quantity | Sodium (mg.) | —Fats in grams— | | | Choles- terol (mg.) |
|---|---|---|---|---|---|---|
| | | | Total | Satu- rated | Unsatu- rated | |
| Coconut almond (Pillsbury) | | | | | | |
| *Frosting Supreme* | 1/12 of pkg. | 60 | 9.0 | | | |
| Coconut pecan (Pillsbury) | | | | | | |
| *Frosting Supreme* | 1/12 of pkg. | 60 | 10.0 | | | |
| Cream cheese: | | | | | | |
| (Betty Crocker) *Creamy* | | | | | | |
| *Deluxe* | 1/12 of pkg. | 100 | 7.0 | | | |
| (Pillsbury) *Frosting Supreme* | 1/12 of pkg. | 115 | 6.0 | | | |
| Double Dutch (Pillsbury) | | | | | | |
| *Frosting Supreme* | 1/12 of pkg. | 45 | 6.0 | | | |
| Lemon: | | | | | | |
| (Betty Crocker) *Sunkist,* | | | | | | |
| *Creamy Deluxe* | 1/12 of pkg. | 95 | 6.0 | | | |
| (Pillsbury) *Frosting Supreme* | 1/12 of pkg. | 80 | 6.0 | | | |
| Orange (Betty Crocker) | | | | | | |
| *Creamy Deluxe* | 1/12 of pkg. | 95 | 6.0 | | | |
| Strawberry (Pillsbury) *Frosting* | | | | | | |
| *Supreme* | 1/12 of pkg. | 75 | 6.0 | | | |
| Vanilla: | | | | | | |
| (Betty Crocker) *Creamy* | | | | | | |
| *Deluxe* | 1/12 of pkg. | 95 | 6.0 | | | |
| (Duncan Hines) | 1/12 of pkg. | 86 | 7.0 | | | 7 |
| (Pillsbury) *Frosting Supreme:* | | | | | | |
| Regular | 1/12 of pkg. | 75 | 6.0 | | | |
| Sour cream | 1/12 of pkg. | 80 | 6.0 | | | |
| White: | | | | | | |
| Home recipe (USDA): | | | | | | |
| Boiled | 1 cup (3.3 oz.) | 134 | 0.0 | | | |
| Uncooked [1] | 4 oz. | 56 | 7.5 | 4. | 3. | |
| (Betty Crocker) *Creamy* | | | | | | |
| *Deluxe* | 1/12 of pkg. | 95 | 6.0 | | | |
| **CAKE ICING MIX:** | | | | | | |
| *Banana (Betty Crocker) | | | | | | |
| *Chiquita* | 1/12 of cake's icing | 100 | 6.0 | | | |
| **Butter Brickle* (Betty Crocker) | 1/12 of cake's icing | 115 | 6.0 | | | |
| *Butter pecan (Betty Crocker) | | | | | | |
| deluxe, creamy | 1/12 of pkg. | 100 | 6.0 | | | |
| *Cherry, creamy (Betty Crocker) | 1/12 of cake's icing | 100 | 6.0 | | | |

(USDA): United States Department of Agriculture
*Prepared as Package Directs
[1]Principal sources of fat: butter & milk.

| Food and Description | Measure or Quantity | Sodium (mg.) | — Fats in grams — | | | Choles-terol (mg.) |
|---|---|---|---|---|---|---|
| | | | Total | Satu-rated | Unsatu-rated | |
| *Chocolate: | | | | | | |
| (USDA) fudge: | | | | | | |
| Regular [1] | 4 oz. | 177 | 16.3 | 6.8 | 9.5 | |
| Creamy, prepared with water | 4 oz. | 263 | 7.4 | 2.3 | 5.1 | |
| Creamy, prepared with water & fat [2] | 4 oz. | 364 | 17.2 | 7.9 | 9.3 | |
| (Betty Crocker) creamy: | | | | | | |
| Almond fudge | 1/12 of pkg. | 75 | 7.0 | | | |
| Fudge | 1/12 of pkg. | 75 | 6.0 | | | |
| Fudge, dark | 1/12 of pkg. | 90 | 6.0 | | | |
| Milk | 1/12 of pkg. | 80 | 5.0 | | | |
| Sour cream | 1/12 of pkg. | 75 | 6.0 | | | |
| (Pillsbury) *Frost It Hot* | 1/8 of pkg. | 50 | 0.0 | | | |
| *Coconut almond: | | | | | | |
| (Betty Crocker) creamy | 1/12 of pkg. | 90 | 8.0 | | | |
| (Pillsbury) | 1/12 of pkg. | 85 | 10.0 | | | |
| *Coconut pecan: | | | | | | |
| (Betty Crocker) creamy | 1/12 of pkg. | 100 | 8.0 | | | |
| (Pillsbury) | 1/12 of pkg. | 105 | 7.0 | | | |
| *Cream cheese & nut (Betty Crocker) creamy | 1/12 of pkg. | 100 | 6.0 | | | |
| *Lemon (Betty Crocker) creamy | 1/12 of pkg. | 100 | 6.0 | | | |
| *Vanilla (Pillsbury) *Frosting Supreme,* regular or sour cream | 1/12 of pkg. | 80 | 6.0 | | | |
| *White: | | | | | | |
| (Betty Crocker): | | | | | | |
| Regular, creamy | 1/12 of pkg. | 100 | 6.0 | | | |
| Fluffy | 1/12 of pkg. | 40 | 0.0 | | | |
| (Pillsbury) fluffy: | | | | | | |
| Regular | 1/12 of pkg. | 65 | 0.0 | | | |
| *Frost It Hot* | 1/8 of pkg. | 50 | 0.0 | | | |
| **CAKE MEAL** (Manischewitz) | 1/2 cup (2.6 oz.) | 2 | | | | |
| **CAKE MIX:** | | | | | | |
| Regular: | | | | | | |
| Angel food: | | | | | | |
| *(USDA) | 1/12 of 10″ cake | 77 | 3.0 | | | 0 |

(USDA): United States Department of Agriculture
*Prepared as Package Directs
[1] Principal sources of fat: vegetable shortening & cocoa.
[2] Principal sources of fat: vegetable shortening, butter & cocoa.

| Food and Description | Measure or Quantity | Sodium (mg.) | Total | Saturated | Unsaturated | Cholesterol (mg.) |
|---|---|---|---|---|---|---|
| (Betty Crocker): | | | | | | |
| Chocolate or confetti | 1/12 of pkg. | 275 | 0.0 | | | |
| Lemon custard | 1/12 of pkg. | 265 | 0.0 | | | |
| One-step | 1/12 of pkg. | 250 | 0.0 | | | |
| Strawberry | 1/12 of pkg. | 270 | 0.0 | | | |
| Traditional | 1/12 of pkg. | 140 | 0.0 | | | |
| (Duncan Hines) | 1/12 of pkg. | 119 | .1 | | | 0 |
| *Apple cinnamon (Betty Crocker) Super Moist | 1/12 of cake | 275 | 11.0 | | | |
| *Applesauce raisin (Betty Crocker) Snackin' Cake | 1/9 of cake | 250 | 4.0 | | | |
| *Banana: | | | | | | |
| (Betty Crocker) Super Moist | 1/12 of cake | 255 | 11.0 | | | |
| (Pillsbury) Pillsbury Plus | 1/12 of cake | 290 | 11.0 | | | |
| *Banana walnut (Betty Crocker) Snackin' Cake | 1/9 of cake | 260 | 6.0 | | | |
| *Black forest cherry (Pillsbury) Bundt | 1/16 of cake | 310 | 8.0 | | | |
| *Boston cream (Pillsbury) Bundt | 1/16 of cake | 310 | 10.0 | | | |
| *Butter (Pillsbury) Pillsbury Plus | 1/12 of cake | 370 | 12.0 | | | |
| *Butter Brickle (Betty Crocker) Super Moist | 1/12 of cake | 265 | 11.0 | | | |
| Butter pecan (Betty Crocker): | | | | | | |
| Snackin' Cake | 1/9 of pkg. | 250 | 6.0 | | | |
| *Super Moist | 1/12 of cake | 250 | 11.0 | | | |
| *Carrot (Betty Crocker): | | | | | | |
| Stir 'N Frost, with cream cheese frosting | 1/6 of cake | 200 | 6.0 | | | |
| Super Moist | 1/12 of cake | 255 | 12.0 | | | |
| Carrot nut (Betty Crocker) Snackin' Cake | 1/9 of pkg. | 240 | 6.0 | | | |
| *Carrot & spice (Pillsbury) Pillsbury Plus | 1/12 of cake | 330 | 11.0 | | | |
| *Cheesecake: | | | | | | |
| (Jell-O) | 1/8 of cake | 351 | 12.0 | | | 28 |
| (Royal) No Bake: | | | | | | |
| Lite | 1/8 of cake | 380 | 10.0 | | | |
| Real | 1/8 of cake | 370 | 9.0 | | | |

(USDA): United States Department of Agriculture
*Prepared as Package Directs

| Food and Description | Measure or Quantity | Sodium (mg.) | Total | — Fats in grams —<br>Satu-<br>rated | Unsatu-<br>rated | Choles-<br>terol<br>(mg.) |
|---|---|---|---|---|---|---|
| *Cherry chip (Betty Crocker) | | | | | | |
| Super Moist | 1/12 of cake | 265 | 3.0 | | | |
| Chocolate: | | | | | | |
| (Betty Crocker): | | | | | | |
| Pudding recipe | 1/6 of cake | 255 | 5.0 | | | |
| Snackin' Cake: | | | | | | |
| Almond | 1/9 of pkg. | 215 | 7.0 | | | |
| Fudge chip | 1/9 of pkg. | 205 | 6.0 | | | |
| Coconut pecan | 1/9 of pkg. | 255 | 5.0 | | | |
| Stir'N Frost: | | | | | | |
| Chocolate chip with | | | | | | |
| chocolate frosting | 1/6 of pkg. | 200 | 6.0 | | | |
| Fudge, with vanilla | | | | | | |
| frosting | 1/6 of pkg. | 250 | 6.0 | | | |
| Stir 'N Streusel, | | | | | | |
| German | 1/6 of pkg. | 245 | 7.0 | | | |
| *Super Moist: | | | | | | |
| Chocolate chip | 1/12 of cake | 425 | 12.0 | | | |
| Fudge | 1/12 of cake | 450 | 11.0 | | | |
| German | 1/12 of cake | 420 | 11.0 | | | |
| Milk | 1/12 of cake | 290 | 11.0 | | | |
| Sour cream | 1/12 of cake | 430 | 11.0 | | | |
| *(Pillsbury): | | | | | | |
| Bundt: | | | | | | |
| Fudge, tunnel of | 1/16 of cake | 310 | 11.0 | | | |
| Macaroon | 1/16 of cake | 300 | 10.0 | | | |
| Microwave: | | | | | | |
| Regular: | | | | | | |
| Plain | 1/8 of cake | 260 | 13.0 | | | |
| With chocolate | | | | | | |
| frosting | 1/8 of cake | 310 | 17.0 | | | |
| With vanilla frosting | 1/8 of cake | 300 | 17.0 | | | |
| Double, supreme | 1/8 of cake | 340 | 19.0 | | | |
| Tunnel of Fudge | 1/8 of cake | 320 | 17.0 | | | |
| Pillsbury Plus: | | | | | | |
| Chip | 1/12 of cake | 290 | 14.0 | | | |
| Dark | 1/12 of cake | 380 | 12.0 | | | |
| Fudge, marble | 1/12 of cake | 300 | 12.0 | | | |
| German | 1/12 of cake | 340 | 11.0 | | | |
| Cinnamon: | | | | | | |
| (Betty Crocker) Stir 'N | | | | | | |
| Streusel | 1/6 of pkg. | 230 | 7.0 | | | |

(USDA): United States Department of Agriculture
*Prepared as Package Directs

| Food and Description | Measure or Quantity | Sodium (mg.) | Total | Fats in grams Satu- rated | Unsatu- rated | Choles- terol (mg.) |
|---|---|---|---|---|---|---|
| *(Pillsbury) *Streusel Swirl* | 1/16 of cake | 200 | 11.0 | | | |
| Coconut pecan (Betty Crocker) *Snackin' Cake* | 1/9 of pkg. | 255 | 7.0 | | | |
| *Coffee cake: | | | | | | |
| (USDA) prepared with egg & milk[1] | 2-oz. serving | 244 | 5.4 | 1.1 | 4.3 | |
| (Aunt Jemima) | 1/8 of cake | 34 | .6 | | | |
| (Pillsbury) apple cinnamon | 1/8 of cake | 150 | 7.0 | | | |
| Date nut (Betty Crocker) *Snackin' Cake* | 1/9 of pkg. | 265 | 6.0 | | | |
| Devil's food: | | | | | | |
| *(Betty Crocker) *Super Moist* | 1/12 of cake | 425 | 12.0 | | | |
| (Duncan Hines) | 1/12 of pkg. | 363 | 4.1 | | | 0 |
| *(Pillsbury) *Pillsbury Plus* | 1/12 of cake | 370 | 14.0 | | | |
| Fudge (See Chocolate) | | | | | | |
| Golden chocolate chip (Betty Crocker) *Snackin' Cake* | 1/9 of pkg. | 255 | 5.0 | | | |
| Lemon: | | | | | | |
| (Betty Crocker): | | | | | | |
| *Pudding | 1/6 of cake | 270 | 5.0 | | | |
| *Stir'N Frost,* with lemon frosting | 1/6 of pkg. | 210 | 7.0 | | | |
| *Super Moist* | 1/12 of cake | 260 | 11.0 | | | |
| *(Pillsbury): | | | | | | |
| *Bundt,* tunnel of | 1/16 of cake | 300 | 9.0 | | | |
| Microwave: | | | | | | |
| Regular | 1/8 of cake | 180 | 13.0 | | | |
| With lemon frosting | 1/8 of cake | 220 | 17.0 | | | |
| Supreme, double | 1/8 of cake | 210 | 15.0 | | | |
| *Pillsbury Plus* | 1/12 of cake | 290 | 11.0 | | | |
| *Streusel Swirl* | 1/16 of cake | 340 | 11.0 | | | |
| Marble: | | | | | | |
| (USDA) dry[2] | 1 oz. | 108 | 3.8 | .9 | 3. | 108 |
| *(Betty Crocker) *Super Moist* | 1/12 of cake | 255 | 11.0 | | | |
| *(Pillsbury) fudge, *Streusel Swirl* | 1/16 of cake | 200 | 11.0 | | | |
| *Orange (Betty Crocker) *Super Moist* | 1/12 of cake | 280 | 11.0 | | | |
| *Pineapple creme (Pillsbury) | | | | | | |

(USDA): United States Department of Agriculture
*Prepared as Package Directs
[1]Principal sources of fat: vegetable shortening, egg & milk.
[2]Principal source of fat: vegetable shortening.

| Food and Description | Measure or Quantity | Sodium (mg.) | Fats in grams Total | Satu- rated | Unsatu- rated | Choles- terol (mg.) |
|---|---|---|---|---|---|---|
| *Bundt* | 1/16 of cake | 300 | 9.0 | | | |
| *Pound: | | | | | | |
| (Betty Crocker) golden | 1/12 of cake | 155 | 9.0 | | | |
| (Dromedary) | 1/2" slice | 340 | 6.0 | | | |
| Spice (Betty Crocker): | | | | | | |
| *Snackin' Cake,* raisin | 1/9 of pkg. | 250 | 5.0 | | | |
| *Stir'N Frost,* with vanilla frosting | 1/6 of pkg. | 305 | 8.0 | | | |
| *Super Moist* | 1/12 of cake | 260 | 11.0 | | | |
| *Strawberry: | | | | | | |
| (Betty Crocker) *Super Moist* | 1/12 of cake | 260 | 11.0 | | | |
| (Pillsbury) *Pillsbury Plus* | 1/12 of cake | 300 | 11.0 | | | |
| *Upside down cake (Betty Crocker) pineapple | 1/9 of cake | 215 | 10.0 | | | |
| White: | | | | | | |
| *(USDA) made with egg whites, water and chocolate icing, 2-layers[1] | 1/16 of 9" dia. cake | 161 | 7.6 | 2.8 | 4.8 | 1 |
| (Betty Crocker): | | | | | | |
| *Stir'N Frost,* made with chocolate frosting | 1/6 of pkg. | 235 | 7.0 | | | |
| *Super Moist: | | | | | | |
| Regular | 1/12 of cake | 275 | 9.0 | | | |
| Sour cream | 1/12 of cake | 260 | 3.0 | | | |
| (Duncan Hines) deluxe | 1/12 of pkg. | 251 | 4.0 | | | |
| *(Pillsbury) *Pillsbury Plus* | 1/12 of cake | 290 | 10.0 | | | |
| Yellow: | | | | | | |
| *(USDA) made with eggs, water and chocolate icing | 1/16 of 9" cake | 170 | 8.5 | | | 36 |
| (Betty Crocker): | | | | | | |
| *Stir'N Frost,* with chocolate frosting | 1/6 of pkg. | 210 | 7.0 | | | |
| *Super Moist: | | | | | | |
| Regular | 1/12 of cake | 270 | 12.0 | | | |
| Butter recipe | 1/12 of cake | 350 | 11.0 | | | |
| (Duncan Hines) deluxe | 1/12 of pkg. | 271 | 3.6 | | | 0 |
| *(Pillsbury): | | | | | | |
| Microwave: | | | | | | |

(USDA): United States Department of Agriculture
*Prepared as Package Directs
[1]Principal sources of fat: vegetable shortening, chocolate, egg & milk.

| Food and Description | Measure or Quantity | Sodium (mg.) | Fats in grams — Total | Satu- rated | Unsatu- rated | Choles- terol (mg.) |
|---|---|---|---|---|---|---|
| Regular | ⅛ of cake | 170 | 13.0 | | | |
| With chocolate frosting | ⅛ of cake | 220 | 17.0 | | | |
| *Pillsbury Plus* | ¹⁄₁₂ of cake | 300 | 12.0 | | | |
| Dietetic: | | | | | | |
| Chocolate (Estee) | ¹⁄₁₀ of pkg. | 75 | 3.0 | | | 0 |
| *Devil's food (Betty Crocker) light style | ¹⁄₁₂ of cake | | 3.0 | | | |
| Lemon (Estee) | ¹⁄₁₀ of pkg. | 80 | 2.0 | | | 0 |
| Pound (Estee) | ¹⁄₁₀ of pkg. | 80 | 2.0 | | | 0 |
| *Yellow (Betty Crocker) light style | ¹⁄₁₂ of cake | | 3.0 | | | |

**CANADIAN WHISKY** (See **DISTILLED LIQUOR**)

**CANDIED FRUIT** (See individual kinds)

**CANDY.** The following values of candies from the U. S. Department of Agriculture are representative of the types sold commercially. These values may be useful when individual brands or sizes are not known:

| Almond: | | | | | | |
|---|---|---|---|---|---|---|
| Chocolate-coated[1] | 1 oz. | 17 | 12.4 | 2. | 10. | |
| Chocolate-coated[1] | 1 cup (6.3 oz.) | 106 | 78.7 | 13. | 66. | |
| Sugar-coated or Jordan[2] | 1 oz. | 6 | 5.3 | Tr. | 5. | |
| Butterscotch[3] | 1 oz. | 19 | 1.0 | <1. | Tr. | |
| Candy corn | 1 oz. | 60 | .6 | | | |
| Caramel: | | | | | | |
| Plain[4] | 1 oz. | 64 | 2.9 | 1. | 2. | |
| Plain with nuts[5] | 1 oz. | 58 | 4.6 | 2. | 3. | |
| Chocolate[6] | 1 oz. | 64 | 2.9 | 1. | 2. | |
| Chocolate with nuts[7] | 1 oz. | 58 | 4.6 | 2. | 3. | |

(USDA): United States Department of Agriculture
*Prepared as Package Directs
[1]Principal sources of fat: almonds, chocolate & vegetable shortening.
[2]Principal source of fat: almonds.
[3]Principal source of fat: butter.
[4]Principal sources of fat: animal & vegetable shortening.
[5]Principal sources of fat: vegetable shortening & nuts.
[6]Principal sources of fat: animal & vegetable shortening & chocolate.
[7]Principal sources of fat: chocolate, vegetable shortening & nuts.

| Food and Description | Measure or Quantity | Sodium (mg.) | — Fats in grams — | | | Choles- terol (mg.) |
|---|---|---|---|---|---|---|
| | | | Total | Satu- rated | Unsatu- rated | |
| Chocolate-flavored roll[1] | 1 oz. | 56 | 2.3 | 1. | 1. | |
| Chocolate: | | | | | | |
| Bittersweet[2] | 1 oz. | < 1 | 11.3 | 6. | 5. | |
| Milk: | | | | | | |
| Plain[2] | 1 oz. | 27 | 9.2 | 5. | 4. | |
| With almonds | 1 oz. | 23 | 10.1 | | | |
| With peanuts | 1 oz. | 19 | 10.8 | | | |
| Semisweet[2] | 1 oz. | < 1 | 10.1 | 6. | 4. | |
| Sweet[2] | 1 oz. | 9 | 10.0 | 6. | 4. | |
| Chocolate discs, sugar-coated[3] | 1 oz. | 20 | 5.6 | 3. | 2. | |
| Coconut center, chocolate-coated[3] | 1 oz. | 56 | 5.0 | 3. | 2. | |
| Fondant, plain[4] | 1 oz. | 60 | .6 | Tr. | Tr. | |
| Fondant, chocolate-covered[5] | 1 oz. | 52 | 3.0 | 1. | 2. | |
| Fudge: | | | | | | |
| Chocolate fudge[5] | 1 oz. | 54 | 3.5 | 1. | 2. | |
| Chocolate fudge, chocolate-coated[6] | 1 oz. | 65 | 4.5 | 2. | 3. | |
| Chocolate fudge with nuts[7] | 1 oz. | 48 | 4.9 | 2. | 3. | |
| Chocolate fudge with nuts, chocolate-coated[8] | 1 oz. | 58 | 5.9 | 2. | 4. | |
| Vanilla fudge[1] | 1 oz. | 59 | 3.1 | 1. | 2. | |
| Vanilla fudge with nuts[8] | 1 oz. | 53 | 4.6 | 2. | 3. | |
| With peanuts & caramel, chocolate-coated[9] | 1 oz. | 36 | 6.5 | 2. | 5. | |
| Gum drops | 1 oz. | 10 | .2 | | | |
| Hard | 1 oz. | 9 | .3 | | | |
| Honeycombed hard candy, with peanut butter, chocolate-covered[10] | 1 oz. | 46 | 5.5 | 2. | 4. | |
| Jelly beans | 1 oz. | 3 | .1 | | | |
| Marshmallows | 1 oz. | 11 | Tr. | | | |
| Mints, uncoated | 1 oz. | 60 | .6 | | | |

(USDA): United States Department of Agriculture
*Prepared as Package Directs
[1]Principal sources of fat: animal & vegetable shortening.
[2]Principal sources of fat: chocolate & cacao butter.
[3]Principal sources of fat: chocolate, milk & cacao butter.
[4]Principal source of fat: butter.
[5]Principal sources of fat: animal & vegetable shortening & chocolate.
[6]Principal sources of fat: chocolate & vegetable shortening.
[7]Principal sources of fat: chocolate, animal & vegetable shortening & English walnuts.
[8]Principal sources of fat: animal & vegetable shortening & nuts.
[9]Principal sources of fat: vegetable shortening, chocolate & peanuts.
[10]Principal sources of fat: vegetable shortening, chocolate & peanut butter.

| Food and Description | Measure or Quantity | Sodium (mg.) | Fats in grams Total | Saturated | Unsaturated | Cholesterol (mg.) |
|---|---|---|---|---|---|---|
| Nougat & caramel, chocolate-covered[1] | 1 oz. | 49 | 3.9 | 2. | 2. | |
| Peanut bar[2] | 1 oz. | 3 | 9.1 | 2. | 7. | |
| Peanut brittle, no added salt or soda[2] | 1 oz. | 9 | 2.9 | <1. | 2. | |
| Peanuts, chocolate-covered[3] | 1 oz. | 17 | 11.7 | 3. | 9. | |
| Raisins, chocolate-covered[4] | 1 oz. | 18 | 4.8 | 3. | 2. | |
| Vanilla creams, chocolate-covered[5] | 1 oz. | 52 | 4.8 | 2. | 3. | |
| **CANDY, COMMERCIAL** (See also **CANDY, DIETETIC**): | | | | | | |
| *Almond Joy* (Peter Paul) | 1.55-oz. bar | 90 | 12.0 | | | |
| *Baby Ruth* (Nabisco) | 2-oz. serving | 120 | 12.0 | | | |
| *Bar-None* (Hershey's) | 1.5-oz. serving | 50 | 14.0 | | | 5 |
| *Bonkers!* (Nab) | 1 piece | 0 | 0.0 | | | |
| *Breath Savers* (Nab) any flavor, sugar free | 1 piece | 0 | 0.0 | | | |
| *Bridge Mix* (Nabisco) | 1 piece (2 grams) | 1 | .4 | | | |
| *Butterfinger* (Nab) | 2-oz. serving | 100 | 12.0 | | | |
| *Butternut* (Hollywood) | 2¼-oz. bar | 120 | 16.0 | | | |
| *Caramel Nip* (Pearson) | 1 piece (.25 oz.) | 17 | .7 | | | |
| *Charleston Chew!* | 2 oz. | 80 | 6.0 | | | |
| Cherry, chocolate-covered (Welch's) *Cortina:* | | | | | | |
| Dark | ¾-oz. piece | 10 | 2.5 | | | |
| Milk | ¾-oz. piece | 10 | 2.0 | | | |
| Chocolate bar: | | | | | | |
| Brazil nut, *Cadbury's* (Peter Paul) | 2-oz. serving | 82 | 18.0 | | | |
| Caramello, *Cadbury's* (Peter Paul) | 2-oz. serving | 108 | 13.0 | | | |
| Crunch, *Nestlé* | 1¹⁄₁₆-oz. bar | 50 | 8.0 | | | 5 |
| Fruit & nut, *Cadbury's* (Peter Paul) | 2-oz. serving | 77 | 16.0 | | | |
| Hazelnut, *Cadbury's* (Peter Paul) | 2-oz. serving | 88 | 17.0 | | | |
| Milk chocolate: | | | | | | |
| *Cadbury's* (Peter Paul) | 2-oz. serving | 94 | 16.0 | | | |

(USDA): United States Department of Agriculture
*Prepared as Package Directs
[1]Principal sources of fat: animal & vegetable shortening & chocolate.
[2]Principal source of fat: peanuts.
[3]Principal sources of fat: peanuts, chocolate & vegetable shortening.
[4]Principal sources of fat: chocolate, milk & cacao butter.
[5]Principal sources of fat: chocolate & vegetable shortening.

| Food and Description | Measure or Quantity | Sodium (mg.) | —Fats in grams— Total | Satu- rated | Unsatu- rated | Choles- terol (mg.) |
|---|---|---|---|---|---|---|
| (Hershey's) | 1.65-oz. bar | 45 | 14.0 | | | 12 |
| (Nestlé) | .35-oz. bar | 7 | 2.8 | | | 2 |
| (Nestlé) | 1¹/₁₅-oz. bar | 21 | 8.5 | | | 7 |
| *Special Dark* (Hershey's) | 1.45-oz. bar | 5 | 12.0 | | | 3 |
| Chocolate bar with almonds: | | | | | | |
| *Cadbury's* (Peter Paul) | 2 oz. | 82 | 18.0 | | | |
| (Hershey's) milk | 1.55-oz. bar | 60 | 15.0 | | | 12 |
| (Nestlé) | 1-oz. serving | 15 | 8.0 | | | 7 |
| *Chocolate Parfait* (Pearson) | .25-oz. piece | 17 | .7 | | | |
| Chocolate, Petite (Andes) | 4-gram piece | 4 | 1.5 | .9 | .54 | Tr. |
| *Chuckles,* any flavor | 1 oz. | 10 | 0.0 | | | |
| *Clark* | .65-oz. serving | 17 | 2.8 | | | |
| *Clark* | 1.5-oz. serving | 39 | 6.4 | | | |
| *Coffee Nip* (Pearson) | .25-oz. piece | 17 | .7 | | | |
| *Coffioca* (Pearson) | .25-oz. piece | 17 | .7 | | | |
| *Creme De Menthe's* (Andes) | .2-oz. piece | 3 | 1.5 | 1.4 | .15 | Tr. |
| *Chuckles* (Nabisco) Jelly, | | | | | | |
| licorice or nougat | ½ oz. | 5 | Tr. | | | |
| (Peter Paul): | | | | | | |
| Creme | 1 oz. | | 6.0 | | | |
| Mini | 1 oz. | | 7.0 | | | |
| *5th Avenue* (Hershey's) | 1.93-oz. serving | 110 | 9.0 | | | |
| Fudge (Nabisco): | | | | | | |
| Bar | 1 piece (.7 oz.) | 20 | 2.5 | | | |
| Squares | 1 piece (.5 oz.) | 12 | 2.5 | | | |
| *Good Stuff* (Nab) | 1.89-oz. piece | 90 | 14.0 | | | |
| Halvah (Sahadi) | 1 oz. | 45 | 10.0 | | | |
| Hard (Jolly Rancher): | | | | | | |
| All flavors except | | | | | | |
| butterscotch | 6-gram piece | 3-5 | Tr. | | | |
| Butterscotch | 6-gram piece | 37 | .3 | | | |
| *Holidays* (M&M/Mars): | | | | | | |
| Plain | 1 oz. | 40 | 6.0 | | | |
| Peanut | 1 oz. | 35 | 7.0 | | | |
| Jelly, *Chuckles:* | | | | | | |
| Bar | 1 oz. | 10 | 0.0 | | | |
| Bean | 1 oz. | 30 | 0.0 | | | |
| Rings | 1 oz. | 10 | 1.0 | | | |
| Jujubes (Nabisco) *Chuckles* | ½ oz. | 7 | Tr. | | | |
| *Kisses,* milk chocolate | | | | | | |
| (Hershey's) | 1 piece (5 grams) | 4 | 1.4 | | | |
| *KitKat* (Hershey's) | 1.625-oz. bar | 60 | 13.0 | | | 12 |
| Licorice: | | | | | | |

(USDA): United States Department of Agriculture
*Prepared as Package Directs

| Food and Description | Measure or Quantity | Sodium (mg.) | Fats in grams — Total | Saturated | Unsaturated | Cholesterol (mg.) |
|---|---|---|---|---|---|---|
| *Licorice Nip* (Pearson) | .25-oz. piece | 17 | .7 | | | |
| (Switzer's) bars, bites or stix | 1 oz. | | Tr. | | | |
| *Life Savers* | 1 piece | 5–10 | 0.0 | | | |
| Lollipop, *Life Savers* | 1 piece | 10 | 0.0 | | | |
| *Mars* (M&M/Mars) | 1.76-oz. bar | 85 | 11.0 | | | 7 |
| *Krackel* (Hershey's) | 1.65-oz. bar | 85 | 14.0 | | | |
| *Mary Jane* (Miller): | | | | | | |
| Small | 1 piece (7.3 grams) | 4 | <.1 | Tr. | Tr. | |
| Large | 1 piece (1¼ oz.) | 23 | .4 | Tr. | Tr. | |
| *Milk Shake* (Hollywood) | 2.375-oz. bar | | 2.0 | | | |
| *Milky Way* (M&M/Mars) | 2.24-oz. bar | 150 | 11.0 | | | 10 |
| Mint or peppermint: | | | | | | |
| Mint parfait: | | | | | | |
| (Andes) | .2-oz. piece | 3 | 1.6 | 1.2 | .4 | Tr. |
| (Pearson) | .25-oz. piece | 17 | .7 | | | |
| Pattie: | | | | | | |
| (Nabisco): | | | | | | |
| Regular | 1 piece | 5 | Tr. | | | |
| Chocolate-covered, *Junior* | 2.4-gram piece | Tr. | .2 | | | |
| *York* (Peter Paul) chocolate covered | 1¼-oz. piece | 12 | 4.0 | | | |
| *M&M's* (M&M/Mars): | | | | | | |
| Plain | 1.7-oz. pkg. | 65 | 10.0 | | | |
| Peanut | 1.8-oz. pkg. | 60 | 13.0 | | | |
| *Mounds* (Peter Paul) | 1.65-oz. piece | 87 | 12.0 | | | |
| *Mr. Goodbar* (Hershey's) | 1.85-oz. bar | 20 | 20.0 | | | 12 |
| Naturally Fruit & Nut Bar (Planters): | | | | | | |
| Almond/apricot | 1 oz. | 75 | 7.0 | | | |
| Almond/pineapple | 1 oz. | 80 | 6.0 | | | |
| Peanut/raisin | 1 oz. | 70 | 7.0 | | | |
| Walnut/apple | 1 oz. | 90 | 8.0 | | | |
| Nougat centers, *Chuckles* (Nabisco) | 1 oz. | 10 | Tr. | | | |
| *$100,000* (Nestlé) | 1¼-oz. bar | 50 | 7.5 | | | 2 |
| Orange slice, *Chuckles* (Nabisco) | 1 oz. | 10 | 1.0 | | | |
| *Park Avenue* (Tom's) | 1.8-oz. serving | 120 | 9.0 | | | |
| Peanut bar (Planters) | 1.6-oz. piece | 110 | 14.0 | | | |
| Peanut butter cup (Reese's) | .9-oz. piece | 90 | 8.0 | | | 4 |
| *Peanut Butter Pals* (Tom's) | 1.3-oz. piece | 100 | 11.0 | | | |

(USDA): United States Department of Agriculture
*Prepared as Package Directs

| Food and Description | Measure or Quantity | Sodium (mg.) | — Fats in grams — | | | Cholesterol (mg.) |
|---|---|---|---|---|---|---|
| | | | Total | Saturated | Unsaturated | |
| Peanut parfait: | | | | | | |
| (Andes) | 5-gram piece | 11 | 1.8 | 1.1 | .7 | Tr. |
| (Pearson's) | .25-oz. piece | 17 | .7 | | | |
| *Peanut Plank* (Tom's) | 1.7-oz. serving | 30 | 11.0 | | | |
| Peanut roll (Tom's) | 1¾-oz. serving | 120 | 11.0 | | | |
| *Pom Poms* (Nabisco) caramel | 1 oz. | 70 | 3.0 | | | |
| *Powerhouse* (Peter Paul) | 2-oz. serving | 193 | 11.0 | | | |
| Raisin, chocolate covered | | | | | | |
| (Nabisco) | 1 piece | Tr. | .2 | | | |
| *Reese's Pieces* (Hershey's) | 1.95-oz. pkg. | 95 | 11.0 | | | 2 |
| *Rolo* (Hershey's) | .2-oz. piece | 12 | 1.3 | | | 1 |
| *Royals* (M&M/Mars) | 1.52-oz. pkg. | 34 | 9.0 | | | |
| Sesame crunch bar (Sahadi) | ¾-oz. bar | 55 | 7.0 | | | 0 |
| *Skittles* (M&M/Mars) | 1 oz. | 13 | .9 | | | |
| *Skor* (Hershey's) | 1.4-oz. bar | 125 | 14.0 | | | 21 |
| *Snickers* (M&M/Mars) | 2.16-oz. bar | 170 | 14.0 | | | 10 |
| Spearmint leaves, *Chuckles* | | | | | | |
| (Nabisco) | 1 oz. | 15 | 1.0 | | | |
| Spice flavored strings, | | | | | | |
| *Chuckles* (Nabisco) | 1 oz. | 10 | 1.0 | | | |
| *Starburst* (M&M/Mars) | 1 oz. | 15 | 2.5 | | | |
| *Stars,* chocolate (Nabisco) | 2.2-gram piece | 3 | .6 | | | |
| *Sugar Babies* (Nabisco) | 1⅝-oz. serving | 85 | 2.0 | | | |
| *Sugar Daddy* (Nabisco) | 1⅜-oz. piece | 85 | 1.0 | | | |
| *Sugar Mama* (Nabisco) | ¾-oz. piece | 30 | 3.0 | | | |
| *3 Musketeers* bar (M&M/Mars) | 2.13-oz. bar | 120 | 8.0 | | | 5 |
| *Ting-A-Ling* (Andes) | 1 piece | 7 | 1.3 | .8 | .5 | Tr. |
| *Tootsie Roll:* | | | | | | |
| Regular: | | | | | | |
| Chocolate | 1 oz. | 6 | 2.5 | | | |
| Flavored | .23-oz. piece | 2 | .5 | | | |
| Pop: | | | | | | |
| Caramel | .49-oz. piece | 4 | .5 | | | |
| Chocolate | .49-oz. piece | Tr. | .3 | | | |
| Flavored | .49-oz. piece | Tr. | .3 | | | |
| Pop drop: | | | | | | |
| Caramel | .2-oz. piece | 1 | .2 | | | |
| Chocolate or flavored | .2-oz. piece | Tr. | .1 | | | |
| *Whatchamacallit* | 1.8-oz. bar | 90 | 14.0 | | | |
| *Wispa* (Peter Paul) | 1 oz. | 47 | 8.0 | | | |
| *Y&S Bites* (Hershey's) | 1 oz. | 85 | 1.0 | | | |
| *Zagnut* (Clark) | 1.2-oz. bar | 34 | 5.0 | | | |

(USDA): United States Department of Agriculture
*Prepared as Package Directs

| Food and Description | Measure or Quantity | Sodium (mg.) | Fats in grams — Total | Satu- rated | Unsatu- rated | Choles- terol (mg.) |
|---|---|---|---|---|---|---|
| *Zero* (Hollywood) | 2-oz. bar | | 8.0 | | | |
| **CANDY DIETETIC:** | | | | | | |
| Carob bar, *Joan's Natural:* | | | | | | |
|   Coconut | 3-oz. piece | 117 | 41.8 | | | 27 |
|   Fruit & nut | 3-oz. piece | 115 | 44.1 | | | 26 |
|   Honey bran | 3-oz. piece | 114 | 35.1 | | | 26 |
|   Peanut | 3-oz. piece | 109 | 40.6 | | | 24 |
| Chocolate (Louis Sherry) | | | | | | |
|   bittersweet or milk | .2-oz. piece | | 2.0 | | | |
| Chocolate bar (Estee): | | | | | | |
|   Coconut | .2-oz. square | 5 | 2.5 | | | 1 |
|   Crunch | .2-oz. square | 5 | 1.5 | | | 1 |
|   Fruit & nut or milk | .2-oz. square | 5 | 2.0 | | | 1 |
| *Estee-ets* (Estee) with peanuts | 1 piece | 2 | .4 | | | Tr. |
| Gum drop (Estee) fruit or | | | | | | |
|   licorice | 1 piece | 1 | Tr. | | | 0 |
| *Gummy Bears* (Estee) | 1 piece | 0 | 0.0 | | | 0 |
| Hard: | | | | | | |
|   (Estee) assorted | 1 piece | 2 | 0.0 | | | 0 |
|   (Louis Sherry) | 1 piece | 2 | 0.0 | | | 0 |
| Lollipop (Estee or Louis | | | | | | |
|   Sherry) | 1 piece | 5 | 0.0 | | | 0 |
| Mint (Estee) | 1.1-gram piece | 0 | 1.0 | | | 0 |
| Peanut butter cup (Estee) | 7.7-gram piece | 10 | 3.6 | | | Tr. |
| TV Mix (Estee) | 1.6-gram piece | 2 | .5 | | | Tr. |
| **CANE SYRUP** (See **SYRUP,** Cane) | | | | | | |
| **CANNELLONI,** frozen: | | | | | | |
| (Blue Star) *Dining Lite:* | | | | | | |
|   Cheese | 9-oz. serving | 940 | 6.8 | | | |
|   Veal & vegetable | 9-oz. serving | 790 | 8.0 | | | |
| (Celentano) florentine | 12-oz. pkg. | 540 | 17.0 | | | 75 |
| (Stouffer's): | | | | | | |
|   Beef & pork, with mornay | | | | | | |
|     sauce | 9⅝-oz. pkg. | 940 | 8.0 | | | 50 |
|   Cheese with tomato sauce | 9⅛-oz. pkg. | 885 | 12.0 | | | 45 |
| (Weight Watchers) florentine | 13-oz. meal | 894 | 14.0 | | | |

(USDA): United States Department of Agriculture
*Prepared as Package Directs

| Food and Description | Measure or Quantity | Sodium (mg.) | Fats in grams — Total | Saturated | Unsaturated | Cholesterol (mg.) |
|---|---|---|---|---|---|---|
| **CANTALOUPE, fresh:** | | | | | | |
| Whole | 1 lb. (weighed whole) | 27 | .2 | | | 0 |
| Whole, medium (USDA) | 5″ dia. melon (1⅔ lbs., weighed with skin & cavity contents) | 46 | .4 | | | 0 |
| Cubed (USDA) | ½ cup (2.9 oz.) | 10 | <.1 | | | 0 |
| **CAPE GOOSEBERRY** (See **GROUND-CHERRY**) | | | | | | |
| **CAPERS** (Crosse & Blackwell) | 1 T. (.6 oz.) | 306 | | | | |
| **CAPICOLA OR CAPACOLA SAUSAGE** (USDA) | 1 oz. | | 13.0 | 5. | 8. | |
| **CAP'N CRUNCH,** cereal (Quaker): | | | | | | |
| Regular | ¾ cup (1 oz.) | 185 | 2.6 | | | |
| *Crunch Berries* | ¾ cup (1 oz.) | 166 | 2.6 | | | |
| Peanut butter | ¾ cup (1 oz.) | 210 | 3.8 | | | |
| **CARAMBOLA,** raw (USDA): | | | | | | |
| Whole | 1 lb. (weighed whole) | 9 | 2.1 | | | 0 |
| Flesh only | 4 oz. | 2 | .6 | | | 0 |
| **CARAWAY SEED** (Information supplied by General Mills Laboratory) | 1 oz. | 13 | <1 | | | (0) |
| (Spice Islands) | 1 tsp. | <1 | | | | (0) |
| **CARDAMOM:** | | | | | | |
| Ground (Spice Islands) | 1 tsp. | <1 | | | | (0) |
| Whole (Spice Islands) | 1 seed | Tr. | | | | (0) |
| **CARISSA OR NATAL PLUM,** raw: | | | | | | |
| Whole (USDA) | 1 lb. (weighed whole) | | 5.1 | | | 0 |
| Flesh only (USDA) | 4 oz. | | 1.5 | | | 0 |

(USDA): United States Department of Agriculture
*Prepared as Package Directs

| Food and Description | Measure or Quantity | Sodium (mg.) | —Fats in grams— | | | Choles-terol (mg.) |
|---|---|---|---|---|---|---|
| | | | Total | Satu-rated | Unsatu-rated | |
| **CARNATION-DO-IT-YOUR-SELF DIET PLAN:** | | | | | | |
| Chocolate | 2 scoops (1.1 oz.) | 110 | 1.0 | | | |
| Vanilla | 2 scoops (1.1 oz.) | 110 | .5 | | | |
| | | | | | | |
| **CARL'S JR. RESTAURANT:** | | | | | | |
| Bacon | 2 strips (10 grams) | 200 | 4.0 | 3. | Tr. | 8 |
| Cake, chocolate | 3.2-oz. piece | 335 | 20.0 | | | 70 |
| *California Roast Beef'n Swiss* Sandwich | 7.2-oz. sandwich | 1,070 | 8.0 | | | 130 |
| Cheese: | | | | | | |
| American | .6-oz. slice | 955 | 5.0 | | | 16 |
| Swiss | .6-oz. slice | 221 | 4.0 | | | 16 |
| Chicken sandwich: | | | | | | |
| *Charbroiler BBQ* | 6.3-oz. sandwich | 955 | 5.0 | 50 | | |
| *Charbroiler Club* | 8.2-oz. sandwich | 1,165 | 85 | | | |
| Cookie, chocolate chip | 2¼-oz. piece | 285 | 13.0 | | | 0 |
| Danish | 3.5-oz. piece | 550 | | | | 0 |
| Eggs, scrambled | 2.4-oz. serving | 105 | | | | 245 |
| Fish sandwich, fillet | 7.9-oz. sandwich | 945 | | | | 90 |
| French toast dips, excluding syrup | 4.7-oz. serving | 576 | | | | 54 |
| Hamburger: | | | | | | |
| Plain: | | | | | | |
| Famous Star | 8.1-oz. serving | 890 | | | | 45 |
| Happy Star | 3-oz. serving | 445 | | | | 45 |
| Old Time Star | 5.9-oz. serving | 760 | | | | 80 |
| Super Star | 10.6-oz. serving | 990 | | | | 125 |
| Cheeseburger, Western Bacon: | | | | | | |
| Regular | 7½-oz. serving | 1,415 | 33.0 | | | 105 |
| Double | 10.4-oz. serving | 1,620 | 53.0 | | | 145 |
| Hot cakes, with margarine, excluding syrup | 5.5-oz. serving | 1,190 | 12.0 | | | 15 |
| Milk, 2% lowfat | 10 fl. oz. | 550 | 6.0 | | | 181 |
| Muffins: | | | | | | |
| Blueberry | 3.5-oz. piece | 360 | 7.0 | | | 34 |
| Bran | 4-oz. piece | 300 | 6.0 | | | 50 |
| English, with margarine | 2-oz. piece | 275 | 6.0 | | | 0 |
| Onion rings | 3.2-oz. order | 105 | 15.0 | | | 260 |
| Orange juice, small | 8 fl. oz. | 2 | 1.0 | | | 0 |

(USDA): United States Department of Agriculture
*Prepared as Package Directs

| Food and Description | Measure or Quantity | Sodium (mg.) | —Fats in grams— Total | Satu- rated | Unsatu- rated | Choles- terol (mg.) |
|---|---|---|---|---|---|---|
| **Potato:** | | | | | | |
| **Baked:** | | | | | | |
| Bacon & cheese | 14.1-oz. serving | 1,810 | 34.0 | | | 45 |
| Broccoli & cheese | 14-oz. serving | 690 | 17.0 | | | 10 |
| Cheese | 14.2-oz. serving | 785 | 22.0 | | | 40 |
| Fiesta | 15.2-oz. serving | 1,230 | 23.0 | | | 40 |
| Lite | 9.8-oz. serving | 35 | 3.0 | | | 0 |
| Sour cream & chive | 10.4-oz. serving | 140 | 13.0 | | | 10 |
| French fries | Regular order (6 oz.) | 626 | 17.0 | | | 15 |
| Hash brown nuggets | 3-oz. serving | 350 | 9.0 | | | 10 |
| **Salad dressing:** | | | | | | |
| **Regular:** | | | | | | |
| Blue cheese | 2-oz. serving | 278 | 14.0 | | | 8 |
| House | 2-oz. serving | 329 | 17.0 | | | 7 |
| Thousand island | 2-oz. serving | 435 | 23.0 | | | 0 |
| Dietetic, Italian | 2-oz. serving | 360 | 10.0 | | | 0 |
| Sausage patty | 1.5-oz. piece | 275 | 17.0 | | | 25 |
| Shake | 1 regular size | 255 | 7.0 | | | 178 |
| **Soft drink:** | | | | | | |
| Sweetened | 1 regular size | 37 | 0.0 | | | 0 |
| Dietetic | 1 regular size | 13 | 0.0 | | | 0 |
| **Soup:** | | | | | | |
| Broccoli, cream of | 1 serving | 845 | 6.0 | | | 22 |
| Chicken & noodle | 1 serving | 605 | 1.0 | | | 14 |
| Clam chowder, Boston | 1 serving | 861 | 8.0 | | | 222 |
| Vegetable, mixed | 1 serving | 807 | 2.0 | | | 3 |
| Steak sandwich, *Country Fried* | 7.2-oz. serving | 1,290 | 33.0 | | | 45 |
| *Sunrise Sandwich:* | | | | | | |
| Bacon | 4.5-oz. serving | 750 | 19.0 | | | 120 |
| Sausage | 6.1-oz. serving | 990 | 32.0 | | | 165 |
| Tea, iced | 1 regular drink | 0 | 0.0 | | | 0 |
| Zucchini | 4.3-oz. serving | 480 | 16.0 | | | 10 |
| **CARNATION INSTANT BREAKFAST:** | | | | | | |
| **Bar:** | | | | | | |
| Chocolate chip | 1 bar | 180 | 11.0 | | | Tr. |
| Chocolate crunch | 1 bar | 145 | 10.0 | | | Tr. |
| Honey nut | 1 bar | 155 | 11.0 | | | Tr. |
| Peanut butter with chocolate chips or peanut butter crunch | 1 bar | 170 | 11.0 | | | Tr. |

(USDA): United States Department of Agriculture
*Prepared as Package Directs

| Food and Description | Measure or Quantity | Sodium (mg.) | — Fats in grams — | | | Choles-terol (mg.) |
|---|---|---|---|---|---|---|
| | | | Total | Satu-rated | Unsatu-rated | |
| **Dry:** | | | | | | |
| Chocolate | 1 envelope | 135 | 1.0 | | | 3 |
| *Chocolate | 8 fl. oz. | 145 | 10.0 | | | |
| Chocolate malt | 1 envelope | 160 | 1.0 | | | 3 |
| *Chocolate malt | 8 fl. oz. | | 9.0 | | | |
| Coffee | 1 envelope | 130 | .3 | | | 4 |
| Eggnog | 1 envelope | 185 | .5 | | | 15 |
| Strawberry | 1 envelope | 195 | .2 | | | 4 |
| Vanilla | 1 envelope | 135 | .2 | | | 4 |

**CAROB FLOUR** (See **FLOUR**)

**CARP,** raw (USDA):

| | | | | | | |
|---|---|---|---|---|---|---|
| Whole | 1 lb. (weighed whole) | 68 | 5.7 | | | |
| Meat only | 4 oz. | 57 | 4.8 | | | |

**CARROT:**
Raw (USDA):

| | | | | | | |
|---|---|---|---|---|---|---|
| Whole | 1 lb. (weighed with full tops) | 126 | .5 | | | 0 |
| Partially trimmed | 1 lb. (weighed without tops, with skins) | 175 | .7 | | | 0 |
| Trimmed | 5½″ × 1″ carrot (1.8 oz.) | 24 | .1 | | | 0 |
| Trimmed | 25 thin strips (1.8 oz.) | 24 | .1 | | | 0 |
| Chunks | ½ cup (2.4 oz.) | 32 | .1 | | | 0 |
| Diced | ½ cup (2.5 oz.) | 34 | .1 | | | 0 |
| Grated or shredded | ½ cup (1.9 oz.) | 26 | .1 | | | 0 |
| Slices | ½ cup (2.3 oz.) | 30 | .1 | | | 0 |
| Strips | ½ cup (2 oz.) | 27 | .1 | | | 0 |
| Boiled, without salt (USDA): | | | | | | |
| Chunks, drained | ½ cup (2.9 oz.) | 27 | .2 | | | 0 |
| Diced, drained | ½ cup (2.5 oz.) | 23 | .1 | | | 0 |
| Slices, drained | ½ cup (2.7 oz.) | 25 | .2 | | | 0 |
| Canned, regular pack: (USDA): | | | | | | |
| Diced, solids & liq. | ½ cup (4.3 oz.) | 290 | .2 | | | 0 |
| Diced, drained solids | ½ cup (2.8 oz.) | 189 | .2 | | | 0 |

(USDA): United States Department of Agriculture
*Prepared as Package Directs

CARROT (Continued)

| Food and Description | Measure or Quantity | Sodium (mg.) | —Fats in grams— | | | Choles-terol (mg.) |
|---|---|---|---|---|---|---|
| | | | Total | Satu-rated | Unsatu-rated | |
| Drained liq. | 4 oz. | 268 | 0.0 | | | 0 |
| (Del Monte) diced, sliced or whole, solids & liq. | 4 oz. | 265 | 0.0 | | | |
| (Larsen) *Freshlike,* diced or sliced, solids & liq. | ½ cup (4 oz.) | 300 | 0.0 | | | |
| Canned, dietetic pack: (USDA): | | | | | | |
| Low sodium, solids & liq. (USDA) | 4 oz. (by wt.) | 44 | .1 | | | 0 |
| Low sodium, drained solids (USDA) | ½ cup (2.8 oz.) | 31 | <.1 | | | 0 |
| (Featherweight) | ½ cup (4 oz.) | 30 | 0.0 | | | |
| (Larsen) *Fresh-Lite,* water pack | ½ cup (4.4 oz.) | 40 | 0.0 | | | |
| (S&W) *Nutradiet,* green label | ½ cup | 50 | 0.0 | | | |
| Dehydrated (USDA) | 1 oz. | 76 | .4 | | | 0 |
| Frozen: | | | | | | |
| Nuggets in butter sauce (Green Giant) | ⅓ of 10-oz. pkg. | 350 | 2.4 | | | |
| (Birds Eye) whole, baby, deluxe | ⅓ of 10-oz. pkg. | 46 | .2 | | | 0 |
| (Green Giant) crinkle cut, in butter sauce | ½ cup | 315 | 1.0 | | | |
| (Larsen) | 3.3 oz. | 40 | 0.0 | | | (0) |
| (McKenzie) whole | 3.3 oz. | 56 | 0.0 | | | (0) |
| Sliced, honey glazed (Green Giant) | ⅓ of 10-oz. pkg. | 217 | 1.7 | | | |
| With brown sugar glaze (Birds Eye) | ½ cup (3.3 oz.) | 500 | 2.4 | | | 0 |
| **CASABA MELON,** fresh (USDA): | | | | | | |
| Whole | 1 lb. (weighed whole) | 27 | Tr. | | | 0 |
| Flesh only | 4 oz. | 14 | Tr. | | | 0 |
| **CASHEW NUT:** | | | | | | |
| Salted: | | | | | | |
| (USDA) | 1 oz. | 57 | 13.0 | 2. | 11. | 0 |
| (USDA) | ½ cup (2.5 oz.) | 140 | 32.0 | 6. | 26. | 0 |
| (USDA) | 5 large or 8 med. (.4 oz.) | 21 | 4.9 | <1. | 4. | 0 |

(USDA): United States Department of Agriculture
*Prepared as Package Directs

104

| Food and Description | Measure or Quantity | Sodium (mg.) | Total | Satu- rated | Unsatu- rated | Choles- terol (mg.) |
|---|---|---|---|---|---|---|
| | | | | — Fats in grams — | | |
| (Tom Houston) | 15 nuts (1.1 oz.) | 60 | 13.7 | | | (0) |
| Dry roasted (Flavor House) | 1 oz. | 36 | 13.4 | | | (0) |
| Dry roasted (Planters) | 1 oz. | 340 | 13.0 | 2. | 11. | 0 |
| Dry roasted (Skippy) | 1 oz. | 142 | 13.2 | 3. | 11. | 0 |
| Oil roasted, *Freshnut* | 1 oz. | 140 | 14.5 | 3. | 11. | 0 |
| Oil roasted (Planters) | 1 oz. | 220 | 14.1 | | | 0 |
| Unsalted: | | | | | | |
| (USDA) | 1 oz. | 4 | 13.0 | 2. | 11. | 0 |
| (USDA) | ½ cup (2.5 oz.) | 10 | 32.0 | 6. | 26. | 0 |
| (USDA) | 5 large or 8 med. (.4 oz.) | 2 | 4.9 | <1. | 4. | 0 |

**CATAWBA WINE:**

| Food and Description | Measure or Quantity | Sodium (mg.) | Total | Satu- rated | Unsatu- rated | Choles- terol (mg.) |
|---|---|---|---|---|---|---|
| (Gold Seal) 13-14% alcohol | 3 fl. oz. (3.3 oz.) | 3 | 0.0 | | | (0) |
| (Great Western) pink, 13% alcohol | 3 fl. oz. | 36 | 0.0 | | | 0 |

**CATFISH:**

| Food and Description | Measure or Quantity | Sodium (mg.) | Total | Satu- rated | Unsatu- rated | Choles- terol (mg.) |
|---|---|---|---|---|---|---|
| Raw (USDA) freshwater, fillet | 4 oz. | 68 | 3.5 | | | |
| Frozen (Mrs. Paul's) breaded & fried: | | | | | | |
| Fillet | 3.6-oz. piece | 243 | 12.0 | | | |
| Fingers | ½ of 8-oz. pkg. | 260 | 14.0 | | | |

**CATSUP:**

| Food and Description | Measure or Quantity | Sodium (mg.) | Total | Satu- rated | Unsatu- rated | Choles- terol (mg.) |
|---|---|---|---|---|---|---|
| Regular pack: | | | | | | |
| (USDA) | ½ cup (5 oz.) | 1,469 | .6 | | | 0 |
| (USDA) | 1 T. (.6 oz.) | 188 | <.1 | | | 0 |
| (Del Monte) | 1 T. (.7 oz.) | 181 | <.1 | | | 0 |
| (Heinz) | 1 T. | 180 | Tr. | | | (0) |
| Dietetic pack: | | | | | | |
| (USDA) low sodium | ½ cup (5 oz.) | 7-49 | .6 | | | 0 |
| (USDA) low sodium | 1 T. (.6 oz.) | <6 | <.1 | | | 0 |
| (Del Monte) no salt added | 1 T. (.5 oz.) | 25 | 0.0 | | | (0) |
| (Dia-Mel) | 1 T. | 20 | 0.0 | | | 0 |
| (Featherweight) | 1 T. | 5 | 0.0 | | | (0) |
| (Hunt's) | 1 T. (.5 oz.) | 0 | 0.0 | | | (0) |

**CAULIFLOWER:**

| Food and Description | Measure or Quantity | Sodium (mg.) | Total | Satu- rated | Unsatu- rated | Choles- terol (mg.) |
|---|---|---|---|---|---|---|
| Raw (USDA): | | | | | | |
| Whole | 1 lb. (weighed untrimmed) | 23 | .4 | | | 0 |

(USDA): United States Department of Agriculture
*Prepared as Package Directs

| Food and Description | Measure or Quantity | Sodium (mg.) | — Fats in grams — | | | Cholesterol (mg.) |
|---|---|---|---|---|---|---|
| | | | Total | Saturated | Unsaturated | |
| Flowerbuds | 1 lb. (weighed trimmed) | 59 | .9 | | | 0 |
| Buds | ½ cup (1.8 oz.) | 6 | .1 | | | 0 |
| Slices | ½ cup (1.5 oz.) | 5 | < .1 | | | 0 |
| Boiled, without salt, drained (USDA) | ½ cup (2.2 oz.) | 6 | .1 | | | 0 |
| Frozen: | | | | | | |
| (USDA): | | | | | | |
| Not thawed | 10-oz. pkg. | 31 | .6 | | | 0 |
| Boiled, drained | ½ cup (3.2 oz.) | 9 | .2 | | | 0 |
| (Birds Eye): | | | | | | |
| Regular | ⅓ of 10-oz. pkg. | 17 | .1 | | | 0 |
| With almonds & selected seasonings | ⅓ of 10-oz. pkg. | 221 | 1.7 | | | 0 |
| With cheese sauce | ⅓ of 10-oz. pkg. | 336 | 5.0 | | | 4 |
| Florets, deluxe | ⅓ of 10-oz. pkg. | 18 | .2 | | | 0 |
| (Green Giant): | | | | | | |
| In cheese sauce | ½ cup | 450 | 2.0 | | | |
| In white cheddar cheese sauce | ½ cup | 415 | 3.0 | | | |
| Polybag | ½ cup | 30 | 0.0 | | | (0) |
| (Larsen) | 3.3 oz. | 45 | 0.0 | | | (0) |
| (McKenzie) | 3.3 oz. | 28 | 0.0 | | | (0) |
| (Mrs. Paul's) & cheese, batter fried | ⅓ of 8-oz. pkg. | 650 | 6.4 | | | |
| **CAVATELLI,** frozen (Celentano) | ⅕ of 16-oz. pkg. | 100 | 1.0 | | | 2 |
| **CAVIAR, STURGEON** (USDA): | | | | | | |
| Pressed | 1 oz. | | 4.7 | | | |
| Whole eggs | 1 oz. | 624 | 4.3 | | | > 85 |
| Whole eggs | 1 T. (.6 oz.) | 352 | 2.4 | | | > 48 |
| **CELERIAC ROOT,** raw | | | | | | |
| (USDA): | | | | | | |
| Whole | 1 lb. (weighed unpared) | 390 | 1.2 | | | 0 |
| Pared | 4 oz. | 113 | .3 | | | 0 |
| **CELERY,** all varieties: | | | | | | |
| Raw (USDA): | | | | | | |
| Whole | 1 lb. (weighed untrimmed) | 429 | .3 | | | 0 |

(USDA): United States Department of Agriculture
*Prepared as Package Directs

| Food and Description | Measure or Quantity | Sodium (mg.) | — Fats in grams — | | | Choles- terol (mg.) |
|---|---|---|---|---|---|---|
| | | | Total | Satu- rated | Unsatu- rated | |
| 1 large outer stalk | 8″ × 1½″ at root end (1.4 oz.) | 50 | <.1 | | | 0 |
| 3 small inner stalks | 5″ × ¾″ (1.8 oz.) | 63 | <.1 | | | 0 |
| Diced, chopped or cut in chunks | ½ cup (2.1 oz.) | 76 | <.1 | | | 0 |
| Slices | ½ cup (1.9 oz.) | 67 | <.1 | | | 0 |
| Boiled without salt, drained: | | | | | | |
| Diced or cut in chunks | ½ cup (2.7 oz.) | 67 | <.1 | | | 0 |
| Slices | ½ cup (3 oz.) | 74 | <.1 | | | 0 |
| Frozen (Larsen) | 3½ oz. | 90 | 0.0 | | | |

**CELERY CABBAGE** (See **CABBAGE, CHINESE**)

**CELERY SEASONING**

| | | | | | | |
|---|---|---|---|---|---|---|
| (French's) | 1 tsp. (5 grams) | 1,430 | .1 | | | (0) |

**CELERY SEED:**

| | | | | | | |
|---|---|---|---|---|---|---|
| Ground (Spice Islands) | 1 tsp. | 2 | | | | (0) |
| Whole (Spice Islands) | 1 tsp. | 4 | | | | (0) |

**CEREAL BREAKFAST FOODS**
(See kind of cereal such as **CORN FLAKES** or brand name such as *KIX*)

**CERVELAT** (USDA):

| | | | | | | |
|---|---|---|---|---|---|---|
| Dry | 1 oz. | | 10.7 | | | |
| Soft | 1 oz. | | 6.9 | | | |

**CHABLIS WINE:**

| | | | | | | |
|---|---|---|---|---|---|---|
| (Gold Seal) 12% alcohol | 3 fl. oz. | 3 | 0.0 | | | |
| (Great Western) 12.5% alcohol | 3 fl. oz. | 31 | 0.0 | | | 0 |
| (Great Western) Diamond, 12.5% alcohol | 3 fl. oz. | <1 | 0.0 | | | 0 |

**CHAMPAGNE:**

| | | | | | | |
|---|---|---|---|---|---|---|
| (Gold Seal) brut, or pink, extra dry, 12% alcohol | 3 fl. oz. (3.2 oz.) | 3 | 0.0 | | | (0) |

(USDA): United States Department of Agriculture
*Prepared as Package Directs

| Food and Description | Measure or Quantity | Sodium (mg.) | —Fats in grams— | | | Choles-terol (mg.) |
|---|---|---|---|---|---|---|
| | | | Total | Satu-rated | Unsatu-rated | |
| (Great Western) regular, brut, extra dry, pink or special reserve, 12.5% alcohol | 3 fl. oz. | 31 | 0.0 | | | 0 |
| **CHARD,** Swiss (USDA): | | | | | | |
| Raw, whole | 1 lb. (weighed untrimmed) | 613 | 1.3 | | | 0 |
| Raw, trimmed | 4 oz. | 167 | .3 | | | 0 |
| Boiled without salt, drained | ½ cup (3.4 oz.) | 83 | .2 | | | 0 |
| **CHARLOTTE RUSSE,** with ladyfingers, whipped cream filling, home recipe (USDA)[1] | 4 oz. | 49 | 16.6 | 8. | 9. | |
| **CHAYOTE,** raw (USDA): | | | | | | |
| Whole | 1 lb. (weighed unpared) | 19 | .4 | | | 0 |
| Pared | 4 oz. | 6 | .1 | | | 0 |
| *CHEERIOS,* cereal (General Mills): | | | | | | |
| Regular | 1¼ cups (1 oz.) | 330 | 2.0 | | | |
| Honey nut | ¾ cup (1 oz.) | 255 | 1.0 | | | |
| **CHEESE:** | | | | | | |
| American or cheddar: | | | | | | |
| (USDA): | | | | | | |
| Natural: | | | | | | |
| Regular | 1 oz. | 198 | 9.1 | 5. | 4. | 28 |
| Regular | 1″ cube (.6 oz.) | 119 | 5.5 | 3. | 2. | 17 |
| Grated or shredded | 1 cup (4.6 oz.) | 917 | 42.1 | 24. | 19. | 130 |
| Grated or shredded | 1 T. (7 grams) | 48 | 2.2 | 1. | 1. | 7 |
| Processed: | | | | | | |
| Regular | 1 oz. | 322 | 8.5 | 5. | 4. | 25 |
| Regular | 1″ cube (.6 oz.) | 204 | 5.4 | 3. | 3. | 16 |
| Regular | 3½″ × 3⅜″ × ⅛″ slice (1 oz.) | 322 | 8.5 | 5. | 4. | 25 |
| Reduced sodium | 1 oz. | 184 | 8.5 | 5. | 4. | 25 |
| Reduced sodium | 1 cube (.6 oz.) | 117 | 5.4 | 3. | 3. | 16 |
| (Dorman's) *Chedda-DeLite* | 1 oz. | 100 | 7.0 | | | 25 |
| (Featherweight) low sodium | 1 oz. | 6 | 9.0 | | | 30 |

(USDA): United States Department of Agriculture
*Prepared as Package Directs
[1]Principal sources of fat: cream & egg.

| Food and Description | Measure or Quantity | Sodium (mg.) | Fats in grams — Total | Satu- rated | Unsatu- rated | Choles- terol (mg.) |
|---|---|---|---|---|---|---|
| (Kraft): | | | | | | |
| Regular: | | | | | | |
| American singles | 1 oz. | 310 | | | | |
| Cheddar | 1 oz. | 180 | | | | |
| Cheddar, sharp, *Old* | | | | | | |
| *English* | 1 oz. | 440 | | | | |
| *Laughing Cow,* natural | 1 oz. | 227 | 9.0 | | | 28 |
| (Polly-O) cheddar, shredded | 1 oz. | 180 | 9.0 | | | |
| (Sargento): | | | | | | |
| Crock, sharp | 1 oz. | 274 | 7.0 | | | 18 |
| Midget, regular or sharp | 1 oz. | 176 | 10.0 | | | 30 |
| Shredded, non-dairy | 1 oz. | 269 | 6.0 | | | 2 |
| Bleu or Blue: | | | | | | |
| (USDA) natural: | | | | | | |
| Regular | 1 oz. | | 8.6 | 5. | 4. | 24 |
| Regular | 1″ cube (.6 oz.) | | 5.2 | 3. | 2. | 15 |
| Crumbled | 1 cup (4.8 oz.) | | 41.2 | 23. | 18. | 117 |
| (Frigo) | 1 oz. | 511 | 8.2 | | | |
| (Sargento) | 1 oz. | 396 | 9.1 | | | 21 |
| Bonbino, *Laughing Cow,* | | | | | | |
| natural | 1 oz. | 227 | 9.0 | | | 27 |
| Brick: | | | | | | |
| (USDA) natural | 1 oz. | | 8.6 | 5. | 4. | 26 |
| (Sargento) sliced | 1 oz. | 159 | 8.0 | | | 27 |
| Brie (Sargento) Danish Danko | 1 oz. | 282 | 7.0 | | | 21 |
| Burgercheese (Sargento) sliced | 1 oz. | 406 | 8.0 | | | 27 |
| Camembert, domestic: | | | | | | |
| Natural (USDA) | 1 oz. | | 7.0 | 4. | 3. | 26 |
| Natural (USDA) | 2¼″ × 2⅛″ × 1⅛″ wedge (3 to a 4-oz. pkg.) | | 9.4 | 5. | 4. | 35 |
| Sargento | 1 oz. | 233 | 7.0 | | | 17 |
| Cheddar (See American) | | | | | | |
| *Chedda-Jack* (Dorman's) | | | | | | |
| shredded | 1 oz. | 100 | 7.0 | | | 24 |
| Colby, natural: | | | | | | |
| (USDA) | 1 oz. | | 9.1 | | | 27 |
| (Featherweight) low sodium | 1 oz. | 4 | 9.0 | | | |
| (Fisher's) | 1 oz. | | 9.0 | | | 33 |
| (Kraft) | 1 oz. | 180 | | | | |
| (Sargento) | 1 oz. | 171 | 9.0 | | | 27 |

(USDA): United States Department of Agriculture
*Prepared as Package Directs

109

| Food and Description | Measure or Quantity | Sodium (mg.) | Fats in grams — Total | Satu- rated | Unsatu- rated | Choles- terol (mg.) |
|---|---|---|---|---|---|---|
| Cottage cheese: | | | | | | |
| Creamed, unflavored: | | | | | | |
| (USDA) | 1 oz. | 65 | 1.2 | < 1. | < 1. | 5 |
| (USDA) | 8-oz. pkg. | 520 | 9.5 | 5. | 5. | 43 |
| (USDA) | 1 packed cup (8.6 oz.) | 561 | 10.3 | 5. | 5. | 47 |
| (USDA) | 1 T. (.5 oz.) | 34 | .6 | Tr. | Tr. | 3 |
| (Borden's): | | | | | | |
| Regular, 4% milk fat: | | | | | | |
| Regular | ½ cup | 400 | 5.0 | | | |
| Unsalted | ½ cup | 40 | 5.0 | | | |
| Dry curd, 5% milk fat | ½ cup | 20 | 1.0 | | | |
| *Lite-Line,* 1.5% milk fat | ½ cup | 400 | 2.0 | | | |
| (Breakstone's): | | | | | | |
| Low fat | 4 oz. | 470 | | | | |
| Smooth & creamy | 4 oz. | 370 | | | | |
| Tangy | 4 oz. | 420 | | | | |
| (Friendship) low fat, no salt added | 1 oz. | 7 | .2 | | | |
| (Johanna Farms): | | | | | | |
| Large or small curd | ½ cup | 450 | 4.6 | | | 19 |
| Low fat | ½ cup | 430 | 1.0 | | | Tr. |
| No salt added | ½ cup | 70 | 1.0 | | | Tr. |
| (Light N' Lively) | 4 oz. | 370 | | | | |
| (Sealtest) | 4 oz. | 460 | | | | |
| Uncreamed: | | | | | | |
| (USDA) | 8-oz. pkg. | 658 | .7 | | | 16 |
| (USDA) | 1 oz. | 82 | < .1 | | | 2 |
| (USDA) | 1 packed cup (7 oz.) | 580 | .6 | | | 14 |
| Cream cheese: | | | | | | |
| Plain, unwhipped: | | | | | | |
| (USDA) | 1 oz. | 71 | 10.7 | 6. | 5. | 31 |
| (USDA) | 3-oz. pkg. (2⅞″ × ⅞″) | 212 | 32.0 | 18. | 14. | 94 |
| (USDA) | 8-oz. pkg. | 568 | 85.6 | 48. | 38. | 252 |
| (USDA) | ½ cup (4.1 oz.) | 288 | 43.4 | 24. | 19. | 128 |
| (USDA) | 1″ cube (.6 oz.) | 40 | 6.0 | 3. | 3. | 18 |
| (USDA) | 1 T. (.5 oz.) | 35 | 5.3 | 3. | 2. | 16 |
| (Breakstone's) | 1 oz. | 25 | 9.5 | | | 113 |
| (Breakstone's) | 1 T. (.5 oz.) | 12 | 4.8 | | | 56 |
| (Kraft) | 1 oz. | 113 | 9.7 | | | |
| (Sealtest) | 1 oz. | 114 | 9.5 | | | |

(USDA): United States Department of Agriculture
*Prepared as Package Directs

| Food and Description | Measure or Quantity | Sodium (mg.) | — Fats in grams — | | | Choles-terol (mg.) |
|---|---|---|---|---|---|---|
| | | | Total | Satu-rated | Unsatu-rated | |
| *Hostess* (Kraft) | 1 oz. | 113 | 9.5 | | | |
| *Philadelphia Brand* (Kraft) | 1 oz. | 113 | 9.7 | | | |
| *Philadelphia Brand,* imitation (Kraft) | 1 oz. | 204 | 3.4 | | | |
| Plain, whipped (Breakstone's): | | | | | | |
| *Temp-Tee* | 1 oz. | 25 | 9.5 | | | 113 |
| *Temp-Tee* | 1 T. (9 grams) | 8 | 3.1 | | | 37 |
| Flavored, unwhipped: | | | | | | |
| Chive (Kraft) *Hostess* | 1 oz. | 170 | 8.0 | | | |
| Chive (Kraft) *Philadelphia Brand* | 1 oz. | 170 | 8.0 | | | |
| Olive-pimento (Kraft) *Hostess* | 1 oz. | 193 | 8.3 | | | |
| Pimento (Kraft) *Hostess* | 1 oz. | 170 | 8.2 | | | |
| Pimento (Kraft) *Philadelphia Brand* | 1 oz. | 170 | 8.2 | | | |
| Pineapple (Kraft) *Hostess* | 1 oz. | 125 | 7.8 | | | |
| Roquefort (Kraft) *Hostess* | 1 oz. | 261 | 7.5 | | | |
| Flavored, whipped (Kraft): | | | | | | |
| Bacon & horseradish | 1 oz. | 159 | 9.4 | | | |
| Blue | 1 oz. | 169 | 9.3 | | | |
| *Catalina* | 1 oz. | 261 | 9.1 | | | |
| Chive | 1 oz. | 170 | 8.8 | | | |
| Onion | 1 oz. | 180 | 8.8 | | | |
| Pimento | 1 oz. | 181 | 8.6 | | | |
| Salami | 1 oz. | 126 | 8.3 | | | |
| Smoked salmon | 1 oz. | 170 | 8.2 | | | |
| Edam: | | | | | | |
| Natural (USDA) | 1 oz. | | 7.9 | | | 29 |
| (Kaukauna) natural | 1 oz. | 275 | 8.0 | | | 25 |
| *Laughing Cow* | 1 oz. | 227 | 8.0 | | | 26 |
| (Sargento) | 1 oz. | 274 | 8.0 | | | 25 |
| Farmer: | | | | | | |
| (Kaukauna) natural | 1 oz. | | | | | 25 |
| (Sargento) | 1 oz. | 132 | 5.0 | | | 16 |
| Feta (Sargento) Danish, cups | 1 oz. | 316 | 6.0 | | | 25 |
| Gjetost (Sargento) Norwegian | 1 oz. | 170 | | | | |
| Gouda: | | | | | | |
| (Kaukauna) natural, regular, with caraway seeds or hickory smoked | 1 oz. | 230 | 8.0 | | | 30 |

(USDA): United States Department of Agriculture
*Prepared as Package Directs

| Food and Description | Measure or Quantity | Sodium (mg.) | —Fats in grams—<br>Total | Satu-rated | Unsatu-rated | Choles-terol (mg.) |
|---|---|---|---|---|---|---|
| *Laughing Cow,* natural: | | | | | | |
| Regular | 1 oz. | 227 | 9.0 | | | 28 |
| Mini, waxed | ¾ oz. | 170 | 6.4 | | | 21 |
| (Sargento) | 1 oz. | 232 | 8.0 | | | 32 |
| *Wispride* | 1 oz. | 298 | 8.0 | | | 24 |
| Grated: | | | | | | |
| (Kraft) Italian blend | 1 oz. | 435 | | | | |
| (Polly-O) | 1 oz. | 530 | 10.0 | | | 25 |
| Gruyère (Swiss Knight) | 1 oz. | 362 | 8.0 | | | 24 |
| Havarti (Sargento) creamy: | | | | | | |
| Regular | 1 oz. | 198 | 7.0 | | | 21 |
| 60% milk | 1 oz. | 198 | 10.0 | | | 21 |
| Jarlsberg (Sargento) Norwegian | 1 oz. | 130 | 7.0 | | | 16 |
| Kettle Morain (Sargento) | 1 oz. | 17 | 8.0 | | | 9 |
| Limburger: | | | | | | |
| Natural (USDA) | 1 oz. | | 7.9 | 4. | 4. | 28 |
| Natural (Sargento) | 1 oz. | 227 | 7.0 | | | 26 |
| Monterey Jack: | | | | | | |
| (Kaukauna) natural | 1 oz. | 150 | 9.0 | | | 25 |
| (Kraft) | 1 oz. | 190 | | | | |
| (Sargento) midget, Longhorn | 1 oz. | 152 | 8.0 | | | |
| Mozzarella: | | | | | | |
| Low moisture, natural (USDA) | 1 oz. | | 7.5 | | | 27 |
| Low moisture, part-skim, natural (USDA) | 1 oz. | | 5.9 | | | 18 |
| (Dorman's) shredded, lite, low sodium | 1 oz. | 90 | 5.0 | | | 15 |
| (Kraft) | 1 oz. | 190 | | | | |
| (Polly-O): | | | | | | |
| Fior de Latte | 1 oz. | 20 | 6.0 | | | 20 |
| Lite | 1 oz. | 200 | 4.0 | | | 16 |
| Part skim milk: | | | | | | |
| Regular | 1 oz. | 280 | 5.0 | | | 15 |
| Shredded | 1 oz. | 280 | 6.0 | | | |
| Smoked | 1 oz. | 240 | 7.0 | | | 25 |
| Whole milk: | | | | | | |
| Regular | 1 oz. | 280 | 6.0 | | | 20 |
| Old fashioned: | | | | | | |
| Regular | 1 oz. | 200 | 4.0 | | | 15 |
| Shredded | 1 oz. | 220 | 6.0 | | | |
| Shredded or sliced | 1 oz. | 220 | 6.0 | | | |

(USDA): United States Department of Agriculture
*Prepared as Package Directs

| Food and Description | Measure or Quantity | Sodium (mg.) | —Fats in grams— | | | Cholesterol (mg.) |
|---|---|---|---|---|---|---|
| | | | Total | Saturated | Unsaturated | |
| **(Sargento):** | | | | | | |
| Bar, rounds, sliced or square | 1 oz. | 150 | 5.0 | | | 15 |
| Shredded, with spices | 1 oz. | 150 | 9.0 | | | 15 |
| Sliced, for pizza | 1 oz. | 150 | 6.0 | | | 15 |
| Whole milk | 1 oz. | 106 | 7.0 | | | 22 |
| **Muenster:** | | | | | | |
| Natural (USDA) | 1 oz. | | 8.6 | | | 25 |
| (Sargento) red rind | 1 oz. | 178 | 9.0 | | | 27 |
| *Wispride* | 1 oz. | 129 | 8.0 | | | 26 |
| Neufchâtel, natural (USDA) | 2⅞″ × 2″ × ⅞″ pkg. (3 oz.) | | 20.4 | | | 64 |
| **Parmesan:** | | | | | | |
| (USDA) natural: | | | | | | |
| Regular | 1 oz. | 208 | 7.4 | 4. | 3. | 27 |
| Grated | 1 oz. | 247 | 9.4 | | | 32 |
| Grated | 1 cup loosely packed (3.7 oz.) | 923 | 35.2 | | | 110 |
| Grated | 1 cup pressed down (4.9 oz.) | 1,219 | 46.5 | | | 158 |
| Grated | 1 T. loosely packed (7 grams) | 58 | 2.2 | | | 8 |
| Grated | 1 T. pressed down (9 grams) | 78 | 3.0 | | | 10 |
| (Polly-O) grated | 1 oz. | 530 | 9.0 | | | 20 |
| (Sargento) | 1 oz. | 445 | 7.0 | | | 3 |
| Pizza (Sargento) | 1 oz. | 306 | 6.0 | | | 2 |
| Pot (Sargento) | 1 oz. | <1 | 0.0 | | | 0 |
| Provolone (Sargento) sliced | 1 oz. | 248 | 8.0 | | | 20 |
| **Ricotta:** | | | | | | |
| (USDA): | | | | | | |
| Natural | 1 oz. | | 3.7 | | | 14 |
| Part skim, natural | 1 oz. | | 2.3 | | | 9 |
| (Polly-O): | | | | | | |
| Lite | 1 oz. | 32 | 2.0 | 5. | | |
| Old fashioned | 1 oz. | 25 | 4.0 | | | 15 |
| Part skim milk: | | | | | | |
| Regular | 1 oz. | 22 | 3.0 | | | 10 |
| No salt added | 1 oz. | 10 | 3.0 | | | 10 |
| Whole milk: | | | | | | |
| Regular | 1 oz. | 22 | 3.5 | | | 17 |
| No salt added | 1 oz. | 10 | 3.5 | | | 17 |

(USDA): United States Department of Agriculture
*Prepared as Package Directs

CHEESE (Continued)

| Food and Description | Measure or Quantity | Sodium (mg.) | Total | Saturated | Unsaturated | Cholesterol (mg.) |
|---|---|---|---|---|---|---|
| | | | — Fats in grams — | | | |
| (Sargento): | | | | | | |
| Part skim milk | 1 oz. | 35 | 3.0 | | | 9 |
| Whole milk | 1 oz. | 24 | 4.0 | | | 14 |
| Romano: | | | | | | |
| (Polly-O) grated | 1 oz. | 530 | 10.0 | | | 30 |
| (Sargento) wedge | 1 oz. | 340 | 8.0 | | | 29 |
| Roquefort, natural: | | | | | | |
| (USDA) | 1 oz. | | 8.6 | 4. | 4. | |
| (USDA) | 1″ cube (.6 oz.) | | 5.2 | 3. | 2. | |
| Samsoe (Sargento) Danish | 1 oz. | 198 | 8.0 | | | 24 |
| Semi-soft: | | | | | | |
| Bel Paese | 1 oz. | 196 | 7.4 | | | |
| Laughing Cow: | | | | | | |
| Babybel: | | | | | | |
| Regular | 1 oz. | 227 | 7.0 | | | 22 |
| Mini | 3/4 oz. | 170 | 6.2 | | | 18 |
| Bonbel: | | | | | | |
| Regular | 1 oz. | 3378 | 8.2 | | | 24 |
| Mini | 3/4 oz. | 170 | 6.2 | | | 18 |
| Reduced calorie | 1 oz. | 170 | 2.5 | | | 8 |
| Slim Jack (Dorman's) | 1 oz. | 70 | 7.0 | | | 22 |
| String (Sargento) | 1 oz. | 150 | 6.0 | | | 15 |
| Swiss: | | | | | | |
| (USDA): | | | | | | |
| Natural | 1 oz. | 201 | 7.9 | 4. | 4. | 28 |
| Natural | 1″ cube (.5 oz.) | 106 | 4.2 | 2. | 2. | 15 |
| Natural | 1 1/4-oz. slice | 248 | 9.8 | 5. | 5. | 35 |
| Process: | | | | | | |
| Regular | 1-oz. slice | 331 | 7.6 | 4. | 3. | 26 |
| Regular | 1″ cube (.6 oz.) | 210 | 4.8 | 3. | 2. | 17 |
| Reduced sodium | 1-oz. slice | 193 | 7.6 | 4. | 3. | 26 |
| Reduced sodium | 1″ cube (.6 oz.) | 126 | 4.8 | 3. | 2. | 17 |
| (Dorman's) light, no salt added | 1 oz. | 8 | 8.0 | | | 26 |
| (Sargento): | | | | | | |
| Domestic | 1 oz. | 74 | 7.0 | | | 26 |
| Imported | 1 oz. | 74 | 8.0 | | | 24 |
| Taco (Sargento) shredded | 1 oz. | 47 | 9.0 | | | 30 |

**CHEESE CAKE** (See **CAKE,** Cheese)

(USDA): United States Department of Agriculture
*Prepared as Package Directs

114

| Food and Description | Measure or Quantity | Sodium (mg.) | Fats in grams | | | Choles- terol (mg.) |
|---|---|---|---|---|---|---|
| | | | Total | Satu- rated | Unsatu- rated | |

**CHEESE DIP** (See **DIP**)

**CHEESE FONDUE:**

| Food and Description | Measure or Quantity | Sodium (mg.) | Total | Satu- rated | Unsatu- rated | Choles- terol (mg.) |
|---|---|---|---|---|---|---|
| Home recipe (USDA) | 4 oz. | 615 | 20.8 | 10. | 10. | |
| *Swiss Knight* | 1 oz. | 186 | 5.0 | | | 14 |

**CHEESE FOOD,** process:

American or cheddar:

| Food and Description | Measure or Quantity | Sodium (mg.) | Total | Satu- rated | Unsatu- rated | Choles- terol (mg.) |
|---|---|---|---|---|---|---|
| (USDA) | 1-oz. slice (3½" × 3⅜" × ⅛") | | 6.8 | 4. | 3. | 20 |
| (USDA) | 1" cube (.6 oz.) | | 4.3 | 2. | 2. | 13 |
| (USDA) | 1 T. (.5 oz.) | | 3.0 | 2. | 2. | 10 |
| (Borden's) *Lite-Line:* | | | | | | |
|   American | 1 oz. | 410 | | | | |
|   Cheddar, sharp | 1 oz. | 440 | | | | |
| (Fisher's) substitute, | | | | | | |
|   Ched-O-Mate or | | | | | | |
|   Sandwich-Mate | 1 oz. | 450 | 7.0 | | | 5 |
| (Sargento) | 1 oz. | 274 | 7.0 | | | 18 |
| *Wispride,* cheddar: | | | | | | |
|   Regular | 1 oz. | 180 | 8.0 | | | 20 |
|   & port wine | 1 oz. | 190 | 7.0 | | | 20 |
| *Cheez-ola* (Fisher's): | | | | | | |
|   Regular | 1 oz. | 400-430 | 7.0 | | | Tr. |
|   Low sodium | 1 oz. | 150-170 | 7.0 | | | Tr. |
| *Chef's Delight* (Fisher's) | 1 oz. | 420-450 | 4.0 | | | 6 |
| *Count Down* (Fisher's) | 1 oz. | 400-430 | 1.0 | | | Tr. |
| Cracker snack (Sargento) | | | | | | |
|   sliced | 1 oz. | 406 | 7.0 | | | 27 |
| Garlic & herbs, *Wispride* | 1 oz. | 180 | 7.0 | | | 20 |
| Jalapeño (Borden's) *Lite-Line* | 1 oz. | 430 | | | | |
| Low sodium (Borden's) | | | | | | |
|   *Lite-Line* | 1 oz. | 200 | | | | |
| *Pizza-Mate* (Fisher's) | 1 oz. | 330-350 | 7.0 | | | Tr. |
| Swiss (Kraft) light, natural | 1 oz. | 55 | | | | 20 |

**CHEESE SPREAD:**

American, process:

| Food and Description | Measure or Quantity | Sodium (mg.) | Total | Satu- rated | Unsatu- rated | Choles- terol (mg.) |
|---|---|---|---|---|---|---|
| (USDA) regular | 1 oz. (2¾" × 2¼" × ¼") | 461 | 6.1 | | | 18 |
| (USDA) regular | 1 T. (.5 oz.) | 228 | 3.0 | | | 9 |

(USDA): United States Department of Agriculture
*Prepared as Package Directs

| Food and Description | Measure or Quantity | Sodium (mg.) | —Fats in grams— | | | Choles- terol (mg.) |
|---|---|---|---|---|---|---|
| | | | Total | Satu- rated | Unsatu- rated | |
| (USDA) regular shredded | 1 packed cup (4 oz.) | 1,836 | 24.2 | | | 72 |
| (USDA) reduced sodium | 1 oz. (2¾″ × 2¼″ × ¼″) | 323 | 6.1 | | | 18 |
| (USDA) reduced sodium | 1 T. (.5 oz.) | 159 | 3.0 | | | 9 |
| (USDA) reduced sodium | 1 packed cup (4 oz.) | 1287 | 24.2 | | | 72 |
| (Nabisco) *Easy Cheese* | 1 tsp. (5 grams) | 70 | 1.0 | | | |
| Bleu, *Laughing Cow* | 1 oz. | 312 | 6.0 | | | 18 |
| Cheddar: | | | | | | |
| *Laughing Cow* | 1 oz. | 312 | 6.0 | | | 18 |
| (Nabisco) *Easy Cheese:* | | | | | | |
| Regular | 1 tsp. (.2 oz.) | 74 | 1.2 | | | |
| Chive | 1 tsp. (.2 oz.) | 68 | 1.1 | | | |
| Sharp | 1 tsp. (.2 oz.) | 64 | 1.2 | | | |
| Cheese & bacon (Nabisco) *Easy Cheese* | 1 tsp. (.2 oz.) | 70 | 1.2 | | | |
| *Cheez Whiz,* process (Kraft) | 1 oz. | 473 | 4.5 | | | 17 |
| Gruyere, *Laughing Cow, La Vache Qui Rit:* | | | | | | |
| Regular | 1 oz. | 312 | 6.0 | | | 18 |
| Reduced calorie | 1 oz. | 312 | 2.6 | | | 7 |
| Nacho (Nabisco) *Easy Cheese* | 1 tsp. (.2 oz.) | 68 | 1.2 | | | |
| Pimento (Prince's) | 1 oz. | 335 | 6.0 | | | 15 |
| Provolone, *Laughing Cow* | 1 oz. | 312 | 6.0 | | | 18 |
| *Velveeta* (Kraft): | | | | | | |
| Regular | 1 oz. | 430 | 5.0 | | | |
| Mexican, with jalapeño peppers | 1 oz. | 440 | | | | |
| **CHEESE STRAW** (USDA): | | | | | | |
| Made with lard[1] | 1 oz. | 204 | 8.5 | 4. | 5. | 9 |
| Made with lard[1] | 5″ × ⅜″ × ⅜″ piece (6 grams) | 43 | 1.8 | <1. | 1. | 2 |
| Made with vegetable shortening[2] | 1 oz. | 204 | 8.5 | 3. | 6. | |
| **CHELOIS WINE** (Great Western) 12.5% alcohol | 3 fl. oz. | 37 | 0.0 | | | 0 |

(USDA): United States Department of Agriculture
*Prepared as Package Directs
[1]Principal sources of fat: lard & milk.
[2]Principal sources of fat: vegetable shortening, milk & lard.

| Food and Description | Measure or Quantity | Sodium (mg.) | — Fats in grams — | | | Choles- terol (mg.) |
|---|---|---|---|---|---|---|
| | | | Total | Satu- rated | Unsatu- rated | |
| **CHERIMOYA,** raw (USDA): | | | | | | |
| Whole | 1 lb. (weighed with skin & seeds) | | 1.1 | | | 0 |
| Flesh only | 4 oz. | | .5 | | | 0 |
| **CHERRY:** | | | | | | |
| Sour: | | | | | | |
| Fresh (USDA): | | | | | | |
| Whole | 1 lb. (weighed with stems) | 7 | 1.1 | | | 0 |
| Whole | 1 lb. (weighed without stems) | 8 | 1.3 | | | 0 |
| Pitted | ½ cup (2.7 oz.) | 2 | .2 | | | 0 |
| Canned, syrup pack, pitted: (USDA): | | | | | | |
| Light syrup | 4 oz. (with liq.) | 1 | .2 | | | 0 |
| Heavy syrup | 4 oz. (with liq.) | 1 | .2 | | | 0 |
| Heavy syrup | ½ cup (4.6 oz.) | 1 | .3 | | | 0 |
| Extra heavy syrup | 4 oz. (with liq.) | 1 | .2 | | | 0 |
| *Thank You Brand* | ½ cup (4.5 oz.) | 13 | 0.0 | | | 0 |
| Canned, water pack, pitted, solids & liq.: | | | | | | |
| (USDA) | ½ cup (4.3 oz.) | 2 | .2 | | | 0 |
| *Thank You Brand* | ½ cup (4.9 oz.) | <5 | 0.0 | | | 0 |
| Frozen, pitted (USDA): | | | | | | |
| Sweetened | ½ cup (4.6 oz.) | 3 | .5 | | | 0 |
| Unsweetened | 4 oz. | 2 | .5 | | | 0 |
| Sweet: | | | | | | |
| Fresh (USDA): | | | | | | |
| Whole, with stems | 1 lb. (weighed with stems) | 8 | 1.2 | | | 0 |
| Whole, with stems | ½ cup (2.3 oz.) | 1 | .2 | | | 0 |
| Pitted | ½ cup (2.9 oz.) | 2 | .2 | | | 0 |
| Canned, syrup pack, with pits, solids & liq.: | | | | | | |
| Light syrup (USDA) | 4 oz. | 1 | .2 | | | 0 |
| Heavy syrup (USDA) | 4 oz. | 1 | .2 | | | 0 |
| Heavy syrup, dark (Del Monte) | ½ cup (4.3 oz.) | 2 | .6 | | | 0 |
| Heavy syrup, Royal Anne (Del Monte) | ½ cup (4.6 oz.) | 2 | .5 | | | 0 |

(USDA): United States Department of Agriculture
*Prepared as Package Directs

| Food and Description | Measure or Quantity | Sodium (mg.) | Total | — Fats in grams — Satu- rated | Unsatu- rated | Choles- terol (mg.) |
|---|---|---|---|---|---|---|
| Heavy syrup, light or dark (Stokely-Van Camp's) | ½ cup (4.2 oz.) | | .2 | | | (0) |
| Extra heavy syrup (USDA) | 4 oz. | 1 | .2 | | | 0 |
| Canned, syrup pack, pitted, solids & liq.: | | | | | | |
| Light syrup (USDA) | 4 oz. | 1 | .2 | | | 0 |
| Heavy syrup (USDA) | 4 oz. | 1 | .2 | | | 0 |
| Heavy syrup (USDA) | ½ cup (4.2 oz.) | 1 | .2 | | | 0 |
| Heavy syrup (Del Monte) | ½ cup (4.3 oz.) | 6 | 1.5 | | | (0) |
| Extra heavy syrup (USDA) | 4 oz. | 1 | .2 | | | 0 |
| Canned, water pack, with pits, solids & liq. (USDA) | 4 oz. | 1 | .2 | | | 0 |
| Canned, water or dietetic pack, pitted, solids & liq.: | | | | | | |
| (USDA) | 4 oz. | 1 | .2 | | | 0 |
| (Blue Boy) | 4 oz. | 1 | Tr. | | | (0) |
| Royal Anne: | | | | | | |
| (Diet Delight) | ½ cup (4.4 oz.) | 6 | Tr. | | | (0) |
| (S & W) *Nutradiet,* low calorie | 14 whole cherries (3.5 oz.) | 3 | Tr. | | | (0) |
| (S & W) *Nutradiet,* unsweetened | 14 whole cherries (3.5 oz.) | 2 | Tr. | | | (0) |
| (Tillie Lewis) | ½ cup (4.5 oz.) | < 10 | .2 | | | 0 |
| Dark (S & W) *Nutradiet,* low calorie | 4 oz. | 1 | .1 | | | (0) |

**CHERRY, BLACK, SOFT DRINK** (See **SOFT DRINK,** Cherry)

**CHERRY, CANDIED** (USDA)    1 oz.              .6          0

**CHERRY COLA** (See **SOFT DRINK,** Cola)

**CHERRY DRINK:**

| Food and Description | Measure or Quantity | Sodium (mg.) | Total | | | Choles- terol (mg.) |
|---|---|---|---|---|---|---|
| Canned, regular pack: | | | | | | |
| (Hi-C) | 6 fl. oz. | 4 | Tr. | | | 0 |
| *Ssips* (Johanna Farms) | 8.45-fl.-oz. container | 20 | 0.0 | | | |
| *Mix (Hi-C) | 6 fl. oz. | 23 | | | | |

(USDA): United States Department of Agriculture
*Prepared as Package Directs

| Food and Description | Measure or Quantity | Sodium (mg.) | —Fats in grams— | | | Choles-terol (mg.) |
|---|---|---|---|---|---|---|
| | | | Total | Satu-rated | Unsatu-rated | |
| **CHERRY, MARASCHINO** | | | | | | |
| (USDA) | 1 oz. (with liq.) | | < .1 | | | 0 |
| **CHERRY PIE** (See **PIE,** Cherry) | | | | | | |
| **CHERRY PIE FILLING** (See **PIE FILLING,** Cherry) | | | | | | |
| **CHERRY JELLY:** | | | | | | |
| Sweetened (Home Brand) | 1 T. | 15 | 0.0 | | | |
| Dietetic (Featherweight) | 1 T. | 40-50 | 0.0 | | | |
| **CHERRY, MARASCHINO** | | | | | | |
| (USDA) | 1 oz. (without liq.) | | Tr. | | | 0 |
| **CHERRY PRESERVE OR JAM:** | | | | | | |
| Sweetened (Home Brand) | 1 T. (.7 oz.) | 15 | 0 | | | 0 |
| Dietetic or low calorie: | | | | | | |
| (Estee) | 1 T. | < 3 | Tr. | | | 0 |
| (Featherweight) | 1 T. | Tr. | 0.0 | | | 0 |
| (Louis Sherry) | 1 T. | 40-50 | 0.0 | | | 0 |
| **CHERRY SOFT DRINK** (See **SOFT DRINK,** Cherry) | | | | | | |
| **CHERVIL:** | | | | | | |
| Raw (USDA) | 1 oz. | | .3 | | | 0 |
| Dry (Spice Islands) | 1 tsp. | < 1 | | | | (0) |
| **CHESTNUT** (USDA): | | | | | | |
| Fresh, in shell | 1 lb. (weighed in shell) | 22 | 5.5 | | | 0 |
| Fresh, shelled | 4 oz. | 7 | 1.7 | | | 0 |
| Dried, in shell | 1 lb. (weighed in shell) | 45 | 15.3 | | | 0 |
| Dried, shelled | 4 oz. | 14 | 4.6 | | | 0 |
| **CHESTNUT FLOUR** (See **FLOUR, CHESTNUT**) | | | | | | |

(USDA): United States Department of Agriculture
*Prepared as Package Directs

| Food and Description | Measure or Quantity | Sodium (mg.) | Total | Satu- rated | Unsatu- rated | Choles- terol (mg.) |
|---|---|---|---|---|---|---|
| | | | | —Fats in grams— | | |

**CHEWING GUM:**
  Sweetened:

| Food and Description | Measure or Quantity | Sodium (mg.) | Total | Satu- rated | Unsatu- rated | Choles- terol (mg.) |
|---|---|---|---|---|---|---|
| *Beechies* | 1 tablet (2 grams) | <1 | 0.0 | | | (0) |
| *Beech-Nut* | 1 stick (3 grams) | <1 | 0.0 | | | (0) |
| *Doublemint* (Wrigley's) | 1 stick (3 grams) | <1 | Tr. | | | 0 |
| *Juicy Fruit* (Wrigley's) | 1 stick (3 grams) | <1 | Tr. | | | 0 |
| Spearmint (Wrigley's) | 1 stick (3 grams) | <1 | Tr. | | | 0 |
| Unsweetened or dietetic: | | | | | | |
| All flavors (Estee) | 1 stick | | <.1 | | | (0) |
| *Care*Free* (Beech-Nut) | 1 stick (3 grams) | <1 | 0.0 | | | (0) |
| (Harvey's) | 1 stick | Tr. | 0.0 | | | 0 |

**CHEX,** cereal (Ralston Purina):

| Food and Description | Measure or Quantity | Sodium (mg.) | Total | Satu- rated | Unsatu- rated | Choles- terol (mg.) |
|---|---|---|---|---|---|---|
| Corn | 1 cup (1 oz.) | 295 | .2 | | | |
| Rice | 1⅛ cups (1 oz.) | 243 | .3 | | | |
| Wheat | ⅔ cup (1 oz.) | 192 | .3 | | | |
| Wheat & raisin | ¾ cup (1.3 oz.) | 216 | .3 | | | |

**CHICKEN** (See also **CHICKEN, CANNED**) (USDA):

| Food and Description | Measure or Quantity | Sodium (mg.) | Total | Satu- rated | Unsatu- rated | Choles- terol (mg.) |
|---|---|---|---|---|---|---|
| Broiler, cooked, meat only | 4 oz. | 75 | 4.3 | 1. | 3. | 99 |
| Capon, raw, ready-to-cook | 1 lb. (weighed with bones) | | 70.2 | 22. | 48. | 324 |
| Capon, raw, meat with skin | 4 oz. | | 24.9 | | | 92 |
| Fryer: | | | | | | |
| Raw: | | | | | | |
| Ready-to-cook | 1 lb. (weighed with bone) | | 15.1 | 5. | 10. | 310 |
| Meat & skin | 1 lb. | | 23.1 | 7. | 16. | 367 |
| Meat only | 1 lb. | 263 | 12.2 | 4. | 8. | 358 |
| Dark meat with skin | 1 lb. | 304 | 28.6 | 9. | 20. | 399 |
| Light meat with skin | 1 lb. | 227 | 17.7 | 5. | 12. | 304 |
| Dark meat without skin | 1 lb. | 304 | 17.2 | 5. | 12. | 399 |
| Light meat without skin | 1 lb. | 227 | 6.8 | 2. | 5. | 358 |
| Skin only | 4 oz. | | 19.4 | 6. | 14. | |
| Back | 1 lb. (weighed with bone) | | 23.5 | 8. | 16. | 198 |
| Breast | 1 lb. (weighed with bone) | | 8.6 | 3. | 6. | 239 |
| Leg or drumstick | 1 lb. (weighed with bone) | | 10.6 | 3. | 8. | 239 |

(USDA): United States Department of Agriculture
*Prepared as Package Directs

| Food and Description | Measure or Quantity | Sodium (mg.) | Total | Satu-rated | Unsatu-rated | Choles-terol (mg.) |
|---|---|---|---|---|---|---|
| | | | | — Fats in grams — | | |
| Neck | 1 lb. (weighed with bone) | | 20.5 | 7. | 14. | 177 |
| Rib | 1 lb. (weighed with bone) | | 12.5 | 4. | 8. | 187 |
| Thigh | 1 lb. (weighed with bone) | | 19.1 | 6. | 13. | 275 |
| Wing | 1 lb. (weighed with bone) | | 16.5 | 5. | 12. | 180 |
| Fried. A 2½-pound chicken (weighed with bone before cooking) will give you: | | | | | | |
| Back[1] | 1 back (2.2 oz.) | | 8.5 | 3. | 6. | 35 |
| Breast[1] | ½ breast (3.3 oz.) | | 4.9 | 2. | 3. | 61 |
| Leg or drumstick[1] | 1 leg (2 oz.) | | 3.8 | 1. | 3. | 34 |
| Neck[1] | 1 neck (2.1 oz.) | | 7.3 | 3. | 5. | 37 |
| Rib[1] | 1 rib (.7 oz.) | | 2.2 | <1. | 2. | 12 |
| Thigh[1] | 1 thigh (2.3 oz.) | | 5.7 | 2. | 4. | 44 |
| Wing[1] | 1 wing (1¾ oz.) | | 4.3 | 1. | 3. | 25 |
| Fryer: | | | | | | |
| Fried: | | | | | | |
| Meat, skin & giblets[1] | 4 oz. | 88 | 13.4 | 3. | 10. | 91 |
| Meat & skin[1] | 4 oz. | 88 | 13.5 | 3. | 10. | 91 |
| Meat only[1] | 4 oz. | 88 | 8.8 | 3. | 6. | 88 |
| Dark meat with skin[1] | 4 oz. | 100 | 15.4 | 5. | 10. | 103 |
| Light meat with skin[1] | 4 oz. | 77 | 11.2 | 4. | 8. | 90 |
| Dark meat without skin[1] | 4 oz. | 100 | 10.5 | 3. | 7. | 103 |
| Light meat without skin[1] | 4 oz. | 77 | 6.9 | 2. | 5. | 103 |
| Skin only[1] | 1 oz. | | 8.2 | 3. | 6. | |
| Hen & cock: | | | | | | |
| Raw: | | | | | | |
| Ready-to-cook | 1 lb. (weighed with bones) | | 82.1 | 26. | 56. | 324 |
| Meat & skin | 1 lb. | | 85.3 | 27. | 58. | 367 |
| Meat only | 1 lb. | 263 | 31.8 | 10. | 21. | 445 |
| Dark meat without skin | 1 lb. | 304 | 34.0 | 11. | 23. | 399 |
| Light meat without skin | 1 lb. | 227 | 16.8 | 5. | 11. | 304 |
| Stewed: | | | | | | |
| Meat, skin & giblets | 4 oz. | | 25.2 | 8. | 17. | 91 |
| Meat & skin | 4 oz. | | 25.9 | 8. | 18. | 99 |
| Meat only | 4 oz. | 62 | 10.1 | 3. | 7. | 99 |

(USDA): United States Department of Agriculture
*Prepared as Package Directs
[1]Principal source of fat: vegetable shortening.

| Food and Description | Measure or Quantity | Sodium (mg.) | Total | Fats in grams — Saturated | Fats in grams — Unsaturated | Cholesterol (mg.) |
|---|---|---|---|---|---|---|
| Chopped | ½ cup (2.5 oz.) | 40 | 6.4 | 2. | 4. | 63 |
| Diced | ½ cup (2.4 oz.) | 37 | 6.0 | 2. | 4. | 58 |
| Ground | ½ cup (2 oz.) | 31 | 5.0 | 2. | 3. | 49 |
| Roaster: | | | | | | |
| Raw: | | | | | | |
| Ready-to-cook | 1 lb. (weighed with bones) | | 59.3 | 19. | 40. | 324 |
| Meat, skin & giblets | 1 lb. | | 54.0 | 18. | 36. | 445 |
| Meat & skin | 1 lb. | | 57.2 | 19. | 38. | 445 |
| Meat only | 1 lb. | 263 | 20.4 | 7. | 14. | 367 |
| Dark meat without skin | 1 lb. | 304 | 21.3 | 7. | 14. | 399 |
| White meat without skin | 1 lb. | 227 | 14.5 | 5. | 10. | 304 |
| Roasted: | | | | | | |
| Total edible | 4 oz. | | 22.9 | 7. | 16. | 99 |
| Meat, skin & giblets | 4 oz. | | 15.9 | 5. | 11. | 92 |
| Meat & skin | 4 oz. | | 16.7 | 5. | 11. | 99 |
| Meat only | 4 oz. | 87 | 7.1 | 2. | 5. | 99 |
| Dark meat without skin | 4 oz. | 100 | 7.4 | 2. | 5. | 99 |
| Light meat without skin | 4 oz. | 75 | 5.6 | 2. | 3. | 99 |
| **CHICKEN A LA KING:** | | | | | | |
| Home recipe (USDA) | 1 cup (8.6 oz.) | 760 | 34.3 | 12. | 22. | 186 |
| Canned (Swanson) | 5¼-oz. serving | 690 | 12.0 | | | |
| Frozen: | | | | | | |
| (Banquet) | 4-oz. pkg. | 550 | 4.0 | | | 40 |
| (Blue Star) *Dining Lite,* with rice | 9½-oz. serving | 920 | 9.6 | | | |
| (Green Giant) twin pouch, with biscuits | 9-oz. entree | 1,545 | 15.0 | | | |
| (Le Menu) | 10¼-oz. dinner | 1,050 | 13.0 | | | |
| (Morton) light | 8-oz. dinner | 600 | 10.0 | | | |
| (Stouffer's) with rice | 9½-oz. pkg. | 900 | 11.0 | | | |
| (Weight Watchers) boil-in-bag | 9-oz. pkg. | 1,060 | 15.0 | | | |
| **CHICKEN BOUILLION/ BROTH,** cube or powder (See also **CHICKEN SOUP**): | | | | | | |
| Regular: | | | | | | |
| (Herb-Ox): | | | | | | |
| Cube | 1 cube | 950 | .1 | | | |

(USDA): United States Department of Agriculture
*Prepared as Package Directs

| Food and Description | Measure or Quantity | Sodium (mg.) | — Fats in grams — | | | Choles- terol (mg.) |
|---|---|---|---|---|---|---|
| | | | Total | Satu- rated | Unsatu- rated | |
| Packet | 1 packet | 960 | .1 | | | |
| (Maggi) | 1 cube | 746 | 0.0 | | | |
| (Wyler's) | 1 cube or 1 tsp. | 900 | Tr. | | | |
| Low sodium: | | | | | | |
| (Borden's) *Lite-Line,* | | | | | | |
| imitation | 1 tsp. | 5 | Tr. | | | |
| (Featherweight) | 1 tsp. | 5 | 1.0 | | | |
| **CHICKEN, CANNED, BONED:** | | | | | | |
| (USDA) | 4 oz. | | 13.3 | 5. | 9. | |
| (USDA) | 1/2 cup (3 oz.) | | 9.9 | 3. | 7. | |
| (Featherweight) low sodium | 5-oz. serving | 99 | 18.0 | | | |
| (Hormel) chunk style: | | | | | | |
| Breast | 6 3/4-oz. serving | 855 | 20.0 | | | |
| Dark | 6 3/4-oz. serving | 933 | 18.0 | | | |
| White & dark | 6 3/4-oz. serving | 857 | 20.0 | | | |
| White & dark, no salt added | 6 3/4-oz. serving | 75 | 18.0 | | | |
| (Swanson) chunk style: | | | | | | |
| Regular | 2 1/2-oz. serving | 240 | 3.0 | | | |
| Mixin' style | 2 1/2-oz. serving | 225 | 8.0 | | | |
| White | 2 1/2-oz. serving | 230 | 2.0 | | | |
| **CHICKEN DINNER OR ENTREE:** | | | | | | |
| Canned: | | | | | | |
| (Hunt's) *Minute Gourmet* | | | | | | |
| Microwave Entree Maker: | | | | | | |
| Barbecue, without chicken | 3.1-oz. serving | 1,040 | Tr. | | | |
| *Barbecue | 6.8-oz. serving | 1,110 | 4.0 | | | |
| Cacciatore, without chicken | 4.6-oz. serving | 780 | 3.0 | | | |
| *Cacciatore | 8.3-oz. serving | 840 | 6.0 | | | |
| Sweet & sour, without chicken | 4.1-oz. serving | 360 | Tr. | | | |
| *Sweet & sour | 7.8-oz. serving | 420 | Tr. | | | |
| (Swanson) & dumplings | 7 1/2-oz. serving | 960 | 12.0 | | | |
| Frozen: | | | | | | |
| (Armour): | | | | | | |
| *Classic Lite:* | | | | | | |
| Breast medallions marsala | 11-oz. serving | 970 | 7.0 | | | 85 |
| Burgundy | 11 1/4-oz. serving | 1,220 | 5.0 | | | 70 |

(USDA): United States Department of Agriculture
*Prepared as Package Directs

| Food and Description | Measure or Quantity | Sodium (mg.) | — Fats in grams — | | | Cholesterol (mg.) |
|---|---|---|---|---|---|---|
| | | | Total | Saturated | Unsaturated | |
| Oriental | 10-oz. serving | 880 | 6.0 | | | 65 |
| Sweet & sour | 11-oz. serving | 640 | 3.0 | | | 70 |
| *Dinner Classics:* | | | | | | |
| Fricassee | 11¾-oz. serving | 1,210 | 12.0 | | | 70 |
| Hawaiian | 11½-oz. serving | 700 | 10.0 | | | 75 |
| Milan | 11½-oz. serving | 1,310 | 12.0 | | | 75 |
| Sweet & sour | 11-oz. serving | 1,240 | 20.0 | | | 65 |
| (Banquet): | | | | | | |
| Dinner: | | | | | | |
| American Favorites, fried | 11-oz. dinner | 1,831 | 11.0 | | | |
| Family Favorites, & dumplings | 9-oz. dinner | 944 | 13.0 | | | |
| Entree: | | | | | | |
| Family Entrees, & dumplings | 32-oz. pkg. | 3,712 | 100.0 | | | |
| Gourmet Entree: | | | | | | |
| Cacciatore | 10-oz. entree | 510 | 5.0 | | | |
| French | 10-oz. entree | 850 | 4.0 | | | |
| (Blue Star) *Dining Lite:* | | | | | | |
| Glazed, with vegetables & rice | 8½-oz. serving | 880 | 6.0 | | | |
| With vegetables & vermicelli | 12⅔-oz. serving | 960 | 6.8 | | | |
| (Celentano): | | | | | | |
| Parmigiana, cutlets | 9-oz. pkg. | 750 | 5.0 | | | 85 |
| Primavera | 11½-oz. pkg. | 650 | 9.0 | | | 45 |
| (Conagra) *Light & Elegant:* | | | | | | |
| Cheese | 8¾-oz. entree | 800 | 11.0 | | | 50 |
| Glazed | 8-oz. entree | 660 | 4.0 | | | 75 |
| Parmigiana | 8-oz. entree | 680 | 6.0 | | | |
| (La Choy) almond, Fresh & lite | 9¾-oz. entree | 820 | 12.0 | | | |
| (Le Menu): | | | | | | |
| Cordon bleu | 11-oz. dinner | 870 | 19.0 | | | |
| Florentine | 11½-oz. dinner | 880 | 23.0 | | | |
| Parmigiana, heart of | 11½-oz. dinner | 890 | 18.0 | | | |
| Sweet & sour | 11¼-oz. dinner | 980 | 22.0 | | | |
| (Morton) dinner: | | | | | | |
| Regular: | | | | | | |
| Boneless | 11-oz. dinner | 500 | 11.8 | | | |
| Boneless | 17-oz. dinner | 1,400 | 22.9 | | | |

(USDA): United States Department of Agriculture
*Prepared as Package Directs

| Food and Description | Measure or Quantity | Sodium (mg.) | —Fats in grams— | | | Choles- terol (mg.) |
|---|---|---|---|---|---|---|
| | | | Total | Satu- rated | Unsatu- rated | |
| Fried | 11-oz. dinner | 900 | 6.9 | | | |
| Light, boneless | 11-oz. dinner | 1,150 | 7.0 | | | |
| (Stouffer's): | | | | | | |
| Regular, divan | 8½-oz. pkg. | 830 | 22.0 | | | |
| *Lean Cuisine:* | | | | | | |
| Glazed, with vegetables & rice | 8½-oz. pkg. | 830 | 8.0 | | | 55 |
| & vegetables with vermicelli | 12¾-oz. pkg. | 1,220 | 7.0 | | | 40 |
| (Swanson): | | | | | | |
| Regular, 4-compartment, fried: | | | | | | |
| Barbecue flavor | 9¼-oz. meal | 960 | 30.0 | | | |
| Breast portion | 10¾-oz. meal | 1,580 | 33.0 | | | |
| Dark meat | 10¼-oz. meal | 1,390 | 32.0 | | | |
| *Hungry-Man:* | | | | | | |
| Boneless | 17½-oz. dinner | 1,640 | 27.0 | | | |
| Fried: | | | | | | |
| Breast portion | 11¾-oz. entree | 1,760 | 37.0 | | | |
| Dark portion with whipped potatoes | 11-oz. entree | 1,370 | 36.0 | | | |
| Parmesan | 20-oz. dinner | 2,080 | 51.0 | | | |
| (Weight Watchers): | | | | | | |
| Cacciatore, boil-in-bag | 10-oz. serving | 1,110 | 8.0 | | | |
| Imperial | 9¼-oz. serving | 840 | 4.0 | | | |
| Parmigiano | 8-oz. serving | 960 | 16.0 | | | |
| Southern fried party | 6½-oz. serving | 787 | 17.0 | | | |
| Sweet & sour with oriental vegetables | 9-oz. serving | 800 | 4.0 | | | |

**CHICKEN & DUMPLINGS**
(See **CHICKEN DINNER**)

| | | | | | | |
|---|---|---|---|---|---|---|
| **CHICKEN FRICASSEE,** home recipe (USDA)[1] | 1 cup (8.5 oz.) | 370 | 22.3 | 7. | 15. | 96 |

**CHICKEN, FRIED,** frozen:
(Banquet):

| | | | | | | |
|---|---|---|---|---|---|---|
| Assorted | 32-oz. pkg. | 6,005 | 95.0 | | | |
| Breast portion | 22-oz. pkg. | 3,860 | 60.0 | | | |
| Drum Snackers | 12-oz. pkg. | 2,128 | 40.0 | | | |
| *Hot 'n' Spicy* | 32-oz. pkg. | 6,005 | 95.0 | | | |

(USDA): United States Department of Agriculture
*Prepared as Package Directs
[1]Principal source of fat: chicken.

| Food and Description | Measure or Quantity | Sodium (mg.) | Total | — Fats in grams — Satu- rated | Unsatu- rated | Choles- terol (mg.) |
|---|---|---|---|---|---|---|
| Thigh & drumstick | 25-oz. pkg. | 4,460 | 80.0 | | | |
| Wings | 12-oz. pkg. | 2,128 | 40.0 | | | |
| (Swanson) *Plump & Juicy:* | | | | | | |
| Assorted: | | | | | | |
| Regular | 3¼-oz. serving | 600 | 17.0 | | | |
| Take-out | 3¼-oz. serving | 660 | 17.0 | | | |
| Breast | 4½-oz. serving | 830 | 21.0 | | | |
| Cutlets | 3½-oz. serving | 440 | 13.0 | | | |
| *Dipsters* | 3-oz. serving | 400 | 14.0 | | | |
| Drumlets | 3-oz. serving | 400 | 14.0 | | | |
| *Nibblers* | 3¼-oz. serving | 640 | 20.0 | | | |
| Thigh & drumstick | 3¼-oz. serving | 550 | 19.0 | | | |
| **CHICKEN GIBLETS** (USDA): | | | | | | |
| Capon, raw | 2 oz. | | 8.3 | | | |
| Fryer, raw | 2 oz. | | 1.8 | | | |
| Fryer, fried, from a 2½-lb. chicken | 1 heart, gizzard & liver (2.1 oz.) | | 6.7 | | | |
| Hen & cock, raw | 2 oz. | | 6.6 | | | |
| Roaster, raw | 2 oz. | | 2.7 | | | |
| **CHICKEN GIZZARD** (USDA): | | | | | | |
| Raw | 2 oz. | 37 | 1.5 | | | 82 |
| Simmered | 2 oz. | 32 | 1.9 | | | 111 |
| **CHICKEN & NOODLES:** | | | | | | |
| Home recipe (USDA)[1] | 1 cup (8.5 oz.) | 600 | 18.5 | 5. | 14. | 96 |
| Frozen (Stouffer's) | 5¾-oz. serving | 720 | 15.0 | | | |
| **CHICKEN NUGGETS,** frozen (Banquet) breaded & fried: | | | | | | |
| Regular | 12-oz. pkg. | 2,292 | 56.0 | | | |
| & cheddar | 12-oz. pkg. | | 76.0 | | | |
| *Hot 'n' Spicy* | 11-oz. pkg. | | 56.0 | | | |
| **CHICKEN, PACKAGED:** | | | | | | |
| (Carl Buddig) smoked, sliced | 1 oz. | 340 | 3.0 | .7 | 1.3 | 12 |
| (Eckrich) breast, sliced | 1 slice | 210 | .5 | | | |
| (Louis Rich) breast, oven roasted | 1-oz. slice | | 2.0 | | | |

(USDA): United States Department of Agriculture
*Prepared as Package Directs
[1]Principal sources of fat: chicken & egg.

| Food and Description | Measure or Quantity | Sodium (mg.) | Fats in grams | | | Choles-terol (mg.) |
|---|---|---|---|---|---|---|
| | | | Total | Satu-rated | Unsatu-rated | |
| **CHICKEN PATTIES,** frozen | | | | | | |
| (Banquet) breaded & fried | 12-oz. pkg. | 2,052 | 56.0 | | | |
| | | | | | | |
| **CHICKEN PIE:** | | | | | | |
| Baked, home recipe (USDA)[1] | 4¼" pie (8 oz.) | 581 | 30.6 | 11. | 19. | 70 |
| Baked, home recipe (USDA)[1] | ⅓ of 9" pie (8.2 oz.) | 594 | 31.3 | 12. | 20. | 72 |
| Frozen: | | | | | | |
| Commercial, unheated (USDA)[2] | 8-oz. pie | 933 | 26.1 | 7. | 19. | 29 |
| (Banquet) | 8-oz. pie | 966 | 24.0 | | | |
| (Stouffer's) | 10-oz. pie | 1,530 | 28.0 | | | |
| (Swanson): | 8-oz. pie | 981 | 24.4 | | | |
| Regular | 8-oz. pie | 840 | 24.0 | | | |
| *Chunky* | 10-oz. pie | 850 | 33.0 | | | |
| *Hungry-Man* | 16-oz. pie | 1,670 | 37.0 | | | |
| | | | | | | |
| **CHICKEN, POTTED** (USDA) | 1 oz. | | 5.4 | | | |
| | | | | | | |
| **CHICKEN SALAD OR SPREAD,** canned: | | | | | | |
| (Carnation) *Spreadable* | ¼ of 7½-oz. can | 230 | 8.8 | | | |
| (Hormel): | | | | | | |
| Regular | 1 oz. | 304 | 4.0 | | | |
| Lunche loaf | 1 oz. | 252 | 5.0 | | | |
| Sandwich Makin's | 1 oz. | 252 | 4.0 | | | |
| (Swanson) | 1 oz. | 140 | 4.0 | | | |
| (Underwood) | ½ of 4¾-oz. can | 575 | 10.9 | | | |
| | | | | | | |
| **CHICKEN SOUP,** canned (See **SOUP,** Chicken) | | | | | | |
| | | | | | | |
| **CHICKEN SOUP MIX** (See **SOUP, MIX,** Chicken) | | | | | | |
| | | | | | | |
| **CHICKEN STEW,** canned | | | | | | |
| (Swanson) | 7⅝ oz. serving | 960 | 7.0 | | | |

(USDA): United States Department of Agriculture
\*Prepared as Package Directs
[1]Principal sources of fat: vegetable shortening, cream, chicken & butter.
[2]Principal sources of fat: vegetable shortening, chicken, cream & corn oil.

| Food and Description | Measure or Quantity | Sodium (mg.) | — Fats in grams — | | | Cholesterol (mg.) |
|---|---|---|---|---|---|---|
| | | | Total | Saturated | Unsaturated | |

**CHICKEN STICKS,** frozen

(Banquet) breaded & fried — 12-oz. pkg. — 2,264 — 52.0

**CHICKEN STOCK BASE**

(French's) — 1 tsp. (3 grams) — 475 — .2

*CHICK-FIL-A:*

| Food and Description | Measure or Quantity | Sodium (mg.) | Total | Cholesterol (mg.) |
|---|---|---|---|---|
| Brownie, fudge, with nuts | 2.8-oz. piece | 213 | 19.1 | |
| Carrot-raisin salad: | | | | |
| Small | 2.7-oz. cup | 8 | 4.8 | 6 |
| Large | 13.1-oz. cup | 37 | 23.7 | 30 |
| Chargrill: | | | | |
| Without bun | 3.6-oz. serving | 770 | 2.5 | 41 |
| With bun | 5¾-oz. serving | 1,027 | 13.7 | 46 |
| Chicken salad cup | 3.4-oz. serving | 543 | 28.2 | 21 |
| Chicken salad plate | 11.8-oz. serving | 1,839 | 63.4 | 97 |
| Chicken salad sandwich | 5.7-oz. serving | 888 | 26.5 | 50 |
| Chicken soup, hearty, breast of, small | 8.5-oz. serving | 530 | 2.7 | 46 |
| *Chick-fil-A:* | | | | |
| Without bun | 3.6-oz. serving | 552 | 6.8 | 42 |
| With bun | 5.7-oz. serving | 1,174 | 8.8 | 66 |
| *Chick-fil-A Nuggets:* | | | | |
| 8-pack | 4-oz. serving | 1,326 | 15.1 | 61 |
| 11-pack | 6-oz. serving | 1,989 | 22.6 | 92 |
| Cole slaw: | | | | |
| 1 cup | 3.7 oz. | 158 | 14.0 | 13 |
| 1 pint | 15¼ oz. | 648 | 67.6 | 52 |
| *Icedream* | 4½ oz. | 51 | 4.8 | 24 |
| Lemonade | Regular order | Tr. | Tr. | Tr. |
| Orange juice | 6 fl. oz. | 2 | Tr. | 0 |
| Pie, lemon | 4.1-oz. slice | 300 | 5.1 | 7 |
| Potato salad | 3.8-oz. cup | 337 | 15.0 | 5 |
| Potato fries, waffle | 3-oz. order | 45 | 13.5 | 7 |
| Tea, iced, unsweetened | 9 fl. oz. | 0 | Tr. | 0 |

*CHICK'N QUICK,* frozen

(Tyson):

| Food and Description | Measure or Quantity | Total Fat |
|---|---|---|
| Breast fillet | 3 oz. | 8.0 |
| Kiev | 5 oz. | 31.0 |
| *Chick'n Cheddar* | 3 oz. | 17.0 |

(USDA): United States Department of Agriculture
*Prepared as Package Directs

| Food and Description | Measure or Quantity | Sodium (mg.) | —Fats in grams— | | | Cholesterol (mg.) |
|---|---|---|---|---|---|---|
| | | | Total | Saturated | Unsaturated | |
| **CHICK PEA OR GARBANZO:** | | | | | | |
| Dry (USDA) | 1 lb. | 118 | 21.8 | 2. | 20. | 0 |
| Dry (USDA) | 1 cup (7.1 oz.) | 52 | 9.6 | Tr. | 10. | 0 |
| Canned, regular pack, solids & liq.: | | | | | | |
| (Allen) | ½ cup | 330 | 3.0 | | | (0) |
| (Furman's) | ⅓ cup (2.6 oz.) | 275 | .7 | | | (0) |
| **CHICORY GREENS,** raw (USDA): | | | | | | |
| Untrimmed | ½ lb. (weighed untrimmed) | | .6 | | | 0 |
| Trimmed | 4 oz. | | .3 | | | 0 |
| **CHICORY, WITLOOF,** Belgian or French endive, raw, bleached head (USDA): | | | | | | |
| Untrimmed | ½ lb. (weighed untrimmed) | 14 | .2 | | | 0 |
| Trimmed, cut | ½ cup (.9 oz.) | 2 | < .1 | | | 0 |
| **CHILI OR CHILI CON CARNE:** | | | | | | |
| Canned, beans only: | | | | | | |
| (Comstock) | ½ cup (4.4 oz.) | 540 | 0.0 | | | |
| (Hormel) in sauce | 5 oz. | 453 | 3.0 | | | |
| Canned, with beans, regular: | | | | | | |
| (USDA) | 1 cup (8.8 oz.) | 1,328 | 15.2 | 8. | 8. | |
| (Gebhardt) hot | ½ of 15-oz. can | 1,000 | 22.0 | | | |
| (Hormel): | | | | | | |
| Regular | ½ of 15-oz. can | 1,127 | 17.0 | | | |
| Hot | ½ of 15-oz. can | 1,121 | 16.0 | | | |
| (Libby's) | ½ of 15-oz. can | 810 | 13.0 | | | |
| (Old El Paso) | 1 cup | 907 | 21.4 | | | |
| Canned, without beans, dietetic: | | | | | | |
| (Estee) | 7½-oz. can | 130 | 28.0 | | | |
| (Featherweight) | 7½-oz. can | 85 | 13.0 | | | |
| Canned without beans: | | | | | | |
| (USDA) not less than 60% meat nor more than 8% cereal & seasonings[1] | 1 cup (9 oz.) | | 37.7 | 18. | 20. | |

(USDA): United States Department of Agriculture
*Prepared as Package Directs
[1]Principal source of fat: beef.

CHILI OR CHILI CON CARNE (Continued)

| Food and Description | Measure or Quantity | Sodium (mg.) | Fats in grams — Total | Satu- rated | Unsatu- rated | Choles- terol (mg.) |
|---|---|---|---|---|---|---|
| (Gebhardt) | 7½ oz. | 1,040 | 32.0 | | | |
| (Hormel): | | | | | | |
| Regular | 7½-oz. serving | 1,101 | 32.0 | | | |
| Hot | ½ of 15-oz. can | 985 | 28.0 | | | |
| *Short Orders* | 7½-oz. can | 961 | 27.0 | | | |
| (Libby's) | ½ of 15-oz. can | | 30.0 | | | |
| Frozen, with beans (Stouffer's) | 8¾-oz. bag | 1,265 | 10.0 | | | |
| **CHILI MAC** (Hormel) *Short Orders* | 7½-oz. can | 1,418 | 10.0 | | | |
| **CHILI POWDER,** with added seasoning (USDA) | 1 T. (.5 oz.) | 236 | 1.9 | | | |
| **CHILI SAUCE:** | | | | | | |
| (USDA) | ½ cup (4.4 oz.) | 1,659 | .4 | | | |
| (USDA) | 1 T. (.5 oz.) | 201 | <.1 | | | |
| (USDA) low sodium | ½ cup (4.4 oz.) | 6-43 | .4 | | | |
| (USDA) low sodium | 1 T. (.5 oz.) | <1-5 | <.1 | | | |
| (Del Monte) | ¼ cup | 835 | 0.0 | | | |
| (El Molino) green, mild | 1 T. | 105 | 0.0 | | | |
| (Featherweight) low sodium | 1 T. | 10 | 0.0 | | | |
| (Ortega): | | | | | | |
| Hot or medium | 1 oz. | 181 | .1 | | | 0 |
| Mild | 1 oz. | 180 | .1 | | | 0 |
| **CHILI SEASONING MIX:** | | | | | | |
| *(Durkee) | 1 cup | 979 | 25.0 | | | |
| (French's) *Chili-O:* | | | | | | |
| Plain | ⅙ of pkg. | 630 | 0.0 | | | |
| With onion | ⅙ of pkg. | 710 | 0.0 | | | |

**CHINESE DATE** (See **JUJUBE**)

**CHINESE DINNER,** (See individual dinners such as Chow Mein)

**CHINESE VEGETABLES** (See **VEGETABLES, MIXED**)

**CHIPS** (See **CRACKERS** for corn chips and **POTATO CHIPS**)

(USDA): United States Department of Agriculture
*Prepared as Package Directs

130

| Food and Description | Measure or Quantity | Sodium (mg.) | — Fats in grams — | | | Choles- terol (mg.) |
|---|---|---|---|---|---|---|
| | | | Total | Satu- rated | Unsatu- rated | |
| **CHIVES,** raw (USDA) | 1 oz. | | <.1 | | | 0 |
| *CHOCO-DILES* (Hostess) | 2-oz. cake | 284 | 10.2 | | | 20 |
| **CHOCOLATE, BAKING:** | | | | | | |
| Bitter or unsweetened: | | | | | | |
| (USDA) | 1 oz. | 1 | 15.0 | 9. | 6. | 0 |
| Grated (USDA) | ½ cup (2.3 oz.) | 3 | 35.0 | 20. | 15. | 0 |
| (Baker's) | 1-oz. sq. | 1 | 15.0 | | | Tr. |
| (Hershey's) | 1 oz. | 5 | 16.0 | | | 4 |
| Sweetened: | | | | | | |
| Bittersweet (USDA) | 1 oz. | <1 | 11.3 | 7. | 5. | 0 |
| Chips, milk (Hershey's) | 1 oz. | 35 | 8.0 | | | |
| Chips, semisweet (Baker's) | ¼ cup (1.5 oz.) | 9 | 10.5 | | | Tr. |
| Chips, semisweet (Hershey's) | 1 oz. | 3 | 8.0 | | | 5 |
| *German's,* sweet (Baker's) | 4½" sq. (1 oz.) | <1 | 9.3 | | | Tr. |
| Morsels, milk (Nestlé's) | 1 oz. | 20 | 9.0 | | | 5 |
| Morsels, semisweet (Nestlé's) | 6-oz. pkg. | 4 | 47.6 | | | |
| Morsels, semisweet (Nestlé's) | 1 oz. | 0 | 8.0 | | | 0 |
| Semisweet, small pieces (USDA) | ½ cup (3 oz.) | 2 | 30.3 | 17. | 13. | |

**CHOCOLATE CAKE** (See
  **CAKE,** Chocolate)

**CHOCOLATE CAKE MIX** (See
  **CAKE MIX,** Chocolate)

**CHOCOLATE CANDY** (See
  **CANDY**)

**CHOCOLATE, HOT,** home
recipe (USDA)  1 cup (8.8 oz.)  120  12.5  8.  5.  31

**CHOCOLATE ICE CREAM**
  (See **ICE CREAM,** Chocolate)

**CHOCOLATE PIE** (See **PIE,**
  Chocolate)

(USDA): United States Department of Agriculture
*Prepared as Package Directs

131

| Food and Description | Measure or Quantity | Sodium (mg.) | Fats in grams — Total | Satu- rated | Unsatu- rated | Choles- terol (mg.) |
|---|---|---|---|---|---|---|
| **CHOCOLATE PIE FILLING** (See **PUDDING OR PIE FILLING,** Chocolate) | | | | | | |
| **CHOCOLATE PUDDING** (See **PUDDING or PIE FILLING,** Chocolate) | | | | | | |
| **CHOCOLATE SOFT DRINK** (See **SOFT DRINK,** Chocolate) | | | | | | |
| **CHOCOLATE SYRUP** (See **SYRUP,** Chocolate) | | | | | | |
| **CHOP SUEY:** | | | | | | |
| Home recipe, with meat (USDA)[1] | 1 cup (8.8 oz.) | 1,052 | 17.0 | 7. | 10. | 64 |
| Canned, with meat (USDA)[2] | 1 cup (8.8 oz.) | 1,378 | 8.0 | 2. | 6. | 7 |
| Frozen: | | | | | | |
| (Banquet) beef: | | | | | | |
| *Buffet Supper* | 32-oz. pkg. | 5,336 | 11.8 | | | |
| *Cookin' Bag* | 7-oz. pkg. | 1,140 | 1.4 | | | |
| Dinner | 12-oz. dinner | 1,802 | 8.2 | | | |
| (Stouffer's) beef, with rice | 12-oz. pkg. | 2,040 | 10.0 | | | |
| **\*CHOP SUEY SEASONING MIX** (Durkee) | 1¾ cups | 5,582 | 32.4 | | | |
| **CHOP SUEY VEGETABLES** (See **VEGETABLES, MIXED**) | | | | | | |
| **CHOW CHOW:** | | | | | | |
| Sour (USDA) | 1 oz. | 379 | .4 | | | 0 |
| Sweet (USDA) | 1 oz. | 149 | .3 | | | 0 |
| **CHOW MEIN:** | | | | | | |
| Home recipe, chicken, without noodles (USDA)[3] | 4 oz. | 325 | 4.5 | 1. | 3. | |
| Canned: | | | | | | |
| (Chun King) Divider-Pak: | | | | | | |

(USDA): United States Department of Agriculture
\*Prepared as Package Directs
[1]Principal sources of fat: butter, beef & pork.
[2]Principal sources of fat: pork, beef & corn oil.
[3]Principal sources of fat: chicken, corn oil & soybeans.

132

| Food and Description | Measure or Quantity | Sodium (mg.) | — Fats in grams — | | | Choles- terol (mg.) |
|---|---|---|---|---|---|---|
| | | | Total | Satu- rated | Unsatu- rated | |
| Chicken | ¼ of pkg. | 821 | 3.6 | | | 13 |
| Pork | ¼ of pkg. | 490 | 3.8 | | | 23 |
| Shrimp | ¼ of pkg. | 258 | 2.1 | | | 28 |
| (La Choy): | | | | | | |
| Regular: | | | | | | |
| Beef | ¾ cup | 890 | 1.0 | | | <20 |
| Chicken | ¾ cup | 800 | 2.0 | | | <20 |
| Meatless | ¾ cup | 780 | 1.0 | | | Tr. |
| Shrimp | ¾ cup | 820 | 1.0 | | | <50 |
| *Bi-pack: | | | | | | |
| Beef | ¾ cup | 840 | 1.0 | | | <20 |
| Chicken | ¾ cup | 970 | 3.0 | | | <20 |
| Shrimp | ¾ cup | 860 | 1.0 | | | <35 |
| Frozen: | | | | | | |
| (Armour) chicken, *Classic Lite* | 10½-oz. pkg. | 1,180 | 4.0 | | | 60 |
| (Blue Star) *Dining Lite* | 11¼-oz. pkg. | 1,450 | 1.3 | | | |
| (La Choy): | | | | | | |
| Regular, chicken | 12-oz. dinner | 1,740 | 4.0 | | | |
| Fresh & Lite, Imperial chicken | 11-oz. entree | 950 | 7.0 | | | |
| (Morton) chicken, light | 11-oz. dinner | 700 | 5.0 | | | |
| (Stouffer's) chicken with rice, *Lean Cuisine* | 11¼-oz. pkg. | 1,155 | 4.0 | | | 25 |
| (Van de Kamp's) Mandarin: | | | | | | |
| Beef | 11-oz. pkg. | 1,700 | 10.0 | | | |
| Chicken | 11-oz. pkg. | 1,180 | 10.0 | | | |
| **CHOW MEIN NOODLES** (See **NOODLES, CHOW MEIN**) | | | | | | |
| **CHOW MEIN SEASONING MIX** (Kikkoman) | 1⅛-oz. pkg. | 3 | .8 | | | <1 |
| **CHOW MEIN VEGETABLES** (See **VEGETABLES, MIXED**) | | | | | | |
| **CHUB,** raw (USDA): | | | | | | |
| Whole | 1 lb. (weighed whole) | | 13.2 | | | |
| Meat only | 4 oz. | | 10.0 | | | |

(USDA): United States Department of Agriculture
*Prepared as Package Directs

| Food and Description | Measure or Quantity | Sodium (mg.) | —Fats in grams— | | | Choles-terol (mg.) |
|---|---|---|---|---|---|---|
| | | | Total | Satu-rated | Unsatu-rated | |
| **CHURCH'S FRIED CHICKEN:** | | | | | | |
| Chicken, fried: | | | | | | |
| Breast | 4.3 oz. | 560 | 17.3 | | | |
| Leg | 2.9 oz. | 286 | 8.6 | | | |
| Thigh | 4.2 oz. | 448 | 21.6 | | | |
| Wing-breast | 4.8 oz. | 583 | 19.7 | | | |
| Corn, with butter oil | 1 ear | 20 | 9.3 | | | |
| French fries | 1 regular order | 126 | 5.5 | | | |
| | | | | | | |
| **CIDER** (See **APPLE CIDER**) | | | | | | |
| | | | | | | |
| **CINNAMON:** | | | | | | |
| Ground (Information supplied by General Mills Laboratory) | 1 oz. | | 1.0 | | | (0) |
| Stick (Spice Islands) | 1 stick | <1 | | | | (0) |
| With sugar (French's) | 1 tsp. (4 grams) | | Tr. | | | (0) |
| | | | | | | |
| **CITRON, CANDIED** (USDA) | 1 oz. | 82 | <.1 | | | 0 |
| | | | | | | |
| *****CITRUS BERRY BLEND,** mix dietetic (Sunkist) | 8 fl. oz. | 20 | 0.0 | | | |
| | | | | | | |
| **CITRUS COOLER** (Hi-C) | 6 fl. oz. (6.3 oz.) | 4 | Tr. | | | 0 |
| | | | | | | |
| **CLAM:** | | | | | | |
| Raw, all kinds, meat & liq. (USDA) | 4 oz. | | 1.0 | | | |
| Raw, all kinds, meat only (USDA) | 4 med. clams (3 oz.) | 102 | 1.4 | | | 42 |
| Raw, hard or round (USDA): | | | | | | |
| Meat & liq. | 1 lb. (weighed in shell) | | .6 | | | |
| Meat only | 1 cup (7 round chowders, 8 oz.) | 465 | 2.0 | | | 114 |
| Raw, soft (USDA): | | | | | | |
| Meat & liq. | 1 lb. (weighed in shell) | | 2.6 | | | |
| Meat only | 1 cup (19 large, 8 oz.) | 82 | 4.3 | | | 114 |
| Canned, all kinds: | | | | | | |
| Solids & liq. (USDA) | 4 oz. | | .8 | | | |

(USDA): United States Department of Agriculture
*Prepared as Package Directs

| Food and Description | Measure or Quantity | Sodium (mg.) | — Fats in grams — | | | Choles-terol (mg.) |
|---|---|---|---|---|---|---|
| | | | Total | Satu-rated | Unsatu-rated | |
| Meat only (USDA) | ½ cup (2.8 oz.) | | 2.0 | | | 50 |
| Minced, drained solids | | | | | | |
| (Gorton's) | 1 can | 1,280 | 20.0 | | | |
| Frozen, fried: | | | | | | |
| Strips, crunchy (Gorton's) | 1 pkg. | 920 | 30.0 | | | |
| Light (Mrs. Paul's) | 5-oz. pkg. | 770 | 26.0 | | | |

**CLAM CHOWDER** (See **SOUP,** Chowder, Clam)

**CLAM FRITTERS,** (See **FRITTERS,** Clam)

**CLAM SANDWICH,** frozen,

| (Mrs. Paul's) | 4½-oz. piece | | 16.1 | | | |
|---|---|---|---|---|---|---|

**CLARET WINE** (Gold Seal) 12% alcohol

| alcohol | 3 fl. oz. (3.1 oz.) | 3 | 0.0 | | | (0) |
|---|---|---|---|---|---|---|

**CLOVE:**

| Ground (Spice Islands) | 1 tsp. | <1 | | | | (0) |
|---|---|---|---|---|---|---|
| Whole (Spice Islands) | 1 clove | <1 | | | | (0) |

**CLUB SODA SOFT DRINK** (See **SOFT DRINK,** Club)

**COCOA,** dry:
Plain (USDA):

| Low fat | ½ cup (1.5 oz.) | 3 | 3.4 | 2. | 2. | 0 |
|---|---|---|---|---|---|---|
| Low fat | 1 T. (5 grams) | <1 | .4 | Tr. | Tr. | 0 |
| Medium-low fat | ½ cup (1.5 oz.) | 3 | 5.5 | 3. | 2. | 0 |
| Medium-low fat | 1 T. (5 grams) | <1 | .7 | Tr. | Tr. | 0 |
| Medium-high fat | ½ cup (1.5 oz.) | 3 | 8.2 | 5. | 3. | 0 |
| Medium-high fat | 1 T. (5 grams) | <1 | 1.0 | <1. | Tr. | 0 |
| High-fat | ½ cup (1.5 oz.) | 3 | 10.2 | 6. | 5. | 0 |
| High-fat | 1 T. (5 grams) | <1 | 1.3 | <1. | <1. | 0 |

Processed with alkali (USDA):

| Medium-low fat | ½ cup (1.5 oz.) | 308 | 5.5 | 3. | 2. | 0 |
|---|---|---|---|---|---|---|
| Medium-low fat | 1 T. (5 grams) | 39 | .7 | Tr. | Tr. | 0 |
| Medium-high fat | ½ cup (1.5 oz.) | 308 | 8.2 | 5. | 3. | 0 |
| Medium-high fat | 1 T. (5 grams) | 39 | 1.0 | <1. | Tr. | 0 |
| High-fat | ½ cup (1.5 oz.) | 308 | 10.2 | 6. | 5. | 0 |

(USDA): United States Department of Agriculture
*Prepared as Package Directs

| Food and Description | Measure or Quantity | Sodium (mg.) | Total | Fats in grams — Saturated | Fats in grams — Unsaturated | Cholesterol (mg.) |
|---|---|---|---|---|---|---|
| High-fat | 1 T. (5 grams) | 39 | 1.3 | < 1. | < 1. | 0 |
| Unsweetened (Hershey's) | 1/3 cup (1 oz.) | 10 | 4.0 | | | 0 |
| **COCOA, HOME RECIPE** | | | | | | |
| (USDA) | 1 cup (8.8 oz.) | 128 | 11.5 | 8. | 4. | 35 |
| ***COCOA KRISPIES,*** cereal | | | | | | |
| (Kellogg's) | 3/4 cup (1 oz.) | 195 | 0.0 | | | (0) |
| **COCOA MIX:** | | | | | | |
| Regular: | | | | | | |
| (USDA): | | | | | | |
| With nonfat dry milk[1] | 1 oz. | 149 | .8 | < 1. | Tr. | |
| Without nonfat dry milk[2] | 1 oz. | 76 | .6 | Tr. | Tr. | 0 |
| (Carnation) chocolate with mini-marshmallows, milk chocolate or rich chocolate[3] | 1-oz. packet | 120 | 1.0 | | | 2 |
| (Hershey's) instant | 1 T. | 15 | .3 | | | Tr. |
| (Nestlé) | 1 1/4 oz. | 110 | 4.0 | | | 0 |
| (Swiss Miss): | | | | | | |
| Regular: | | | | | | |
| Double rich | 1 envelope | 160 | 3.0 | | | |
| Milk chocolate | 1 envelope or 3-4 heaping tsp. | 170 | 3.0 | | | |
| European creme: | | | | | | |
| Amaretto, creme de menthe or mocha | 1 1/4-oz. env. | 120 | 4.0 | | | |
| Chocolate | 1 1/4-oz. env. | 180 | 4.0 | | | |
| Dietetic: | | | | | | |
| (Carnation): | | | | | | |
| *70 Calorie* | .73-oz. packet | 125 | 0.0 | | | 2 |
| Sugar free | .5-oz. packet | 160 | < 1.0 | | | 2 |
| *(Estee) | 6 fl. oz. | 75 | Tr. | | | |
| (Swiss Miss): | | | | | | |
| Lite | 1 envelope | 210 | Tr. | | | |
| Milk chocolate or with sugar free mini marshmallows | 1 envelope | 190 | Tr. | | | |
| ***COCOA PUFFS,*** cereal | | | | | | |
| (General Mills) | 1 cup (1 oz.) | 205 | 1.0 | | | (0) |

(USDA): United States Department of Agriculture
*Prepared as Package Directs
[1]Principal sources of fat: cocoa & milk.
[2]Principal source of fat: cocoa.
[3]Principal sources of fat: milk, cocoa & modified coconut oil.

| Food and Description | Measure or Quantity | Sodium (mg.) | —Fats in grams— | | | Choles- terol (mg.) |
|---|---|---|---|---|---|---|
| | | | Total | Satu- rated | Unsatu- rated | |
| **COCONUT:** | | | | | | |
| Fresh (USDA): | | | | | | |
| Whole | 1 lb. (weighed in shell) | 54 | 83.3 | 72. | 11. | 0 |
| Meat only | 4 oz. | 26 | 40.0 | 34. | 6. | 0 |
| Meat only | 2″ × 2″ × ½″ piece (1.6 oz.) | 10 | 15.9 | 14. | 2. | 0 |
| Grated or shredded | 1 firmly packed cup (4.6 oz.) | 30 | 45.9 | 39. | 7. | 0 |
| Grated | 1 lightly packed cup (2.9 oz.) | 18 | 28.2 | 24. | 4. | 0 |
| Cream, liq. expressed from grated coconut | 4 oz. | 5 | 36.5 | 32. | 5. | 0 |
| Milk, liq. expressed from mixture of grated coconut & water | 4 oz. | | 28.2 | 25. | 3. | 0 |
| Water, liq. from coconut | 1 cup (8.5 oz.) | 60 | .5 | | | 0 |
| Dried, canned or packaged: | | | | | | |
| Sweetened, shredded (USDA) | ½ lightly packed cup (1.6 oz.) | | 18.0 | 16. | 2. | 0 |
| Unsweetened (USDA) | ½ lightly packed cup (1.6 oz.) | | 30.0 | 26. | 4. | 0 |
| *Angel-Flake* (Baker's) | ½ cup (1.3 oz.) | 86 | 11.8 | | | 0 |
| Cookie (Baker's) | ½ cup (2 oz.) | 136 | 18.6 | | | 0 |
| Cream of (Coco Lopez) | 1 T. | 5 | 2.5 | | | (0) |
| Crunchies (Baker's) | ½ cup (2.1 oz.) | 144 | 30.2 | | | 0 |
| Premium shred (Baker's) | ½ cup (1.5 oz.) | 100 | 13.8 | | | 0 |
| Southern-style (Baker's) | ½ cup (1.5 oz.) | | 13.4 | | | 0 |
| ***COCO WHEATS,*** cereal | 2 T. (.6 oz.) | 1 | .6 | | | (0) |
| **COD:** | | | | | | |
| Raw, whole (USDA) | 1 lb. (weighed whole) | 98 | .4 | | | 70 |
| Raw, meat only (USDA) | 4 oz. | 79 | .3 | | | 57 |
| Raw, meat rinsed in brine (USDA) | 4 oz. | 289 | .3 | | | 57 |
| Broiled (USDA) | 4 oz. | 125 | 6.0 | | | |
| Canned (USDA) | 4 oz. | | .3 | | | |
| Dehydrated, lightly salted (USDA) | 4 oz. | 9,185 | 3.2 | | | |

(USDA): United States Department of Agriculture
*Prepared as Package Directs

| Food and Description | Measure or Quantity | Sodium (mg.) | — Fats in grams — | | Choles- terol (mg.) |
|---|---|---|---|---|---|
| | | | Total | Satu- rated   Unsatu- rated | |
| Dried, salted (USDA) | 4 oz. | | .8 | | 93 |
| Dried, salted (USDA) | 5½" × 1½" × ½" (2.8 oz.) | | .6 | | 66 |
| Frozen (Gorton's) | 4 oz. | 70 | 1.0 | | |

**COD DINNER OR ENTREE,**
frozen:

| | | | | | |
|---|---|---|---|---|---|
| (Armour) *Dinner Classics,* almondine | 12-oz. dinner | 1,440 | 15.0 | | 95 |
| (Blue Star) *Dining Lite,* fillet | 10-oz. meal | 570 | 5.7 | | |
| (Frionor) *Norway Gourmet:* | | | | | |
| With dill sauce | 4.5-oz. piece | 169 | 0.0 | | 0 |
| With toasted bread crumbs | 4.5-oz. piece | 359 | 8.0 | | 14 |

**CODFISH CAKE** (See **FISH CAKE**)

**COFFEE:**
Regular:

| | | | | | |
|---|---|---|---|---|---|
| *Max-Pax | ¾ cup | 1 | Tr. | | 0 |
| *(Maxwell House) | ¾ cup | Tr. | Tr. | | 0 |
| *(Yuban) | ¾ cup | Tr. | Tr. | | 0 |
| Instant: | | | | | |
| Dry (USDA) | 1 oz. | 20 | Tr. | | 0 |
| Dry (USDA) | 1 rounded tsp. (2 grams) | 2 | Tr. | | 0 |
| *(USDA) | 1 cup (8.4 oz.) | 2 | Tr. | | 0 |
| *(Maxwell House) | ¾ cup | Tr. | Tr. | | 0 |
| *(Yuban) | ¾ cup | Tr. | Tr. | | 0 |
| Decaffeinated: | | | | | |
| *Decaf* | 1 tsp. (2 grams) | Tr. | 0.0 | | (0) |
| *Sanka regular | ¾ cup | Tr. | Tr. | | 0 |
| *Sanka instant | ¾ cup | Tr. | Tr. | | 0 |
| *Siesta | ¾ cup | 1 | Tr. | | 0 |
| Freeze-dried: | | | | | |
| *Maxim | ¾ cup | Tr. | Tr. | | 0 |
| *Sanka | ¾ cup | Tr. | Tr. | | 0 |

**COFFEE SOUTHERN,** liqueur,

| | | | | | |
|---|---|---|---|---|---|
| 55 proof | 1 fl. oz. | Tr. | 0.0 | | 0 |

(USDA): United States Department of Agriculture
*Prepared as Package Directs

| Food and Description | Measure or Quantity | Sodium (mg.) | Total | Satu- rated | Unsatu- rated | Choles- terol (mg.) |
|---|---|---|---|---|---|---|
| **COLA SOFT DRINK** (See **SOFT DRINK,** Cola) | | | | | | |
| **COLESLAW,** not drained (USDA): | | | | | | |
| Prepared with commercial French dressing [1] | 4 oz. | 304 | 8.3 | 1. | 7. | |
| Prepared with homemade French dressing, using corn oil [2] | 4 oz. | 149 | 13.9 | 1. | 13. | |
| Prepared with homemade French dressing, using cottonseed oil [3] | 4 oz. | 149 | 13.9 | 3. | 10. | |
| Prepared with mayonnaise [2] | 4 oz. | 136 | 15.9 | 2. | 14. | |
| Prepared with mayonnaise-type salad dressing [2] | 4 oz. | 141 | 9.0 | 1. | 8. | |
| **COLLARDS:** | | | | | | |
| Raw (USDA): | | | | | | |
| Leaves, including stems | 1 lb. | 195 | 3.2 | | | 0 |
| Leaves only | ½ lb. | | 1.2 | | | 0 |
| Boiled without salt, drained (USDA): | | | | | | |
| Leaves, cooked in large amount of water | ½ cup (3.4 oz.) | | .7 | | | 0 |
| Leaves & stems, cooked in small amount of water | 4 oz. | 28 | .7 | | | 0 |
| Leaves, cooked in small amount of water | ½ cup (3.4 oz.) | | .7 | | | 0 |
| Canned, chopped, solids & liq.: | | | | | | |
| (Allen) | ½ cup (4 oz.) | 15 | Tr. | | | (0) |
| (Sunshine) | ½ cup (4.1 oz.) | 378 | .4 | | | (0) |
| Frozen: | | | | | | |
| Not thawed (USDA) | 10-oz. pkg. | 51 | 1.1 | | | 0 |
| Boiled, chopped, drained (USDA) | ½ cup (3 oz.) | 14 | .3 | | | 0 |
| (Birds Eye) chopped | ⅓ of 10-oz. pkg. | 45 | .4 | | | 0 |
| (Frosty Acres) | ⅓ of 10-oz. pkg. | 45 | 0.0 | | | (0) |
| (McKenzie) | ⅓ of 10-oz. pkg. | 56 | 0.0 | | | (0) |
| (Southland) | ⅕ of 16-oz. pkg. | 45 | Tr. | | | (0) |

(USDA): United States Department of Agriculture
*Prepared as Package Directs
[1]Principal sources of fat: soybean oil, cottonseed oil & corn oil.
[2]Principal source of fat: corn oil.
[3]Principal source of fat: cottonseed oil.

| Food and Description | Measure or Quantity | Sodium (mg.) | —Fats in grams— | | | Choles-terol (mg.) |
|---|---|---|---|---|---|---|
| | | | Total | Satu-rated | Unsatu-rated | |
| **CONCORD WINE:** | | | | | | |
| (Gold Seal) 13-14% alcohol | 3 fl. oz. (3.3 oz.) | 3 | 0.0 | | | (0) |
| (Pleasant Valley) red. 12.5% alcohol | 3 fl. oz. | 23 | 0.0 | | | 0 |
| | | | | | | |
| **COOKIE, COMMERCIAL:** | | | | | | |
| Almond Supreme (Pepperidge Farm) | 1 piece | 21 | 5.0 | | | |
| Animal: | | | | | | |
| (Dixie Belle) | 1 piece | 7 | .2 | | | |
| (Nabisco) *Barnum's Animals* | 1 piece | 11 | .4 | | | |
| (Sunshine) | 1 piece | 13 | .3 | | | 0 |
| (Tom's) | 1/2 oz. | 200 | 5.0 | | | |
| Apricot Raspberry (Pepperidge Farm) | 1 piece | 26 | 2.0 | | | |
| Assortment: (Nabisco) *Mayfair:* | | | | | | |
| Crown creme sandwich | 1 piece | | 2.3 | | | |
| Fancy shortbread biscuit | 1 piece | | 1.7 | | | |
| Filigree creme sandwich | 1 piece | | 2.5 | | | |
| *Mayfair* creme sandwich | 1 piece | | 3.0 | | | |
| Tea rose creme | 1 piece | | 2.3 | | | |
| (Pepperidge Farm): | | | | | | |
| Butter | 1 piece | 25 | 3.0 | | | |
| *Champagne* | 1 piece | 18 | 1.3 | | | |
| Chocolate lace & Pirouette | 1 piece | 15 | 2.0 | | | |
| Seville | 1 piece | 25 | 3.0 | | | |
| *Southport* | 1 piece | 35 | 4.5 | | | |
| Blueberry (Pepperidge Farm) | 1 piece | 23 | 2.5 | | | |
| *Blueberry Newtons* (Nabisco) | 1 piece | 53 | 1.3 | | | |
| *Bordeaux* (Pepperidge Farm) | 1 piece | 23 | 1.6 | | | |
| Brown edge wafer (Nabisco) | 1 piece | 16 | 1.5 | | | |
| Brownie: | | | | | | |
| (Hostess) | 1 1/4-oz. piece | 76 | 6.0 | | | 11 |
| (Nabisco) *Almost Home* | 1 1/4-oz. piece | 75 | 7.0 | | | |
| (Pepperidge Farm) chocolate nut | .4-oz. piece | 27 | 3.3 | | | |
| *Brussels* (Pepperidge Farm) | 1 piece | 32 | 2.6 | | | |
| *Brussels Mint* (Pepperidge Farm) | 1 piece | 40 | 3.3 | | | |
| Butter (Sunshine) | 1 piece | 37 | 1.0 | | | < 1 |
| *Cappucino* (Pepperidge Farm) | 1 piece | 20 | 3.0 | | | |
| *Chessman* (Pepperidge Farm) | 1 piece | 26 | 2.0 | | | |

(USDA): United States Department of Agriculture
*Prepared as Package Directs

| Food and Description | Measure or Quantity | Sodium (mg.) | — Fats in grams — | | | Cholesterol (mg.) |
|---|---|---|---|---|---|---|
| | | | Total | Saturated | Unsaturated | |
| Chocolate & chocolate-covered: | | | | | | |
| (Keebler) stripes | 1 piece | 50 | 3.0 | | | |
| (Nabisco): | | | | | | |
| Pin Wheel, cake | 1 piece | 35 | 5.0 | | | |
| Snap | 1 piece | 20 | .6 | | | |
| (Sunshine) nuggets | 1 piece | 18 | 1.0 | | | < 1 |
| Chocolate chip: | | | | | | |
| (Keebler) Rich 'n Chips | 1 piece | 70 | 4.0 | | | |
| (Nabisco): | | | | | | |
| Almost Home, fudge | 1 piece | 65 | 2.5 | | | |
| Chips Ahoy: | | | | | | |
| Regular | 1 piece | 32 | 2.3 | | | |
| Chewy | 1 piece | 55 | 3.0 | | | |
| Snaps | 1 piece | 17 | .7 | | | |
| (Pepperidge Farm): | | | | | | |
| Regular | 1 piece | 30 | 2.6 | | | |
| Chocolate | 1 piece | 25 | 3.0 | | | |
| Mocha | 1 piece | 22 | 2.0 | | | |
| (Sunshine): | | | | | | |
| Chip-A-Roos, regular | 1 piece | 50 | 3.0 | | | Tr. |
| Chippy Chews | 1 piece | 35 | 2.0 | | | 0 |
| (Tom's) | 1.7-oz. serving | 120 | 9.0 | | | |
| Cinnamon Raisin (Nabisco) Almost Home | 1 piece | 47 | 3.5 | | | |
| Coconut bars (USDA)[1] | 1 oz. | 42 | 6.9 | 2. | 5. | |
| Creme stick (Dutch Twin) | 1 piece | 3 | 2.1 | | | |
| Danish (Nabisco) Imported | 1 piece | 14 | 1.6 | | | |
| Date Nut Granola (Pepperidge Farm) | 1 piece | 32 | 3.0 | | | |
| Fig bar: | | | | | | |
| (Nabisco) Fig Newtons | 1 piece | 50 | 1.0 | | | |
| (Sunshine) Chewies | 1 piece | 30 | 1.0 | | | 0 |
| (Tom's) | 1.8-oz. serving | 130 | 2.0 | | | |
| Fruit Stick (Nabisco) Almost Home: | | | | | | |
| Apple | 1 piece | 30 | 2.5 | | | |
| Blueberry | 1 piece | 90 | 2.0 | | | |
| Cherry | 1 piece | 100 | 2.0 | | | |
| Iced dutch apple | 1 piece | 40 | 1.0 | | | |
| Gingerman (Pepperidge Farm) | 1 piece | 25 | 1.3 | | | |

(USDA): United States Department of Agriculture
*Prepared as Package Directs
[1]Principal sources of fat: butter, egg & coconut

| Food and Description | Measure or Quantity | Sodium (mg.) | Fats in grams — Total | Saturated | Unsaturated | Cholesterol (mg.) |
|---|---|---|---|---|---|---|
| Ginger Snap: | | | | | | |
| (Nabisco) | 1 piece | 50 | .7 | | | |
| (Sunshine) | 1 piece | 23 | .7 | | | 0 |
| Golden Fruit Raisin (Sunshine) | 1 piece | 40 | 1.0 | | | 0 |
| Hazelnut (Pepperidge Farm) | 1 piece | 37 | 3.0 | | | |
| Ladyfinger (USDA)[1] | 3¼″ × 1⅜″ × 1⅛″ | 8 | .9 | .2 | .7 | 40 |
| *Lemon Coolers* (Sunshine) | 1 piece | 22 | 1.3 | | | Tr. |
| Lemon nut (Pepperidge Farm) | 1 piece | 25 | 3.3 | | | |
| *Lido* (Pepperidge Farm) | 1 piece | 42 | .5 | | | |
| Macaroon, coconut (Nabisco) | 1 piece | 65 | 9.0 | | | |
| *Mallopuffs* (Sunshine) | 1 piece | 60 | 2.0 | | | 0 |
| Marshmallow: | | | | | | |
| (Nabisco) | | | | | | |
| *Mallomars* | 1 piece | 17 | 3.0 | | | |
| Puffs, cocoa covered | 1 piece | 55 | 4.0 | | | |
| Sandwich | 1 piece | 20 | .8 | | | |
| *Twirl* cakes | 1 piece | 55 | 5.0 | | | |
| *Milano* (Pepperidge Farm) | 1 piece | 26 | 3.3 | | | |
| *Mint Milano* (Pepperidge Farm) | 1 piece | 35 | 4.3 | | | |
| Molasses (Nabisco) *Pantry* | 1 piece | 65 | 2.0 | | | |
| Molasses Crisp (Pepperidge Farm) | 1 piece | 25 | 1.6 | | | |
| *Nilla* wafer (Nabisco) | 1 piece | 14 | .6 | | | |
| Oatmeal: | | | | | | |
| (Keebler) old fashioned | 1 piece | 115 | 3.0 | | | |
| (Nabisco) *Bakers Bonus* | 1 piece | 45 | 2.5 | | | |
| (Pepperidge Farm): | | | | | | |
| Irish | 1 piece | 40 | 2.3 | | | |
| Raisin | 1 piece | 57 | 2.7 | | | |
| (Sunshine) Country | 1 piece | 60 | 2.0 | | | 0 |
| *Orange Milano* (Pepperidge Farm) | 1 piece | 35 | 4.3 | | | |
| *Orbits* (Sunshine) butter | 1 piece | 19 | .5 | | | Tr. |
| Peanut & peanut butter (Nabisco): | | | | | | |
| *Almost Home,* regular | 1 piece | 47 | 3.5 | | | |
| *Nutter-Butter,* sandwich | 1 piece | 50 | 3.0 | | | |
| Pecan Sandies (Keebler) | 1 piece | 75 | 5.0 | | | |
| Raisin: | | | | | | |
| (Nabisco) *Almost Home:* | | | | | | |
| Fudge chocolate chip | 1 piece | 42 | 2.5 | | | |
| Iced applesauce | 1 piece | 35 | 4.0 | | | |

(USDA): United States Department of Agriculture
*Prepared as Package Directs

| Food and Description | Measure or Quantity | Sodium (mg.) | — Fats in grams — | | | Choles- terol (mg.) |
|---|---|---|---|---|---|---|
| | | | Total | Satu- rated | Unsatu- rated | |
| (Pepperidge Farm) bran | 1 piece | 27 | 2.7 | | | |
| Raisin bran (Pepperidge Farm) *Kitchen Hearth* | 1 piece | 26 | 2.7 | | | |
| Sandwich: | | | | | | |
| (Keebler): | | | | | | |
| Fudge creme | 1 piece | 30 | 3.0 | | | |
| *Pitter Patter* | 1 piece | 120 | 4.0 | | | |
| (Nabisco): | | | | | | |
| Regular: | | | | | | |
| *Baronet* | 1 piece | 25 | 2.0 | | | |
| *Gaity* | 1 piece | 28 | 1.7 | | | |
| *Giggles,* chocolate | 1 piece | 35 | 3.0 | | | |
| *I Screams* | 1 piece | 35 | 3.5 | | | |
| *Oreo,* regular | 1 piece | 57 | 2.0 | | | |
| *Almost Home,* fudge | 1 piece | 120 | 6.0 | | | |
| (Sunshine): | | | | | | |
| Regular, *Hydrox* | 1 piece | 45 | 2.0 | | | 0 |
| *Chips 'n Middles,* fudge | 1 piece | 65 | 3.0 | | | Tr. |
| *Tru-Blu* | 1 piece | 75 | 3.0 | | | 0 |
| Shortbread or shortcake: | | | | | | |
| (Nabisco): | | | | | | |
| *Lorna Doone* | 1 piece | 33 | 1.7 | | | |
| Pecan | 1 piece | 40 | 4.5 | | | |
| (Pepperidge Farm) | 1 piece | 43 | 4.0 | | | |
| *Social Tea,* biscuit (Nabisco) | 1 piece | 18 | .7 | | | |
| Sprinkles (Sunshine) | 1 piece | 65 | 2.0 | | | 0 |
| Sugar cookie (Nabisco) rings, *Bakers Bonus* | 1 piece | 50 | 2.5 | | | |
| Sugar wafer: | | | | | | |
| (Dutch Twin) any flavor | 1 piece | 2 | 1.8 | | | |
| (Nabisco) *Biscos* | 1 piece | 4 | .9 | | | |
| (Sunshine) | 1 piece | 12 | 2.0 | | | 0 |
| Tahiti (Pepperidge Farm) | 1 piece | 25 | 5.5 | | | |
| Toy (Sunshine) | 1 piece | 18 | .4 | | | 0 |
| Vanilla Wafer: | | | | | | |
| (Keebler) | 1 piece | 17 | 1.0 | | | |
| (Sunshine) | 1 piece | 16 | 1.0 | | | 1 |
| (Tom's) | 1.7-oz. serving | 160 | 8.0 | | | |
| Waffle creme (Dutch Twin) | 1 piece | | 2.4 | .5 | 2. | 0 |

**COOKIE CRISP,** cereal:

| | | | | | | |
|---|---|---|---|---|---|---|
| Chocolate chip | 1 cup (1 oz.) | 188 | 1.0 | | | |
| Vanilla | 1 cup (1 oz.) | 200 | 1.1 | | | |

(USDA): United States Department of Agriculture
*Prepared as Package Directs

| Food and Description | Measure or Quantity | Sodium (mg.) | — Fats in grams — | | | Cholesterol (mg.) |
|---|---|---|---|---|---|---|
| | | | Total | Saturated | Unsaturated | |
| **COOKIE, DIETETIC:** | | | | | | |
| Almond chocolate wafer (Estee) | 1 piece | 2 | 1.7 | | | |
| Angel puffs (Stella D'oro) | 1 piece (3 grams) | 2 | 1.0 | | | |
| Apple pastry (Stella D'oro) | 1 piece (.8 oz.) | 42 | 3.9 | | | |
| Assorted (Estee) | 1 piece (6 grams) | 3 | 1.4 | Tr. | 1. | |
| Assorted filled wafers (Estee) | 1 piece (5 grams) | 3 | 1.3 | Tr. | 1. | |
| Banana wafers (Estee) | 1 piece | 12 | 8.5 | | | |
| *Beljuin Treats* (Estee) | 1 piece | 10 | 1.7 | | | |
| Chocolate chip (Estee) | 1 piece (6 grams) | 11 | 1.0 | Tr. | <1. | |
| Chocolate Holland filled wafer (Estee) | 1 piece (3 grams) | 1 | 1.2 | Tr. | <1. | 1 |
| Chocolate & vanilla wafer (Estee) | 1 piece (4 grams) | 3 | 1.3 | Tr. | 1. | |
| Fig pastry (Stella D'oro) | 1 piece (.9 oz.) | 20 | 3.7 | | | |
| Fruit flavored wafer (Estee) | 1 piece (4 grams) | 1 | 1.2 | Tr. | <1. | 1 |
| *Have-A-Heart* (Stella D'oro) | 1 piece (.7 oz.) | 22 | 5.1 | | | |
| Holland bittersweet wafer (Estee) | 1 piece | 3 | 8.3 | | | |
| Holland milk chocolate wafer (Estee) | 1 piece (.8 oz.) | 3 | 8.3 | 3. | 6. | 8 |
| Kichel (Stella D'oro) | 1 piece (1 gram) | 2 | .5 | | | |
| *Monties* (Estee) | 1 piece | 10 | 2.2 | | | |
| Oatmeal raisin (Estee) | 1 piece (7 grams) | 2 | 1.4 | Tr. | 1. | 2 |
| Pastry stick (Estee) | 1 piece (7 grams) | 3 | 2.1 | 2. | Tr. | |
| Peach-apricot pastry (Stella D'oro) | 1 piece (.8 oz.) | 14 | 4.2 | | | |
| Prune pastry (Stella D'oro) | 1 piece (.8 oz.) | 15 | 3.4 | | | |
| *Royal Nuggets* (Stella D'oro) | 1 piece (<1 gram) | 1 | .1 | | | |
| Sandwich, chocolate (Estee) | 1 piece (8 grams) | 3 | 2.1 | <1. | 2. | |
| Sandwich, Duplex (Estee) | 1 piece (9 grams) | 3 | 2.0 | <1. | 1. | |
| **COOKIE DOUGH:** | | | | | | |
| *Refrigerated (Pillsbury): Brownie, Fudge: Regular | 1/24 of pkg. | 115 | 5.0 | | | |

(USDA): United States Department of Agriculture
*Prepared as Package Directs

| Food and Description | Measure or Quantity | Sodium (mg.) | — Fats in grams — | | | Choles- terol (mg.) |
|---|---|---|---|---|---|---|
| | | | Total | Satu- rated | Unsatu- rated | |
| Microwave with chocolate flavored chips | 1/9 of pkg. | 110 | 9.0 | | | |
| Chocolate chip | 1 cookie | 55 | 3.0 | | | |
| Chocolate chocolate chip | 1 cookie | 35 | 3.0 | | | |
| Oatmeal raisin | 1 cookie | 60 | 3.0 | | | |
| Peanut butter | 1 cookie | 70 | 3.0 | | | |
| Sugar | 1 cookie | 70 | 3.0 | | | |
| *Frozen (Rich's): | | | | | | |
| Chocolate chip | 1 cookie | 120 | 5.9 | | | 7 |
| Oatmeal: | | | | | | |
| Regular | 1 cookie | 90 | 5.2 | | | 1 |
| With raisins | 1 cookie | 73 | 4.4 | | | 6 |
| Super jumbo | 1 cookie | 226 | 13.1 | | | 2 |
| Peanut butter | 1 cookie | 185 | 6.5 | | | 2 |
| Ranger | 1 cookie | 90 | 7.0 | | | 5 |
| Sugar | 1 cookie | 111 | 5.4 | | | 6 |

## COOKIE, HOME RECIPE:

| Food and Description | Measure or Quantity | Sodium (mg.) | Total | Satu- rated | Unsatu- rated | Choles- terol (mg.) |
|---|---|---|---|---|---|---|
| Brownie with nuts (USDA): | | | | | | |
| Made with butter[1] | 1 oz. | 71 | 8.5 | 3. | 6. | 24 |
| Made with butter[1] | .7-oz. piece (1¾" × 1¾" × ⅞") | 50 | 6.0 | 2. | 4. | 17 |
| Made with vegetable shortening[2] | 1 oz. | 71 | 8.9 | 2. | 7. | |
| Chocolate Chip (USDA): | | | | | | |
| Made with butter[3] | 1 oz. | 99 | 8.0 | 4. | 4. | |
| Made with vegetable shortening[2] | 1 oz. | 99 | 8.5 | 2. | 6. | |
| Sugar, soft, thick (USDA): | | | | | | |
| Made with butter[4] | 1 oz. | 90 | 4.3 | 2. | 2. | |
| Made with vegetable shortening[5] | 1 oz. | 90 | 4.8 | 1. | 4. | |

## COOKIE MIX:

| Food and Description | Measure or Quantity | Sodium (mg.) | Total | Satu- rated | Unsatu- rated | Choles- terol (mg.) |
|---|---|---|---|---|---|---|
| Plain, dry (USDA)[6] | 1 oz. | 100 | 6.9 | 2. | 5. | |

(USDA): United States Department of Agriculture
*Prepared as Package Directs
[1]Principal sources of fat: pecans, butter, chocolate & egg.
[2]Principal sources of fat: pecans, vegetable shortening, chocolate & egg.
[3]Principal sources of fat: butter, chocolate, walnuts & egg.
[4]Principal sources of fat: butter, egg & milk.
[5]Principal sources of fat: vegetable shortening, egg & milk.
[6]Principal source of fat: vegetable shortening.

| Food and Description | Measure or Quantity | Sodium (mg.) | — Fats in grams — | | | Cholesterol (mg.) |
|---|---|---|---|---|---|---|
| | | | Total | Saturated | Unsaturated | |
| *Plain, prepared with egg & water (USDA)[1] | 1 oz. | 98 | 6.9 | 2. | 5. | |
| *Plain, prepared with milk (USDA)[2] | 1 oz. | 98 | 6.7 | 2. | 5. | |
| Brownie: | | | | | | |
| Dry, with egg (USDA)[3] | 1 oz. | 85 | 3.4 | < 1. | 3. | |
| Dry, without egg (USDA)[4] | 1 oz. | 55 | 4.6 | 1. | 4. | |
| *Dry, with egg, prepared with water & nuts (USDA)[5] | 1 oz. | 62 | 5.3 | < 1. | 4. | |
| *Dry, without egg, prepared with egg, water & nuts (USDA)[5] | 1 oz. | 47 | 5.7 | 1. | 5. | |
| *(Betty Crocker): | | | | | | |
| Fudge: | | | | | | |
| Regular | 1/16 of pkg. | 100 | 6.0 | | | |
| Family size | 1/24 of pkg. | 95 | 5.0 | | | |
| Supreme | 1/24 of pkg. | 80 | 3.0 | | | |
| Golden, Family size | 1/24 of pkg. | 105 | 5.0 | | | |
| Walnut: | | | | | | |
| Regular | 1/16 of pkg. | 100 | 7.0 | | | |
| Family size | 1/24 of pkg. | 85 | 6.0 | | | |
| (Duncan Hines) | 1/24 of pkg. | 98 | 2.8 | | | 0 |
| *(Pillsbury) Fudge: | | | | | | |
| Deluxe: | | | | | | |
| Plain | 2″ square (1/16 pkg.) | 100 | 6.0 | | | |
| Family size | 2″ square (1/24 pkg.) | 95 | 7.0 | | | |
| With walnuts | 2″ square (1/16 pkg.) | 90 | 8.0 | | | |
| Microwave | 1/9 of pkg. | 105 | 9.0 | | | |
| Ultimate: | | | | | | |
| Caramel fudge chunk | 2″ square (1/16 pkg.) | 105 | 7.0 | | | |
| Double | 2″ square (1/16 pkg.) | 105 | 6.0 | | | |

(USDA): United States Department of Agriculture
*Prepared as Package Directs
[1]Principal sources of fat: vegetable shortening & egg.
[2]Principal sources of fat: vegetable shortening & milk.
[3]Principal sources of fat: vegetable shortening, cocoa & egg.
[4]Principal sources of fat: vegetable shortening & cocoa.
[5]Principal sources of fat: walnuts, vegetable shortening, cocoa & egg.

| Food and Description | Measure or Quantity | Sodium (mg.) | Fats in grams — Total | Satu- rated | Unsatu- rated | Choles- terol (mg.) |
|---|---|---|---|---|---|---|
| Rocky road | 2″ square (¹⁄₁₆ pkg) | 95 | 8.0 | | | |
| Chocolate (Duncan Hines) double | ¹⁄₃₆ of pkg. | 38 | 3.1 | | | 0 |
| Chocolate chip: | | | | | | |
| (Betty Crocker) *Big Batch* | 1 cookie | 47 | 3.0 | | | |
| (Duncan Hines) | ¹⁄₃₆ of pkg. | 42 | 3.6 | | | 0 |
| Date bar (Betty Crocker) | ¹⁄₂₄ of pkg. | 50 | 4.0 | | | |
| Macaroon (Betty Crocker) coconut | ¹⁄₂₄ of pkg. | 15 | 4.0 | | | |
| Oatmeal: | | | | | | |
| *(Betty Crocker) *Big Batch* | 1 cookie | 50 | 3.0 | | | |
| (Duncan Hines) Raisin | ¹⁄₃₆ of pkg. | 31 | 3.1 | | | 0 |
| *(Quaker) | 1 cookie | 71 | 2.8 | | | |
| Peanut Butter (Duncan Hines) | ¹⁄₃₆ of pkg. | 31 | 3.1 | | | |
| Sugar: | | | | | | |
| *(Betty Crocker) *Big Batch* | 1 cookie | 47 | 2.5 | | | |
| (Duncan Hines) | ¹⁄₃₆ of pkg. | 33 | 2.5 | | | 0 |
| *Vienna Dream Bar (Betty Crocker) | ¹⁄₂₄ of pkg. | 65 | 5.0 | | | |

**COOKING FATS** (See **FATS**)

**COOKING SPRAY,** *Mazola No Stick*

| | | | | | | |
|---|---|---|---|---|---|---|
| | 2-second spray | | .8 | | | 0 |

**CORIANDER,** whole or ground (Spice Islands)

| | | | | | | |
|---|---|---|---|---|---|---|
| | 1 tsp. | < 1 | | | | (0) |

**CORN:**
Fresh, white or yellow (USDA):

| Food and Description | Measure or Quantity | Sodium | Total | | | Choles |
|---|---|---|---|---|---|---|
| Raw, untrimmed, on cob | 1 lb. (weighed in husk) | Tr. | 1.6 | | | 0 |
| Raw, trimmed, on cob | 1 lb. (husk removed) | Tr. | 2.5 | | | 0 |
| Raw, kernels | 4 oz. | Tr. | 1.1 | | | 0 |
| Boiled without salt, kernels, cut from cob, drained | 1 cup (5.9 oz.) | Tr. | 1.7 | | | 0 |
| Boiled without salt, whole | 1 ear (5″ × 1¾″) (4.9 oz.) | Tr. | .8 | | | 0 |

Canned, regular pack:
Golden or yellow, whole

(USDA): United States Department of Agriculture
*Prepared as Package Directs

| Food and Description | Measure or Quantity | Sodium (mg.) | — Fats in grams — | | | Cholesterol (mg.) |
|---|---|---|---|---|---|---|
| | | | Total | Saturated | Unsaturated | |
| kernel: | | | | | | |
| Solids & liq., vacuum pack (USDA) | 1/2 cup (3.7 oz.) | 250 | .5 | | | 0 |
| Solids & liq., wet pack (USDA) | 1/2 cup (4.5 oz.) | 302 | .8 | | | 0 |
| Drained solids, wet pack (USDA) | 1/2 cup (3 oz.) | 203 | .7 | | | 0 |
| Drained liq., wet pack (USDA) | 4 oz. | 268 | Tr. | | | 0 |
| (Allen) whole kernel, solids and liq. | 1/2 cup (4.2 oz.) | 300 | <1 | | | (0) |
| (Comstock) solids and liq.: | | | | | | |
| Whole kernel | 1/2 cup | 350 | 0.0 | | | (0) |
| Cream style | 1/2 cup | 440 | 0.0 | | | (0) |
| (Del Monte) solids and liq.: | | | | | | |
| Whole kernel, regular or vacuum pack | 1/2 cup | 355 | 1.0 | | | (0) |
| Cream style | 1/2 cup (4 oz.) | 355 | 1.0 | | | (0) |
| (Green Giant) solids and liq.: | | | | | | |
| Cream style | 1/2 of 8 1/2-oz. can | 320 | 1.0 | | | (0) |
| Whole kernel: | | | | | | |
| Regular | 1/4 of 17-oz. can | 270 | 1.0 | | | (0) |
| *Mexicorn* | 1/2 of 7-oz. can | 335 | Tr. | | | (0) |
| Shoepeg | 1/4 of 17-oz. can | 270 | 1.0 | | | (0) |
| Vacuum pack | 1/2 of 7-oz. can | 230 | 0.0 | | | (0) |
| (Larsen) *Freshlike,* solids and liq.: | | | | | | |
| Cream style | 1/2 cup | 290 | 1.0 | | | (0) |
| Whole kernel: | | | | | | |
| Regular | 1/2 cup | 320 | 1.0 | | | (0) |
| Vacuum pack: | | | | | | |
| Plain | 1/2 cup | 260 | 1.0 | | | (0) |
| With peppers | 1/2 cup | 300 | 1.0 | | | |
| White, whole kernel: | | | | | | |
| Solids & liq., wet pack (USDA) | 1/2 cup (4.5 oz.) | 302 | .8 | | | 0 |
| Drained solids, wet pack (USDA) | 1/2 cup (2.8 oz.) | 189 | .6 | | | 0 |
| Drained liq., wet pack (USDA) | 4 oz. | 268 | Tr. | | | 0 |

(USDA): United States Department of Agriculture
*Prepared as Package Directs

| Food and Description | Measure or Quantity | Sodium (mg.) | Total | Fats in grams — Saturated | Unsaturated | Cholesterol (mg.) |
|---|---|---|---|---|---|---|
| (Del Monte) solids and liq.: | | | | | | |
| Cream style | ½ cup | 355 | 0.0 | | | (0) |
| Whole kernel | ½ cup | 355 | 0.0 | | | (0) |
| (Green Giant) solids and | | | | | | |
| liq., vacuum pack | 4 oz. | 315 | Tr. | | | (0) |
| Canned, white or yellow, dietetic pack: | | | | | | |
| Solids & liq., wet pack (USDA) | 4 oz. | 2 | .6 | | | 0 |
| Drained solids (USDA) | 4 oz. | 2 | .8 | | | 0 |
| Drained liq. (USDA) | 4 oz. (by wt.) | 2 | Tr. | | | 0 |
| (Del Monte) no added salt, solids and liq., any style | ½ cup | <10 | 1.0 | | | |
| (Diet Delight) whole kernel, solids and liq. | ½ cup (4.4 oz.) | 5 | 0.0 | | | |
| (Larsen) Fresh-Lite, whole kernel, water pack, solids and liq. | ½ cup (4.5 oz.) | 5 | 1.0 | | | |
| Frozen: | | | | | | |
| (Birds Eye): | | | | | | |
| On the cob: | | | | | | |
| Farmside | 4.4-oz. ear | 4 | 1.0 | | | 0 |
| Little Ears | 2.3-oz. ear | 2 | .5 | | | 0 |
| Whole kernel: | | | | | | |
| Plain | ⅓ of 10-oz. pkg. | 3 | .7 | | | 0 |
| With butter sauce | ⅓ of 10-oz. pkg. | 178 | 1.0 | | | 4 |
| (Frosty Acres): | | | | | | |
| On the cob | 1 whole ear | 0 | .5 | | | (0) |
| Kernels | 3.3 oz. | 5 | 1.0 | | | (0) |
| (Green Giant): | | | | | | |
| On the cob: | | | | | | |
| Nibblers | 2.7-oz. ear | 10 | 1.0 | | | (0) |
| Niblet-Ears | 4.9-oz. ear | 20 | .7 | | | (0) |
| Whole kernel: | | | | | | |
| In cream sauce, Niblets | ½ cup | 295 | 5.0 | | | |
| Harvest Fresh, Niblets | ½ cup | 280 | 0.0 | | | |
| Polybag, Niblets | ½ cup | 5 | 1.0 | | | |
| Shoepeg, white, in butter sauce | ½ cup | 290 | 2.0 | | | |
| (Larsen): | | | | | | |
| On the cob | 3-inch or 5-inch piece | 5 | 1.0 | | | |

(USDA): United States Department of Agriculture
*Prepared as Package Directs

| Food and Description | Measure or Quantity | Sodium (mg.) | Total | Fats in grams Saturated | Unsaturated | Cholesterol (mg.) |
|---|---|---|---|---|---|---|
| Whole kernel (McKenzie): | 3.3 oz. | 5 | 1.0 | | | |
| On the cob | 5-inch ear | 25 | 1.0 | | | |
| Whole kernel | 3.3 oz. | 19 | 1.0 | | | |

**CORNBREAD:**

| Food and Description | Measure or Quantity | Sodium (mg.) | Total | Saturated | Unsaturated | Cholesterol (mg.) |
|---|---|---|---|---|---|---|
| Corn pone, home recipe, prepared with white, whole-ground cornmeal (USDA)[1] | 4 oz. | 449 | 6.0 | 2. | 4. | |
| Corn sticks, frozen (Aunt Jemima) | 3 pieces (1¾ oz.) | 360 | 5.1 | | | |
| Johnnycake, home recipe, prepared with yellow, degermed cornmeal (USDA)[1] | 4 oz. | 782 | 5.9 | 2. | 4. | |
| Southern-style, home recipe, prepared with degermed cornmeal (USDA)[1] | 2½″ × 2½″ × 1⅝″ piece (2.9 oz.) | 491 | 5.0 | 1. | 4. | 58 |
| Southern-style, home recipe, prepared with whole-ground cornmeal (USDA)[1] | 4 oz. | 712 | 8.2 | 2. | 6. | |
| Spoonbread, home recipe, prepared with white, whole-ground cornmeal (USDA)[2] | 4 oz. | 547 | 12.9 | 5. | 8. | |

**CORNBREAD MIX:**

| Food and Description | Measure or Quantity | Sodium (mg.) | Total | Saturated | Unsaturated | Cholesterol (mg.) |
|---|---|---|---|---|---|---|
| Dry (USDA)[3] | 1 oz. | 328 | 3.6 | <1. | 3. | |
| *Prepared with egg & milk: | | | | | | |
| (USDA)[4] | 4 oz. | 844 | 9.5 | 3. | 6. | 78 |
| (USDA)[4] | 2⅜″ muffin (1.4 oz.) | 298 | 3.4 | 1. | 2. | 28 |
| (USDA)[4] | 2½″ × 2½″ × 1⅜″ piece (1.9 oz.) | 409 | 4.6 | 2. | 3. | 38 |

(USDA): United States Department of Agriculture
*Prepared as Package Directs
[1]Principal sources of fat: lard & egg.
[2]Principal sources of fat: lard, egg & milk.
[3]Principal sources of fat: vegetable shortening & egg.
[4]Principal sources of fat: vegetable shortening, milk & egg.

| Food and Description | Measure or Quantity | Sodium (mg.) | Total | Satu- rated | Unsatu- rated | Choles- terol (mg.) |
|---|---|---|---|---|---|---|
| | | | — Fats in grams — | | | |
| *(Aunt Jemima) | ⅙ of cornbread (2.4 oz.) | 600 | 7.0 | | | |
| *(Dromedary) | 2″ × 2″ piece (1.4 oz.) | 480 | 3.0 | | | |
| *(Pillsbury) *Ballard* | ⅛ of pkg. | 570 | 3.0 | | | |
| **CORN *CHEX,*** cereal, dry | 1¼ cups (1 oz.) | 304 | .1 | | | (0) |
| **CORN CHIPS** (See **CRACKERS**) | | | | | | |
| **CORNED BEEF:** | | | | | | |
| Uncooked, boneless, medium fat (USDA) | 1 lb. | 5,897 | 113.4 | 54. | 59. | |
| Cooked, boneless, medium fat (USDA) | 4 oz. | 1,973 | 34.5 | 17. | 17. | |
| Canned: | | | | | | |
| Lean (USDA) | 4 oz. | | 9.1 | 5. | 5. | |
| Medium fat (USDA) | 4 oz. | | 13.6 | 7. | 7. | |
| Fat (USDA) | 4 oz. | | 20.4 | 10. | 10. | |
| (Libby's) | ⅓ of 7-oz. can | 720 | 9.0 | | | |
| Packaged: | | | | | | |
| (Carl Buddig) | 1 oz. | 380 | 2.0 | .9 | .9 | 16 |
| (Eckrich) | 1-oz. serving | 340 | 2.0 | | | |
| (Oscar Mayer) | .7-oz. slice | 248 | .4 | | | 8 |
| **CORNED BEEF HASH,** canned: | | | | | | |
| With potato (USDA)[1] | 4 oz. | 612 | 12.8 | 6. | 7. | |
| (Libby's) | ½ of 15-oz. can | 1,260 | 27.0 | | | |
| *Mary Kitchen* (Hormel): | | | | | | |
| Regular | ½ of 15-oz. can | 1,396 | 24.0 | | | |
| *Short Orders* | 7½-oz. can | 1,368 | 24.0 | | | |
| **CORNED BEEF HASH DINNER,** frozen (Banquet) | 10-oz. dinner | 1,752 | 13.3 | | | |
| **CORNED BEEF SPREAD** (Underwood) | 4½-oz. can | 1,220 | 20.0 | | | |
| **CORN FLAKES,** cereal: | | | | | | |
| Whole (USDA) | 1 cup (1 oz.) | 291 | .1 | | | 0 |

(USDA): United States Department of Agriculture
*Prepared as Package Directs
[1]Principal source of fat: beef.

| Food and Description | Measure or Quantity | Sodium (mg.) | — Fats in grams — | | | Choles- terol (mg.) |
|---|---|---|---|---|---|---|
| | | | Total | Satu- rated | Unsatu- rated | |
| Crushed (USDA) | 1 cup (2.5 oz.) | 704 | .3 | | | 0 |
| Frosted (USDA) | 1 cup (1.4 oz.) | 310 | <.1 | | | 0 |
| (Featherweight) low sodium | 1¼ cups | 10 | 0.0 | | | (0) |
| (General Mills) *Country* | 1 cup (1 oz.) | 310 | <1.0 | | | (0) |
| (Kellogg's): | | | | | | |
| Regular | 1 cup (1 oz.) | 280 | 0.0 | | | (0) |
| Honey and nut | ¾ cup (1 oz.) | 190 | 1.0 | | | (0) |
| Sugar frosted | ¾ cup (1 oz.) | 190 | 0.0 | | | (0) |
| (Ralston Purina): | | | | | | |
| Regular | 1 cup (1 oz.) | 267 | .1 | | | (0) |
| Sugar frosted | ¾ cup (1 oz.) | 179 | .5 | | | (0) |

**CORN FRITTER** (See
**FRITTER,** Corn)

**CORN GRITS** (See **HOMINY**)

**CORNMEAL MIX:**

| Food and Description | Measure or Quantity | Sodium (mg.) | Total | Satu- rated | Unsatu- rated | Choles- terol (mg.) |
|---|---|---|---|---|---|---|
| Bolted (Aunt Jemima) | ¼ cup (1 oz.) | 337 | .7 | | | (0) |
| Self-rising (Aunt Jemima) | ¼ cup (1 oz.) | 382 | .9 | | | (0) |

**CORNMEAL, WHITE OR YELLOW:**

Dry (USDA):

| Food and Description | Measure or Quantity | Sodium (mg.) | Total | Satu- rated | Unsatu- rated | Choles- terol (mg.) |
|---|---|---|---|---|---|---|
| Bolted | 1 cup (4.3 oz.) | 1 | 4.1 | Tr. | 4. | 0 |
| Degermed | 1 cup (4.3 oz.) | 1 | 1.7 | | | 0 |
| Self-rising, degermed | 1 cup (5 oz.) | 1,946 | 1.6 | | | 0 |
| Self-rising, whole-ground | 1 cup (5 oz.) | 1,946 | 4.1 | Tr. | 4. | 0 |
| Whole-ground, unbolted | 1 cup (4.3 oz.) | 1 | 4.8 | Tr. | 5. | 0 |
| Cooked: | | | | | | |
| *Bolted (Aunt Jemina) | ⅔ cup | <1 | .7 | | | (0) |
| Degermed (USDA) | 1 cup (8.5 oz.) | 264 | .5 | | | 0 |
| *Degermed (Albers) | 1 cup | | .5 | | | (0) |
| *Degermed (Aunt Jemima) | ⅔ cup | <1 | .3 | | | (0) |

| Food and Description | Measure or Quantity | Sodium (mg.) | Total | Satu- rated | Unsatu- rated | Choles- terol (mg.) |
|---|---|---|---|---|---|---|
| **CORN POPS,** cereal (Kellogg's) | 1 cup (1 oz.) | 95 | 0.0 | | | |
| **CORN PUDDING,** home recipe (USDA)[1] | 1 cup (8.6 oz.) | 1,068 | 11.5 | 5. | 7. | 103 |
| **CORN SALAD,** raw (USDA): | | | | | | |
| Untrimmed | 1 lb. (weighed untrimmed) | | 1.7 | | | 0 |

(USDA): United States Department of Agriculture
*Prepared as Package Directs
[1]Principal sources of fat: milk, vegetable shortening & egg.

| Food and Description | Measure or Quantity | Sodium (mg.) | — Fats in grams — | | | Choles-terol (mg.) |
|---|---|---|---|---|---|---|
| | | | Total | Satu-rated | Unsatu-rated | |
| Trimmed | 4 oz. | | .5 | | | 0 |
| **CORN SOUFFLE,** frozen | | | | | | |
| (Stouffer's) | 12-oz. pkg. | 1,674 | 22.0 | | | |
| **CORNSTARCH:** | | | | | | |
| (USDA) | 1 cup (4.5 oz.) | Tr. | Tr. | | | 0 |
| (USDA) | 1 T. (8 grams) | Tr. | Tr. | | | 0 |
| (Argo) | 1 T. (10 grams) | Tr. | <.1 | | | 0 |
| (Duryeas) | 1 T. (10 grams) | Tr. | <.1 | | | 0 |
| (Kingsford's) | 1 T. (10 grams) | Tr. | <.1 | | | 0 |
| **CORNSTARCH PUDDING** (See **PUDDING,** Vanilla) | | | | | | |
| **CORN STICK** (See **CORNBREAD**) | | | | | | |
| **CORN *TOTAL,*** cereal (General Mills) | 1 cup (1 oz.) | 310 | 1.0 | | | (0) |
| **COTTAGE PUDDING,** home recipe (USDA)[1]: | | | | | | |
| Without sauce[2] | 2 oz. | 170 | 6.4 | 4. | 3. | |
| With chocolate sauce | 2 oz. | 132 | 5.0 | | | |
| With strawberry sauce | 2 oz. | 132 | 5.0 | | | |
| **COUGH DROP:** | | | | | | |
| (Beech-Nut) | 1 drop (2 grams) | <1 | 0.0 | | | (0) |
| (Estee) | 1 drop | <1 | Tr. | | | (0) |
| (Pine Bros.) | 1 drop (3 grams) | <1 | 0.0 | | | (0) |
| ***COUNT CHOCULA,*** cereal (General Mills) | 1 cup (1 oz.) | 205 | 1.0 | | | (0) |
| **COWPEA,** including black-eyed peas (USDA): Immature seeds: | | | | | | |
| Raw, whole | 1 lb. (weighed in pods) | 5 | 2.0 | | | 0 |

(USDA): United States Department of Agriculture
*Prepared as Package Directs
[1]Made with sodium aluminum sulfate-type baking powder.
[2]Principal sources of fat: butter, egg & milk.

| Food and Description | Measure or Quantity | Sodium (mg.) | —Fats in grams— | | | Cholesterol (mg.) |
|---|---|---|---|---|---|---|
| | | | Total | Saturated | Unsaturated | |
| Raw, shelled | ½ cup (2.5 oz.) | 1 | .6 | | | 0 |
| Boiled without salt, drained | ½ cup (2.9 oz.) | <1 | 1.7 | | | 0 |
| Canned, solids & liq. | 4 oz. | 268 | .3 | | | 0 |
| Frozen (See **BLACK-EYED PEA,** frozen) | | | | | | |
| Young pods with seeds: | | | | | | |
| Raw, whole | 1 lb. (weighed untrimmed) | 17 | 1.2 | | | 0 |
| Boiled without salt, drained | 4 oz. | 3 | .3 | | | 0 |
| Mature seeds, dry: | | | | | | |
| Raw | ½ cup (3 oz.) | 29 | 1.3 | | | 0 |
| Boiled without salt, drained | ½ cup (4.4 oz.) | 10 | .4 | | | 0 |
| **CRAB,** all species: | | | | | | |
| Fresh (USDA): | | | | | | |
| Steamed, whole | 1 lb. (weighed in shell) | | 4.1 | | | 218 |
| Steamed, meat only | 1 cup (4.4 oz.) | | 2.4 | | | 125 |
| Canned: | | | | | | |
| Drained solids (USDA) | 1 packed cup (5.6 oz.) | 1,600 | 4.0 | | | 162 |
| (Del Monte) Alaska King | 7½-oz. can | 1,178 | .6 | | | |
| Frozen (Wakefield's) Alaska King, thawed & drained | 4 oz. | 1 | 1.1 | | | 113 |
| **CRAB APPLE,** fresh (USDA): | | | | | | |
| Whole | 1 lb. (weighed whole) | 4 | 1.3 | | | 0 |
| Flesh only | 4 oz. | 1 | .3 | | | 0 |
| **CRAB AU GRATIN,** frozen | | | | | | |
| (Gorton's) *Light Recipe* | 1 pkg. | 810 | 13.0 | | | |
| **CRAB, DEVILED:** | | | | | | |
| Home recipe (USDA)[1] | 1 cup (8.5 oz.) | 2,081 | 22.6 | | | 245 |
| Frozen (Mrs. Paul's) | 3-oz. piece | 385 | 6.0 | | | |
| Frozen, miniature (Mrs. Paul's) | 3½-oz. serving | 195 | 10.0 | | | |

**CRAB, IMITATION** (See **SURIMI**)

(USDA): United States Department of Agriculture
*Prepared as Package Directs
[1]Prepared with bread cubes, butter, parsley, eggs, lemon juice & catsup.

| Food and Description | Measure or Quantity | Sodium (mg.) | —Fats in grams— | | | Cholesterol (mg.) |
|---|---|---|---|---|---|---|
| | | | Total | Saturated | Unsaturated | |

**CRAB IMPERIAL:**

| Food and Description | Measure or Quantity | Sodium (mg.) | Total | Saturated | Unsaturated | Cholesterol (mg.) |
|---|---|---|---|---|---|---|
| Home recipe (USDA)[1] | 1 cup (7.8 oz.) | 1,602 | 16.7 | | | 308 |
| Frozen (Gorton's) *Light Recipe,* stuffed | 1 pkg. | 950 | 15.0 | | | |

**CRACKERS, PUFFS AND CHIPS:**

| Food and Description | Measure or Quantity | Sodium (mg.) | Total | Saturated | Unsaturated | Cholesterol (mg.) |
|---|---|---|---|---|---|---|
| Arrowroot biscuit (Nabisco) | 1 piece | 13 | .7 | | | |
| Bacon-flavored thins (Nabisco) | 1 piece | 30 | .6 | | | |
| Bran wafer (Featherweight) low salt | 1 piece | < 1 | .2 | | | |
| *Bugles* (Tom's) | 1 oz. | 300 | 8.0 | | | |
| Cafe (Sunshine) | 1 piece | 45 | 1.0 | | | 0 |
| Cheese flavored: | | | | | | |
| *American Heritage* (Sunshine): | | | | | | |
| Cheddar | 1 piece | 30 | .8 | | | < 1 |
| Parmesan | 1 piece | 45 | 1.0 | | | < 1 |
| Cheddar sticks (Flavor Tree) | 1 oz. | 445 | 11.0 | | | |
| Cheese bites (Tom's) | 1½ oz. | 540 | 9.0 | | | |
| *Chee-Tos,* crunchy | 1 oz. | 280 | 10.0 | | | 0 |
| *Cheez Balls* (Planters) | 1 oz. | 270 | 11.0 | | | 0 |
| *Cheez Curls* (Planters) | 1 oz. | 290 | 11.0 | | | 0 |
| *Cheeze-It* (Sunshine) | 1 piece | 11 | .3 | | | 0 |
| Corn Cheese (Tom's) crunchy | 1⅝ oz. | 270 | 18.0 | | | |
| (Dixie Belle) | 1 piece | 10 | .2 | | | |
| *Nips* (Nabisco) | 1 piece | 10 | .2 | | | |
| *Tid-Bit* (Nabisco) | 1 piece | 12 | .3 | | | |
| *Chicken in a Biskit* (Nabisco) | 1 piece | 16 | .6 | | | |
| *Club* cracker (Keebler) | 1 piece | 39 | .7 | | | |
| Corn chips: | | | | | | |
| *Dipsy Doodle* (Wise) | 1 oz. | 180 | | | | |
| (Featherweight) low sodium | 1 oz. | 3 | 11.0 | | | |
| (Flavor Tree) | 1 oz. | 260 | 8.0 | | | |
| *Fritos* (Frito-Lay): | | | | | | |
| Regular | 1 oz. | 230 | 9.0 | | | 0 |
| Barbecue flavor | 1 oz. | 320 | 9.0 | | | 0 |
| (Laura Scudder's) | 1 oz. | 125 | 10.0 | | | 0 |
| (Tom's) regular | 1 oz. | 400 | 17.0 | | | |
| Corn Stick (Flavor Tree) | 1 oz. | 220 | 10.0 | | | |

(USDA): United States Department of Agriculture
*Prepared as Package Directs
[1]Prepared with butter, flour, milk, onion, green pepper, eggs & lemon juice.

| Food and Description | Measure or Quantity | Sodium (mg.) | — Fats in grams — | | | Cholesterol (mg.) |
|---|---|---|---|---|---|---|
| | | | Total | Saturated | Unsaturated | |
| *Crown Pilot* (Nabisco) | 1 piece | 65 | 1.0 | | | |
| *Diggers* (Nabisco) | 1 piece | 7 | 2.5 | | | |
| *English Water Biscuit* | | | | | | |
| (Pepperidge Farm) | 1 piece | 22 | .4 | | | |
| *Escort* (Nabisco) | 1 piece | 37 | 1.1 | | | |
| *Goldfish* (Pepperidge Farm) | | | | | | |
| tiny | 1 piece | 4 | Tr. | | | |
| Graham: | | | | | | |
| *Cinnamon Crisp* (Keebler) | 1 piece | 21 | .5 | | | |
| (Dixie Belle) sugar-honey | | | | | | |
| coated | 1 piece | 26 | .4 | | | |
| *Honeymaid* (Nabisco) | 1 piece | 45 | .5 | | | |
| (Sunshine) cinnamon | 1 piece | 24 | .7 | | | 0 |
| Graham, chocolate or | | | | | | |
| cocoa-covered: | | | | | | |
| (Keebler) | 1 piece | 25 | 2.0 | | | |
| (Nabisco) | 1 piece | | 2.7 | | | |
| *Great Crisps!* (Nabisco): | | | | | | |
| French onion | 1 piece | 13 | .6 | | | |
| Nacho | 1 piece | 31 | .5 | | | |
| Real bacon | 1 piece | 26 | .4 | | | |
| *Hi-Ho* (Sunshine) | 1 piece | 31 | 1.2 | | | <1 |
| *Meal Mates* (Nabisco) | 1 piece | 47 | 1.0 | | | |
| Melba Toast (See **MELBA TOAST**) | | | | | | |
| *Nachips* (Old El Paso) | 1 piece | 11 | 1.0 | | | |
| Nacho rings (Tom's) | 1 oz. | 330 | 11.0 | | | |
| Onion rings (Wise) | 1 oz. | 360 | | | | |
| Oyster: | | | | | | |
| (Dixie Belle) | 1 piece | 11 | .1 | | | |
| (Nabisco) *Dandy* or | | | | | | |
| *Oysterettes* | 1 piece | 11 | Tr. | | | |
| (Sunshine) | 1 piece | 12 | .1 | | | 0 |
| Party (Estee) | ½ oz. | 50 | 4.0 | | | 0 |
| Party mix (Flavor Tree) | 1 oz. | 400 | 11.0 | | | |
| Pizza Crunchies (Planters) | 1 oz. | 160 | 10.0 | | | |
| *Ritz* (Nabisco) | 1 piece | 30 | 1.0 | | | |
| *Roman Meal Wafer,* boxed | 1 piece | 20 | .5 | | | Tr. |
| *Royal Lunch* (Nabisco) | 1 piece | 80 | 2.0 | | | |
| Rusk, *Holland* (Nabisco) | 1 piece | 35 | 1.0 | | | |
| Rye toast (Keebler) | 1 piece | 29 | .8 | | | |

(USDA): United States Department of Agriculture
*Prepared as Package Directs

| Food and Description | Measure or Quantity | Sodium (mg.) | Total | Satu-rated | Unsatu-rated | Choles-terol (mg.) |
|---|---|---|---|---|---|---|
| *Ry-Krisp:* | | | | | | |
| Natural | 1 triple cracker | 48 | .1 | | | |
| Seasoned | 1 triple cracker | 65 | .4 | | | |
| Sesame | 1 triple cracker | 75 | .7 | | | |
| Saltine: | | | | | | |
| (Dixie Belle) regular | 1 piece | 36 | .3 | | | (0) |
| *Krispy* (Sunshine) | 1 piece | 42 | .2 | | | 0 |
| *Premium* (Nabisco) unsalted | 1 piece | 23 | .4 | | | (0) |
| *Zesta* (Keebler) | 1 piece | 41 | .4 | | | (0) |
| Sesame: | | | | | | |
| *American Heritage* (Sunshine) | 1 piece | 31 | 1.0 | | | 0 |
| Butter flavored (Nabisco) | 1 piece | | | | | |
| Chip (Flavor Tree) | 1 oz. | 410 | 10.0 | | | |
| Crunch (Flavor Tree) | 1 oz. | 70 | 10.0 | | | 0 |
| (Estee) | ½ oz. | 120 | 4.0 | | | 0 |
| Stick (Flavor Tree): | | | | | | |
| Regular | 1 oz. | 405 | 10.0 | | | |
| With bran | 1 oz. | 370 | 11.0 | | | |
| Toast (Keebler) | 1 piece | 28 | .8 | | | |
| Snackers (Ralston) | 1 piece | 23 | .8 | | | |
| *Snackin Crisp* (Durkee) *D&C* | 1 oz. | 257 | 10.0 | | | |
| Snacks Sticks (Pepperidge Farm): | | | | | | |
| Cheese | 1 piece | 43 | .8 | | | |
| Pumpernickel | 1 piece | 48 | .6 | | | |
| Sesame | 1 piece | 43 | .8 | | | |
| *Sociables* (Nabisco) | 1 piece | 22 | .5 | | | |
| Sour cream-onion stick (Flavor Tree) | 1 oz. | 415 | 10.0 | | | |
| Table Water Cracker (Carr's) small | 1 piece | | .7 | | | |
| Taco chip (Laura Scudder's) | 1 oz. | 200 | 8.0 | | | 0 |
| Tortilla chips: | | | | | | |
| *Doritos:* | | | | | | |
| Regular | 1 oz. | 230 | 6.0 | | | 0 |
| *Cool Ranch:* | | | | | | |
| Regular | 1 oz. | 190 | 7.0 | | | 0 |
| Light | 1 oz. | 240 | 4.0 | | | 0 |
| Nacho cheese: | | | | | | |
| Regular | 1 oz. | 240 | 7.0 | | | 0 |

(USDA): United States Department of Agriculture
*Prepared as Package Directs

| Food and Description | Measure or Quantity | Sodium (mg.) | Total | Fats in grams — Saturated | Unsaturated | Cholesterol (mg.) |
|---|---|---|---|---|---|---|
| Light | 1 oz. | 290 | 4.0 | | | 0 |
| *Salsa Rio* | 1 oz. | 170 | 7.0 | | | 0 |
| Taco | 1 oz. | 220 | 7.0 | | | 0 |
| (Laura Scudder's) | 1 oz. | 90 | 7.0 | | | 0 |
| (Planters) taco | 1 oz. | 150 | 8.0 | | | 0 |
| (Tom's) | 1½ oz. | 260 | 10.0 | | | |
| *Town House* (Keebler) | 1 piece | 29 | 1.0 | | | |
| *Triscuit* (Nabisco) regular | 1 piece | 30 | .7 | | | |
| *Tuc* (Keebler) | 1 piece | 28 | 1.3 | | | |
| *Twigs* (Nabisco) | 1 piece | 40 | .8 | | | |
| *Uneeda Biscuit* (Nabisco) unsalted | 1 piece | 33 | 1.0 | | | |
| Unsalted (Featherweight) | 2 sections (½ cracker) | 3 | 1.0 | | | |
| *Waverly* (Nabisco) | 1 piece | 40 | .7 | | | |
| Wheat (Pepperidge Farm) cracked or hearty | 1 piece | 50 | 1.4 | | | |
| Wheat Nuts (Flavor Tree) | 1 oz. | 185 | 18.0 | | | 0 |
| Wheat Snack (Dixie Belle) | 1 piece | 12 | .4 | | | |
| *Wheatsworth* (Nabisco) | 1 piece | 27 | .6 | | | |
| *Wheat Thins* (Nabisco) cheese | 1 piece | 15 | .4 | | | |
| Wheat Toast (Keebler) | 1 piece | 30 | .8 | | | |

**CRACKER CRUMBS:**

| | | | | | | |
|---|---|---|---|---|---|---|
| Graham (USDA)[1] | 1 cup (3 oz.) | 576 | 8.1 | 2. | 6. | |
| Graham (Keebler) | 3 oz. | 460 | 9.9 | | | |
| Graham (Nabisco) | 1½ cups (4.6 oz. or 9″ pie shell) | 823 | 14.0 | | | |
| Graham (Sunshine) | ½ cup | 495 | 7.0 | | | 0 |

***CRACKER JACK*** (See **POPCORN**)

**CRACKER MEAL:**

| | | | | | | |
|---|---|---|---|---|---|---|
| (USDA)[1] | 3 oz. | 935 | 11.1 | 3. | 8. | |
| (USDA) | 1 T. (.4 oz.) | 110 | 1.3 | Tr. | 1. | |

**CRACKER PIE CRUST MIX** (See **PIECRUST MIX**)

(USDA): United States Department of Agriculture
*Prepared as Package Directs
[1]Principal source of fat: vegetable shortening.

| Food and Description | Measure or Quantity | Sodium (mg.) | —Fats in grams— Total | Satu- rated | Unsatu- rated | Choles- terol (mg.) |
|---|---|---|---|---|---|---|
| **CRANAPPLE** (Ocean Spray): | | | | | | |
| Canned: | | | | | | |
| Regular | ½ cup (4.5 oz.) | 3 | .3 | | | 0 |
| Low calorie | ½ cup (4.2 oz.) | 4 | .1 | | | 0 |
| *Frozen | ½ cup (4.4 oz.) | 2 | Tr. | | | 0 |
| **CRANBERRY:** | | | | | | |
| Fresh: | | | | | | |
| Untrimmed (USDA) | 1 lb. (weighed with stems) | 9 | 3.0 | | | 0 |
| Stems removed (USDA) | 1 cup (4 oz.) | 2 | .8 | | | 0 |
| (Ocean Spray) | 1 oz. | < 1 | .5 | | | 0 |
| Dehydrated (USDA) | 1 oz. | 5 | 1.9 | | | |
| **CRANBERRY JUICE COCKTAIL:** | | | | | | |
| (USDA) approx. 33% cranberry juice | ½ cup (4.4 oz.) | 1 | .1 | | | 0 |
| Canned: | | | | | | |
| Regular (Ocean Spray) | ½ cup (4.4 oz.) | 2 | < .1 | | | 0 |
| Low calorie (Ocean Spray) | ½ cup (4.4 oz.) | 5 | < .1 | | | 0 |
| *Frozen (Ocean Spray) | ½ cup (4.4 oz.) | 1 | Tr. | | | |
| **CRANBERRY-ORANGE RELISH:** | | | | | | |
| Uncooked (USDA) | 4 oz. | 1 | .5 | | | 0 |
| (Ocean Spray) | 4 oz. | 12 | .4 | | | 0 |
| **CRANBERRY SAUCE:** | | | | | | |
| Home recipe, sweetened, unstrained (USDA) | 4 oz. | 1 | .3 | | | 0 |
| Canned: | | | | | | |
| Sweetened, strained (USDA) | ½ cup (4.8 oz.) | 1 | .3 | | | 0 |
| Jellied (Ocean Spray) | 4 oz. | | 1.5 | | | 0 |
| Whole berry (Ocean Spray) | 4 oz. | | .4 | | | 0 |
| **CRANORANGE RELISH** | | | | | | |
| (Ocean Spray) | 2 oz. | 18 | .1 | | | |
| **CRANPRUNE** (Ocean Spray) | ½ cup (4.4 oz.) | 3 | .1 | | | 0 |
| **CRAPPIE,** white, raw, meat only | | | | | | |
| (USDA) | 4 oz. | | .9 | | | |

(USDA): United States Department of Agriculture
*Prepared as Package Directs

| Food and Description | Measure or Quantity | Sodium (mg.) | — Fats in grams — | | | Choles- terol (mg.) |
|---|---|---|---|---|---|---|
| | | | Total | Satu- rated | Unsatu- rated | |
| **CRAYFISH,** freshwater (USDA): | | | | | | |
| Raw, in shell | 1 lb. (weighed in shell) | | .3 | | | |
| Raw, meat only | 4 oz. | | .6 | | | |
| **CRAZY COW,** cereal (General Mills) | 1 cup (1 oz.) | 185 | 1.0 | | | |
| **CREAM:** | | | | | | |
| Half & half: | | | | | | |
| (USDA) | 1 cup (8.5 oz.) | 111 | 28.3 | 15. | 14. | 104 |
| (USDA) | 1 T. (.5 oz.) | 7 | 1.8 | <1. | <1. | 6 |
| (Johanna Farms) | 1 T. (.5 oz.) | 6 | 1.7 | | | 6 |
| Light, table, or coffee: | | | | | | |
| (USDA) | 1 cup (8.5 oz.) | 103 | 49.4 | 26. | 23. | 158 |
| (USDA) | 1 T. (.5 oz.) | 6 | 3.1 | 2. | 1. | 10 |
| 18% butterfat (Johanna Farms) | 1 T. (.5 oz.) | 6 | 2.9 | | | 10 |
| Light whipping: | | | | | | |
| (USDA) | 1 cup (8.4 oz.) | 86 | 74.8 | 41. | 34. | |
| (USDA) | 1 T. (.5 oz.) | 5 | 4.7 | 3. | 2. | |
| 30% fat (Sealtest) | 1 T. (.5 oz.) | 5 | 4.5 | | | |
| Heavy whipping: | | | | | | |
| Unwhipped (USDA) | 1 cup (8.4 oz. or 2 cups whipped) | 76 | 89.5 | 50. | 40. | 317 |
| Unwhipped (USDA) | 1 T. (.5 oz.) | 5 | 5.6 | 3. | 2. | 20 |
| 36% butterfat (Johanna Farms) | 1 T. (.5 oz.) | 6 | 5.6 | | | 21 |
| Sour: | | | | | | |
| (USDA) | 1 cup (8.1 oz.) | 99 | 47.4 | 25. | 22. | 152 |
| (USDA) | 1 T. (.4 oz.) | 5 | 2.5 | 1. | 1. | 8 |
| (Borden's) | 1 cup (8.6 oz.) | 96 | 43.2 | | | |
| (Borden's) | 1 T. (.5 oz.) | 6 | 2.7 | | | |
| (Breakstone's) | 8-oz. container | 112 | 41.5 | | | 112 |
| (Breakstone's) | 1 T. (.5 oz.) | 8 | 2.8 | | | 8 |
| (Sealtest) | 1 T. (.5 oz.) | 6 | 2.7 | | | |
| Half & half (Sealtest) | 1 T. (.5 oz.) | 6 | 1.8 | | | |
| Imitation: | | | | | | |
| (Sealtest) nondairy | 1 T. (.5 oz.) | 16 | 2.7 | | | |
| *Sour Treat* (Delite) | 1 T. (.5 oz.) | 6 | 2.2 | | | |
| *Zest* (Borden's) 13.5% vegetable fat | 1 T. | 16 | 2.0 | | | |

(USDA): United States Department of Agriculture
*Prepared as Package Directs

| Food and Description | Measure or Quantity | Sodium (mg.) | — Fats in grams — | | | Cholesterol (mg.) |
|---|---|---|---|---|---|---|
| | | | Total | Saturated | Unsaturated | |
| Sour cream, dried (Data from General Mills) | 1 oz. | 87 | 16.2 | | | |
| Sour dairy dressing (Sealtest) | 1 T. (.5 oz.) | 7 | 1.8 | | | |
| Sour dressing or sour cream, made with nonfat dry milk: | | | | | | |
| (USDA) | 1 cup (8.3 oz.) | | 38.0 | 35. | 3. | |
| (USDA) | 1 T. (.4 oz.) | | 2.0 | 2. | Tr. | |
| Sour dressing, cultured (Breakstone's) | 1 T. (.5 oz.) | 9 | 2.4 | | | 0 |
| Whipped (See **TOPPING,** Whipped) | | | | | | |
| **CREAM PUFF,** home recipe, with custard filling (USDA)[1] | 3½″ × 2″ (4.6 oz.) | 108 | 18.1 | 5. | 13. | 187 |
| *CREAM OF RICE,* cereal, no salt added | 1 oz. | 0 | 0.0 | | | |
| **CREAM OR CREME SOFT DRINK** (See **SOFT DRINK,** Cream) | | | | | | |
| **CREAM SUBSTITUTE:** | | | | | | |
| Liquid, frozen (USDA) | 1 cup (8.6 oz.) | | 27.0 | 25. | 2. | |
| Liquid, frozen (USDA) | 1 tsp. (5 grams) | | .6 | <1. | Tr. | |
| Powdered (USDA) | 1 cup (3.3 oz.) | | 33.0 | 31. | 2. | |
| Powdered (USDA) | 1 tsp. (2 grams) | | 1.0 | <1. | Tr. | |
| *Coffee-Mate* (Carnation)[2] | 1 oz.-packet | 5 | 1.1 | | | <1 |
| *Coffee Rich* (Rich's) | ½ oz. | 7 | 1.4 | .9 | .5 | 0 |
| *Cremora* (Borden's) | 1 tsp. | 5 | .4 | | | |
| *N-Rich* (Swiss Miss) | 1 tsp. | 5 | <1.0 | | | 0 |
| **CREAM OF TARTAR** (Spice Islands) | 1 tsp. | 8 | | | | (0) |
| *CREAM OF WHEAT,* cereal: | | | | | | |
| *Instant | 1 oz. (¾ cup cooked) | 0 | 0.0 | | | |
| Mix 'n Eat: | | | | | | |
| *Regular | 3½ T. (1 oz.) | 180 | 0.0 | | | |

(USDA): United States Department of Agriculture
*Prepared as Package Directs
[1]Principal sources of fat: vegetable shortening, egg & milk.
[2]Principal source of fat: modified coconut oil.

| Food and Description | Measure or Quantity | Sodium (mg.) | Total | — Fats in grams — Saturated | Unsaturated | Cholesterol (mg.) |
|---|---|---|---|---|---|---|
| Baked apple & cinnamon, dry | 3¾ T. (1¼ oz.) | 240 | 0.0 | | | |
| Maple & brown sugar, dry | 3¾ T. (1¼ oz.) | 180 | 0.0 | | | |
| Quick, dry | 1 oz. (¾ cup cooked) | 30 | 0.0 | | | |
| Regular, dry | 1 oz. (¾ cup cooked) | 0 | 0.0 | | | |
| **CREPE, FROZEN:** | | | | | | |
| (Mrs. Paul's): | | | | | | |
| Crab | ½ of 5½-oz. pkg. | 578 | 5.9 | | | |
| Shrimp | ½ of 5½-oz. pkg. | 523 | 5.9 | | | |
| (Stouffer's): | | | | | | |
| Chicken with mushroom sauce | 8¼-oz. pkg. | 1,040 | 22.0 | | | |
| Ham and asparagus | 6¼-oz. pkg. | 840 | 20.0 | | | |
| Ham and swiss cheese with cheddar cheese sauce | 7½-oz. pkg. | 905 | 25.0 | | | |
| Spinach with cheddar cheese sauce | 9½-oz. pkg. | 995 | 25.0 | | | |
| **CRESS, GARDEN** (USDA): | | | | | | |
| Raw, whole | 1 lb. (weighed untrimmed) | 45 | 2.3 | | | 0 |
| Boiled without salt, in small amount of water, short time, drained (USDA) | 1 cup (6.3 oz.) | 14 | 1.1 | | | 0 |
| Boiled without salt, large amount of water, long time, drained (USDA) | 1 cup (6.3 oz.) | 14 | 1.1 | | | 0 |
| **CRISPIX,** cereal (Kellogg's) | ¾ cup (1 oz.) | 230 | 0.0 | | | |
| **CRISP RICE,** cereal: | | | | | | |
| (Featherweight) low sodium | 1 cup (1 oz.) | <10 | 0.0 | | | |
| (Ralston Purina) | 1 cup (1 oz.) | 206 | .1 | | | |
| **CRISPY WHEATS'N RAISINS,** cereal (General Mills) | ¾ cup (1 oz.) | 180 | 1.0 | | | |

(USDA): United States Department of Agriculture
*Prepared as Package Directs

| Food and Description | Measure or Quantity | Sodium (mg.) | —Fats in grams— Total | Satu-rated | Unsatu-rated | Choles-terol (mg.) |
|---|---|---|---|---|---|---|
| **CROAKER** (USDA): | | | | | | |
| Atlantic: | | | | | | |
| Raw, whole | 1 lb. (weighed whole) | 134 | 3.4 | | | |
| Raw, meat only | 4 oz. | 99 | 2.5 | | | |
| Baked | 4 oz. | 136 | 3.6 | | | |
| White, raw, meat only | 4 oz. | | .9 | | | |
| Yellowfin, raw, meat only | 4 oz. | | .9 | | | |
| **CROUTON:** | | | | | | |
| (Kellogg's) *Croutettes* | ⅔ cup (.7 oz.) | 260 | 0.0 | | | |
| (Pepperidge Farm): | | | | | | |
| Cheese and garlic | ¹⁄₁₂ of 6-oz. box | 180 | 3.0 | | | |
| Onion and garlic | ¹⁄₁₂ of 6-oz. box | 160 | 3.0 | | | |
| Seasoned | ¹⁄₁₂ of 6-oz. box | 210 | 3.0 | | | |
| **CRULLER** (See **DOUGHNUT**) | | | | | | |
| **CUCUMBER,** fresh (USDA): | | | | | | |
| Eaten with skin | ½ lb. (weighed with skin) | 13 | .2 | | | 0 |
| Eaten without skin | ½ lb. (weighed with skin) | 10 | .2 | | | 0 |
| Not pared, 10-oz. cucumber | 7½" × 2" pared cucumber (7.3 oz.) | 12 | .2 | | | 0 |
| Pared | 6 slices (2" × ⅛", 1.8 oz.) | 3 | <.1 | | | 0 |
| Pared & diced | ½ cup (2.5 oz.) | 4 | <.1 | | | 0 |
| **CUMIN SEED,** whole or ground (Spice Islands) | 1 tsp. | <1 | | | | (0) |
| **CUPCAKE:** | | | | | | |
| Home recipe (USDA)[1]: | | | | | | |
| Made with butter, without icing[2] | 2¾" cupcake (1.4 oz.) | 120 | 5.1 | 3. | 2. | |
| Made with vegetable shortening, without icing[3] | 2¾" cupcake (1.4 oz.) | 120 | 5.6 | 2. | 4. | |

(USDA): United States Department of Agriculture
*Prepared as Package Directs
[1]Made with sodium aluminum sulfate-type baking powder.
[2]Principal sources of fat: butter, egg & milk.
[3]Principal sources of fat: vegetable shortening, egg & milk.

| Food and Description | Measure or Quantity | Sodium (mg.) | Fats in grams — Total | Satu- rated | Unsatu- rated | Choles- terol (mg.) |
|---|---|---|---|---|---|---|
| With chocolate icing | 2¾" cupcake (1.8 oz.) | 114 | 7.0 | | | |
| With boiled white icing | 2¾" cupcake (1.8 oz.) | 131 | 5.2 | | | |
| With uncooked white icing | 2¾" cupcake (1.8 oz.) | 114 | 5.9 | | | |
| Commercial (Hostess): | | | | | | |
| Chocolate | 1¾-oz. piece | 249 | 4.5 | | | 5 |
| Orange | 1½-oz. piece | 170 | 4.3 | | | 13 |
| **CUPCAKE MIX:** | | | | | | |
| (USDA)[1] | 4 oz. | 676 | 15.4 | 3. | 12. | |
| *Prepared with eggs, milk, without icing (USDA)[2] | 2½" cupcake (.9 oz.) | 113 | 3.0 | <1. | 2. | |
| *Prepared with eggs, milk, with chocolate icing (USDA)[3] | 2½" cupcake (1.2 oz.) | 121 | 4.5 | 2. | 3. | |
| *(Flako) | 1 large cupcake (1.3 oz., ¹⁄₁₂ of pkg.) | 195 | 5.0 | | | |
| **CURRANT:** | | | | | | |
| Fresh (USDA): | | | | | | |
| Black European: | | | | | | |
| Whole | 1 lb. (weighed with stems) | 13 | .4 | | | 0 |
| Stems removed | 4 oz. | 3 | .1 | | | 0 |
| Red & white: | | | | | | |
| Whole | 1 lb. (weighed with stems) | 9 | .9 | | | 0 |
| Stems removed | 1 cup (3.9 oz.) | 2 | .2 | | | 0 |
| Dried, Zante: | | | | | | |
| (Del Monte) | ½ cup (2.4 oz.) | <10 | 0.0 | | | |
| (Sun-Maid) | ½ cup (2.5 oz.) | 18 | 0.0 | | | |
| **CURRY POWDER:** | | | | | | |
| (Crosse & Blackwell) | 1 T. (6 grams) | | .2 | | | (0) |
| (Spice Islands) | 1 tsp. | 1 | | | | (0) |

(USDA): United States Department of Agriculture
*Prepared as Package Directs
[1]Principal source of fat: vegetable shortening.
[2]Principal sources of fat: vegetable shortening, egg & milk.
[3]Principal sources of fat: vegetable shortening, chocolate, egg & milk.

| Food and Description | Measure or Quantity | Sodium (mg.) | — Fats in grams — Total | Satu- rated | Unsatu- rated | Choles- terol (mg.) |
|---|---|---|---|---|---|---|
| **CUSK** (USDA): | | | | | | |
| Raw, drawn | 1 lb. (weighed drawn, head & tail on) | | .5 | | | |
| Raw, meat only | 4 oz. | | .2 | | | |
| Steamed | 4 oz. | 84 | .8 | | | |
| **CUSTARD:** | | | | | | |
| Home recipe, baked (USDA) | ½ cup (4.7 oz.) | 104 | 7.3 | 4. | 3. | 139 |
| Canned (Thank You Brand) egg | ½ cup | 195 | 5.2 | | | 71 |
| Chilled (Swiss Miss): | | | | | | |
| Chocolate | 4 oz. | 149 | 6.0 | | | 3 |
| Egg | 4 oz. | 180 | 6.0 | | | 3 |
| **CUSTARD APPLE,** bullock's heart, fresh (USDA): | | | | | | |
| Whole | 1 lb. (weighed with skin & seeds) | | 1.6 | | | 0 |
| Flesh only | 4 oz. | | .7 | | | 0 |
| **CUSTARD, FROZEN** (See **ICE CREAM**) | | | | | | |
| **C.W. POST,** cereal (Post): | | | | | | |
| Plain | ¼ cup (1 oz.) | 49 | 4.4 | | | |
| Raisin | ¼ cup (1 oz.) | 44 | 4.1 | | | |

# D

| Food and Description | Measure or Quantity | Sodium (mg.) | Total | Satu- rated | Unsatu- rated | Choles- terol (mg.) |
|---|---|---|---|---|---|---|
| **DAIQUIRI COCKTAIL:** | | | | | | |
| (National Distillers) *Duet,* 12½% alcohol | 8 fl.-oz. can | Tr. | 0.0 | | | (0) |
| Mix (Holland House): | | | | | | |
| Liquid: | | | | | | |
| Regular | 1 oz. | 111 | 0.0 | | | |
| Raspberry | 1 oz. | 4 | 0.0 | | | |
| Strawberry | 1 oz. | 3 | 0.0 | | | |
| Instant | .56-oz. serving | 21 | 0.0 | | | |

(USDA): United States Department of Agriculture
*Prepared as Package Directs

| Food and Description | Measure or Quantity | Sodium (mg.) | —Fats in grams— | | | Cholesterol (mg.) |
|---|---|---|---|---|---|---|
| | | | Total | Saturated | Unsaturated | |
| **DAIRY CRISP,** cereal (Pet) | ¼ cup | 140 | 4.0 | | | |
| | | | | | | |
| **DAIRY QUEEN:** | | | | | | |
| Banana split | 13.5-oz. serving | 150 | 11.0 | | | 30 |
| *Brownie Delight,* hot fudge | 9.4-oz. serving | 225 | 25.0 | | | 20 |
| *Buster Bar* | 5¼-oz. piece | 175 | 29.0 | | | 7 |
| Chicken sandwich | 7.8-oz. sandwich | 870 | 41.0 | | | 77 |
| Cone: | | | | | | |
| Plain, any flavor, regular | 5-oz. cone | 80 | 7.0 | | | 14 |
| Dipped, chocolate, regular | 5½-oz. cone | 100 | 16.0 | | | 16 |
| *Dilly Bar* | 3-oz. piece | 50 | 13.0 | | | 8 |
| *Double Delight* | 9-oz. serving | 150 | 20.0 | | | 26 |
| *DQ Sandwich* | 2.1-oz. sandwich | 40 | 4.0 | | | 6 |
| Fish sandwich: | | | | | | |
| Plain | 6-oz. sandwich | 875 | 17.0 | | | 60 |
| With cheese | 6¼-oz. sandwich | 1,035 | 21.0 | | | 71 |
| Float | 14-oz. serving | 85 | 7.0 | | | 20 |
| Freeze, vanilla | 12-oz. serving | 180 | 12.0 | | | 20 |
| French fries: | | | | | | |
| Regular | 2½-oz. serving | 115 | 10.0 | | | 11 |
| Large | 4-oz. serving | 181 | 16.0 | | | 17 |
| Hamburger: | | | | | | |
| Plain: | | | | | | |
| Single | 5.2-oz. burger | 630 | 16.0 | | | 45 |
| Double | 7.4-oz. burger | 660 | 28.0 | | | 85 |
| Triple | 9.6-oz. burger | 690 | 45.0 | | | 135 |
| With cheese: | | | | | | |
| Single | 5.7-oz. burger | 790 | 20.0 | | | 50 |
| Double | 8.4-oz. burger | 980 | 37.0 | | | 95 |
| Triple | 10.63-oz. burger | 1,010 | 50.0 | | | 145 |
| Hot dog: | | | | | | |
| Regular: | | | | | | |
| Plain | 3.5-oz. serving | 830 | 16.0 | | | 45 |
| With cheese | 4-oz. serving | 990 | 21.0 | | | 55 |
| With chili | 4½-oz. serving | 985 | 20.0 | | | 55 |
| Super: | | | | | | |
| Plain | 6.2-oz. serving | 1,365 | 27.0 | | | 80 |
| With cheese | 6.9-oz. serving | 1,605 | 34.0 | | | 100 |
| With chili | 7.7-oz. serving | 1,595 | 32.0 | | | 100 |
| Malt, chocolate: | | | | | | |
| Large | 20¾-oz. serving | 360 | 25.0 | | | 70 |
| Regular | 14¾-oz. serving | 260 | 18.0 | | | 50 |

(USDA): United States Department of Agriculture
*Prepared as Package Directs

| Food and Description | Measure or Quantity | Sodium (mg.) | — Fats in grams — | | | Choles- terol (mg.) |
|---|---|---|---|---|---|---|
| | | | Total | Satu- rated | Unsatu- rated | |
| Small | 10¼-oz. serving | 180 | 13.0 | | | 35 |
| *Mr. Misty:* | | | | | | |
| Plain: | | | | | | |
| Large | 15½-oz. serving | <10 | 0.0 | | | 0 |
| Regular | 11.64-oz. serving | <10 | 0.0 | | | 0 |
| Small | 8¼-oz. serving | <10 | 0.0 | | | 0 |
| Kiss | 3.14-oz. serving | <10 | 0.0 | | | 0 |
| Float | 14.5-oz. serving | 95 | 7.0 | | | 20 |
| Freeze | 14.5-oz. serving | 140 | 12.0 | | | 30 |
| Onion rings | 3-oz. serving | 140 | 16.0 | | | 15 |
| Parfait | 10-oz. serving | 140 | 8.0 | | | 30 |
| *Peanut Buster Parfait* | 10¾-oz. serving | 250 | 34.0 | | | 30 |
| Shake, chocolate: | | | | | | |
| Large | 20¾-oz. serving | 360 | 26.0 | | | 70 |
| Regular | 14¾-oz. serving | 260 | 19.0 | | | 50 |
| Small | 10¼-oz. serving | 180 | 13.0 | | | 35 |
| Strawberry shortcake | 11-oz. serving | 215 | 11.0 | | | 25 |
| Sundae, chocolate: | | | | | | |
| Large | 8¾-oz. serving | 165 | 10.0 | | | 30 |
| Regular | 6¼-oz. serving | 120 | 8.0 | | | 20 |
| Small | 3¾-oz. serving | 75 | 4.0 | | | 10 |
| Tomato | ½ oz. | <10 | 0.0 | | | 0 |

**DAMSON PLUM** (See **PLUM**)

**DANDELION GREENS,** raw
(USDA):

| Food and Description | Measure or Quantity | Sodium (mg.) | Total | | | Choles- terol (mg.) |
|---|---|---|---|---|---|---|
| Trimmed | 1 lb. | 345 | 3.2 | | | 0 |
| Boiled without salt, drained | ½ cup (3.2 oz.) | 40 | .5 | | | 0 |

**DANISH PASTRY** (See
**COFFEE CAKE**)

**DANNY** (See **YOGURT**)

**DATE,** dry:
Domestic:

| Food and Description | Measure or Quantity | Sodium (mg.) | Total | | | Choles- terol (mg.) |
|---|---|---|---|---|---|---|
| With pits (USDA) | 1 lb. (weighed with pits) | 4 | 2.0 | | | 0 |
| Without pits (USDA) | 4 oz. | 1 | .6 | | | 0 |
| Without pits, chopped (USDA) | 1 cup (6.1 oz.) | 2 | .9 | | | 0 |

(USDA): United States Department of Agriculture
*Prepared as Package Directs

167

| Food and Description | Measure or Quantity | Sodium (mg.) | —Fats in grams— | | | Choles-terol (mg.) |
|---|---|---|---|---|---|---|
| | | | Total | Satu-rated | Unsatu-rated | |
| Whole (Cal-Date) | 1 date (.8 oz.) | <1 | .1 | | | |
| Diced (Cal-Date) | 4 oz. | 1 | .7 | | | |
| Chopped (Dromedary) | 1 cup (5 oz.) | 17 | 2.5 | | | |
| Pitted (Dromedary) | 1 cup (5 oz.) | 17 | 1.3 | | | |
| Imported, Iraq (Bordo): | | | | | | |
| Whole | 4 average dates (.9 oz.) | 52 | .6 | | | |
| Diced | ¼ cup (2 oz.) | 114 | 1.4 | | | |
| **DELAWARE WINE:** | | | | | | |
| (Gold Seal) 12% alcohol | 3 fl. oz. (3.2 oz.) | 3 | 0.0 | | | (0) |
| (Great Western) 12.5% alcohol | 3 fl. oz. | 2 | 0.0 | | | |
| ***DEVIL DOGS*** (Drake's) | 1 piece (1.6 oz.) | | 7.6 | | | |
| **DEVIL'S FOOD CAKE** (See **CAKE,** Devil's Food) | | | | | | |
| **DEWBERRY,** fresh (See **BLACKBERRY,** fresh) | | | | | | |
| **DEWBERRY PRESERVE** | | | | | | |
| (Bama) | 1 T. (.7 oz.) | 1 | <.1 | | | |
| **DILL:** | | | | | | |
| Seed (Data from General Mills) | 1 oz. | 28 | | | | (0) |
| Seed (Spice Islands) | 1 tsp. | <1 | | | | (0) |
| Weed (Spice Islands) | 1 tsp. | <1 | | | | (0) |
| ***DING DONG*** (Hostess) | 1 piece (1.3 oz.) | 132 | 9.1 | | | 7 |
| **DINNER,** frozen (See individual listings such as **BEEF DINNER, CHICKEN DINNER, CHINESE DINNER, ENCHILADA DINNER,** etc.) | | | | | | |
| **DIP:** | | | | | | |
| Acapulco (Ortega): | | | | | | |
| Plain | 1 oz. | 1 | .1 | | | 0 |
| American cheese | 1 oz. | 172 | 4.6 | | | 24 |

(USDA): United States Department of Agriculture
*Prepared as Package Directs

| Food and Description | Measure or Quantity | Sodium (mg.) | — Fats in grams — | | | Choles- terol (mg.) |
|---|---|---|---|---|---|---|
| | | | Total | Satu- rated | Unsatu- rated | |
| Cheddar cheese | 1 oz. | 106 | 4.9 | | | 24 |
| Monterey jack cheese | 1 oz. | 124 | 4.5 | | | 15 |
| Blue cheese (Breakstone's) | 1 oz. | 207 | 5.2 | | | 14 |
| Jalapeño: | | | | | | |
| *Fritos* | 1 oz. | 88 | 1.7 | | | |
| (Hain) natural | 1 oz. | | 2.1 | | | 0 |
| (Wise) | 1 T. | 50 | 0.0 | | | Tr. |
| Onion (Thank You Brand) | 1 T. | 191 | 3.6 | | | 0 |
| Onion bean (Hain) | 1 oz. | | 2.0 | | | 0 |
| Picante sauce (Wise) | 1 T. | 65 | 0.0 | | | |
| Taco: | | | | | | |
| (Thank You Brand) | 1 T. | 129 | 3.6 | | | Tr. |
| (Wise) | 1 T. | 57 | 0.0 | | | |
| **DIP 'UM SAUCE,** canned (French's): | | | | | | |
| Barbecue | 1 T. | 180 | 0.0 | | | |
| Hot mustard | 1 T. | 275 | .5 | | | |
| Sweet'n sour | 1 T. | 12 | 0.0 | | | |
| **DISTILLED LIQUOR,** 80 proof to 100 proof (USDA) | 1 fl. oz. (1 oz.) | <1 | | | | 0 |
| **DOCK,** including **SHEEP SORREL** (USDA): | | | | | | |
| Raw, whole | 1 lb. (weighed untrimmed) | 16 | 1.0 | | | 0 |
| Raw, trimmed | 4 oz. | 6 | .3 | | | 0 |
| Boiled, without salt, drained | 4 oz. | 3 | .2 | | | 0 |
| **DOGFISH,** Spiny, raw, meat only (USDA) | 4 oz. | | 10.2 | | | |
| **DOLLY VARDEN,** raw, meat & skin (USDA) | 4 oz. | | 7.4 | | | |
| **DOUGHNUT:** | | | | | | |
| (USDA)[1] | | | | | | |
| Cake type | 1.1-oz. piece | 160 | 6.0 | 1. | 5. | |
| Yeast leavened | 2 oz. | 133 | 15.1 | 3. | 12. | |
| (Hostess): | | | | | | |
| Regular: | | | | | | |
| Chocolate coated | 1-oz. piece | 151 | 8.5 | | | 4 |

(USDA): United States Department of Agriculture
*Prepared as Package Directs
[1]Principal sources of fat: vegetable shortening & egg.

| Food and Description | Measure or Quantity | Sodium (mg.) | —Fats in grams— | | | Choles- terol (mg.) |
|---|---|---|---|---|---|---|
| | | | Total | Satu- rated | Unsatu- rated | |
| Cinnamon | 1-oz. piece | 111 | 5.7 | | | 6 |
| Old-fashioned, glazed | 2-oz. piece | 199 | 11.9 | | | 11 |
| Powdered sugar | 1-oz. piece | 153 | 6.0 | | | 7 |
| *Donettes:* | | | | | | |
| Frosted | .45-oz. piece | 50 | 3.5 | | | 5 |
| Powdered sugar | .33-oz. piece | 51 | 2.0 | | | 2 |
| (Morton) frozen: | | | | | | |
| Regular: | | | | | | |
| Bavarian cream or chocolate iced | 1 piece | 75 | 9.0 | | | 11 |
| Glazed | 1½-oz. piece | 75 | 7.0 | | | 10 |
| Jelly | 1.8-oz. piece | 75 | 8.0 | | | 11 |
| *Donut Holes:* | | | | | | |
| Devil's food | ⅕ of 7¾-oz. pkg. | 105 | 8.0 | | | 5 |
| Vanilla | ⅕ of 7¾-oz. pkg. | 123 | 8.0 | | | 5 |
| *Morning Light:* | | | | | | |
| Chocolate | 2-oz. serving | 177 | 10.0 | | | 6 |
| Glazed | 2-oz. serving | 176 | 10.0 | | | 6 |
| Jelly | 2.6-oz. serving | 193 | 11.0 | | | 8 |

**DRUM,** raw (USDA):
| | | | | | | |
|---|---|---|---|---|---|---|
| Freshwater: | | | | | | |
| Whole | 1 lb. (weighed whole) | 83 | 6.1 | | | |
| Meat only | 4 oz. | 79 | 5.9 | | | |
| Red: | | | | | | |
| Whole | 1 lb. (weighed whole) | 102 | .7 | | | |
| Meat only | 4 oz. | 62 | .5 | | | |

**DUCK,** raw (USDA):
| | | | | | | |
|---|---|---|---|---|---|---|
| Domesticated: | | | | | | |
| Ready-to-cook | 1 lb. (weighed with bones) | | 106.4 | | | |
| Meat & skin | 4 oz. | | 32.4 | | | |
| Meat only | 4 oz. | 84 | 9.3 | | | |
| Wild: | | | | | | |
| Dressed | 1 lb. (weighed dressed) | | 41.6 | | | |

(USDA): United States Department of Agriculture
*Prepared as Package Directs

170

| Food and Description | Measure or Quantity | Sodium (mg.) | — Fats in grams — | | | Choles- terol (mg.) |
|---|---|---|---|---|---|---|
| | | | Total | Satu- rated | Unsatu- rated | |
| Meat, skin and giblets | 4 oz. | | 17.9 | | | |
| Meat only | 4 oz. | | 5.9 | | | |
| **DUMPLINGS,** stuffed, canned, dietetic (Featherweight) with chicken | 7½-oz. serving | 117 | 5.0 | | | |

# E

| Food and Description | Measure or Quantity | Sodium (mg.) | Total | Satu- rated | Unsatu- rated | Choles- terol (mg.) |
|---|---|---|---|---|---|---|
| **ECLAIR,** home recipe, with custard filling & chocolate icing (USDA)[1] | 4 oz. | 93 | 15.4 | 5. | 11. | |
| **EEL** (USDA): | | | | | | |
| Raw, meat only | 4 oz. | | 20.8 | 5. | 16. | |
| Smoked, meat only | 4 oz. | | 31.5 | 7. | 25. | |
| **EGG, CHICKEN** (USDA): | | | | | | |
| Raw: | | | | | | |
| White only | 1 large egg (1.2 oz.) | 48 | Tr. | | | 0 |
| White only | 1 cup (9 oz.) | 372 | Tr. | | | 0 |
| Yolk only | 1 large egg (.6 oz.) | 9 | 5.2 | 2. | 4. | 250 |
| Yolk only | 1 cup (8.5 oz.) | 125 | 73.4 | 24. | 49. | 3552 |
| Whole, small | 1 egg (1.3 oz.) | 45 | 4.3 | 1. | 3. | 186 |
| Whole, medium | 1 egg (1.5 oz.) | 53 | 5.0 | 2. | 3. | 220 |
| Whole | 1 cup (8.8 oz.) | 306 | 28.9 | 10. | 19. | 1265 |
| Whole, large | 1 egg (1.8 oz.) | 61 | 5.7 | 2. | 4. | 251 |
| Whole, extra large | 1 egg (2 oz.) | 70 | 6.6 | 2. | 4. | 289 |
| Whole, jumbo | 1 egg (2.3 oz.) | 79 | 7.4 | 3. | 5. | 325 |
| Cooked: | | | | | | |
| Boiled without salt | 1 large egg (1.8 oz.) | 61 | 5.7 | 2. | 4. | 251 |
| Fried in butter[2] | 1 large egg (1.6 oz.) | 155 | 7.9 | 3. | 5. | |
| Omelet, mixed with milk & cooked in fat[3] | 1 large egg (2.2 oz.) | 159 | 8.0 | 3. | 5. | |

(USDA): United States Department of Agriculture
*Prepared as Package Directs
[1]Principal sources of fat: vegetable shortening, egg, milk, chocolate & butter.
[2]Principal sources of fat: egg & butter.
[3]Principal sources of fat: egg, milk & vegetable fat.

| Food and Description | Measure or Quantity | Sodium (mg.) | Total | Fats in grams — Satu- rated | Fats in grams — Unsatu- rated | Choles- terol (mg.) |
|---|---|---|---|---|---|---|
| Poached | 1 large egg (1.7 oz.) | 130 | 5.6 | 2. | 4. | 242 |
| Scrambled, mixed with milk & cooked in fat [1] | 1 cup (7.8 oz.) | 565 | 28.4 | 11. | 17. | 904 |
| Scrambled, mixed with milk & cooked in fat [1] | 1 large egg (2.3 oz.) | 164 | 8.3 | 3. | 5. | 263 |
| Dried: | | | | | | |
| White, flakes | 1 oz. | 293 | <.1 | | | |
| White, powder | 1 oz. | 313 | <.1 | | | |
| Yolk | 1 cup (3.4 oz.) | 96 | 54.3 | 17. | 37. | 2525 |
| Whole | 1 cup (3.8 oz.) | 461 | 44.5 | 14. | 30. | 2052 |
| Whole, glucose reduced | 1 oz. | 126 | 12.2 | 4. | 8. | |
| Frozen, whole, raw | 1 oz. | 35 | 3.3 | 1. | 2. | |
| **EGG, DUCK,** raw (USDA) | 1 egg (2.8 oz.) | 98 | 11.6 | | | |
| **EGG, GOOSE,** raw (USDA) | 1 egg (5.8 oz.) | | 21.8 | | | |
| **EGG, TURKEY,** raw (USDA) | 1 egg (3.1 oz.) | | 10.4 | | | |
| **EGG BREAKFAST OR ENTREE,** frozen (Swanson): | | | | | | |
| Omelet: | | | | | | |
| With cheese & ham | 7-oz. meal | 1,160 | 31.0 | | | |
| Spanish style | 7¾-oz. meal | 840 | 17.0 | | | |
| Scrambled, with sausage & hash brown potatoes | 6¼-oz. meal | 790 | 33.0 | | | |
| *EGG FOO YUNG, canned: | | | | | | |
| (Chun King) stir fry | 5-oz. serving | 517 | 8.2 | | | 142 |
| (La Choy) | 1 patty & ¼ cup sauce | 760 | 7.0 | | | |
| **EGG NOG,** dairy (Borden's) [2] | ½ cup (4.2 oz.) | 80 | 9.0 | | | |
| **EGG NOG COCKTAIL,** (Mr. Boston) 15% alcohol | 3 fl. oz. | 71 | 2.1 | | | |
| **EGGPLANT:** | | | | | | |
| Raw, whole (USDA) | 1 lb. (weighed untrimmed) | 7 | .7 | | | 0 |

(USDA): United States Department of Agriculture
*Prepared as Package Directs
[1]Principal sources of fat: egg, milk & vegetable fat.
[2]Principal sources of fat: milk and egg yolk.

| Food and Description | Measure or Quantity | Sodium (mg.) | Fats in grams — Total | Satu- rated | Unsatu- rated | Choles- terol (mg.) |
|---|---|---|---|---|---|---|
| Boiled without salt, drained (USDA) | 4 oz. | 1 | .2 | | | 0 |
| Boiled without salt, drained, diced (USDA) | 1 cup (7.1 oz.) | 2 | .4 | | | 0 |
| Frozen: | | | | | | |
| (Celentano): | | | | | | |
| Parmigiana | ½ of 16-oz. pkg. | 405 | 22.0 | | | 60 |
| Rollettes | 11-oz. pkg. | 510 | 30.0 | | | 105 |
| (Weight Watchers) | | | | | | |
| parmigiana | 13-oz. pkg. | 1,073 | 13.0 | | | |
| | | | | | | |
| **EGG ROLL,** frozen: | | | | | | |
| (Chun King): | | | | | | |
| Chicken | .8-oz. piece | 139 | 1.5 | | | 2 |
| Meat & shrimp | .8-oz. piece | 133 | 1.6 | | | 4 |
| Meat & shrimp | 3.45-oz. piece | 589 | 6.0 | | | 14 |
| Shrimp | .8-oz. piece | 134 | 1.3 | | | 3 |
| (La Choy): | | | | | | |
| Almond chicken | 2 pieces | 1,020 | 21.0 | | | |
| Beef & broccoli | 2 pieces | 1,060 | 13.0 | | | |
| Chicken | .5-oz. piece | 62 | 1.0 | | | |
| Lobster | 3-oz. piece | 485 | 5.0 | | | |
| Meat & shrimp | .24-oz. piece | 42 | .5 | | | |
| Meat & shrimp | .5-oz. piece | 73 | .7 | | | |
| Shrimp | .5-oz. piece | 70 | .7 | | | |
| Shrimp | 3-oz. piece | 575 | 4.0 | | | |
| | | | | | | |
| **EGG SUBSTITUTE:** | | | | | | |
| *Egg Beaters* (Fleischmann's): | | | | | | |
| Cholesterol-free | ¼ cup | 80 | 0.0 | | | 0 |
| With cheese, 99% real egg product | ½ cup | 440 | 6.0 | | | 5 |
| *Egg Magic* (Featherweight) | ½ envelope (1 egg) | 123 | 4.0 | 1. | 3. | 15 |
| *Scramblers* (Morningstar Farms) | 1 egg equivalent | 75 | 1.5 | | | 0 |
| | | | | | | |
| **ELDERBERRY,** fresh (USDA): | | | | | | |
| Whole | 1 lb. (weighed with stems) | | 2.1 | | | 0 |
| Stems removed | 4 oz. | | .6 | | | 0 |

(USDA): United States Department of Agriculture
*Prepared as Package Directs

| Food and Description | Measure or Quantity | Sodium (mg.) | Total | Satu- rated | Unsatu- rated | Choles- terol (mg.) |
|---|---|---|---|---|---|---|
| | | | | —Fats in grams— | | |

**ENCHILADA OR ENCHILADA DINNER,** frozen:
Beef:
  (Banquet):

| | | | | | | |
|---|---|---|---|---|---|---|
| Dinner | 12-oz. meal | 1,805 | 15.0 | | | |
| Entree | 2-lb. pkg. | 5,908 | 32.0 | | | |
| (Hormel) | 1 enchilada | 573 | 5.0 | | | |
| (Morton) | | | | | | |
| (Van de Kamp's): | | | | | | |
| Dinner, regular | 11-oz. dinner | 2,177 | 15.0 | | | |
| Entree, shredded | 5½-oz. serving | 930 | 10.0 | | | |
| Cheese: | | | | | | |
| (Banquet) | 12-oz. dinner | 2,166 | 19.0 | | | |
| (Van de Kamp's) | 12-oz. dinner | 1,664 | 20.0 | | | |
| Chicken (Van de Kamp's) | 7½-oz. pkg. | 1,108 | 10.0 | | | |

**ENCHILADA SAUCE:**
Canned, *Old El Paso:*

| | | | | | | |
|---|---|---|---|---|---|---|
| Green chili | ¼ cup | 400 | .2 | | | |
| Mild | ¼ cup | 250 | .9 | | | |
| *Mix (Durkee) | 1 cup | 96 | .6 | | | |

**ENDIVE, BELGIAN OR FRENCH** (See **CHICORY, WITLOOF**)

**ENDIVE, CURLY, OR ESCAROLE,** raw (USDA):

| | | | | | | |
|---|---|---|---|---|---|---|
| Untrimmed | 1 lb. (weighed untrimmed) | 56 | .4 | | | 0 |
| Trimmed | ½ lb. | 32 | .2 | | | 0 |
| Cut up or shredded | 1 cup (2.5 oz.) | 10 | <.1 | | | 0 |

**ESCAROLE** (See **ENDIVE**)

**EULACHON OR SMELT,** raw, meat only (USDA) | 4 oz. | | 7.0 |

(USDA): United States Department of Agriculture
*Prepared as Package Directs

| Food and Description | Measure or Quantity | Sodium (mg.) | — Fats in grams — | | | Choles-terol (mg.) |
|---|---|---|---|---|---|---|
| | | | Total | Satu-rated | Unsatu-rated | |

# F

**FARINA** (See also **CREAM OF WHEAT**):
Regular:
Dry:

| Food and Description | Measure or Quantity | Sodium (mg.) | Total | Satu-rated | Unsatu-rated | Choles-terol (mg.) |
|---|---|---|---|---|---|---|
| (USDA) | 1 cup (6 oz.) | 3 | 1.5 | | | 0 |
| Cream, enriched (H-O) | 1 cup (6.1 oz.) | 8 | 1.2 | | | 0 |

Cooked:

| | | | | | | |
|---|---|---|---|---|---|---|
| (USDA) | 1 cup (8.4 oz.) | 343 | .2 | | | 0 |
| (Pillsbury) | ⅔ cup (1 oz. dry) | 270 | .2 | | | (0) |

Quick-cooking (USDA):

| | | | | | | |
|---|---|---|---|---|---|---|
| Dry | 1 oz. | 71 | .3 | | | 0 |
| Cooked | 1 cup (8.6 oz.) | 466 | .2 | | | 0 |

Instant-cooking (USDA):

| | | | | | | |
|---|---|---|---|---|---|---|
| Dry | 1 oz. | 2 | .3 | | | 0 |
| Cooked | 4 oz. | 213 | .1 | | | 0 |

**FAT, COOKING:**

| | | | | | | |
|---|---|---|---|---|---|---|
| Lard (USDA) | 1 lb. | 0 | 454.0 | 172 | 282. | 431 |
| Lard (USDA) | 1 cup (7.2 oz.) | 0 | 205.0 | 78. | 127. | 195 |
| Lard (USDA) | 1 T. (.5 oz.) | 0 | 13.0 | 5. | 8. | 12 |
| Vegetable (USDA) | 1 cup (7.1 oz.) | 0 | 200.0 | 50. | 150. | 0 |
| Vegetable (USDA) | 1 T. (.4 oz.) | 0 | 12.0 | 3. | 9. | 0 |
| *Crisco* | 1 T. (.4 oz.) | 0 | 11.7 | 3. | 9. | 0 |
| *Fluffo* | 1 T. (.4 oz.) | 0 | 11.7 | 4. | 7. | Tr. |
| *Light Spry* | 1 T. (.4 oz.) | 0 | 10.6 | 3. | 8. | 0 |
| *Light Spry* | ¼ lb. | 0 | 113.4 | 32. | 82. | 0 |

**FENNEL LEAVES,** raw, (USDA):

| | | | | | | |
|---|---|---|---|---|---|---|
| Untrimmed | 1 lb. (weighed untrimmed) | | 1.7 | | | 0 |
| Trimmed | 4 oz. | | .5 | | | 0 |

**FENNEL SEED** (Spice Islands)

| | | | | | | |
|---|---|---|---|---|---|---|
| | 1 tsp. | 1 | | | | (0) |

**FIG:**
Fresh:

| | | | | | | |
|---|---|---|---|---|---|---|
| (USDA) | 1 lb. | 9 | 1.4 | | | 0 |
| Small (USDA) | 1.3-oz. fig (1½″) | <1 | .1 | | | 0 |
| Candied (USDA) | 1 oz. | | <.1 | | | 0 |

(USDA): United States Department of Agriculture
*Prepared as Package Directs

| Food and Description | Measure or Quantity | Sodium (mg.) | Total | Saturated | Unsaturated | Cholesterol (mg.) |
|---|---|---|---|---|---|---|
| | | | | — Fats in grams — | | |
| Candied (Bama) | 1 T. (.7 oz.) | <1 | <.1 | | | |
| Canned, regular pack, solids & liq.: | | | | | | |
| Light syrup (USDA) | 4 oz. | 2 | .2 | | | 0 |
| Heavy syrup: | | | | | | |
| (USDA) | ½ cup (4.4 oz.) | 3 | .3 | | | 0 |
| (USDA) | 3 figs & 2 T. syrup | 2 | .2 | | | 0 |
| (Del Monte) | ½ cup (4.4 oz.) | 1 | .4 | | | ·0 |
| (Stokely-Van Camp's) | ½ cup (4.2 oz.) | | .2 | | | (0) |
| Extra heavy syrup (USDA) | 4 oz. | 2 | .2 | | | 0 |
| Canned, unsweetened or dietetic pack, solids & liq.: | | | | | | |
| Water pack (USDA) | 4 oz. | 2 | .2 | | | 0 |
| Kadota (Diet Delight) | ½ cup (4.4 oz.) | 4 | .1 | | | (0) |
| (Tillie Lewis) | ½ cup (4.5 oz.) | <10 | .2 | | | (0) |
| Whole: | | | | | | |
| (S & W) *Nutradiet,* low calorie | 6 whole figs (3.5 oz.) | 2 | .1 | | | (0) |
| (S & W) *Nutradiet,* unsweetened | 6 whole figs (3.5 oz.) | 2 | 1 | | | (0) |
| Dried: | | | | | | |
| Chopped (USDA) | 1 cup (6 oz.) | 58 | 2.2 | | | 0 |
| (USDA) | .7-oz. fig (2″ × 1″) | 7 | .3 | | | 0 |
| Calimyrna (Sun-Maid) | ½ cup | <20 | 2.0 | | | (0) |
| Mission (Del Monte) | 1 cup (5.4 oz.) | 30 | 3.5 | | | (0) |
| **FIG JUICE,** canned (Sunsweet) | 6 fl. oz. | 24 | 0 | | | |
| *FIGURINES* (Pillsbury): | | | | | | |
| Chocolate, *S'mores* or vanilla | 1 bar | 45 | 5.0 | | | |
| Chocolate caramel or chocolate peanut butter | 1 bar | 45 | 6.0 | | | |
| **FILBERT OR HAZELNUT** (USDA): | | | | | | |
| Whole | 1 lb. (weighed in shell) | 4 | 130.2 | 7. | 123. | 0 |
| Shelled | 1 oz. | <1 | 17.7 | <1. | 17. | 0 |

(USDA): United States Department of Agriculture
*Prepared as Package Directs

| Food and Description | Measure or Quantity | Sodium (mg.) | — Fats in grams — | | | Choles-terol (mg.) |
|---|---|---|---|---|---|---|
| | | | Total | Satu-rated | Unsatu-rated | |
| **FINNAN HADDIE** (See **HADDOCK, SMOKED**) | | | | | | |
| | | | | | | |
| **FISH** (See individual listings) | | | | | | |
| | | | | | | |
| **FISH CAKE:** | | | | | | |
| Home recipe, fried (USDA) [1] | 2 oz. | | 4.5 | | | |
| Frozen: | | | | | | |
| Fried, reheated (USDA) | 2 oz. | | 10.1 | | | |
| (Mrs. Paul's) | 1 cake | 335 | 4.0 | | | |
| Thins (Mrs. Paul's) | 1 cake | 510 | 7.5 | | | |
| | | | | | | |
| **FISH & CHIPS,** frozen: | | | | | | |
| (Gorton's) | 1 pkg. | 1,380 | 72.0 | | | |
| (Mrs. Paul's) | 14-oz. pkg. | | 21.4 | | | |
| (Swanson): | | | | | | |
| Regular | 5½-oz. serving | 600 | 17.0 | | | |
| *Hungry-Man* | 14¾-oz. serving | 1,350 | 36.0 | | | |
| (Van de Kamp's) | 7-oz. serving | 640 | 25.0 | | | |
| | | | | | | |
| **FISH DINNER OR ENTREE,** frozen: | | | | | | |
| (Banquet) | 8¾-oz. dinner | 927 | 33.0 | | | |
| (Morton) | 10-oz. dinner | 1,400 | 7.1 | | | |
| (Mrs. Paul's): | | | | | | |
| Regular, parmesan | 5-oz. serving | 540 | 11.0 | | | |
| Light: | | | | | | |
| Dijon | 8½-oz. serving | 650 | 14.0 | | | |
| Mornay | 10-oz. serving | 665 | 10.0 | | | |
| (Stouffer's) *Lean Cuisine:* | | | | | | |
| Divan | 12⅜-oz. pkg. | 785 | 10.0 | | | 85 |
| Florentine | 9-oz. pkg. | 815 | 8.0 | | | 100 |
| (Van de Kamp's) | 12-oz. dinner | 1,820 | 10.0 | | | |
| (Weight Watchers): | | | | | | |
| Au gratin | 9¼-oz. meal | 910 | 7.0 | | | |
| Oven fried | 6¾-oz. serving | 470 | 12.0 | | | |
| | | | | | | |
| **FISH FILLET,** frozen: | | | | | | |
| (Gorton's): | | | | | | |
| Regular, crunchy | 1 piece | 220 | 13.0 | | | |
| Light recipe: | | | | | | |
| Lightly breaded | 1 piece | 380 | 7.0 | | | |
| Tempura | 1 piece | 400 | 12.0 | | | |

(USDA): United States Department of Agriculture
*Prepared as Package Directs
[1] Prepared with canned flaked fish, potato & egg.

| Food and Description | Measure or Quantity | Sodium (mg.) | Total | —Fats in grams—<br>Satu-<br>rated | Unsatu-<br>rated | Choles-<br>terol (mg.) |
|---|---|---|---|---|---|---|
| (Mrs. Paul's): | | | | | | |
| Batter fried: | | | | | | |
| Regular | 1 fillet | 415 | 9.5 | | | |
| Supreme light | 1 fillet | 505 | 10.0 | | | |
| Breaded: | | | | | | |
| Crispy, crunchy | 1 fillet | 325 | 8.0 | | | |
| Light, fried | 1 fillet | 770 | 13.0 | | | |
| Buttered | 1 fillet | 390 | 6.5 | | | |
| (Van de Kamp's): | | | | | | |
| Batter dipped, french fried | 3-oz. piece | 230 | 10.0 | | | |
| Light & crunchy | 2-oz. piece | 175 | 15.0 | | | |
| **FISH FLAKES,** canned (USDA) | 4 oz. | | .7 | | | |
| **FISH KABOB,** frozen: | | | | | | |
| (Mrs. Paul's) | ⅓ of 10-oz. pkg. | 429 | 9.6 | | | |
| (Van de Kamp's) | 1 piece | 430 | 15.0 | | | |
| **FISH LOAF,** home recipe (USDA)[1] | 4 oz. | | 4.2 | | | |
| **FISH STICK,** frozen: | | | | | | |
| Cooked, commercial, 3¾″ × 1″ × ½″ sticks (USDA) | 10 sticks (8-oz. pkg.) | | 20.2 | | | |
| (Gorton's): | | | | | | |
| Batter dipped, crispy | 1 piece | 140 | 3.5 | | | |
| Breaded | 1 piece | 120 | 2.2 | | | |
| Potato crisp | 1 piece | 100 | 5.0 | | | |
| Value pack | 1 piece | 105 | 2.7 | | | |
| (Mrs. Paul's): | | | | | | |
| Batter fried | .87-oz. piece | 199 | 3.8 | | | |
| Breaded & fried | ¾-oz. piece | 114 | 2.5 | | | |
| (Van de Kamp's) Batter dipped, *Light & Crispy* | .9-oz. piece | 75 | 5.0 | | | |
| **FLOUNDER:** | | | | | | |
| Raw (USDA): | | | | | | |
| Whole | 1 lb. (weighed whole) | 117 | 1.2 | | | 75 |
| Meat only | 4 oz. | 88 | .9 | | | 57 |
| Baked (USDA) | 4 oz. | 269 | 9.3 | | | |

(USDA): United States Department of Agriculture
*Prepared as Package Directs
[1]Prepared with canned flaked fish, bread crumbs, eggs, tomatoes, onion & fat.

| Food and Description | Measure or Quantity | Sodium (mg.) | Fats in grams — Total | Satu- rated | Unsatu- rated | Choles- terol (mg.) |
|---|---|---|---|---|---|---|
| Frozen: | | | | | | |
| (Gorton's): | | | | | | |
| *Fishmarket Fresh* | 4 oz. | 140 | 1.0 | | | |
| Light recipe, stuffed | 1 pkg. | 880 | 14.0 | | | |
| (Le Menu) with salmon | | | | | | |
| mousse | 10½-oz. pkg. | 1,060 | 18.0 | | | |
| (Mrs. Paul's) crispy, crunchy | 2-oz. piece | 400 | 7.5 | | | |
| (Van de Kamp's) *Today's* | | | | | | |
| *Catch* | 4 oz. | 130 | 0.0 | | | |
| **FLOUR:** | | | | | | |
| Buckwheat, dark, sifted | | | | | | |
| (USDA) | 1 cup (3.5 oz.) | | 2.4 | | | 0 |
| Buckwheat, light, sifted | | | | | | |
| (USDA) | 1 cup (3.5 oz.) | | 1.2 | | | 0 |
| Carob or St. John's-bread | | | | | | |
| (USDA) | 1 oz. | | .4 | | | 0 |
| Chestnut (USDA) | 1 oz. | 3 | 1.0 | | | 0 |
| Corn, sifted (USDA) | 1 cup (3.9 oz.) | 1 | 2.9 | Tr. | 3. | 0 |
| Cottonseed (USDA) | 1 oz. | | 1.9 | <1. | 1. | 0 |
| Cottonseed (Data from General | | | | | | |
| Mills) | 1 oz. | 8 | 1.2 | | | (0) |
| Rye: | | | | | | |
| Light (USDA): | | | | | | |
| Unsifted, spooned | 1 cup (3.6 oz.) | 1 | 1.0 | | | 0 |
| Sifted, spooned | 1 cup (3.1 oz.) | <1 | .9 | | | 0 |
| Medium (USDA) | 1 oz. | <1 | .5 | | | 0 |
| Dark (USDA): | | | | | | |
| Unstirred | 1 cup (4.5 oz.) | 1 | 3.3 | | | 0 |
| Stirred | 1 cup (4.5 oz.) | 1 | 3.3 | | | 0 |
| Soybean (USDA): | | | | | | |
| Defatted, stirred | 1 cup (3.6 oz.) | 1 | .9 | | | 0 |
| Low fat, stirred | 1 cup (3.1 oz.) | <1 | 5.9 | <1. | 5. | 0 |
| Full fat, stirred | 1 cup (2.5 oz.) | <1 | 14.6 | 2. | 12. | 0 |
| High fat | 1 oz. | <1 | 3.4 | <1. | 3. | 0 |
| Sunflower seed, partially | | | | | | |
| defatted (USDA) | 1 oz. | 16 | 1.0 | Tr. | 1. | 0 |
| Tapioca, unsifted, spooned | | | | | | |
| (USDA) | 1 cup (3.8 oz.) | 3 | .2 | | | 0 |
| Wheat: | | | | | | |
| All-purpose: | | | | | | |
| (USDA) | 1 oz. | <1 | .3 | | | 0 |

(USDA): United States Department of Agriculture
*Prepared as Package Directs

| Food and Description | Measure or Quantity | Sodium (mg.) | Fats in grams — Total | Saturated | Unsaturated | Cholesterol (mg.) |
|---|---|---|---|---|---|---|
| Unsifted, dipped | 1 cup (5 oz.) | 3 | 1.4 | | | 0 |
| Unsifted, spooned | 1 cup (4.4 oz.) | 3 | 1.3 | | | 0 |
| Sifted, spooned | 1 cup (4.1 oz.) | 2 | 1.2 | | | 0 |
| Bread: | | | | | | |
| (USDA) | 1 oz. | <1 | .3 | | | 0 |
| Unsifted, dipped | 1 cup (4.8 oz.) | 3 | 1.5 | | | 0 |
| Unsifted, spooned | 1 cup (4.3 oz.) | 2 | 1.4 | | | 0 |
| Sifted, spooned | 1 cup (4.1 oz.) | 2 | 1.3 | | | 0 |
| Cake or pastry: | | | | | | |
| (USDA) | 1 oz. | <1 | .2 | | | 0 |
| Unsifted, dipped | 1 cup (4.2 oz.) | 2 | 1.0 | | | 0 |
| Unsifted, spooned | 1 cup (3.9 oz.) | 2 | .9 | | | 0 |
| Sifted, spooned | 1 cup (3.5 oz.) | 2 | .8 | | | 0 |
| Gluten: | | | | | | |
| (USDA) | 1 oz. | <1 | .5 | | | 0 |
| Unsifted, dipped | 1 cup (5 oz.) | 3 | 2.7 | | | 0 |
| Unsifted, spooned | 1 cup (4.8 oz.) | 3 | 2.6 | | | 0 |
| Sifted, spooned | 1 cup (4.8 oz.) | 3 | 2.6 | | | 0 |
| Self-rising: | | | | | | |
| (USDA) | 1 oz. | 306 | .3 | | | 0 |
| Unsifted, dipped | 1 cup (4.6 oz.) | 1,403 | 1.3 | | | 0 |
| Unsifted, spooned | 1 cup (4.5 oz.) | 1,370 | 1.3 | | | 0 |
| Sifted, spooned | 1 cup (3.7 oz.) | 1,144 | 1.1 | | | 0 |
| Whole wheat: | | | | | | |
| (USDA) | 1 oz. | <1 | .6 | | | 0 |
| Stirred, spooned | 1 cup (4.8 oz.) | 4 | 2.7 | | | 0 |
| Aunt Jemima, self-rising | | | | | | |
| (Quaker) | 1 cup (4 oz.) | 1,400 | 1.2 | | | (0) |
| Gold Medal (Betty Crocker): | | | | | | |
| Regular | 1 cup | 3 | 1.4 | | | (0) |
| Better-for-bread | 1 cup | 3 | 1.4 | | | (0) |
| Self-rising | 1 cup | 1,743 | 1.3 | | | (0) |
| Wondra | 1 cup | 3 | 1.4 | | | (0) |
| Presto, self-rising | 1 cup (3.9 oz.) | 1,320 | .9 | | | 0 |
| (Quaker) | 1 cup (4 oz.) | 4 | 1.2 | | | (0) |
| Softasilk for cakes (Betty Crocker) | 1 cup | 2 | .9 | | | (0) |
| | | | | | | |
| FRANKENBERRY, cereal | | | | | | |
| (General Mills) | 1 cup (1 oz.) | 205 | 1.0 | | | (0) |

(USDA): United States Department of Agriculture
*Prepared as Package Directs

| Food and Description | Measure or Quantity | Sodium (mg.) | —Fats in grams— | | | Choles-terol (mg.) |
|---|---|---|---|---|---|---|
| | | | Total | Satu-rated | Unsatu-rated | |
| **FRANKFURTER OR WIENER:** | | | | | | |
| Raw: | | | | | | |
| All kinds (USDA) | 1.6-oz. frankfurter | 499 | 12.5 | | | |
| All meat (USDA) | 1.6-oz. frankfurter | | 11.6 | | | 29 |
| With cereal (USDA) | 1.6-oz. frankfurter | | 9.3 | | | |
| With nonfat dry milk (USDA) | 1.6-oz. frankfurter | | 11.6 | | | |
| With nonfat dry milk & cereal (USDA) | 1.6-oz. frankfurter | | 9.8 | | | |
| (Eckrich): | | | | | | |
| Beef | 1.6-oz. frankfurter | 480 | 13.0 | | | |
| Beef, jumbo | 2-oz. frankfurter | 620 | 17.0 | | | |
| Meat | 1.2-oz. frankfurter | 360 | 11.0 | | | |
| (Hormel): | | | | | | |
| Beef | 1.6-oz. frankfurter | 362 | 10.0 | | | |
| *Range Brand, Wranglers,* smoked | 1 frankfurter | 619 | 15.0 | | | |
| (Hygrades) beef, *Ball Park* | 2-oz. frankfurter | | 15.6 | | | |
| (Louis Rich) turkey | 1.5-oz. frankfurter | | 8.0 | | | |
| (Oscar Mayer): | | | | | | |
| Bacon & cheddar | 1.6-oz. frankfurter | 509 | 12.7 | | | 30 |
| Beef | 1.6-oz. frankfurter | 460 | 13.5 | | | 28 |
| Cheese: | | | | | | |
| Regular | 1.6-oz. frankfurter | 474 | 13.2 | | | 30 |
| Nacho | 1.6-oz. frankfurter | 549 | 12.5 | | | 30 |
| Little Wiener | 2" frankfurter | 92 | 2.6 | | | 5 |
| Wiener | 1.6-oz. frankfurter | 459 | 13.5 | | | 24 |
| Cooked, all kinds, 10 per lb. raw (USDA) | 1 frankfurter | | 12.2 | | | 28 |
| Canned (USDA) | 2 oz. | | 10.3 | | | |
| **FRANKS & BEANS** (See **BEANS & FRANKS**) | | | | | | |
| ***FRANKS-N-BLANKETS,*** frozen (Durkee) | 1 piece (.4 oz.) | | 3.8 | | | |
| **FRENCH TOAST,** frozen: | | | | | | |
| (Aunt Jemima) regular | 1 slice (1.5 oz.) | 216 | 2.2 | | | |
| (Swanson) plain | 6½-oz. breakfast | 770 | 26.0 | | | |
| **FRITTERS:** | | | | | | |
| Apple, frozen (Mrs. Paul's) | 2-oz. fritter | 385 | 7.5 | | | |

(USDA): United States Department of Agriculture
*Prepared as Package Directs

| Food and Description | Measure or Quantity | Sodium (mg.) | —Fats in grams— | | | Choles-terol (mg.) |
|---|---|---|---|---|---|---|
| | | | Total | Satu-rated | Unsatu-rated | |
| Clam, home recipe (USDA) | 1 fritter (1.4 oz.) | | 6.0 | | | 52 |
| Corn: | | | | | | |
| Home recipe (USDA) | 1 fritter (1.2 oz.) | 541 | 24.4 | 5.7 | 18.7 | |
| Frozen (Mrs. Paul's) | 2-oz. piece | 363 | 6.0 | | | |
| **FROG LEGS,** raw (USDA): | | | | | | |
| Bone in | 1 lb. (weighed with bone) | | .9 | | | 147 |
| Meat only | 4 oz. | | .3 | | | 57 |
| *FROOT LOOPS,* cereal (Kellogg's) | 1 cup (1 oz.) | 135 | 1.0 | | | (0) |
| *FROSTED RICE,* cereal (Ralston Purina) | 1 cup (1 oz.) | 151 | .4 | | | (0) |
| **FROSTING** (See **CAKE ICING**) | | | | | | |
| **FROZEN CUSTARD** (See **ICE CREAM**) | | | | | | |
| **FROZEN DESSERT** (See also *TOFUTTI*): | | | | | | |
| (Baskin-Robbins) Low, Lite 'n Luscious, chunky banana | ½ cup | 50 | 1.0 | | | 3 |
| (Borden's) ice milk, strawberry or vanilla | ½ cup | 65 | 2.0 | | | |
| *Eskimo* bar, chocolate covered | 2½-fl.-oz. bar | 40 | 7.0 | | | |
| *FRUIT N' APPLE,* juice (Tree Top) canned or frozen | 6 fl. oz. | 10 | 0.0 | | | 0 |
| *FRUIT N' BERRY,* juice (Tree Top) canned or frozen | 6 fl. oz. | 10 | 0.0 | | | 0 |
| *FRUIT BITS* (Sun-Maid) | 1 oz. | 24 | .3 | | | |
| **FRUIT COCKTAIL:** | | | | | | |
| Canned, regular pack, solids & liq.: | | | | | | |
| Light syrup (USDA) | 4 oz. | 6 | .1 | | | 0 |
| Heavy syrup (USDA) | ½ cup (4.5 oz.) | 6 | .1 | | | 0 |

(USDA): United States Department of Agriculture
*Prepared as Package Directs

| Food and Description | Measure or Quantity | Sodium (mg.) | — Fats in grams — | | | Choles-terol (mg.) |
|---|---|---|---|---|---|---|
| | | | Total | Satu-rated | Unsatu-rated | |
| Heavy syrup (Del Monte) | ½ cup (4.3 oz.) | <10 | .1 | | | (0) |
| Heavy syrup (Libby's) | ½ cup | 8 | .1 | | | (0) |
| Heavy syrup (Stokely-Van Camp's) | ½ cup (4 oz.) | | .1 | | | (0) |
| Extra heavy syrup (USDA) | 4 oz. | 6 | .1 | | | 0 |
| Canned, unsweetened or dietetic pack, solids & liq.: | | | | | | |
| Water pack (USDA) | 4 oz. | 6 | .1 | | | 0 |
| (S & W) *Nutradiet* | 4 oz. | 3 | .1 | | | (0) |
| **FRUIT COMPOTE** (Rokeach) | ½ cup (4 oz.) | 4 | 1.0 | | | |
| ***FRUIT & FIBRE,*** cereal (Post): | | | | | | |
| Apple & cinnamon | ½ cup (1 oz.) | 195 | .3 | | | 0 |
| Dates, raisins & walnuts | ½ cup (1 oz.) | 170 | .7 | | | 0 |
| ***FRUIT N' GRAPE,*** juice (Tree Top) | 6 fl. oz. | 10 | 0.0 | | | 0 |
| ***FRUIT 'N JUICE BAR*** (Dole): | | | | | | |
| Orange or strawberry | 2½-fl.-oz. bar | 6 | Tr. | | | |
| Pineapple | 2½-fl.-oz. bar | 4 | Tr. | | | |
| **FRUIT, MIXED:** | | | | | | |
| Canned: | | | | | | |
| (Hunt's) *Snack-Pak* | 5-oz. container | 5 | <1.0 | | | |
| (Libby's) lite | ½ cup | 10 | 1.0 | | | |
| Dried: | | | | | | |
| (Del Monte) | 2 oz. | 10 | 0.0 | | | |
| (Sun-Maid/Sunsweet) | 2 oz. | 11 | Tr. | | | |
| Frozen (Birds Eye) | 5 oz. | 4 | .3 | | | 0 |
| **FRUIT & NUT MIX** (Carnation): | | | | | | |
| All fruit | .9-oz. packet | 10 | Tr. | | | |
| Deluxe trail mix | .9-oz. packet | 10 | 8.0 | | | |
| Raisins & nuts | .9-oz. packet | 10 | 7.0 | | | |
| Tropical fruit & nuts | .9-oz. packet | 10 | 3.0 | | | |
| **FRUIT PUNCH:** | | | | | | |
| Canned: | | | | | | |
| (Hi-C) | 6 fl. oz. | <1 | Tr. | | | (0) |
| (Lincoln) party | 6 fl. oz. | 30 | 0.0 | | | (0) |

(USDA): United States Department of Agriculture
*Prepared as Package Directs

| Food and Description | Measure or Quantity | Sodium (mg.) | — Fats in grams — | | | Cholesterol (mg.) |
|---|---|---|---|---|---|---|
| | | | Total | Saturated | Unsaturated | |
| *Mix, dietetic: | | | | | | |
|   *Crystal Light* | 6 fl. oz. | <1 | Tr. | | | 0 |
|   (Sunkist) | 6 fl. oz. | 15 | 0.0 | | | (0) |
| **FRUIT ROLLS:** | | | | | | |
|   (Betty Crocker) *Fruit Roll-Ups* | .5-oz. piece | 5 | <1.0 | | | |
|   (Flavor Tree) | ¾-oz. piece | 15 | Tr. | | | |
|   (Sunkist) | .5-oz. piece | 10 | Tr. | | | |
| **FRUIT SALAD:** | | | | | | |
|   Bottled, chilled (Kraft) | 4 oz. | 115 | .1 | | | (0) |
|   Canned, regular pack, solids & liq.: | | | | | | |
|     Light syrup (USDA) | 4 oz. | 1 | .1 | | | 0 |
|     Heavy syrup (USDA) | ½ cup (4.3 oz.) | 1 | .1 | | | 0 |
|     Heavy syrup (Del Monte): | | | | | | |
|       Fruits for salad | ½ cup (4.3 oz.) | 10 | 0.0 | | | 0 |
|       Tropical | ½ cup (4.4 oz.) | <10 | 0.0 | | | 0 |
|     Extra heavy syrup (USDA) | 4 oz. | 1 | .1 | | | 0 |
|   Canned, unsweetened or dietetic pack: | | | | | | |
|     Water pack (USDA) | 4 oz. | 1 | .1 | | | 0 |
|     (Diet Delight) | ½ cup (4.4 oz.) | 5 | 0.0 | | | (0) |
| **FRUIT SQUARES** (Pepperidge Farm): | | | | | | |
|   Apple | 2½-oz. piece | 175 | 12.0 | | | |
|   Blueberry | 2½-oz. piece | 190 | 11.0 | | | |
|   Cherry | 2½-oz. piece | 185 | 12.0 | | | |

# G

| Food and Description | Measure or Quantity | Sodium (mg.) | Total | Saturated | Unsaturated | Cholesterol (mg.) |
|---|---|---|---|---|---|---|
| **GARBANZO,** dry (See **CHICK PEA,** dry) | | | | | | |
| **GARLIC,** raw (USDA): | | | | | | |
|   Whole | 2 oz. (weighed with skin) | 10 | .1 | | | 0 |
|   Peeled | 1 oz. | 5 | <.1 | | | 0 |

(USDA): United States Department of Agriculture
*Prepared as Package Directs

| Food and Description | Measure or Quantity | Sodium (mg.) | —Fats in grams— | | | Choles-terol (mg.) |
|---|---|---|---|---|---|---|
| | | | Total | Satu-rated | Unsatu-rated | |
| **GARLIC:** | | | | | | |
| Dried, chips (Spice Islands) | 1 tsp. | 1 | | | | (0) |
| Powdered (Spice Islands) | 1 tsp. | 1 | | | | (0) |
| **GARLIC SPREAD** (Lawry's) | 1 T. (.5 oz.) | | 8.2 | | | |
| **GEFILTE FISH:** | | | | | | |
| (Mother's) any type | 4 oz. | | 1.0 | | | |
| (Rokeach): | | | | | | |
| Natural broth | 2-oz. piece | | .8 | | | |
| Jelled | 1 piece | | .6 | | | |
| **GELATIN,** unflavored, dry: | | | | | | |
| (USDA) | 1 envelope (7 grams) | | Tr. | | | 0 |
| (Knox) | 1 envelope (7 grams) | 0 | 0.0 | | | (0) |
| **GELATIN DESSERT POWDER:** | | | | | | |
| Regular: | | | | | | |
| Dry (USDA) | 3-oz. pkg. | 270 | 0.0 | | | 0 |
| Dry (USDA) | ½ cup (3.3 oz.) | 297 | 0.0 | | | 0 |
| *Prepared with water (USDA) | ½ cup (4.2 oz.) | 61 | 0.0 | | | 0 |
| *Prepared with fruit added (USDA) | ½ cup (4.3 oz.) | 41 | .2 | | | 0 |
| *(Jell-O): | | | | | | |
| Apricot, black cherry, mixed fruit, orange, peach, raspberry, strawberry or strawberry vanilla | ½ cup | 55 | Tr. | | | 0 |
| Blackberry | ½ cup | 54 | Tr. | | | 0 |
| Cherry | ½ cup | 77 | Tr. | | | 0 |
| Grape | ½ cup | 40 | Tr. | | | 0 |
| Lemon or wild strawberry | ½ cup | 81 | Tr. | | | 0 |
| Lime | ½ cup | 62 | Tr. | | | 0 |
| Raspberry, black | ½ cup | 39 | Tr. | | | 0 |
| *(Royal): | | | | | | |
| Apple, blackberry, cherry, lemon-lime, orange, raspberry, strawberry | | | | | | |

(USDA): United States Department of Agriculture
*Prepared as Package Directs

| Food and Description | Measure or Quantity | Sodium (mg.) | —Fats in grams— | | | Cholesterol (mg.) |
|---|---|---|---|---|---|---|
| | | | Total | Saturated | Unsaturated | |
| banana or tropical fruit | ½ cup | 95 | 0.0 | | | 0 |
| Lemon, peach or strawberry | ½ cup | 100 | 0.0 | | | 0 |
| Lime or pineapple | ½ cup | 90 | 0.0 | | | 0 |
| *Dietetic, all flavors (D-Zerta) | ½ cup (4.3 oz.) | 5 | Tr. | | | 0 |
| **GELATIN DRINK,** plain or flavored (Knox) | 1 envelope (.7 oz.) | 20 | 0.0 | | | (0) |
| **GINGER** (Spice Islands): | | | | | | |
| Whole | 1 average piece | 1 | | | | (0) |
| Ground | 1 tsp. | 1 | | | | (0) |
| **GINGER ALE,** soft drink (See **SOFT DRINK, GINGER ALE**) | | | | | | |
| **GINGERBREAD,** home recipe (USDA)[1]: | | | | | | |
| Made with butter[2] | 1.9-oz. piece (2″ × 2″ × 2″) | 130 | 5.3 | 3. | 3. | |
| Made with vegetable shortening[3] | 1.9-oz. piece (2″ × 2″ × 2″) | 130 | 5.9 | 2. | 4. | |
| **GINGERBREAD MIX:** | | | | | | |
| Dry (USDA)[4] | 1 oz. | 131 | 2.9 | <1. | 2. | |
| *Prepared with water (USDA)[5] | ⅑ of 8″ sq. (2.2 oz.) | 192 | 4.3 | <1. | 4. | <1 |
| *(Betty Crocker) | ⅑ of cake | 325 | 7.0 | | | |
| *(Dromedary) | 1.2-oz. piece (2″ × 2″) | 190 | 2.0 | | | |
| **GINGER ROOT,** fresh (USDA): | | | | | | |
| With skin | 1 oz. | 2 | .3 | | | 0 |
| Without skin | 1 oz. | 2 | .3 | | | 0 |

(USDA): United States Department of Agriculture
*Prepared as Package Directs
[1]Made with sodium aluminum sulfate-type baking powder.
[2]Principal sources of fat: butter, egg & milk.
[3]Principal sources of fat: vegetable shortening, egg & milk.
[4]Principal source of fat: vegetable shortening.
[5]Principal sources of fat: vegetable shortening & egg.

| Food and Description | Measure or Quantity | Sodium (mg.) | —Fats in grams— | | | Choles- terol (mg.) |
|---|---|---|---|---|---|---|
| | | | Total | Satu- rated | Unsatu- rated | |
| **GOOD HUMOR** (See **ICE CREAM**) | | | | | | |
| **GOOSE,** domesticated (USDA): | | | | | | |
| Raw, ready-to-cook | 1 lb. (weighed with bones) | | 104.3 | | | |
| Raw, total edible | 1 lb. | | 142.9 | | | |
| Raw, meat & skin | 1 lb. | | 152.4 | | | |
| Raw, meat only | 1 lb. | | 32.2 | | | |
| Roasted, total edible | 4 oz. | | 40.8 | | | |
| Roasted, meat & skin | 4 oz. | | 43.2 | | | |
| Roasted, meat only | 4 oz. | 141 | 11.1 | | | |
| **GOOSEBERRY** (USDA): | | | | | | |
| Fresh | 1 lb | 5 | .9 | | | 0 |
| Fresh | 1 cup (5.3 oz.) | 2 | .3 | | | 0 |
| Canned, solids & liq.: | | | | | | |
| Regular pack, heavy or extra heavy syrup | 4 oz. | 1 | .1 | | | 0 |
| Water pack | 4 oz. | 1 | .1 | | | 0 |
| **GOOSE, GIBLET,** raw (USDA) | 4 oz. | | 7.9 | | | |
| **GOOSE GIZZARD,** raw (USDA) | 4 oz. | | 6.0 | | | |
| **GRANOLA BAR:** | | | | | | |
| *Nature Valley:* | | | | | | |
| Regular: | | | | | | |
| Almond | .8-oz. piece | 80 | 4.0 | | | |
| Cinnamon or oats & honey | .8-oz. piece | 65 | 4.0 | | | |
| Coconut | .8-oz. piece | 65 | 6.0 | | | |
| Chewey: | | | | | | |
| Apple | 1 bar | 65 | 5.0 | | | |
| Chocolate chip | 1 bar | 85 | 7.0 | | | |
| Peanut butter | 1 bar | 80 | 7.0 | | | |
| Raisin | 1 bar | 65 | 5.0 | | | |
| *New Trail* (Hershey's) chocolate covered: | | | | | | |
| Chocolate chip | 1.2-oz. piece | 60 | 11.0 | | | |
| Cocoa creme | 1.3-oz. piece | 70 | 9.0 | | | |
| Cookies & creme | 1.3-oz. piece | 85 | 11.0 | | | |

(USDA): United States Department of Agriculture
*Prepared as Package Directs

| Food and Description | Measure or Quantity | Sodium (mg.) | Fats in grams — Total | Satu- rated | Unsatu- rated | Choles- terol (mg.) |
|---|---|---|---|---|---|---|
| Peanut butter | 1.3-oz. piece | 90 | 11.0 | | | |

*GRANOLA BAR MIX, chewey,
*Nature Valley, Bake-A-Bar:*
Chocolate chip, oats & honey

| | | | | | | |
|---|---|---|---|---|---|---|
| or raisins & spice | 1/24 pkg. | 40 | 4.0 | | | |
| Peanut butter | 1/24 pkg. | 60 | 4.0 | | | |

## GRANOLA CEREAL:
*Nature Valley:*
Cinnamon & raisin, fruit &

| | | | | | | |
|---|---|---|---|---|---|---|
| nut or toasted oats | 1/3 cup (1 oz.) | 35 | 5.0 | | | |
| Coconut & honey | 1/3 cup (1 oz.) | 35 | 7.0 | | | |

*Sun Country* (Kretschmer):

| | | | | | | |
|---|---|---|---|---|---|---|
| With almonds | 1/4 cup (1 oz.) | 10 | 4.8 | | | |
| With raisins | 1/4 cup (1 oz.) | 10 | 4.5 | | | |

## GRANOLA CLUSTER, *Nature Valley:*

| | | | | | | |
|---|---|---|---|---|---|---|
| Almond | 1 piece | 140 | 3.0 | | | |
| Apple-cinnamon | 1 piece | 125 | 4.0 | | | |
| Caramel | 1 piece | 95 | 3.0 | | | |
| Chocolate chip | 1 piece | 100 | 4.0 | | | |
| Raisin | 1 piece | 110 | 3.0 | | | |

## GRANOLA & FRUIT BAR,
*Nature Valley:*

| | | | | | | |
|---|---|---|---|---|---|---|
| Apple or raspberry | 1 bar | 150 | 5.0 | | | |
| Date | 1 bar | 135 | 5.0 | | | |

## GRANOLA SNACK, *Kudos*
(M&M/Mars):

| | | | | | | |
|---|---|---|---|---|---|---|
| Chocolate chip | 1 1/4-oz. serving | 60 | 9.0 | | | |
| Nutty fudge | 1.3-oz. serving | 60 | 11.0 | | | |
| Peanut butter | 1.3-oz. serving | 70 | 12.0 | | | |

## GRAPE:
Fresh:
American type (slip skin),
Concord, Delaware,
Niagara, Catawba &
Scuppernong, pulp only:

(USDA): United States Department of Agriculture
*Prepared as Package Directs

| Food and Description | Measure or Quantity | Sodium (mg.) | —Fats in grams— | | | Choles-terol (mg.) |
|---|---|---|---|---|---|---|
| | | | Total | Satu-rated | Unsatu-rated | |
| (USDA) | ½ lb. (weighed with stem, skin & seeds) | 4 | 1.4 | | | 0 |
| (USDA) | ½ cup (2.7 oz.) | 2 | .8 | | | 0 |
| (USDA) | 3½" × 3" bunch (3.5 oz.) | 2 | .6 | | | 0 |
| European type (adherent skin), Malaga, Muscat, Thompson seedless, Emperor & Flame Tokay, with skin: | | | | | | |
| (USDA) | ½ lb. (weighed with stems & seeds) | 6 | .6 | | | 0 |
| Whole (USDA) | 20 grapes (¾" dia.) | 2 | .2 | | | 0 |
| Whole (USDA) | ½ cup (3.1 oz.) | 3 | .3 | | | 0 |
| Halves (USDA) | ½ cup (3 oz.) | 3 | .3 | | | 0 |
| Canned, solids & liq. (USDA): | | | | | | |
| Thompson seedless, heavy syrup | 4 oz. | 5 | .1 | | | 0 |
| Thompson seedless, water pack | 4 oz. | 5 | .1 | | | 0 |

**GRAPE DRINK:**
Canned:

| Food and Description | Measure or Quantity | Sodium (mg.) | Total | | | |
|---|---|---|---|---|---|---|
| *Capri Sun* | 6¾ fl. oz. | 19 | 0.0 | | | |
| (Lincoln) | 6 fl. oz. | 30 | 0.0 | | | |
| (Welchade) | 6 fl. oz. | 20 | 0.0 | | | |
| Chilled (Sunkist) | 8.45-fl.-oz. container | 0 | 0.0 | | | |
| *Mix: | | | | | | |
| Regular (Hi-C) | 6 fl. oz. | 42 | 0.0 | | | |
| Dietetic (Sunkist) | 8 fl. oz. | 25 | 0.0 | | | |

**GRAPE JAM:**

| Food and Description | Measure or Quantity | Sodium (mg.) | Total | | | Choles-terol (mg.) |
|---|---|---|---|---|---|---|
| (Bama) | 1 T. (.7 oz.) | 3 | <.1 | | | (0) |
| (Smucker's) | 1 T. (.7 oz.) | 5 | <.1 | | | (0) |

**GRAPE JELLY,** low calorie:

| Food and Description | Measure or Quantity | Sodium (mg.) | Total | | | Choles-terol (mg.) |
|---|---|---|---|---|---|---|
| (Kraft) | 1 oz. | 37 | <.1 | | | (0) |
| (Diet Delight) Concord | 1 T. (.6 oz.) | 21 | Tr. | | | (0) |

(USDA): United States Department of Agriculture
*Prepared as Package Directs

| Food and Description | Measure or Quantity | Sodium (mg.) | —Fats in grams— | | | Choles-terol (mg.) |
|---|---|---|---|---|---|---|
| | | | Total | Satu-rated | Unsatu-rated | |
| (S & W) *Nutradiet,* Concord | 1 T. (.5 oz.) | | <.1 | | | (0) |
| (Slenderella) | 1 T. (.7 oz.) | 34 | <.1 | | | (0) |
| (Smucker's) | 1 T. (.7 oz.) | Tr. | Tr. | | | (0) |
| (Tillie Lewis) | 1 T. (.5 oz.) | 4 | Tr. | | | 0 |
| **GRAPE JUICE:** | | | | | | |
| Canned: | | | | | | |
| (USDA) | ½ cup (4.4 oz.) | | Tr. | | | 0 |
| (Heinz) | 5½-fl.-oz. can | 2 | .2 | | | (0) |
| (S & W) *Nutradiet* | 4 oz. (by wt.) | 2 | .1 | | | (0) |
| Frozen, concentrate, sweetened: | | | | | | |
| (USDA) | 6-fl.-oz. can (7.6 oz.) | 6 | Tr. | | | 0 |
| Diluted with 3 parts water | | | | | | |
| (USDA) | ½ cup (4.4 oz.) | 1 | Tr. | | | 0 |
| *(Minute Maid) | ½ cup (4.2 oz.) | 1 | Tr. | | | 0 |
| *(Snow Crop) | ½ cup (4.2 oz.) | 1 | Tr. | | | 0 |
| **GRAPE JUICE DRINK,** canned (USDA) approximately 30% grape juice | 1 cup (8.8 oz.) | 2 | Tr. | | | 0 |
| *GRAPE-NUTS,* cereal (Post) | ¼ cup (1 oz.) | 147 | .1 | | | 0 |
| *GRAPE-NUTS FLAKES,* cereal (Post) | ¼ cup (1 oz.) | 197 | .1 | | | 0 |
| **GRAPEFRUIT:** | | | | | | |
| Fresh, pulp only: | | | | | | |
| Pink & red: | | | | | | |
| Seeded type (USDA) | 1 lb. (weighed with seeds and skin) | 2 | .2 | | | 0 |
| Seeded type (USDA) | ½ med. grapefruit (3¾", 8.5 oz.) | 1 | .1 | | | 0 |
| Seedless type (USDA) | 1 lb. (weighed with skin) | 2 | .2 | | | 0 |
| Seedless type (USDA) | ½ med. grapefruit (8.5 oz.) | 1 | .1 | | | 0 |

(USDA): United States Department of Agriculture
*Prepared as Package Directs

| Food and Description | Measure or Quantity | Sodium (mg.) | — Fats in grams — | | | Cholesterol (mg.) |
|---|---|---|---|---|---|---|
| | | | Total | Satu-rated | Unsatu-rated | |
| **White:** | | | | | | |
| Seeded type (USDA) | 1 lb. (weighed with seeds & skin) | 2 | .2 | | | 0 |
| Seeded type (USDA) | ½ med. grapefruit (3¾", 8.5 oz.) | 1 | .1 | | | 0 |
| Seedless type (USDA) | 1 lb. (weighed with skin) | 2 | .2 | | | 0 |
| Seedless type, sections (USDA) | 1 cup (7 oz.) | 2 | .2 | | | 0 |
| Seedless type (USDA) | ½ med. grapefruit (3¾", 8.5 oz.) | 1 | .1 | | | 0 |
| (Sunkist) | ½ grapefruit (8.5 oz.) | 1 | Tr. | | | 0 |
| Bottled, chilled, sweetened sections (Kraft) | 4 oz. | 115 | .1 | | | (0) |
| Bottled, chilled, unsweetened sections (Kraft) | 4 oz. | 115 | .1 | | | (0) |
| Canned, sections, syrup pack, solids & liq.: | | | | | | |
| (USDA) | ½ cup (4.5 oz.) | 1 | .1 | | | 0 |
| (Del Monte) | ½ cup (4.5 oz.) | 2 | | | | 0 |
| Light syrup (Stokely-Van Camp's) | ½ cup (4 oz.) | | .1 | | | (0) |
| Canned, sections, unsweetened or dietetic pack, solids & liq.: | | | | | | |
| Water pack (USDA) | ½ cup (4.2 oz.) | 5 | .1 | | | 0 |
| Juice pack (Del Monte) | ½ cup (4.5 oz.) | 1 | .5 | | | 0 |
| (Diet Delight) unsweetened | ½ cup (4.3 oz.) | 5 | <.1 | | | (0) |
| (S & W) *Nutradiet* | 4 oz. | 2 | .1 | | | (0) |
| **GRAPEFRUIT JUICE:** | | | | | | |
| Fresh, pink, red or white, all varieties (USDA) | ½ cup (4.3 oz.) | 1 | .1 | | | 0 |
| Bottled, chilled, sweetened (Kraft) | ½ cup (4.3 oz.) | 1 | .1 | | | (0) |
| Bottled, chilled, unsweetened (Kraft) | ½ cup (4.3 oz.) | 1 | .1 | | | (0) |

(USDA): United States Department of Agriculture
*Prepared as Package Directs

| Food and Description | Measure or Quantity | Sodium (mg.) | — Fats in grams — | | | Choles- terol (mg.) |
|---|---|---|---|---|---|---|
| | | | Total | Satu- rated | Unsatu- rated | |
| Canned: | | | | | | |
| Sweetened: | | | | | | |
| (USDA) | ½ cup (4.4 oz.) | 1 | .1 | | | 0 |
| (Del Monte) | ½ cup (4.3 oz.) | 1 | Tr. | | | 0 |
| Unsweetened: | | | | | | |
| (USDA) | ½ cup (4.4 oz.) | 1 | .1 | | | 0 |
| (Del Monte) | ½ cup (4.3 oz.) | 5 | .2 | | | 0 |
| (Diet Delight) | ½ cup (4 oz.) | 7 | Tr. | | | (0) |
| Frozen, concentrate: | | | | | | |
| Sweetened: | | | | | | |
| (USDA) | 6-fl.-oz. can (7.4 oz.) | 6 | .6 | | | 0 |
| *Diluted with 3 parts water (USDA) | ½ cup (4.4 oz.) | 1 | .1 | | | 0 |
| *(Minute Maid) | ½ cup (4.2 oz.) | <1 | Tr. | | | 0 |
| *(Snow Crop) | ½ cup (4.2 oz.) | <1 | Tr. | | | 0 |
| Unsweetened: | | | | | | |
| (USDA) | 6-fl.-oz. can (7.3 oz.) | 8 | .8 | | | 0 |
| *Diluted with 3 parts water (USDA) | ½ cup (4.4 oz.) | 1 | .1 | | | 0 |
| *(Minute Maid) | ½ cup (4.2 oz.) | <1 | Tr. | | | 0 |
| *(Snow Crop) | ½ cup (4.2 oz.) | <1 | Tr. | | | 0 |
| Dehydrated, crystals: | | | | | | |
| (USDA) | 4-oz. can | 11 | 1.1 | | | 0 |
| *Reconstituted (USDA) | ½ cup (4.4 oz.) | 1 | .1 | | | 0 |
| **GRAPEFRUIT-ORANGE JUICE** (See **ORANGE-GRAPEFRUIT JUICE**) | | | | | | |
| **GRAPEFRUIT PEEL, CANDIED** (USDA) | 1 oz. | | <.1 | | | 0 |
| **GRAVY,** canned: | | | | | | |
| Au jus (Franco-American) | 2 oz. | 290 | 0.0 | | | |
| Beef (Franco-American) | 2 oz. | 310 | 1.0 | | | |
| Brown: | | | | | | |
| (Estee) dietetic | ¼ cup | 85 | 0.0 | | | |
| (Franco-American) with onion | 2 oz. | 340 | 1.0 | | | |
| Chicken (Franco-American): | | | | | | |
| Regular | 2 oz. | 320 | 4.0 | | | |

(USDA): United States Department of Agriculture
*Prepared as Package Directs

| Food and Description | Measure or Quantity | Sodium (mg.) | — Fats in grams — | | | Choles- terol (mg.) |
|---|---|---|---|---|---|---|
| | | | Total | Satu- rated | Unsatu- rated | |
| Giblet | 2 oz. | 320 | 2.0 | | | |
| Mushroom (Franco-American) | 2 oz. | 320 | 1.0 | | | |
| Pork (Franco-American) | 2 oz. | 350 | 3.0 | | | |
| Turkey (Franco-American) | 2 oz. | 300 | 2.0 | | | |
| **GRAVY MASTER** | 1 fl. oz. (1.3 oz.) | 746 | Tr. | | | 0 |
| **GRAVY WITH MEAT OR TURKEY,** frozen: | | | | | | |
| (Banquet): | | | | | | |
| Entree for one: | | | | | | |
| & sliced beef | 4 oz. | 426 | 3.0 | | | 40 |
| & sliced turkey | 5 oz. | 586 | 5.0 | | | 45 |
| *Family Entrees:* | | | | | | |
| & salisbury steak | 32-oz. pkg. | 5,100 | 90.0 | | | |
| & sliced beef | 32-oz. pkg. | 3,600 | 54.0 | | | |
| & sliced turkey | 32-oz. pkg. | 4,040 | 32.0 | | | |
| (Morton) light, entrees: | | | | | | |
| Beef | 8 oz. | 490 | 9.0 | | | |
| Chicken | 8 oz. | 600 | 9.0 | | | |
| Salisbury steak | 8 oz. | 570 | 11.0 | | | |
| Turkey | 8 oz. | 1,310 | 4.0 | | | |
| (Swanson) & beef | 8-oz. meal | 760 | 6.0 | | | |
| **GRAVY MIX:** | | | | | | |
| *Au jus (Durkee) | 1 cup | 913 | .1 | | | |
| *Au jus (French's) | 1/4 cup | 260 | 0.0 | | | |
| Brown: | | | | | | |
| *(Durkee) | 1 cup (.8-oz. pkg.) | 1,037 | .3 | | | |
| *(French's) | 1/4 cup | 250 | 1.0 | | | |
| (McCormick) | 7/8-oz. pkg. | 680 | 1.2 | | | |
| *(Pillsbury) | 1/4 cup | 300 | 0.0 | | | |
| Chicken: | | | | | | |
| *(Durkee) | 1 cup (1-oz. pkg.) | 1,710 | 2.3 | | | |
| *(French's) | 1/4 cup | 270 | 1.2 | | | |
| *(McCormick) | 2-oz. serving | 325 | 3.0 | | | |
| *Homestyle (French's) | 1/4 cup | 250 | 1.0 | | | 2 |
| Mushroom: | | | | | | |
| *(Durkee) | 1 cup (.8-oz. pkg.) | 1,170 | 1.0 | | | |
| *(French's) | 1/4 cup | 250 | .5 | | | |

(USDA): United States Department of Agriculture
*Prepared as Package Directs

193

| Food and Description | Measure or Quantity | Sodium (mg.) | Fats in grams — Total | Satu- rated | Unsatu- rated | Choles- terol (mg.) |
|---|---|---|---|---|---|---|
| Onion: | | | | | | |
| *(Durkee) | 1 cup (1-oz. pkg.) | 953 | .5 | | | |
| *Pork (French's) | ¼ cup | 250 | 1.0 | | | |
| *Turkey: | | | | | | |
| (Durkee) | ¼ cup | 330 | .5 | | | |
| (French's) | ¼ cup | 290 | 1.0 | | | |

**GREEN PEA** (See **PEA**)

**GREENS, MIXED,** canned, solids & liq.:

| | | | | | | |
|---|---|---|---|---|---|---|
| (Allen) | ½ cup (4 oz.) | 100 | < 1.0 | | | |
| (Sunshine) | ½ cup | 468 | .4 | | | |

**GRITS** (See **HOMINY GRITS**)

**GROUND-CHERRY,** Poha or Cape Gooseberry, fresh (USDA):

| | | | | | | |
|---|---|---|---|---|---|---|
| Whole | 1 lb. (weighed with husks & stems) | | 2.9 | | | 0 |
| Flesh only | 4 oz. | | .8 | | | 0 |

**GROUPER,** raw (USDA):

| | | | | | | |
|---|---|---|---|---|---|---|
| Whole | 1 lb. (weighed whole) | | 1.0 | | | |
| Meat only | 4 oz. | | .6 | | | |

**GUAVA, COMMON,** fresh (USDA):

| | | | | | | |
|---|---|---|---|---|---|---|
| Whole | 1 lb. (weighed untrimmed) | 18 | 2.6 | | | 0 |
| Whole | 1 guava (2.8 oz.) | 3 | .5 | | | 0 |
| Flesh only | 4 oz. | 5 | .7 | | | 0 |

**GUAVA NECTAR,** canned

| | | | | | | |
|---|---|---|---|---|---|---|
| (Libby's) | 6 fl. oz. | 5 | 0.0 | | | |

**GUAVA, STRAWBERRY,** fresh (USDA):

| | | | | | | |
|---|---|---|---|---|---|---|
| Whole | 1 lb. (weighed untrimmed) | 18 | 2.7 | | | 0 |

(USDA): United States Department of Agriculture
*Prepared as Package Directs

| Food and Description | Measure or Quantity | Sodium (mg.) | — Fats in grams — | | | Choles- terol (mg.) |
|---|---|---|---|---|---|---|
| | | | Total | Satu- rated | Unsatu- rated | |
| Flesh only | 4 oz. | 5 | .7 | | | 0 |
| **GUINEA HEN,** raw (USDA): | | | | | | |
| Ready-to-cook | 1 lb. (weighed with bones) | | 24.4 | | | |
| Meat & skin | 4 oz. | | 7.3 | | | |
| Giblets | 2 oz. | | 4.0 | | | |

**GUM** (See **CHEWING GUM**)

# H

| | | | | | | |
|---|---|---|---|---|---|---|
| **HADDOCK:** | | | | | | |
| Raw (USDA): | | | | | | |
| Whole | 1 lb. (weighed whole) | 133 | .2 | | | 131 |
| Meat only | 4 oz. | 69 | .1 | | | 68 |
| Fried, dipped in egg, milk & bread crumbs (USDA) | 4″ × 3″ × ½″ fillet (3.5 oz.) | 177 | 6.4 | | | |
| Frozen: | | | | | | |
| (Gorton's): | | | | | | |
| *Fishmarket Fresh* | 4 oz. | 100 | 1.0 | | | |
| Light recipe | 1 piece | 570 | 10.0 | | | |
| (Mrs. Paul's): | | | | | | |
| Batter fried, crunchy light | 2 oz. | 400 | 7.5 | | | |
| Breaded & fried, light & natural | 6 oz. | 960 | 14.0 | | | |
| (Van de Kamp's) batter dipped | 2 oz. | 215 | 5.0 | | | |
| Smoked, canned or not (USDA) | 4 oz. | | .5 | | | |
| **HAKE,** raw (USDA): | | | | | | |
| Whole | 1 lb. (weighed whole) | 144 | .8 | | | |
| Meat only | 4 oz. | 84 | .5 | | | |

**HALF & HALF,** milk & cream (See **CREAM**)

(USDA): United States Department of Agriculture
*Prepared as Package Directs

| Food and Description | Measure or Quantity | Sodium (mg.) | Fats in grams — Total | Satu- rated | Unsatu- rated | Choles- terol (mg.) |
|---|---|---|---|---|---|---|
| **HALIBUT:** | | | | | | |
| Atlantic & Pacific: | | | | | | |
| Raw (USDA): | | | | | | |
| Whole | 1 lb. (weighed whole) | 145 | 3.2 | | | 134 |
| Meat only, not dipped in brine | 4 oz. | 61 | 1.4 | | | 57 |
| Meat only, dipped in brine (USDA) | 4 oz. | 408 | 1.4 | | | 57 |
| Broiled with vegetable shortening (USDA) | 6½" × 2½" × 8" or 4" × 3" × ½" steak (4.4 oz.) | 168 | 8.8 | | | 75 |
| Smoked (USDA) | 4 oz. | | 17.0 | | | |
| California, raw, meat only (USDA) | 4 oz. | | 1.6 | | | |
| **HAM** (See also **PORK**): | | | | | | |
| Boiled: | | | | | | |
| Luncheon meat (USDA)[1] | 1 oz. | | 4.8 | 2. | 3. | |
| Luncheon meat, chopped (USDA)[1] | 1 cup (4.8 oz.) | | 23.1 | 8. | 15. | |
| Luncheon meat, diced (USDA)[1] | 1 cup (5 oz.) | | 24.0 | 8. | 16. | |
| (Hormel) | 1 oz. | 319 | 1.4 | Tr. | <1. | 15 |
| Chopped, sliced (Hormel) | 1 oz. | 289 | 5.8 | | | |
| Minced (Oscar Mayer) | 1 slice (10 per ½ lb.) | 251 | 4.4 | | | |
| Smoked (Oscar Mayer) | 1 slice (8 per 6 oz.) | 246 | 1.5 | | | |
| Smoked, thin sliced (Oscar Mayer) | 1 slice (10 per 3 oz.) | 87 | .6 | | | |
| Canned: | | | | | | |
| (USDA) | 1 oz. | 312 | 3.5 | 1. | 2. | |
| (Armour Star) | 1 oz. | | 3.5 | | | |
| (Hormel) | 1 oz. (8-lb. can) | | 4.2 | | | |
| (Hormel) | 1 oz. (6-lb. can) | | 2.6 | | | |
| (Hormel) | 1 oz. (4-lb. can) | | 3.1 | | | |
| (Hormel) | 1 oz. (1-lb. 8-oz. can) | | 3.1 | | | |

(USDA): United States Department of Agriculture
*Prepared as Package Directs
[1]Principal source of fat: pork.

| Food and Description | Measure or Quantity | Sodium (mg.) | — Fats in grams — | | | Choles- terol (mg.) |
|---|---|---|---|---|---|---|
| | | | Total | Satu- rated | Unsatu- rated | |
| (Oscar Mayer) *Jubilee,* bone in | 1 lb. | 5,307 | 54.4 | | | |
| (Oscar Mayer) *Jubilee,* boneless | 1 lb. | 5,307 | 54.4 | | | |
| (Oscar Mayer) *Jubilee,* boneless | ½-lb. slice | 2,654 | 15.9 | | | |
| (Oscar Mayer) *Jubilee,* special trim, as purchased | 1 oz. | 276 | 2.3 | | | |
| (Oscar Mayer) *Jubilee,* special trim, cooked | 1 oz. | 298 | 1.4 | < 1. | < 1. | 8 |
| (Oscar Mayer) steak | 1 slice (8 to lb.) | 663 | 3.4 | | | |
| (Swift) | 1¾-oz. slice (5″ × 2¼″ × ¼″) | 422 | 7.8 | | | |
| (Swift) *Hostess* | 1 oz. (4-lb. can) | 269 | 1.6 | | | |
| Chopped or minced, canned: | | | | | | |
| (USDA)[1] | 1 oz. | | 4.8 | 2. | 3. | |
| (Hormel) | 1 oz. (8-lb. can) | 369 | 7.9 | 3. | 5. | 13 |
| (Oscar Mayer) | 1-oz. slice | 310 | 4.8 | | | |
| Chopped, spiced or unspiced, canned: | | | | | | |
| (USDA)[1] | 1 oz. | 350 | 7.1 | 3. | 5. | |
| Chopped (USDA)[1] | 1 cup (4.8 oz.) | 1,678 | 33.9 | 12. | 22. | |
| Diced (USDA)[1] | 1 cup (5 oz.) | 1,740 | 35.1 | 13. | 22. | |
| (Hormel) | 1 oz. (5-lb. can) | | 6.6 | | | |
| Deviled, canned: | | | | | | |
| (USDA)[1] | 1 oz. | | 9.2 | 3. | 6. | |
| (USDA)[1] | 1 T. (.5 oz.) | | 4.2 | 2. | 3. | |
| (Hormel) | 1 oz. (3-oz. can) | | 6.1 | | | |
| (Underwood) | 4½-oz. can | 1,156 | 40.8 | | | |
| (Underwood) | 1 T. (.5 oz.) | 122 | 4.3 | | | |
| Packaged: | | | | | | |
| (Carl Buddig) smoked, sliced | 1 oz. | 400 | 3.0 | .8 | 2. | 20 |
| (Eckrich): | | | | | | |
| Chopped: | | | | | | |
| Regular | 1-oz. slice | 330 | 2.0 | | | |
| *Smorgas Pak* | ¾-oz. slice | 250 | 2.0 | | | |
| Cooked | 1.2-oz. slice | 470 | 1.0 | | | |
| Imported, Danish | 1.3-oz. slice | 487 | 1.2 | | | |
| Loaf | 1-oz. slice | 330 | 6.0 | | | |
| Smoked, sweet: | | | | | | |
| Regular | ¾-oz. slice | 270 | 1.0 | | | |
| Slender-sliced | 1-oz. serving | 360 | 3.0 | | | |

(USDA): United States Department of Agriculture
*Prepared as Package Directs
[1]Principal source of fat: pork.

| Food and Description | Measure or Quantity | Sodium (mg.) | — Fats in grams — | | | Cholesterol (mg.) |
|---|---|---|---|---|---|---|
| | | | Total | Saturated | Unsaturated | |
| (Hormel): | | | | | | |
| Black-peppered, *Light & Lean* | 1 slice | | 1.0 | | | |
| Chopped | 1 slice | 347 | 2.5 | | | |
| Cooked, *Light & Lean* | 1 slice | | 1.0 | | | |
| Glazed, *Light & Lean* | 1 slice | | 1.0 | | | |
| Red peppered, *Light & Lean* | 1 slice | | 1.0 | | | |
| (Ohse): | | | | | | |
| Chopped | 1 oz. | 260 | 5.0 | | | |
| Cooked | 1 oz. | 260 | 1.0 | | | |
| Smoked: | | | | | | |
| Regular | 1 oz. | 320 | 3.0 | | | |
| 95% fat free | 1 oz. | 310 | 1.0 | | | |
| Turkey ham | 1 oz. | 370 | 1.0 | | | |
| (Oscar Mayer): | | | | | | |
| Chopped | 1-oz. slice | 378 | 4.5 | | | 14 |
| Slice, boneless, *Jubilee* | 4-oz. serving | 1,396 | 4.4 | | | 52 |
| Smoked, cooked | ¾-oz. slice | 383 | 1.1 | | | 10 |
| Smoked, cooked | 1-oz. slice | 382 | 1.4 | | | 14 |
| Steak, boneless, 95% fat free, *Jubilee* | 2-oz. serving | 711 | 2.2 | | | 27 |
| **HAM & CHEESE:** | | | | | | |
| Canned (Hormel): | | | | | | |
| Loaf | 3 oz. | 1,135 | 22.0 | | | |
| Patties | 1 patty | 468 | 18.0 | | | |
| Packaged: | | | | | | |
| (Eckrich) loaf | 1-oz. slice | 350 | 5.0 | | | |
| (Hormel) loaf | 1 slice | 334 | 4.5 | | | |
| (Oscar Mayer) loaf | 1-oz. slice | 370 | 6.2 | | | |
| **HAM CROQUETTE,** home recipe (USDA)[1] | 4 oz. | 388 | 17.1 | 7. | 10 | |
| **HAM DINNER:** | | | | | | |
| Frozen: | | | | | | |
| (Banquet) | 10-oz. dinner | 1148 | 22.0 | | | |
| (Morton) | 10-oz. dinner | 700 | 4.5 | | | |
| **HAM SPREAD,** salad: | | | | | | |
| (Carnation) *Spreadable* | ¼ of 7½-oz. can | 335 | 8.0 | | | 15 |
| (Oscar Mayer) | 1 oz. | 259 | 4.4 | | | 10 |

(USDA): United States Department of Agriculture
*Prepared as Package Directs
[1]Principal sources of fat: butter, ham & vegetable shortening.

| Food and Description | Measure or Quantity | Sodium (mg.) | Total | —Fats in grams—<br>Satu-<br>rated | Unsatu-<br>rated | Choles-<br>terol (mg.) |
|---|---|---|---|---|---|---|
| **\*HAMBURGER SEASONING MIX:** | | | | | | |
| *Hamburger Helper:* | | | | | | |
| Beef noodle | ⅕ of pkg. | 970 | 15.0 | | | |
| Beef romanoff | ⅕ of pkg. | 1,095 | 16.0 | | | |
| Cheeseburger macaroni | ⅕ of pkg. | 1,025 | 18.0 | | | |
| Hash | ⅕ of pkg. | 920 | 15.0 | | | |
| (Durkee) | 1 cup | 1,012 | 50.5 | | | |
| **HAWAIIAN PUNCH,** canned: | | | | | | |
| Regular: | | | | | | |
| Apple or grape | 6 fl. oz. | 13 | 0.0 | | | (0) |
| Cherry or fruit juicy red | 6 fl. oz. | 17 | 0.0 | | | (0) |
| Island fruit cocktail, orange or wild fruit | 6 fl. oz. | 19 | 0.0 | | | (0) |
| Tropical fruit | 6 fl. oz. | 8 | 0.0 | | | (0) |
| *Very Berry* | 6 fl. oz. | 22 | 0.0 | | | (0) |
| Dietetic, punch | 6 fl. oz. | 20 | 0.0 | | | (0) |
| **HAWS, SCARLET,** raw (USDA): | | | | | | |
| Whole | 1 lb. (weighed with core) | | 2.5 | | | 0 |
| Flesh & skin | 4 oz. | | .8 | | | 0 |
| **HAZELNUT** (See **FILBERT**) | | | | | | |
| **HEADCHEESE:** | | | | | | |
| (USDA)[1] | 1 oz. | | 6.2 | 2. | 4. | |
| (Oscar Mayer) | 1-oz. slice | 338 | 4.1 | | | 21 |
| **HEART** (USDA): | | | | | | |
| Beef: | | | | | | |
| Lean, raw | 1 lb. | 390 | 16.3 | | | 680 |
| Lean, braised | 4 oz. | 118 | 6.5 | | | 311 |
| Lean, braised, chopped or diced | 1 cup (5.1 oz.) | 151 | 8.3 | | | 397 |
| Lean with visible fat, raw | 1 lb. | | 93.9 | | | |
| Lean with visible fat, braised | 4 oz. | | 32.9 | | | |
| Calf, raw | 1 lb. | 426 | 26.8 | | | |
| Calf, braised | 4 oz. | 128 | 10.3 | | | |
| Chicken, raw | 1 lb. | 358 | 27.2 | | | 771 |
| Chicken, simmered | 1 heart (5 grams) | 3 | .4 | | | 12 |

(USDA): United States Department of Agriculture
\*Prepared as Package Directs
[1]Principal source of fat: pork.

| Food and Description | Measure or Quantity | Sodium (mg.) | — Fats in grams — | | | Choles-terol (mg.) |
|---|---|---|---|---|---|---|
| | | | Total | Satu-rated | Unsatu-rated | |
| Chicken, simmered, chopped or diced | 1 cup (5.1 oz.) | 100 | 10.4 | | | 335 |
| Hog, raw | 1 lb. | 245 | 20.0 | | | |
| Hog, braised | 4 oz. | 74 | 7.8 | | | |
| Lamb, raw | 1 lb. | | 43.5 | | | |
| Lamb, braised | 4 oz. | | 16.3 | | | |
| Turkey, raw | 1 lb. | 313 | 50.8 | | | 680 |
| Turkey, simmered | 4 oz. | 69 | 15.0 | | | 270 |
| Turkey, simmered, chopped or diced | 1 cup (5.1 oz.) | 88 | 19.1 | | | 345 |
| **HEARTLAND,** cereal (Pet) | 1 oz. | | 3.7 | | | (0) |
| **HERRING:** | | | | | | |
| Raw (USDA): | | | | | | |
| Atlantic, whole | 1 lb. (weighed whole) | | 26.1 | 5. | 21. | 197 |
| Atlantic, meat only | 4 oz. | | 12.8 | 2. | 11. | 96 |
| Pacific, meat only | 4 oz. | 84 | 2.9 | Tr. | 3. | |
| Canned: | | | | | | |
| Plain, solids & liq. (USDA) | 4 oz. | | 15.4 | | | 110 |
| Plain, solids & liq. (USDA) | 15-oz. can | | 57.8 | | | 412 |
| Pickled, Bismarck type (USDA) | 4 oz. | | 17.1 | | | |
| Salted or brined (USDA) | 4 oz. | | 17.2 | | | |
| Smoked (USDA): | | | | | | |
| Bloaters | 4 oz. | | 14.1 | | | |
| Hard | 4 oz. | 7,066 | 17.9 | | | |
| Kippered | 4 oz. | | 14.6 | | | |
| **HICKORY NUT** (USDA): | | | | | | |
| Whole | 1 lb. (weighed in shell) | | 109.1 | 9. | 100. | 0 |
| Shelled | 4 oz. | | 77.9 | 7. | 71. | 0 |
| **HO-HOS** (Hostess) | 1-oz. piece | 85 | 6.0 | | | 13 |
| **HOMINY GRITS:** | | | | | | |
| Dry: | | | | | | |
| Degermed (USDA) | ½ cup (2.8 oz.) | <1 | .6 | | | 0 |
| Instant (Quaker) | .8-oz. packet | 347 | .1 | | | |
| Cooked: | | | | | | |
| Degermed (USDA) | 1 cup (8.6 oz.) | 502 | .2 | | | 0 |
| (Albers) | 1 cup | | .2 | | | |
| (Aunt Jemima) | ⅔ cup | <1 | .2 | | | |

(USDA): United States Department of Agriculture
*Prepared as Package Directs

| Food and Description | Measure or Quantity | Sodium (mg.) | —Fats in grams— | | | Cholesterol (mg.) |
|---|---|---|---|---|---|---|
| | | | Total | Satu-rated | Unsatu-rated | |
| **HONEY,** strained: | | | | | | |
| (USDA) | ½ cup (5.7 oz.) | 8 | 0.0 | | | 0 |
| (USDA) | 1 T. (.7 oz.) | 1 | 0.0 | | | 0 |
| *HONEYCOMB,* cereal (Post) | 1⅓ cups (1 oz.) | 214 | .5 | | | 0 |
| **HONEYDEW,** fresh (USDA): | | | | | | |
| Whole | 1 lb. (weighed whole) | 34 | .9 | | | 0 |
| Wedge | 2″ × 7″ wedge (5.3 oz.) | 11 | .3 | | | 0 |
| Flesh only | 4 oz. | 14 | .3 | | | 0 |
| Flesh only, diced | 1 cup (5.9 oz.) | 20 | .5 | | | 0 |
| *HONEY SMACKS,* cereal | | | | | | |
| (Kellogg's) | ¾ cup | 70 | 0.0 | | | |
| **HORSERADISH:** | | | | | | |
| Raw (USDA): | | | | | | |
| Whole | 1 lb. (weighed unpared) | 26 | 1.0 | | | 0 |
| Pared | 1 oz. | 2 | <.1 | | | 0 |
| Dehydrated (Heinz) | 1 T. | 95 | .2 | | | (0) |
| Dry (Spice Islands) | 1 tsp. | <1 | | | | (0) |
| Prepared (USDA) | 1 oz. | 27 | <.1 | | | 0 |
| *HOSTESS O'S* (Hostess) | 2¼-oz. piece | 428 | 10.9 | | | 14 |
| **HYACINTH BEAN** (USDA): | | | | | | |
| Young pod, raw: | | | | | | |
| Whole | 1 lb. (weighed untrimmed) | 8 | 1.2 | | | 0 |
| Trimmed | 4 oz. | 2 | .3 | | | 0 |
| Dry seeds | 4 oz. | | 1.7 | | | 0 |

# I

| | | | | | | |
|---|---|---|---|---|---|---|
| **ICE CREAM** (Listed by type, such as sandwich, or *Whammy,* or by flavor. See also **FROZEN DESSERT**): | | | | | | |
| Almond amaretto (Baskin-Robbins) | 4 fl. oz. | 30 | 17.0 | | | 43 |

(USDA): United States Department of Agriculture
*Prepared as Package Directs

| Food and Description | Measure or Quantity | Sodium (mg.) | Fats in grams — Total | Satu-rated | Unsatu-rated | Choles-terol (mg.) |
|---|---|---|---|---|---|---|
| Bar: | | | | | | |
| (Good Humor) vanilla, chocolate coated | 3-fl.-oz. piece | 40 | 11.0 | | | |
| (Häagen-Dazs): | | | | | | |
| Chocolate, dark chocolate coating | 1 piece | 50 | 25.0 | | | |
| Vanilla, milk chocolate coated | 1 bar | 60 | 23.0 | | | |
| *Bon Bons* (Carnation) vanilla | 1 piece | 11 | 2.4 | | | |
| Brandied black cherry (Häagen-Dazs) | 4 fl. oz. | 55 | 14.0 | | | |
| Butter Almond (Breyers) | ½ cup | 125 | | | | |
| Butter pecan: | | | | | | |
| (Breyers) | ¼ pt. | 125 | | | | |
| (Good Humor) bulk | 4 fl. oz. | | 9.0 | | | |
| (Häagen-Dazs) | 4 fl. oz. | 100 | 24.0 | | | |
| Cappuccino: | | | | | | |
| (Baskin-Robbins) chip | 4 fl. oz. | 40 | 19.0 | | | 45 |
| (Häagen-Dazs) | 4 fl. oz. | 65 | 16.0 | | | |
| Chocolate: | | | | | | |
| (Baskin-Robbins): | | | | | | |
| Regular | 4 fl. oz. | 128 | 12.6 | | | |
| Mousse royale | 4 fl. oz. | 150 | 13.6 | | | |
| (Breyers) | ½ cup | 35 | | | | |
| (Good Humor) bulk | 4 fl. oz. | | 7.0 | | | |
| (Häagen-Dazs) mint | 4 fl. oz. | 50 | 26.0 | | | |
| (Howard Johnson's) | ½ cup | | 15.9 | | | |
| Chocolate chip (Häagen-Dazs) | 4 fl. oz. | 55 | 18.0 | | | |
| Chocolate chip cookie (Good Humor) | 1 sandwich | | | | | |
| Chocolate eclair (Good Humor) bar | 3-fl.-oz. piece | 70 | 9.0 | | | |
| Chocolate malt bar (Good Humor) | 3-fl. oz. bar | 50 | 13.0 | | | |
| Chocolate raspberry truffle (Baskin-Robbins) | 4 fl. oz. | 40 | 19.0 | | | 40 |
| Coffee: | | | | | | |
| (Breyers) | ½ cup | 50 | | | | |
| (Häagen-Dazs) chip | 4 fl. oz. | 68 | 18.0 | | | |
| Cookies & cream: | | | | | | |
| (Breyers) | ½ cup | 60 | | | | |
| (Häagen-Dazs) | 4 fl. oz. | 90 | 17.2 | | | |
| (Sealtest) | ½ cup | 75 | | | | |

(USDA): United States Department of Agriculture
*Prepared as Package Directs

| Food and Description | Measure or Quantity | Sodium (mg.) | Fats in grams — Total | Satu-rated | Unsatu-rated | Choles-terol (mg.) |
|---|---|---|---|---|---|---|
| Cookie sandwich (Good Humor) | 2.7-fl. oz. piece | 195 | 11.0 | | | |
| *Eskimo Pie*, vanilla with chocolate coating | 3-fl.-oz. bar | | 12.0 | | | |
| *Eskimo, Thin Mint,* with chocolate coating | 2-fl.-oz. bar | | 12.0 | | | |
| *Fat Frog* (Good Humor) | 3-fl.-oz. pop | 45 | 7.0 | | | |
| Fudge royal (Sealtest) | 1/2 cup | 55 | | | | |
| Grand marnier (Baskin-Robbins) | 4 fl. oz. | 50 | 12.0 | | | 50 |
| *Heart* (Good Humor) | 4-fl.-oz. pop | 60 | 12.0 | | | |
| Honey (Häagen-Dazs) | 4 fl. oz. | 65 | 16.9 | | | |
| *Jamoca* (Baskin-Robbins) | 1 scoop (2 1/2 fl. oz.) | 64 | 8.0 | | | |
| Key lime & cream (Häagen-Dazs) | 4 fl. oz. | 30 | 7.2 | | | |
| Macadamia nut (Häagen-Dazs) | 4 fl. oz. | 114 | 24.0 | | | |
| Maple walnut (Häagen-Dazs) | 4 fl. oz. | 55 | 25.2 | | | |
| Mint chocolate chip (Breyers) | 1/2 cup | 45 | | | | |
| *Oreo,* cookies 'n cream: | | | | | | |
| Bulk | 3 fl. oz. | 100 | 8.0 | | | |
| Sandwich | 1 piece | 300 | 11.0 | | | |
| Peach (Häagen-Dazs) | 4 fl. oz. | 50 | 14.0 | | | |
| Pralines 'n cream (Baskin-Robbins) | 1 scoop (2 1/2 fl. oz.) | 266 | 13.1 | | | |
| Rocky road (Baskin-Robbins) | 4 fl. oz. | 123 | 11.2 | | | |
| Rum raisin (Häagen-Dazs) | 4 fl. oz. | 65 | 16.0 | | | |
| Sandwich (Good Humor) | 2 1/2-oz. piece | 120 | 5.0 | | | |
| *Sharks* (Good Humor) | 3-fl.-oz. pop | 0 | 0.0 | | | |
| Strawberry: | | | | | | |
| (Baskin-Robbins) wild, light | 4 fl. oz. | 70 | 1.2 | | | |
| (Breyers) | 1/2 cup | 40 | | | | |
| (Häagen-Dazs) | 4 fl. oz. | 55 | 15.2 | | | |
| (Howard Johnson's) | 1/2 cup | | 12.4 | | | |
| Toasted almond bar (Good Humor) | 3-fl.-oz. piece | 30 | 8.0 | | | |
| Vanilla: | | | | | | |
| (Baskin-Robbins) regular | 4 fl. oz. | 91 | 13.1 | | | |
| (Häagen-Dazs) | 4 fl. oz. | 65 | 17.2 | | | |
| (Howard Johnson's) | 1/2 cup | | 16.5 | | | |
| (Meadow Gold) | 1/2 cup | | 7.0 | | | |
| (Sealtest) | 1/2 cup | 50 | | | | |

(USDA): United States Department of Agriculture
*Prepared as Package Directs

ICE CREAM (Continued)

| Food and Description | Measure or Quantity | Sodium (mg.) | Fats in grams — Total | Saturated | Unsaturated | Cholesterol (mg.) |
|---|---|---|---|---|---|---|
| Vanilla slice (Good Humor): | | | | | | |
| Regular | 3.2-fl.-oz. slice | 45 | 6.1 | | | |
| Calorie controlled | 3.2-fl.-oz. slice | 45 | 1.0 | | | |
| Vanilla swiss almond (Häagen-Dazs) | 4 fl. oz. | 60 | 22.0 | | | |
| *Whammy* (Good Humor) assorted | 1.6-oz. piece | 25 | 6.0 | | | |
| **ICE CREAM CONE,** cone only: | | | | | | |
| (Baskin-Robbins): | | | | | | |
| Cake | .2-oz. piece | 26 | .3 | | | |
| Sugar | .5-oz. piece | 45 | 1.0 | | | |
| (Comet) sugar | .4-oz. piece | 35 | 0.0 | | | |
| **ICE CREAM CUP,** cup only | | | | | | |
| (Comet) regular or chocolate | 1 cup | 5 | 0.0 | | | |
| *ICE CREAM MIX (Salada): | | | | | | |
| Dutch chocolate | 1 cup | 75 | 19.0 | | | |
| Peach, vanilla or wild strawberry | 1 cup | 60 | 19.0 | | | |
| **ICE MILK:** | | | | | | |
| (USDA): | | | | | | |
| Hardened, with salt added | 1 cup (4.6 oz.) | 89 | 6.7 | 4. | 3. | 26 |
| Soft serve, with salt added | 1 cup (6.2 oz.) | 119 | 8.9 | 3. | 4. | 35 |
| (Sealtest) coffee | ½ cup | 55 | 2.0 | | | |
| **ICING** (See **CAKE ICING**) | | | | | | |
| **INCONNU OR SHEEFISH,** raw: | | | | | | |
| Whole (USDA) | 1 lb. (weighed whole) | | 19.4 | | | |
| Meat only (USDA) | 4 oz. | | 7.7 | | | |

**INSTANT BREAKFAST** (See individual brand name or company listings)

**IRISH WHISKEY** (See **DISTILLED LIQUOR**)

(USDA): United States Department of Agriculture
*Prepared as Package Directs

| Food and Description | Measure or Quantity | Sodium (mg.) | Total | — Fats in grams — Satu- rated | Unsatu- rated | Choles- terol (mg.) |
|---|---|---|---|---|---|---|

# J

**JACKFRUIT,** fresh (USDA):

| Food and Description | Measure or Quantity | Sodium (mg.) | Total | Satu-rated | Unsatu-rated | Choles-terol (mg.) |
|---|---|---|---|---|---|---|
| Whole | 1 lb. (weighed with seeds & skin) | 3 | .4 | | | 0 |
| Flesh only | 4 oz. | 2 | .3 | | | 0 |

***JACK IN THE BOX:***

| | | | | | | |
|---|---|---|---|---|---|---|
| Breakfast Jack | 4.4-oz. serving | 871 | 13.0 | | | 203 |
| Burger: | | | | | | |
|   Regular | 3.6-oz. serving | 556 | 13.0 | | | 26 |
|   Cheeseburger: | | | | | | |
|     Regular | 4-oz. serving | 746 | 14.0 | | | 41 |
|     Bacon | 8.1-oz. serving | 1,127 | 39.0 | | | 85 |
|     Ultimate | 9.9-oz. serving | 1,176 | 69.0 | | | 127 |
|     Ham & swiss | 9.1-oz. serving | 1,217 | 49.0 | | | 106 |
|   *Jumbo Jack:* | | | | | | |
|     Regular | 7.8-oz. serving | 733 | 34.0 | | | 73 |
|     With cheese | 8.5-oz. serving | 1,090 | 40.0 | | | 102 |
|     Monterey Burger | 9.9-oz. serving | 1,124 | 57.0 | | | 152 |
|     Mushroom | 6.4-oz. serving | 910 | 24.0 | | | 64 |
|     Swiss & bacon | 6.6-oz. serving | 1,458 | 47.0 | | | 92 |
| Canadian crescent | 4.7-oz. serving | 851 | 31.0 | | | 226 |
| Cheesecake | 3.5-oz. serving | 208 | 17.5 | | | 63 |
| Chicken strips | 1 piece | 177 | 3.5 | | | 17 |
| Chicken supreme sandwich | 8.1-oz. serving | 1,535 | 36.0 | | | 62 |
| Club pita sandwich, excluding | | | | | | |
|   sauce | 6.3-oz. serving | 931 | 8.0 | | | 43 |
| Coffee, black | 8 fl. oz. | 26 | 0.0 | | | 0 |
| Egg, scrambled, platter | 8.8-oz. serving | 1,188 | 40.0 | | | 354 |
| Egg roll | 1 piece | 301 | 6.3 | | | 10 |
| Fish supreme sandwich | 8-oz. sandwich | 1,047 | 32.0 | | | 66 |
| French fries: | | | | | | |
|   Regular | 2.4-oz. order | 164 | 12.0 | | | 8 |
|   Large | 3.8-oz. order | 262 | 19.0 | | | 13 |
|   Jumbo | 4.8-oz. order | 328 | 24.0 | | | 16 |
| Jelly, grape | .5-oz. serving | 3 | 0.0 | | | 0 |
| Ketchup | 1 serving | 99 | 0.0 | | | 0 |
| Mayonnaise | 1 serving | 127 | 17.0 | | | 10 |
| Milk, low fat | 8 fl. oz. | 122 | 5.0 | | | 18 |
| Milk shake: | | | | | | |
|   Chocolate | 11.4-oz. serving | 270 | 7.0 | | | 25 |

(USDA): United States Department of Agriculture
*Prepared as Package Directs

| Food and Description | Measure or Quantity | Sodium (mg.) | — Fats in grams — | | | Cholesterol (mg.) |
|---|---|---|---|---|---|---|
| | | | Total | Saturated | Unsaturated | |
| Strawberry | 11.4-oz. serving | 240 | 7.0 | | | 25 |
| Vanilla | 11.2-oz. serving | 230 | 6.0 | | | 25 |
| Mustard | 1 serving | 138 | .5 | | | 0 |
| Nachos: | | | | | | |
| Cheese | 6-oz. serving | 1,154 | 35.0 | | | 37 |
| Supreme | 11.9-oz. serving | 2,194 | 45.0 | | | 59 |
| Onion rings | 3.8-oz. serving | 407 | 23.0 | | | 27 |
| Orange juice | 6.5-oz. serving | 0 | 0.0 | | | 0 |
| Pancake platter | 8.1-oz. serving | 888 | 22.0 | | | 99 |
| Salad: | | | | | | |
| Chef | 11.7-oz. salad | 900 | 18.0 | | | 142 |
| Side | 3.9-oz. salad | 84 | 3.0 | | | Tr. |
| Taco | 14.8-oz. salad | 1,670 | 38.0 | | | 91 |
| Salad dressing: | | | | | | |
| Regular: | | | | | | |
| Blue cheese | 1.2-oz. serving | 459 | 11.0 | | | 9 |
| Buttermilk | 1.2-oz. serving | 347 | 18.0 | | | 10 |
| Thousand island | 1.2-oz. serving | 350 | 15.0 | | | 11 |
| Dietetic or low calorie, | | | | | | |
| French | 1.2-oz. serving | 300 | 4.0 | | | 0 |
| Sauce: | | | | | | |
| A-1 | 1.8-oz. serving | 809 | Tr. | | | 0 |
| Barbecue | .9-oz. serving | 300 | Tr. | | | 0 |
| Guacamole | .9-oz. serving | 130 | 5.0 | | | 0 |
| Mayo-mustard | .8-oz. serving | 247 | 13.0 | | | 10 |
| Mayo-onion | .8-oz. serving | 140 | 15.0 | | | 20 |
| Salsa | .9-oz. serving | 129 | Tr. | | | 0 |
| Seafood cocktail | 1-oz. serving | 206 | Tr. | | | 0 |
| Sweet & sour | 1-oz. serving | 160 | Tr. | | | 0 |
| Sausage crescent | 5.5-oz. serving | 1,012 | 43.0 | | | 187 |
| Shrimp | 1 piece (.3 oz.) | 67 | 1.6 | | | 8 |
| Soft drink: | | | | | | |
| Sweetened: | | | | | | |
| Coca-Cola Classic | 12 fl. oz. | 14 | 0.0 | | | 0 |
| Dr. Pepper | 12 fl. oz. | 18 | 0.0 | | | 0 |
| Root beer, Ramblin | 12 fl. oz. | 20 | 0.0 | | | 0 |
| Sprite | 12 fl. oz. | 46 | 0.0 | | | 0 |
| Diet, Coca-Cola | 12 fl. oz. | 26 | 0.0 | | | 0 |
| Supreme crescent | 5.1-oz. serving | 1,053 | 40.0 | | | 178 |
| Syrup, pancake | 1.5-oz. serving | 6 | 0.0 | | | 0 |
| Taco: | | | | | | |
| Regular | 2.9-oz. serving | 406 | 11.0 | | | 21 |
| Super | 4.8-oz. serving | 765 | 17.0 | | | 37 |

(USDA): United States Department of Agriculture
*Prepared as Package Directs

| Food and Description | Measure or Quantity | Sodium (mg.) | — Fats in grams — | | | Choles- terol (mg.) |
|---|---|---|---|---|---|---|
| | | | Total | Satu- rated | Unsatu- rated | |
| Tea, iced, plain | 12 fl. oz. | 4 | 0.0 | | | 0 |
| Turnover, hot apple | 4.2-oz. piece | 350 | 24.0 | | | 15 |
| **JACK MACKEREL,** raw, meat only (USDA) | 4 oz. | | 6.4 | | | |
| **JAM,** sweetened (See also individual listings by flavor): | | | | | | |
| (USDA) | 1 oz. | 3 | <.1 | | | 0 |
| (USDA) | 1 T. (.7 oz.) | 2 | Tr. | | | 0 |
| **JELLY,** sweetened (See also individual listings by flavor): | | | | | | |
| (USDA) | 1 oz. | 5 | <.1 | | | 0 |
| (USDA) | 1 T. (.6 oz.) | 3 | Tr. | | | 0 |
| ***JELL-O FRUIT & CREAM BAR:*** | | | | | | |
| Blueberry, raspberry or strawberry | 1.7-oz. bar | 98 | 2.8 | | | 5 |
| Peach | 1.7-oz. bar | 109 | 2.8 | | | 5 |
| ***JELL-O PUDDING POPS:*** | | | | | | |
| Banana, butterscotch or vanilla | 2-oz. bar | 63 | 2.6 | | | 1 |
| Chocolate or chocolate fudge | 2-oz. bar | 99 | 2.7 | | | 1 |
| Chocolate & caramel swirl | 2-oz. bar | 83 | 2.6 | | | 1 |
| **JERUSALEM ARTICHOKE** (USDA): | | | | | | |
| Unpared | 1 lb. (weighed with skin) | | .3 | | | 0 |
| Pared | 4 oz. | | .1 | | | 0 |
| **JORDAN ALMOND** (See **CANDY**) | | | | | | |
| **JUICE** (See individual flavors) | | | | | | |
| **JUJUBE or CHINESE DATE** (USDA): | | | | | | |
| Fresh, whole | 1 lb. (weighed with seeds) | 13 | .8 | | | 0 |
| Fresh, flesh only | 4 oz. | 3 | .2 | | | 0 |

(USDA): United States Department of Agriculture
*Prepared as Package Directs

| Food and Description | Measure or Quantity | Sodium (mg.) | Fats in grams Total | Satu- rated | Unsatu- rated | Choles- terol (mg.) |
|---|---|---|---|---|---|---|
| Dried, whole | 1 lb. (weighed with seeds) | | 4.4 | | | 0 |
| Dried, flesh only | 1 oz. | | .3 | | | 0 |

**JUNIOR FOOD** (See **BABY FOOD**)

# K

***KABOOMS,*** cereal (General Mills) | 1 cup (1 oz.) | 370 | 6.0 | | | (0)

**KALE:**

| | | | | | | |
|---|---|---|---|---|---|---|
| Raw, leaves only (USDA) | 1 lb. (weighed untrimmed) | 218 | 2.3 | | | 0 |
| Raw, leaves including stems (USDA) | 1 lb. (weighed trimmed) | 252 | 2.7 | | | 0 |
| Boiled without salt, leaves only (USDA) | 4 oz. | 49 | .8 | | | 0 |
| Boiled without salt, including stems (USDA) | ½ cup (1.9 oz.) | 24 | .4 | | | 0 |
| Canned (Allen) chopped, solids & liq. | ½ cup | 15 | <1.0 | | | |
| Frozen, chopped: | | | | | | |
| Not thawed (USDA) | 4 oz. | 29 | .6 | | | 0 |
| Boiled, drained (USDA) | ½ cup (3.2 oz.) | 19 | .5 | | | 0 |
| (Birds Eye) | ⅓ of 10-oz. pkg. | 14 | .4 | | | 0 |
| (Frosty Acres) | 3.3 oz. | 15 | 0.0 | | | (0) |
| (McKenzie) | 3.3 oz. | 28 | 0.0 | | | (0) |
| (Southland) | ⅕ of 16-oz. pkg. | 15 | .4 | | | (0) |

***KARO,*** syrup (See **SYRUP**)

**KASHA** (See **BUCKWHEAT, Groats**)

**KETCHUP** (See **CATSUP**)

(USDA): United States Department of Agriculture
*Prepared as Package Directs

| Food and Description | Measure or Quantity | Sodium (mg.) | Fats in grams Total | Satu- rated | Unsatu- rated | Choles- terol (mg.) |
|---|---|---|---|---|---|---|
| **KIDNEY** (USDA): | | | | | | |
| Beef, raw | 4 oz. | 200 | 7.6 | | | 425 |
| Beef, braised | 4 oz. | 287 | 13.6 | | | 912 |
| Beef braised, ¼″ slices | 1 cup (4.9 oz.) | 354 | 16.8 | | | 1126 |
| Calf, raw | 4 oz. | | 5.2 | | | 425 |
| Hog, raw | 4 oz. | 130 | 4.1 | | | 425 |
| Lamb, raw | 4 oz. | 257 | 3.7 | | | 425 |
| **KIELBASA** (Oscar Mayer) | 6-oz. link | 1,658 | 4.4 | | | |
| **KINGFISH,** raw (USDA): | | | | | | |
| Whole | 1 lb. (weighed whole) | 166 | 6.0 | | | |
| Meat only | 4 oz. | 94 | 3.4 | | | |
| ***KING VITAMAN,*** cereal (Quaker) | 1¼ cups (1 oz.) | 251 | 1.2 | | | (0) |
| **KIPPERS** (See **HERRING**) | | | | | | |
| ***KIX,*** cereal (General Mills) | 1½ cups (1 oz.) | 315 | 1.0 | | | (0) |
| **KNOCKWURST,** (USDA) | 1 oz. | | 6.6 | | | |
| **KOHLRABI** (USDA): | | | | | | |
| Raw, whole | 1 lb. (weighed with skin, without leaves) | 26 | .3 | | | 0 |
| Raw, diced | 1 cup (4.9 oz.) | 11 | .1 | | | 0 |
| Boiled without salt, drained | 1 cup (5.5 oz.) | 9 | .2 | | | 0 |
| ***KOOL-AID** (General Foods): | | | | | | |
| Regular | 1 cup (9.3 oz.) | 13 | Tr. | | | 0 |
| Sugar sweetened | 1 cup (9.3 oz.) | 13 | Tr. | | | 0 |
| **KUMQUAT,** fresh (USDA): | | | | | | |
| Whole | 1 lb. (weighed with seeds) | 30 | .4 | | | 0 |
| Flesh & skin | 4 oz. | 8 | .1 | | | 0 |

(USDA): United States Department of Agriculture
*Prepared as Package Directs

| Food and Description | Measure or Quantity | Sodium (mg.) | — Fats in grams — | | | Choles- terol (mg.) |
|---|---|---|---|---|---|---|
| | | | Total | Satu- rated | Unsatu- rated | |

# L

**LAKE COUNTRY,** wine
(Taylor):

| | | | | | | |
|---|---|---|---|---|---|---|
| Red dinner, 12½% alcohol | 3 fl. oz. | | | | | 0 |
| White dinner, 12½% alcohol | 3 fl. oz. | | | | | 0 |

**LAKE HERRING,** raw (USDA):

| | | | | | | |
|---|---|---|---|---|---|---|
| Whole | 1 lb. (weighed whole) | 111 | 5.4 | | | |
| Meat only | 4 oz. | 53 | 2.6 | | | |

**LAKE TROUT,** raw (USDA):

| | | | | | | |
|---|---|---|---|---|---|---|
| Drawn | 1 lb. (weighed with head, fins & bone) | | 16.8 | | | |
| Meat only | 4 oz. | | 11.3 | | | |

**LAKE TROUT OR SISCOWET,**
raw (USDA):

| | | | | | | |
|---|---|---|---|---|---|---|
| Less than 6.5 lb. whole | 1 lb. (weighed whole) | | 33.4 | | | |
| Less than 6.5 lb. whole | 4 oz. (meat only) | | 22.6 | | | |
| More than 6.5 lb. whole | 1 lb. (weighed whole) | | 88.8 | | | |
| More than 6.5 lb. whole | 4 oz. (meat only) | | 61.7 | | | |

**LAMB,** choice grade (USDA):
Chop, broiled:
  Loin. One 5-oz. chop
  (weighed with bone before
  cooking) will give you:

| | | | | | | |
|---|---|---|---|---|---|---|
| Lean & fat | 2.8 oz. | 55 | 22.9 | 13. | 10. | 76 |
| Lean only | 2.3 oz. | 46 | 4.9 | 3 | 2 | 65 |

  Rib. One 5-oz. chop
  (weighed with bone before
  cooking) will give you:

| | | | | | | |
|---|---|---|---|---|---|---|
| Lean & fat | 2.9 oz. | 57 | 29.2 | 16. | 13. | 80 |
| Lean only | 2 oz. | 39 | 5.9 | 3. | 3. | 56 |
| Fat, separable, cooked | 1 oz. | | 21.4 | 12. | 10. | |

Leg:

| | | | | | | |
|---|---|---|---|---|---|---|
| Raw, lean & fat | 1 lb. (weighed with bone) | 280 | 61.7 | 35. | 27. | 271 |

(USDA): United States Department of Agriculture
*Prepared as Package Directs

| Food and Description | Measure or Quantity | Sodium (mg.) | — Fats in grams — | | | Choles- terol (mg.) |
| --- | --- | --- | --- | --- | --- | --- |
| | | | Total | Satu- rated | Unsatu- rated | |
| Roasted, lean & fat | 4 oz. | 79 | 21.4 | 12. | 9. | 111 |
| Roasted, lean only | 4 oz. | 79 | 7.9 | 4. | 4. | 113 |
| Shoulder: | | | | | | |
| Raw, lean & fat | 1 lb. (weighed with bone) | 280 | 92.0 | 52. | 40. | 274 |
| Roasted, lean & fat | 4 oz. | 79 | 30.8 | 17. | 14. | 111 |
| Roasted, lean only | 4 oz. | 79 | 11.3 | 6. | 5. | 113 |

**LAMB'S QUARTERS** (USDA):
| | | | | | | |
| --- | --- | --- | --- | --- | --- | --- |
| Raw, trimmed | 1 lb. | | 3.6 | | | 0 |
| Boiled, drained | 4 oz. | | .8 | | | 0 |

**LARD** (See **FAT, COOKING**)

**LASAGNE:**
| | | | | | | |
| --- | --- | --- | --- | --- | --- | --- |
| Canned (Hormel) *Short Orders* | 7½-oz. can | 1,083 | 14.0 | | | |
| Frozen: | | | | | | |
| (Armour) *Dinner Classics* | 10-oz. meal | 1,110 | 16.0 | | | 70 |
| (Banquet) *Family Entrees,* with meat sauce | 32-oz. pkg. | 6,000 | 66.0 | | | |
| (Blue Star) *Dining Lite:* | | | | | | |
| Vegetable | 11-oz. meal | 720 | 7.1 | | | |
| Zucchini | 11-oz. meal | 780 | 7.0 | | | |
| (Celentano): | | | | | | |
| Regular | ½ of 16-oz. pkg. | 410 | 16.0 | | | 77 |
| Primavera | 11-oz. pkg. | 500 | 9.0 | | | 50 |
| (Conagra) *Light & Elegant,* florentine | 11¼-oz. entree | 980 | 5.0 | | | 25 |
| (Le Menu) vegetable | 11-oz. dinner | 1,010 | 20.0 | | | |
| (Stouffer's) *Lean Cuisine,* zucchini | 11-oz. serving | 1,000 | 5.0 | | | 20 |
| (Swanson) *Hungry-Man* | 18¾-oz. dinner | 1,510 | 26.0 | | | |
| (Weight Watchers): | | | | | | |
| Regular | 12-oz. serving | 1,097 | 11.0 | | | |
| Italian cheese | 12-oz. serving | 1,420 | 16.0 | | | |

**LEEKS,** raw (USDA):
| | | | | | | |
| --- | --- | --- | --- | --- | --- | --- |
| Whole | 1 lb. (weighed untrimmed) | 12 | .7 | | | 0 |
| Trimmed | 4 oz. | 6 | .3 | | | 0 |

**LEMON,** fresh (USDA):
| | | | | | | |
| --- | --- | --- | --- | --- | --- | --- |
| Fruit, including peel | 1 lb. (weighed whole) | 13 | 1.3 | | | 0 |

(USDA): United States Department of Agriculture
*Prepared as Package Directs

| Food and Description | Measure or Quantity | Sodium (mg.) | Fats in grams — Total | Satu- rated | Unsatu- rated | Choles- terol (mg.) |
|---|---|---|---|---|---|---|
| Fruit, including peel | 2⅛" lemon (3.8 oz., seeds removed) | 3 | .3 | | | 0 |
| Peeled fruit | 1 med. lemon (2⅛") | 1 | .2 | | | 0 |

**LEMONADE:**
Canned:

| Food and Description | Measure or Quantity | Sodium (mg.) | Total | Satu- rated | Unsatu- rated | Choles- terol (mg.) |
|---|---|---|---|---|---|---|
| *Capri Sun* | 6¾ fl. oz. | 2 | 0.0 | | | (0) |
| *Country Time* | 8 fl. oz. | 61 | 0.0 | | | 0 |
| (Hi-C) | 6 fl. oz. | 6 | Tr. | | | (0) |
| Chilled (Minute Maid) | 6 fl. oz. | <1 | Tr. | | | (0) |

Frozen:
(USDA):

| Food and Description | Measure or Quantity | Sodium (mg.) | Total | Satu- rated | Unsatu- rated | Choles- terol (mg.) |
|---|---|---|---|---|---|---|
| Undiluted | 6-fl.-oz. can | 4 | .2 | | | 0 |
| *Diluted with 4⅓ parts water | ½ cup (4.4 oz.) | Tr. | Tr. | | | 0 |
| *Country Time* | 8 fl. oz. | 26 | Tr. | | | 0 |
| *(Sunkist) | 6 fl. oz. | Tr. | Tr. | | | (0) |

*Mix:
Regular:

| Food and Description | Measure or Quantity | Sodium (mg.) | Total | Satu- rated | Unsatu- rated | Choles- terol (mg.) |
|---|---|---|---|---|---|---|
| *Country Time,* presweetened | 8 fl. oz. | 29 | Tr. | | | 0 |
| *Kool-Aid* | 8 fl. oz. | <1 | Tr. | | | 0 |

Dietetic:

| Food and Description | Measure or Quantity | Sodium (mg.) | Total | Satu- rated | Unsatu- rated | Choles- terol (mg.) |
|---|---|---|---|---|---|---|
| *Crystal Light* | 8 fl. oz. | <1 | 0.0 | | | 0 |
| *Kool-Aid* | 8 fl. oz. | <1 | Tr. | | | 0 |
| (Sunkist) | 8 fl. oz. | 35 | 0.0 | | | (0) |

**LEMON JUICE:**
Fresh:

| Food and Description | Measure or Quantity | Sodium (mg.) | Total | Satu- rated | Unsatu- rated | Choles- terol (mg.) |
|---|---|---|---|---|---|---|
| (USDA) | ½ cup (4.3 oz.) | 1 | .2 | | | 0 |
| (USDA) | 1 T. (.5 oz.) | <1 | <.1 | | | 0 |
| (Sunkist) | 1 lemon (3.9 oz.) | 1 | Tr. | | | 0 |
| (Sunkist) | 1 T. (.5 oz.) | Tr. | Tr. | | | 0 |

Canned, unsweetened:

| Food and Description | Measure or Quantity | Sodium (mg.) | Total | Satu- rated | Unsatu- rated | Choles- terol (mg.) |
|---|---|---|---|---|---|---|
| (USDA) | ½ cup (4.3 oz.) | 1 | .1 | | | 0 |
| (USDA) | 1 T. (.5 oz.) | <1 | <.1 | | | 0 |

Plastic container:

| Food and Description | Measure or Quantity | Sodium (mg.) | Total | Satu- rated | Unsatu- rated | Choles- terol (mg.) |
|---|---|---|---|---|---|---|
| (USDA) | ½ cup (4 oz.) | 1 | .1 | | | 0 |
| (ReaLemon) | 1 T. (.5 oz.) | 4 | Tr. | | | (0) |

Frozen, unsweetened:

| Food and Description | Measure or Quantity | Sodium (mg.) | Total | Satu- rated | Unsatu- rated | Choles- terol (mg.) |
|---|---|---|---|---|---|---|
| Concentrate (USDA) | ½ cup (5.1 oz.) | 7 | 1.3 | | | 0 |

(USDA): United States Department of Agriculture
*Prepared as Package Directs

| Food and Description | Measure or Quantity | Sodium (mg.) | Fats in grams — Total | Satu- rated | Unsatu- rated | Choles- terol (mg.) |
|---|---|---|---|---|---|---|
| Single strength (USDA) | ½ cup (4.3 oz.) | 1 | .2 | | | 0 |
| Full strength, already reconstituted (Minute Maid) | ½ cup (4.2 oz.) | 1 | <.1 | | | 0 |
| Full strength, already reconstituted (Snow Crop) | ½ cup (4.2 oz.) | 1 | <.1 | | | 0 |
| **LEMON-LIMEADE,** sweetened, concentrate, frozen: | | | | | | |
| *(Minute Maid) | ½ cup | 5 | Tr. | | | (0) |
| *(Snow Crop) | ½ cup | Tr. | Tr. | | | 0 |
| **LEMON PEEL:** | | | | | | |
| Raw (USDA) | 1 oz. | 2 | <.1 | | | 0 |
| Dried (Spice Islands) | 1 tsp. | <1 | | | | (0) |
| Candied (USDA) | 1 oz. | | <.1 | | | 0 |
| **LEMON & PEPPER SEASONING** (French's) | 1 tsp. | 800 | Tr. | | | |
| **LEMON PIE** (See **PIE,** Lemon) | | | | | | |
| **LEMON PIE FILLING MIX** (See **PUDDING MIX,** Lemon) | | | | | | |
| **LENTIL:** | | | | | | |
| Whole: | | | | | | |
| Dry: | | | | | | |
| (USDA) | ½ lb. | 68 | 2.5 | | | 0 |
| (USDA) | 1 oz. | 9 | .3 | | | 0 |
| (USDA) | 1 cup (6.7 oz.) | 57 | 2.1 | | | 0 |
| Cooked, drained (USDA) | ½ cup (3.6 oz.) | | Tr. | | | 0 |
| Split, dry, without seed coat (USDA) | ½ lb. | | 2.0 | | | 0 |
| **LETTUCE** (USDA): | | | | | | |
| Bibb, untrimmed | 1 lb. (weighed untrimmed) | 30 | .7 | | | 0 |
| Bibb, untrimmed | 7.8-oz. head (4" dia.) | 15 | .3 | | | 0 |
| Boston, untrimmed | 1 lb. (weighed untrimmed) | 30 | .7 | | | 0 |
| Boston, untrimmed | 7.8-oz. head (4" dia.) | 15 | .3 | | | 0 |

(USDA): United States Department of Agriculture
*Prepared as Package Directs

LETTUCE (Continued)

| Food and Description | Measure or Quantity | Sodium (mg.) | Fats in grams — Total | Satu- rated | Unsatu- rated | Choles- terol (mg.) |
|---|---|---|---|---|---|---|
| Butterhead varieties (See Bibb) | | | | | | |
| Cos (See Romaine) | | | | | | |
| Dark green (See Romaine) | | | | | | |
| Grand Rapids | 1 lb. (weighed untrimmed) | 26 | .9 | | | 0 |
| Grand Rapids | 2 large leaves (1.8 oz.) | 4 | .2 | | | 0 |
| Great Lakes, untrimmed | 1 lb. (weighed untrimmed) | 39 | .4 | | | 0 |
| Great Lakes, trimmed | 1-lb. head (4¾" dia., weighed trimmed) | 41 | .5 | | | 0 |
| Iceberg: | | | | | | |
| Untrimmed | 1 lb. (weighed untrimmed) | 39 | .4 | | | 0 |
| Trimmed | 1-lb. head (4¾" dia., weighed trimmed) | 41 | .5 | | | 0 |
| Leaves | 1 cup (2.3 oz.) | 6 | <.1 | | | 0 |
| Chopped | 1 cup (2 oz.) | 5 | <.1 | | | 0 |
| Chunks | 1 cup (2.6 oz.) | 7 | <.1 | | | |
| Loose leaf varieties (See Salad Bowl): | | | | | | |
| New York | 1 lb. (weighed untrimmed) | 39 | .4 | | | 0 |
| New York | 1-lb. head (4¾" dia., weighed trimmed) | 41 | .5 | | | 0 |
| Romaine: | | | | | | |
| Untrimmed | 1 lb. (weighed untrimmed) | 26 | .9 | | | 0 |
| Shredded & broken into pieces | ½ cup (.8 oz.) | 2 | <.1 | | | 0 |
| Salad Bowl: | | | | | | |
| Untrimmed | 1 lb. (weighed untrimmed) | 26 | .9 | | | 0 |
| Trimmed | 2 large leaves (1.8 oz.) | 4 | .2 | | | 0 |
| Simpson: | | | | | | |
| Untrimmed | 1 lb. (weighed untrimmed) | 26 | .9 | | | 0 |
| Trimmed | 2 large leaves (1.8 oz.) | 4 | .2 | | | 0 |
| White Paris (See Romaine) | | | | | | |

(USDA): United States Department of Agriculture
*Prepared as Package Directs

| Food and Description | Measure or Quantity | Sodium (mg.) | Fats in grams — Total | Satu- rated | Unsatu- rated | Choles- terol (mg.) |
|---|---|---|---|---|---|---|
| **LIFE,** cereal (Quaker) regular | ⅔ cup (1 oz.) | 163 | .5 | | | (0) |
| **LI'L ANGELS** (Hostess) | 1-oz. piece | 92 | 2.0 | | | 2 |
| **LIMA BEAN** (See **BEAN, LIMA**) | | | | | | |
| **LIME,** fresh, whole: | | | | | | |
| (USDA) | 1 lb. (weighed with skin & seeds) | 8 | .8 | | | 0 |
| (USDA) | 1 med. (2″ dia., 2.4 oz.) | 1 | .1 | | | 0 |
| **LIMEADE,** concentrate, sweetened, frozen: | | | | | | |
| (USDA) | 6-fl.-oz. can (7.7 oz.) | Tr. | .2 | | | 0 |
| *Diluted with 4⅓ parts water | | | | | | |
| (USDA) | ½ cup (4.4 oz.) | Tr. | Tr. | | | 0 |
| (ReaLemon) | 6-oz. can | 4 | .2 | | | |
| *(Minute Maid) | ½ cup (4.2 oz.) | Tr. | Tr. | | | 0 |
| **LIME ICE,** home recipe (USDA) | 8 oz. (by wt.) | Tr. | Tr. | | | 0 |
| **LIME JUICE:** | | | | | | |
| Fresh (USDA) | 1 cup (8.7 oz.) | 2 | .2 | | | 0 |
| Canned or bottled, unsweetened: | | | | | | |
| (USDA) | 1 T. (.5 oz.) | Tr. | Tr. | | | 0 |
| (USDA) | 1 cup (8.7 oz.) | 2 | .2 | | | 0 |
| *ReaLime* | 1 T. | 5 | Tr. | | | (0) |
| **LINGCOD,** raw (USDA): | | | | | | |
| Whole | 1 lb. (weighed whole) | 91 | 1.2 | | | |
| Meat only | 4 oz. | 67 | .9 | | | |
| **LITCHI NUT** (USDA): | | | | | | |
| Fresh: | | | | | | |
| Whole | 4 oz. (weighed in shell with seeds) | 2 | .2 | | | 0 |
| Flesh only | 4 oz. | 3 | .3 | | | 0 |

(USDA): United States Department of Agriculture
*Prepared as Package Directs

LITCHI NUT (Continued)

| Food and Description | Measure or Quantity | Sodium (mg.) | Total | Satu-rated | Unsatu-rated | Choles-terol (mg.) |
|---|---|---|---|---|---|---|
| | | | | — Fats in grams — | | |
| Dried: | | | | | | |
| Whole | 4 oz. (weighed in shell with seeds) | 2 | .6 | | | 0 |
| Flesh only | 2 oz. | 2 | .7 | | | 0 |
| **LIVER:** | | | | | | |
| Beef, raw (USDA) | 1 lb. | 617 | 17.2 | | | 1361 |
| Beef, fried (USDA) | 4 oz. | 209 | 12.0 | | | 497 |
| Beef, fried (USDA) | 6½″ × 2⅜″ × ⅜″ slice (3 oz.) | 150 | 9.0 | | | 372 |
| Calf, raw (USDA) | 1 lb. | 331 | 21.3 | | | 1361 |
| Calf, fried (USDA) | 4 oz. | 134 | 15.0 | | | 497 |
| Calf, fried (USDA) | 6½″ × 2⅜″ × ⅜″ slice (3 oz.) | 100 | 11.2 | | | 372 |
| Chicken, raw (USDA) | 1 lb. | 318 | 16.8 | | | 2517 |
| Chicken, raw, frozen (Swanson) | 8-oz. pkg. | 138 | 6.1 | | | |
| Chicken, simmered (USDA) | 4 oz. | 69 | 5.0 | | | 846 |
| Chicken, simmered (USDA) | 2″ × 2″ × ⅝″ liver (.9 oz.) | 15 | 1.1 | | | 186 |
| Goose, raw (USDA) | 1 lb. | 635 | 45.4 | | | |
| Hog, raw (USDA) | 1 lb. | 331 | 16.8 | 6. | 11. | 1301 |
| Hog, fried (USDA) | 4 oz. | 126 | 13.0 | 3. | 10. | 497 |
| Hog, fried (USDA) | 6½″ × 2⅜″ × ⅜″ slice (3 oz.) | 94 | 9.8 | 3. | 7. | 372 |
| Lamb, raw (USDA) | 1 lb. | 236 | 17.7 | | | 1361 |
| Lamb, broiled (USDA) | 4 oz. | 96 | 14.1 | | | 497 |
| Lamb, broiled (USDA) | 6½″ × 2⅜″ × ⅜″ slice (3 oz.) | 72 | 10.5 | | | 372 |
| Turkey, raw (USDA) | 1 lb. | 286 | 18.1 | | | 1973 |
| Turkey, simmered (USDA) | 4 oz. | 62 | 5.4 | | | 679 |
| Turkey, simmered, chopped (USDA) | 1 cup (4.9 oz.) | 77 | 6.7 | | | 839 |

**LIVER PÂTÉ** (See **PÂTÉ**)

**LIVER SAUSAGE OR LIVERWURST:**

| Food and Description | Measure or Quantity | Sodium (mg.) | Total | Satu-rated | Unsatu-rated | Choles-terol (mg.) |
|---|---|---|---|---|---|---|
| Fresh (USDA) | 1 oz. | | 7.3 | | | |
| Sliced (Oscar Mayer) | .9-oz. slice (10 slices to 9 oz.) | 264 | 8.8 | | | |
| Ring (Oscar Mayer) | 1 oz. | 287 | 7.9 | | | |
| Smoked (USDA) | 1 oz. | | 7.8 | | | |

(USDA): United States Department of Agriculture
*Prepared as Package Directs

| Food and Description | Measure or Quantity | Sodium (mg.) | —Fats in grams— | | | Cholesterol (mg.) |
|---|---|---|---|---|---|---|
| | | | Total | Saturated | Unsaturated | |

**LIVERWURST SPREAD:**

| | | | | | | |
|---|---|---|---|---|---|---|
| (Hormel) | 1 oz. | | 6.0 | | | |
| (Underwood) | 1 oz. | 237 | 7.9 | | | |

**LOBSTER** (USDA):
Raw:

| | | | | | | |
|---|---|---|---|---|---|---|
| Whole | 1 lb. (weighed whole) | | 2.2 | | | |
| Meat only | 4 oz. | 238 | 2.2 | | | 96 |
| Cooked, meat only | 4 oz. | | 1.7 | | | |
| Cooked, meat only | 1 cup (½″ cubes, 5.1 oz.) | 304 | 2.2 | | | 123 |
| Canned, meat only | 4 oz. | 238 | 1.7 | | | |

**LOBSTER NEWBURG:**

| | | | | | | |
|---|---|---|---|---|---|---|
| Home recipe (USDA)[1] | 4 oz. | 260 | 12.0 | | | 206 |
| Home recipe (USDA)[1] | 1 cup (8.8 oz.) | 572 | 26.5 | | | 455 |

**LOBSTER PASTE,** canned

| | | | | | | |
|---|---|---|---|---|---|---|
| (USDA) | 1 oz. | | 2.7 | | | |

**LOBSTER SALAD,** home

| | | | | | | |
|---|---|---|---|---|---|---|
| recipe (USDA) | 4 oz. | 141 | 7.3 | | | |

**LOGANBERRY** (USDA):
Fresh:

| | | | | | | |
|---|---|---|---|---|---|---|
| Untrimmed | 1 lb. (weighed with caps) | 4 | 2.6 | | | 0 |
| Trimmed | 1 cup (5.1 oz.) | 1 | .9 | | | 0 |
| Canned, solids & liq.: | | | | | | |
| Water pack | 4 oz. | 1 | .5 | | | 0 |
| Juice pack | 4 oz. | 1 | .6 | | | 0 |
| Light syrup | 4 oz. | 1 | .5 | | | 0 |
| Heavy syrup | 4 oz. | 1 | .5 | | | 0 |
| Extra heavy syrup | 4 oz. | 1 | .5 | | | 0 |

**LONGAN** (USDA):
Fresh:

| | | | | | | |
|---|---|---|---|---|---|---|
| Whole | 1 lb. (weighed with shell & seeds) | | .2 | | | 0 |
| Flesh only | 4 oz. | | .1 | | | 0 |

(USDA): United States Department of Agriculture
*Prepared as Package Directs
[1]Prepared with butter, egg yolks, sherry & cream.

217

| Food and Description | Measure or Quantity | Sodium (mg.) | —Fats in grams— | | | Cholesterol (mg.) |
|---|---|---|---|---|---|---|
| | | | Total | Saturated | Unsaturated | |
| Dried: | | | | | | |
| Whole | 1 lb. (weighed with shell & seeds) | | .7 | | | 0 |
| Flesh | 4 oz. | | .5 | | | 0 |
| *LONG JOHN SILVER'S:* | | | | | | |
| Catfish fillet | 2.7-oz. piece | 469 | 12.0 | | | 49 |
| Catsup | .4 oz. | 136 | Tr. | | | |
| *Chicken Plank* | 1.4-oz. piece | 295 | 6.0 | | | 10 |
| Chicken sandwich | 6.1-oz. sandwich | 1,159 | 32.0 | | | 44 |
| Chowder, clam | 1 order | 611 | 5.0 | | | 17 |
| Clams, breaded | 4.7-oz. order | 1,170 | 31.0 | | | 2 |
| Coleslaw | 3½ oz. (drained on fork) | 367 | 15.0 | | | 12 |
| Corn on the cob | 5.3-oz. ear | | 4.0 | | | |
| Cracker | 1 piece | 36 | .5 | | | |
| Drinks: | | | | | | |
| Regular, carbonated or noncarbonated | 10 fl. oz. | | 0.0 | | | 0 |
| Dietetic | 10 fl. oz. | | 0.0 | | | 0 |
| Fish fillet: | | | | | | |
| Baked, with sauce | 5.5-oz. serving | 361 | 2.0 | | | 90 |
| Batter fried | 3-oz. piece | 673 | 12.0 | | | 31 |
| Kitchen breaded | 2-oz. piece | 374 | 6.0 | | | 25 |
| Fish sandwich | 6.4-oz. sandwich | 1,243 | 33.0 | | | 48 |
| Fryer | 3-oz. serving | 6 | 12.0 | | | 13 |
| Hush puppies | .85-oz. piece | 202 | 3.5 | | | <1 |
| Oyster, breaded, fried | .7-oz. piece | 65 | 3.0 | | | 5 |
| Peg leg, battered | 1-oz. piece | 225 | 7.0 | | | 17 |
| Pie: | | | | | | |
| Apple | 4-oz. piece | 247 | 11.0 | | | 10 |
| Cherry | 4-oz. piece | 251 | 11.0 | | | 10 |
| Lemon meringue | 3½-oz. piece | 254 | 6.0 | | | 5 |
| Pecan | 4-oz. piece | 435 | 22.0 | | | 92 |
| Pumpkin | 4-oz. piece | 242 | 11.0 | | | 35 |
| Scallop, batter fried | .7-oz. piece | 201 | 3.0 | | | 2 |
| Seafood salad | 5.8-oz. serving | 833 | 29.0 | | | 168 |
| Seafood sauce | 1.2-oz. serving | 358 | 0.0 | | | 0 |
| Shrimp: | | | | | | |
| Batter fried | .6-oz. piece | 154 | 3.0 | | | 17 |
| Breaded, fried | 4.7-oz. order | 1,229 | 23.0 | | | 96 |
| Chilled | .2-oz. piece | 19 | Tr. | | | 12 |

(USDA): United States Department of Agriculture
*Prepared as Package Directs

| Food and Description | Measure or Quantity | Sodium (mg.) | Fats in grams — Total | Satu- rated | Unsatu- rated | Choles- terol (mg.) |
|---|---|---|---|---|---|---|
| Tartar sauce | 1-oz. serving | | 11.0 | | | |
| Vegetables, mixed | 4-oz. serving | 570 | 2.0 | | | Tr. |
| **LOQUAT,** fresh (USDA): | | | | | | |
| Whole | 1 lb. (weighed with seeds) | | .7 | | | 0 |
| Flesh only | 4 oz. | | .2 | | | 0 |
| ***LUCKY CHARMS,*** cereal (General Mills) | 1 cup (1 oz.) | 185 | 1.0 | | | (0) |
| **LUNCHEON MEAT** (See also individual listings, e.g., **BOLOGNA**): | | | | | | |
| All meat (Oscar Mayer) | 1-oz. slice | 346 | 9.2 | | | 16 |
| Banquet loaf (Eckrich) | ¾-oz. slice | 250 | 4.0 | | | |
| Barbecue Loaf: | | | | | | |
| (Eckrich) | 1-oz. slice | 370 | 2.0 | | | |
| (Oscar Mayer) | 1-oz. slice | 346 | 2.5 | | | 13 |
| Beef, jellied (Hormel) loaf | 1 slice | 450 | 2.0 | | | |
| Gourmet loaf (Eckrich): | | | | | | |
| Regular | 1-oz. slice | 390 | 1.0 | | | |
| Smorgas-Pac | ¾-oz. slice | 300 | 1.0 | | | |
| Ham roll sausage (Oscar Mayer) | 1-oz. slice | 329 | 2.2 | | | 13 |
| Honey loaf: | | | | | | |
| (Eckrich) | 1-oz. slice | 350 | 2.0 | | | |
| (Hormel) | 1 slice | 292 | 2.5 | | | |
| (Oscar Mayer) | 1-oz. slice | 366 | 1.2 | | | |
| Iowa brand (Hormel) | 1 slice | 303 | 3.0 | | | |
| Liver cheese (Oscar Mayer) | 1.3-oz. slice | 433 | 10.0 | | | |
| Liver loaf (Hormel) | 1 slice | 352 | 6.5 | | | |
| Luncheon roll sausage (Oscar Mayer) | .8-oz. slice | 222 | 1.7 | | | 11 |
| Luxury loaf (Oscar Mayer) | 1-oz. slice | 300 | 1.2 | | | 13 |
| Macaroni & cheese loaf (Eckrich) | 1-oz. slice | 370 | 6.0 | | | |
| Meat loaf (USDA) | 1 oz. | | 3.7 | | | |
| New England brand: | | | | | | |
| (Eckrich) | 1-oz. slice | 440 | 2.0 | | | |
| (Oscar Mayer) | 1-oz. slice | 360 | 2.2 | | | 17 |

(USDA): United States Department of Agriculture
*Prepared as Package Directs

| Food and Description | Measure or Quantity | Sodium (mg.) | — Fats in grams — | | | Cholesterol (mg.) |
|---|---|---|---|---|---|---|
| | | | Total | Saturated | Unsaturated | |
| Old fashioned loaf: | | | | | | |
| (Eckrich): | | | | | | |
| Regular | 1-oz. slice | 330 | 6.0 | | | |
| *Smorgas-Pac* | 1-oz. slice | 340 | 6.0 | | | |
| (Oscar Mayer) | 1-oz. slice | 321 | 4.2 | | | 14 |
| Olive loaf: | | | | | | |
| (Eckrich) | 1-oz. slice | 370 | 7.0 | | | |
| (Hormel) | 1 slice | 405 | 3.5 | | | |
| (Oscar Mayer) | 1-oz. slice | 395 | 4.4 | | | 13 |
| Peppered loaf: | | | | | | |
| (Eckrich) | 1-oz. slice | 390 | 2.0 | | | |
| (Oscar Mayer) | 1-oz. slice | 361 | 2.1 | | | 13 |
| Pickle loaf (Eckrich) | 1-oz. slice | 320 | 7.0 | | | |
| Pickle & pimiento loaf (Oscar Mayer) | 1-oz. slice | 394 | 4.2 | | | 12 |
| Picnic loaf (Oscar Mayer) | 1-oz. slice | 330 | 4.4 | | | 12 |
| **LUNG,** raw (USDA): | | | | | | |
| Beef | 1 lb. | | 10.4 | | | |
| Calf | 1 lb. | | 17.2 | | | |
| Lamb | 1 lb. | | 10.4 | | | |

# M

| Food and Description | Measure or Quantity | Sodium (mg.) | Total | Saturated | Unsaturated | Cholesterol (mg.) |
|---|---|---|---|---|---|---|
| **MACADAMIA NUT** (USDA): | | | | | | |
| Whole | 1 lb. (weighed in shell) | | 100.7 | | | 0 |
| Shelled | 4 oz. | | 81.2 | | | 0 |

**MACARONI.** Plain macaroni products are essentially the same in caloric value and carbohydrate content on the same weight basis. The longer they are cooked, the more water is absorbed and this affects the nutritive values.[1]

| Food and Description | Measure or Quantity | Sodium (mg.) | Total | Saturated | Unsaturated | Cholesterol (mg.) |
|---|---|---|---|---|---|---|
| Dry: | | | | | | |
| (USDA) | 1 oz. | < 1 | .3 | | | 0 |
| Elbow type | 1 cup (4.8 oz.) | 3 | 1.6 | | | 0 |
| 1-inch pieces | 1 cup (3.8 oz.) | 2 | 1.3 | | | 0 |
| 2-inch pieces | 1 cup (3 oz.) | 2 | 1.0 | | | 0 |

(USDA): United States Department of Agriculture
*Prepared as Package Directs
[1]Cholesterol applies to this plain macaroni which is made without milk.

| Food and Description | Measure or Quantity | Sodium (mg.) | — Fats in grams — | | | Choles-terol (mg.) |
| --- | --- | --- | --- | --- | --- | --- |
| | | | Total | Satu-rated | Unsatu-rated | |
| Cooked (USDA): | | | | | | |
| 8-10 minutes, firm | 4 oz. | 1 | .6 | | | 0 |
| 8-10 minutes, firm | 1 cup (4.6 oz.) | 1 | .6 | | | 0 |
| 14-20 minutes, tender | 1 cup (4.9 oz.) | 1 | .6 | | | 0 |
| 14-20 minutes, tender | (4 oz.) | 1 | .5 | | | 0 |
| Canned (Franco-American): | | | | | | |
| BeefyOs, & beef in tomato sauce | 7½-oz. can | 1,250 | 8.0 | | | |
| PizzzOs, in pizza sauce | 7½-oz. can | 1,060 | 2.0 | | | |
| Frozen: | | | | | | |
| (Morton) & beef | 10-oz. dinner | 800 | 6.1 | | | |
| (Stouffer's) & beef with tomatoes | ½ of 11½-oz. pkg. | 810 | 8.0 | | | |
| (Swanson) & beef | 12-oz. dinner | 850 | 14.0 | | | |

**MACARONI & CHEESE:**

| Food and Description | Measure or Quantity | Sodium | Total | Satu-rated | Unsatu-rated | Choles-terol |
| --- | --- | --- | --- | --- | --- | --- |
| Home recipe, baked (USDA)[1] | 1 cup (7.1 oz.) | 1,086 | 22.2 | 10. | 12. | 42 |
| Canned: | | | | | | |
| (USDA)[2] | 1 cup (8.5 oz.) | 730 | 9.6 | 5. | 5. | |
| (Franco-American) | 7⅜-oz. can | 960 | 5.0 | | | |
| (Hormel) | 7½-oz. can | 917 | 6.0 | | | |
| Frozen: | | | | | | |
| (Banquet): | | | | | | |
| Casserole | 8-oz. meal | 930 | 17.0 | | | |
| Dinner, Family Favorites | 9-oz. meal | 940 | 16.0 | | | |
| (Celentano) baked | ½ of 11-oz. pkg. | 425 | 13.0 | | | 37 |
| (Conagra) Light & Elegant | 9-oz. entree | 1,010 | 9.0 | | | 5 |
| (Morton): | | | | | | |
| Casserole | 20-oz. pkg. | 2,600 | 19.9 | | | |
| Dinner | 11-oz. dinner | 1,000 | 7.3 | | | |
| (Stouffer's) | ½ of 12-oz. pkg. | 780 | 12.0 | | | |
| (Swanson) | 12-oz. entree | 1,850 | 16.0 | | | |

**MACARONI & CHEESE MIX:**

| Food and Description | Measure or Quantity | Sodium | Total | | | |
| --- | --- | --- | --- | --- | --- | --- |
| (Golden Grain) | ¼ of pkg. | 430 | 2.0 | | | |
| *(Kraft): | | | | | | |
| Regular | ¼ of pkg. | 420 | | | | |
| Velveeta | ¼ of pkg. | 720 | | | | |
| *(Lipton) | ¼ of pkg. | | 10.0 | | | |

(USDA): United States Department of Agriculture
*Prepared as Package Directs
[1]Principal sources of fat: cheese, margarine, milk & butter.
[2]Principal sources of fat: cheese, corn oil & milk.

| Food and Description | Measure or Quantity | Sodium (mg.) | — Fats in grams — | | | Choles-terol (mg.) |
|---|---|---|---|---|---|---|
| | | | Total | Satu-rated | Unsatu-rated | |
| **MACARONI & CHEESE PIE,** frozen (Swanson) | 7-oz. pie | 880 | 9.0 | | | |
| **MACE,** ground (Spice Islands) | 1 tsp. | 2 | | | | (0) |
| **MACKEREL** (USDA): | | | | | | |
| Atlantic: | | | | | | |
| Raw: | | | | | | |
| Whole | 1 lb. (weighed whole) | | 29.9 | | | 233 |
| Meat only | 4 oz. | | 13.8 | | | 108 |
| Broiled with butter or margarine | 8½″ × 2½″ × ½″ fillet (3.7 oz.) | | 16.6 | | | |
| Broiled with vegetable shortening | 8½″ × 2½″ × ½″ fillet (3.7 oz.) | | 16.6 | | | 106 |
| Canned, solids & liq. | 4 oz. | | 12.6 | | | 107 |
| Canned, solids & liq. | 15-oz. can | | 47.2 | | | 400 |
| Pacific: | | | | | | |
| Raw: | | | | | | |
| Dressed | 1 lb. (weighed with bones & skin) | | 23.8 | | | |
| Meat only | 4 oz. | | 8.3 | | | |
| Canned, solids & liq. | 4 oz. | | 11.3 | | | |
| Salted | 4 oz. | | 28.5 | | | |
| Smoked | 4 oz. | | 14.7 | | | |
| **MACKEREL, JACK** (See **JACK MACKEREL**) | | | | | | |
| **MAI TAI COCKTAIL,** dry mix (Holland House) | 1 serving (.6 oz.) | 4 | 0.0 | | | |
| **MALT,** dry (USDA) | 1 oz. | | .5 | | | (0) |
| **MALTED MILK MIX:** | | | | | | |
| Dry powder, "unfortified" (USDA) | 1 oz. (3 heaping tsps.) | 125 | 2.4 | | | |
| *Prepared with whole milk (USDA) | 1 cup (8.3 oz.) | 214 | 10.3 | | | |

(USDA): United States Department of Agriculture
*Prepared as Package Directs

| Food and Description | Measure or Quantity | Sodium (mg.) | Total | Satu- rated | Unsatu- rated | Choles- terol (mg.) |
|---|---|---|---|---|---|---|
| | | | — Fats in grams — | | | |
| Chocolate, instant (Borden's) | 2 heaping tsps. (.7 oz.) | 64 | .9 | | | |
| Chocolate (Carnation)[1] | 3 heaping tsps. (.7 oz.) | 98 | 1.7 | Tr. | Tr. | 4 |
| **MALT EXTRACT,** dried (USDA) | 1 oz. | 23 | Tr. | | | (0) |
| **MALT LIQUOR:** | | | | | | |
| Colt 45 | 6 fl. oz. | 7 | 0.0 | | | 0 |
| Kingsbury, non-alcoholic | 6 fl. oz. | 10 | 0.0 | | | 0 |
| Mickeys | 6 fl. oz. | 7 | 0.0 | | | 0 |
| *MALT-O-MEAL, cereal | 1 T. | <1 | 0.0 | | | 0 |
| **MAMEY OR MAMMEE APPLE,** fresh (USDA): | | | | | | |
| Whole | 1 lb. (weighed with skin & seeds) | 42 | 1.4 | | | 0 |
| Fresh only | 4 oz. | 17 | .6 | | | 0 |
| **MANDARIN ORANGE, CANNED:** | | | | | | |
| Light syrup (Del Monte) | 1/2 cup (4.5 oz.) | 8 | Tr. | | | 0 |
| Low calorie, solids & liq. (Diet Delight) | 1/2 cup (4.3 oz.) | 5 | Tr. | | | (0) |
| Unsweetened, solids & liq. (S & W) Nutradiet | 4 oz. | 2 | Tr. | | | (0) |
| **MANDARIN ORANGE, FRESH** (See **TANGERINE**) | | | | | | |
| **MANGO,** fresh (USDA): | | | | | | |
| Whole | 1 lb. (weighed with seeds & skin) | 21 | 1.2 | | | 0 |
| Whole | 1 med. (7.1 oz.) | 9 | .5 | | | 0 |
| Flesh only, diced or sliced | 1/2 cup (2.9 oz.) | 6 | 3.0 | | | 0 |
| **MANICOTTI,** frozen (Celentano): | | | | | | |
| Without sauce | 1 piece (7 oz.) | 420 | 18.0 | | | |
| With sauce | 2 pieces (8 oz.) | 435 | 15.0 | | | 86 |

(USDA): United States Department of Agriculture
*Prepared as Package Directs
[1]Principal sources of fat: wort solids, milk, cocoa & lecithin.

| Food and Description | Measure or Quantity | Sodium (mg.) | Total | Satu-rated | Unsatu-rated | Choles-terol (mg.) |
|---|---|---|---|---|---|---|
| | | | | — Fats in grams — | | |

*MANWICH* (Hunt's):

| Food and Description | Measure or Quantity | Sodium (mg.) | Total | Satu-rated | Unsatu-rated | Choles-terol (mg.) |
|---|---|---|---|---|---|---|
| Original | 5.8-oz. serving | 630 | 13.0 | | | |
| Mexican flavor | 5.8-oz. serving | 690 | 14.0 | | | |

**MAPLE SYRUP** (See **SYRUP, MAPLE**)

**MARGARINE:**

Salted:

Made with hydrogenated fat, regular or soft:

| Food and Description | Measure or Quantity | Sodium (mg.) | Total | Satu-rated | Unsatu-rated | Choles-terol (mg.) |
|---|---|---|---|---|---|---|
| (USDA) | 1 lb. | 4,477 | 367.4 | 82. | 286. | 0 |
| (USDA) | 4 oz. (1 stick) | 1,119 | 91.9 | 20. | 70. | 0 |
| (USDA) | 1 cup or 1 tub (8 oz.) | 2,239 | 183.7 | 41. | 143. | 0 |
| (USDA) | 1 T. (1/8 of stick, .5 oz.) | 138 | 11.3 | 3. | 9. | 0 |
| (USDA) | 1 pat (1″ × 1/3″ × 1″, 5 grams) | 49 | 4.0 | <1. | 3. | 0 |

Made with liquid oil, regular or soft:

| Food and Description | Measure or Quantity | Sodium (mg.) | Total | Satu-rated | Unsatu-rated | Choles-terol (mg.) |
|---|---|---|---|---|---|---|
| (USDA) | 1 lb. | 4,477 | 367.4 | 86. | 281. | 0 |
| (USDA) | 4 oz. (1 stick) | 1,119 | 91.9 | 22. | 70. | 0 |
| (USDA) | 1 cup or 1 tub (8 oz.) | 2,239 | 183.7 | 43. | 141. | 0 |
| (USDA) | 1 T. (.5 oz.) | 138 | 11.3 | 3. | 9. | 0 |
| (USDA) | 1 pat (1″ × 1/3″ × 1″, 5 grams) | 49 | 4.0 | <1. | 3. | 0 |

Made with two-thirds animal fat & one-third vegetable fat:

| Food and Description | Measure or Quantity | Sodium (mg.) | Total | Satu-rated | Unsatu-rated | Choles-terol (mg.) |
|---|---|---|---|---|---|---|
| (USDA) | 1 lb. | 4,477 | 367.4 | | | 227 |
| (USDA) | 4 oz. (1 stick) | 1,119 | 91.9 | | | 57 |
| (USDA) | 1 cup or 1 tub (8 oz.) | 2,239 | 183.7 | | | 113 |
| (USDA) | 1 T. (1/8 of stick, .5 oz.) | 138 | 11.3 | | | 7 |
| (USDA) | 1 pat (1″ × 1/3″ × 1″, 5 grams) | 49 | 4.0 | | | 2 |
| (Blue Bonnet) regular | 1 T. (.5 oz.) | 99 | 11.2 | 2. | 9. | 0 |
| (Blue Bonnet) soft | 1 T. (.5 oz.) | 99 | 11.2 | 2. | 9. | 0 |
| (Borden's) Danish flavor | 1 T. (.5 oz.) | 112 | 11.2 | 8. | 3. | |

(USDA): United States Department of Agriculture
*Prepared as Package Directs

| Food and Description | Measure or Quantity | Sodium (mg.) | Total | Satu- rated | Unsatu- rated | Choles- terol (mg.) |
|---|---|---|---|---|---|---|
| | | | | — Fats in grams — | | |
| (Fleischmann's) regular or soft | 1 T. (.5 oz.) | 95 | 11.0 | 2. | 9. | 0 |
| (Golden Glow) | 1 T. (.4 oz.) | 86 | 10.0 | | | |
| (Good Luck) soft | 1 T. (.4 oz.) | 86 | 10.0 | 2. | 8. | 0 |
| (Holiday) | 1 T. (.5 oz.) | 165 | 11.4 | | | 0 |
| (Imperial) stick | 1 T. (.5 oz.) | 112 | 11.2 | 2. | 9. | 0 |
| (Imperial) *Sof-Spread* | 1 T. (.5 oz.) | 96 | 11.2 | 2. | 9. | 0 |
| (Mazola)[1] | 1 T. (.5 oz.) | 119 | 11.2 | 2. | 9. | 0 |
| (Miracle) corn oil | 1 T. (9 grams) | 74 | 7.4 | | | |
| (Nucoa)[1] | 1 T. (.5 oz.) | 165 | 11.2 | 3. | 9. | 0 |
| (Nucoa) soft[1] | 1 T. (.4 oz.) | 130 | 10.0 | 2. | 8. | 0 |
| (Parkay) regular | 1 T. (.5 oz.) | 112 | 11.2 | | | |
| (Parkay) soft cup | 1 T. (.5 oz.) | 106 | 10.6 | | | |
| (Parkay) corn oil deluxe | 1 T. (.5 oz.) | 112 | 11.2 | | | |
| (Parkay) corn oil soft | 1 T. (.5 oz.) | 106 | 10.6 | | | |
| (Parkay) safflower oil, soft | 1 T. (.5 oz.) | 106 | 10.6 | | | |
| (Parkay) squeeze | 1 T. (.5 oz.) | 112 | 11.2 | | | |
| (Phenix) | 1 T. (.5 oz.) | 112 | 11.2 | | | |
| (Promise) soft or stick | 1 T. (.5 oz.) | 96 | 10.0 | 2. | 8. | 0 |
| (Saffola) cube | 1 T. (.5 oz.) | 120 | 11.2 | 2. | 9. | 0 |
| (Saffola) soft | 1 T. (.5 oz.) | 114 | 11.2 | 2. | 9. | 0 |
| Unsalted: | | | | | | |
| Made with hydrogenated fat, regular or soft: | | | | | | |
| (USDA) | 1 lb. | 45 | 367.4 | 82. | 286. | 0 |
| (USDA) | 4 oz. (1 stick) | 11 | 91.9 | 20. | 71. | 0 |
| (USDA) | 1 cup or 1 tub (8 oz.) | 23 | 183.7 | 41. | 143. | 0 |
| (USDA) | 1 T. (1/8 of stick, .5 oz.) | 1 | 11.3 | 3. | 9. | 0 |
| (USDA) | 1 pat (1″ × 1/3″ × 1″, 5 grams) | <1 | 4.0 | <1. | 3. | 0 |
| Made with liquid oil, regular or soft: | | | | | | |
| (USDA) | 1 lb. | 45 | 367.4 | 86. | 281 | 0 |
| (USDA) | 4 oz. (1 stick) | 11 | 91.9 | 22. | 70. | 0 |
| (USDA) | 1 cup or 1 tub (8 oz.) | 23 | 183.7 | 43. | 141. | 0 |
| (USDA) | 1 T. (1/8 stick, .5 oz.) | 1 | 11.3 | 3. | 9. | 0 |
| (USDA) | 1 pat (1″ × 1/3″ × 1″, 5 grams) | <1 | 4.0 | <1. | 3. | 0 |

(USDA): United States Department of Agriculture
*Prepared as Package Directs
[1]Principal source of fat: vegetable oil.

| Food and Description | Measure or Quantity | Sodium (mg.) | — Fats in grams — | | | Choles- terol (mg.) |
|---|---|---|---|---|---|---|
| | | | Total | Satu- rated | Unsatu- rated | |
| Made with two-thirds animal fat & one-third vegetable fat: | | | | | | |
| (USDA) | 1 lb. | 45 | 367.4 | | | 227 |
| (USDA) | 4 oz. (1 stick) | 11 | 91.9 | | | 57 |
| (USDA) | 1 cup or 1 tub (8 oz.) | 23 | 183.7 | | | 113 |
| (USDA) | 1 T. (⅛ stick, .5 oz.) | 1 | 11.3 | | | 7 |
| (USDA) | 1 pat (1″ × ⅓″ × 1″, 5 grams) | <1 | 4.0 | | | 2 |
| (Fleischmann's) regular | 1 T. (.5 oz.) | 1 | 11.2 | 2. | 9. | 0 |
| (Mazola)[1] | 1 T. (.5 oz.) | Tr. | 11.3 | 2. | 9. | 0 |

## MARGARINE, IMITATION,
diet, salted:

| | | | | | | |
|---|---|---|---|---|---|---|
| (Fleischmann's) | 1 T. (.5 oz.) | 100 | 6.0 | 1. | 5. | 0 |
| (Imperial) | 1 T. (.5 oz.) | 136 | 5.5 | Tr. | 5. | (0) |
| (Mazola) | 1 cup (8.3 oz.) | 2,338 | 92.6 | 17. | 76. | 0 |
| (Mazola) | 1 T. (.5 oz.) | 130 | 5.7 | 1. | 5. | 0 |
| (Parkay) | 1 T. (.5 oz.) | 120 | 5.9 | | | |

## MARGARINE, WHIPPED:
Salted:

| | | | | | | |
|---|---|---|---|---|---|---|
| (USDA) | 1 stick or ½ cup (2.7 oz.) | 750 | 61.6 | 14. | 48. | 0 |
| (Blue Bonnet) | 1 T. (9 grams) | 70 | 7.4 | 2. | 6. | 0 |
| (Imperial) | 1 T. (9 grams) | 62 | 7.2 | 1. | 6. | (0) |
| (Miracle) cottonseed-soybean | 1 T. (9 grams) | 74 | 7.4 | | | |
| (Parkay) cup | 1 T. (9 grams) | 74 | 7.4 | | | |
| Unsalted (USDA) | 1 stick or ½ cup (2.7 oz.) | 8 | 61.6 | 14. | 47. | 0 |

## MARGARITA COCKTAIL MIX
(Holland House):
Liquid:

| | | | | | | |
|---|---|---|---|---|---|---|
| Regular | 1 oz. | 92 | 0.0 | | | |
| Strawberry | 1 oz. | 3 | 0.0 | | | |
| Instant: | | | | | | |
| Regular | .5-oz. packet | 4 | 0.0 | | | |
| Strawberry | .6-oz. packet | <1 | 0.0 | | | |

(USDA): United States Department of Agriculture
*Prepared as Package Directs
[1]Principal source of fat: vegetable oil.

| Food and Description | Measure or Quantity | Sodium (mg.) | Total | Satu-rated | Unsatu-rated | Choles-terol (mg.) |
|---|---|---|---|---|---|---|
| **MARINADE MIX, MEAT:** | | | | | | |
| (Durkee) | 1-oz. pkg. | 4,101 | .7 | | | (0) |
| (French's) | 1-oz. pkg. | 4,320 | 0.0 | | | (0) |
| (Kikkoman) | 1-oz. pkg. | 4,000 | .4 | | | 0 |
| **MARJORAM** (Spice Islands) | 1 tsp. | <1 | | | | (0) |
| **MARMALADE:** | | | | | | |
| Sweetened: | | | | | | |
| (USDA) | 1 T. (.7 oz.) | 3 | <.1 | | | 0 |
| (Bama) | 1 T. (.7 oz.) | 2 | <.1 | | | (0) |
| (Kraft) | 1 oz. | <1 | <.1 | | | (0) |
| (Smucker's) | 1 T. (.7 oz.) | 0 | Tr. | | | (0) |
| Low calorie: | | | | | | |
| (Estee) | 1 T. | <3 | 0.0 | | | (0) |
| (S & W) *Nutradiet* | 1 T. (.5 oz.) | | <.1 | | | (0) |
| **MARMALADE PLUM** (See **SAPOTE**) | | | | | | |
| ***MARSHMALLOW FLUFF*** | 1 heaping tsp. | 5 | .1 | | | 0 |
| ***MARSHMALLOW KRISPIES,*** cereal (Kellogg's) | 1¼ cups | 285 | 0.0 | | | (0) |
| **MATZO** (Manischewitz): | | | | | | |
| Regular: | | | | | | |
| Plain | 1-oz. piece | <5 | 3.0 | | | 0 |
| American | 1-oz. board | 175 | 1.2 | | | 0 |
| Egg | 1 matzo | <10 | 2.0 | | | 20 |
| Egg & onion | 1-oz. piece | 180 | .9 | | | Tr. |
| Miniature | 2-gram matzo | Tr. | Tr. | | | 0 |
| Tea, thin | 1 matzo | <5 | .3 | | | 0 |
| *Tam Tam:* | | | | | | |
| Regular | 2.3-gram matzo | 17 | .8 | | | |
| Garlic | 2.3-gram matzo | 16 | .8 | | | |
| Onion | 2.9-gram matzo | 16 | .8 | | | |
| Wheat | 2.9-gram matzo | 18 | .8 | | | |
| Wheat | 2-gram matzo | Tr. | Tr. | | | 0 |
| Dietetic: | | | | | | |
| *Tam Tam,* unsalted | 1 piece | Tr. | .7 | | | 0 |
| Thins | 1 piece | <5 | .4 | | | 0 |

(USDA): United States Department of Agriculture
*Prepared as Package Directs

227

| Food and Description | Measure or Quantity | Sodium (mg.) | — Fats in grams — | | | Choles- terol (mg.) |
|---|---|---|---|---|---|---|
| | | | Total | Satu- rated | Unsatu- rated | |
| **MATZO FARFEL** | | | | | | |
| (Manischewitz) | ½ cup | Tr. | .4 | | | 0 |
| **MATZO MEAL** (Manischewitz) | 1 cup (4.1 oz.) | 2 | .9 | | | Tr. |
| **MAYONNAISE:** | | | | | | |
| (USDA)[1] | 1 cup (7.8 oz.) | 1,319 | 176.6 | 31. | 146. | 155 |
| (USDA)[1] | 1 T. (.5 oz.) | 84 | 11.2 | 2. | 9. | 10 |
| (Bama) | 1 T. (.5 oz.) | 16 | 13.2 | | | |
| (Bennett's) | 1 T. (.5 oz.) | 73 | 12.4 | | | 13 |
| (Hellmann's) *Real*[2] | 1 T. (.5 oz.) | 80 | 11.2 | | | 8 |
| (Kraft) | 1 T. (.5 oz.) | 65 | | | | 5 |
| *MAYPO,* cereal, dry, any flavor: | | | | | | |
| Instant | 1 oz. | <1 | 1.3 | | | |
| 1-minute | 1 oz. | <1 | 1.4 | | | |
| *MCDONALD'S:* | | | | | | |
| *Big Mac* | 1 hamburger | 979 | 35.0 | | | 83 |
| Biscuit: | | | | | | |
| Plain | 1 order | 786 | 18.2 | | | 9 |
| With bacon, egg & cheese | 1 order | 1,269 | 31.6 | | | 263 |
| With sausage | 1 order | 1,147 | 30.9 | | | 48 |
| With sausage & egg | 1 order | 1,301 | 39.9 | | | 285 |
| Cheeseburger | 1 cheeseburger | 743 | 16.0 | | | 41 |
| *Chicken McNuggets* | 1 serving | 512 | 21.3 | | | 73 |
| *Chicken McNuggets* Sauce: | | | | | | |
| Barbecue | 1.1-oz. serving | 309 | .4 | | | <1 |
| Honey | .5-oz. serving | 2 | Tr. | | | <1 |
| Hot mustard | 1.1-oz. serving | 259 | 2.4 | | | 3 |
| Cookies: | | | | | | |
| Chocolate chip | 1 package | 313 | 16.3 | | | 18 |
| *McDonaldland* | 1 package | 358 | 10.8 | | | 10 |
| *Egg McMuffin* | 1 serving | 885 | 15.8 | | | 259 |
| Egg, scrambled | 1 serving | 205 | 13.0 | | | 514 |
| English muffin, with butter | 1 muffin | 310 | 5.3 | | | 15 |
| *Filet-O-Fish* | 1 sandwich | 799 | 25.7 | | | 45 |
| Grapefruit juice | 6 fl. oz. | 2 | .2 | | | |
| Hamburger | 1 hamburger | 506 | 11.3 | | | 29 |
| Hot cakes with butter & syrup | 1 serving | 1,070 | 10.3 | | | 47 |
| Pie: | | | | | | |
| Apple | 1 pie | 398 | 14.3 | | | 12 |
| Cherry | 1 pie | 427 | 13.6 | | | 13 |

(USDA): United States Department of Agriculture
*Prepared as Package Directs
[1]Principal sources of fat: soybean oil, cottonseed oil, corn oil & egg.
[2]Principal sources of fat: vegetable oil & egg.

| Food and Description | Measure or Quantity | Sodium (mg.) | — Fats in grams — | | | Choles- terol (mg.) |
|---|---|---|---|---|---|---|
| | | | Total | Satu- rated | Unsatu- rated | |
| Potato: | | | | | | |
| Fried | 1 regular order | 109 | 11.5 | | | 8 |
| Hash browns | 1 order | 325 | 7.0 | | | 7 |
| *Quarter Pounder:* | | | | | | |
| Regular | 1 hamburger | 718 | 23.5 | | | 81 |
| With cheese | 1 hamburger | 1,220 | 31.6 | | | 101 |
| Salads & condiments: | | | | | | |
| Chef's salad | 1 serving | 490 | 13.6 | 5.9 | 7.65 | 152 |
| Garden salad | 1 serving | 160 | 6.8 | 2.9 | 3.9 | 107 |
| Chicken oriental salad | 1 serving | 230 | 3.4 | .9 | 2.4 | 78 |
| Shrimp salad | 1 serving | 480 | 2.8 | .7 | 2.1 | 193 |
| Side salad | 1 serving | 100 | 4.1 | 1.6 | 2.4 | 86 |
| Bacon bits | 1 packet (3 grams) | 95 | 1.2 | | | 0 |
| Chow mein noodles | 1 packet | 60 | 2.2 | .3 | 1.7 | 2 |
| Croutons | 1 packet | 140 | 2.2 | .5 | 1.5 | 0 |
| Dressings: | | | | | | |
| Blue cheese | .5 oz. | 150 | 6.9 | | | 6 |
| French | .5 oz. | 180 | 5.2 | | | 0 |
| Oriental | .5 oz. | 180 | .1 | | | 0 |
| Thousand island | .5 oz. | 100 | 7.5 | | | 8 |
| Lo-cal vinaigrette | .5 oz. | 60 | .5 | | | 0 |
| *Sausage McMuffin:* | | | | | | |
| Plain | 1 sandwich | 830 | 21.9 | 7.8 | 14.1 | 64 |
| With egg | 1 sandwich | 980 | 27.4 | | | 336 |
| Sausage, pork | 1 serving | 350 | 16.3 | 5.9 | 10.4 | 48 |
| Shake: | | | | | | |
| Chocolate | 1 serving | 240 | 10.6 | | | 41 |
| Strawberry | 1 serving | 170 | 10.1 | | | 41 |
| Vanilla | 1 serving | 170 | 10.2 | | | 41 |
| Sundae: | | | | | | |
| Caramel, hot | 1 serving | 160 | 9.1 | | | 35 |
| Hot fudge | 1 serving | 160 | 9.4 | | | 28 |
| Strawberry | 1 serving | 85 | 7.3 | | | 27 |

**MEAL** (See **CORNMEAL** or **CRACKER MEAL** or **MATZO MEAL**)

**MEATBALL DINNER OR ENTREE,** frozen:

| | | | | | | |
|---|---|---|---|---|---|---|
| (Green Giant) sweet & sour | 9.4-oz. entree | 820 | 10.0 | | | |
| (Swanson) | 8 1/2-oz. entree | 900 | 18.0 | | | |

(USDA): United States Department of Agriculture
*Prepared as Package Directs

| Food and Description | Measure or Quantity | Sodium (mg.) | —Fats in grams— | | | Choles- terol (mg.) |
|---|---|---|---|---|---|---|
| | | | Total | Satu- rated | Unsatu- rated | |
| **\*MEATBALL SEASONING** | | | | | | |
| **MIX** (Durkee) Italian style | 1 cup | 1,019 | 48.5 | | | |
| **MEATBALL STEW:** | | | | | | |
| Canned *Dinty Moore* (Hormel) | 7½-oz. serving | | 15.8 | | | |
| Frozen *Lean Cuisine* | | | | | | |
| (Stouffer's) | 10-oz. serving | 1,260 | 7.0 | | | 65 |
| **MEATBALLS, SWEDISH,** | | | | | | |
| frozen: | | | | | | |
| (Armour) *Dinner Classics* | 11½-oz. meal | 1,560 | 28.0 | | | 105 |
| (Stouffer's) with noodles | 11-oz. pkg. | 1,620 | 27.0 | | | |
| **MEAT LOAF DINNER,** frozen: | | | | | | |
| (Banquet): | | | | | | |
| Dinner | 11-oz. dinner | 1,333 | 26.0 | | | |
| Entree for One | 5-oz. | 827 | 15.0 | | | 45 |
| (Morton) | 11-oz. dinner | 1,300 | 17.3 | | | |
| (Swanson) with tomato sauce | 9-oz. entree | 950 | 15.0 | | | |
| **MEAT LOAF SEASONING** | | | | | | |
| **MIX:** | | | | | | |
| \*(Bell's) | 4½ oz. | 700 | 20.0 | | | |
| (Contadina) | 3¾-oz. pkg. | 4,301 | 3.2 | | | |
| **MEAT, POTTED:** | | | | | | |
| (Hormel) | 1 T. | 145 | 2.0 | | | |
| (Libby's) | ⅓ of 5-oz. can | 297 | 8.4 | | | |
| **MEAT TENDERIZER:** | | | | | | |
| Unseasoned (French's) | 1 tsp. | 1,760 | Tr. | | | |
| Seasoned (French's) | 1 tsp. | 1,520 | Tr. | | | |
| **MELBA TOAST:** | | | | | | |
| Garlic (Keebler) | 1 piece (2 grams) | 30 | .2 | | | |
| Garlic, round (Old London) | 1 piece (2 grams) | 42 | .2 | | | |
| Onion (Keebler) | 1 piece (2 grams) | 32 | .2 | | | |
| Onion, round (Old London) | 1 piece (2 grams) | 33 | .3 | | | |
| Plain (Keebler) | 1 piece (2 grams) | 32 | .2 | | | |
| Pumpernickel (Old London) | 1 piece (4 grams) | 72 | <.1 | | | |
| Rye (Old London) | 1 piece (4 grams) | 44 | <.1 | | | |
| Rye, unsalted (Old London) | 1 piece (4 grams) | <1 | <.1 | | | |
| Sesame (Keebler) | 1 piece (2 grams) | 24 | .5 | | | |

(USDA): United States Department of Agriculture
\*Prepared as Package Directs

| Food and Description | Measure or Quantity | Sodium (mg.) | — Fats in grams — | | | Choles- terol (mg.) |
|---|---|---|---|---|---|---|
| | | | Total | Satu- rated | Unsatu- rated | |
| Sesame, rounds (Old London) | 1 piece (2 grams) | 23 | .4 | | | |
| Wheat (Old London) | 1 piece (4 grams) | 35 | <.1 | | | |
| Wheat, unsalted (Old London) | 1 piece (4 grams) | <1 | <.1 | | | |
| White: | | | | | | |
| (Keebler) | 1 piece (4 grams) | 39 | .1 | | | |
| (Old London) | 1 piece (4 grams) | 37 | <.1 | | | |
| Unsalted (Old London) | 1 piece (4 grams) | <1 | <.1 | | | |
| **MELLORINE** (Sealtest) | ¼ pt. (2.3 oz.) | 48 | 6.6 | | | |
| **MELON** (See individual listings, e.g., **CANTALOUPE, WATERMELON,** etc.) | | | | | | |
| **MELON BALL,** in syrup, frozen (USDA) | ½ cup (4.1 oz.) | 10 | .1 | | | 0 |
| **MENHADEN,** Atlantic, canned, solids & liq. (USDA) | 4 oz. | | 11.6 | | | |
| **MENUDO,** canned (Hormel) *Casa Grande* | 7½-oz. can | 1,097 | 2.0 | | | |
| **MEXICALI DOGS,** frozen (Hormel) | 5-oz. serving | 952 | 21.0 | | | |
| **MEXICAN DINNER,** frozen: | | | | | | |
| (Banquet): | | | | | | |
| Regular | 12-oz. dinner | 1,995 | 18.0 | | | |
| Combination | 12-oz. dinner | 1,978 | 17.0 | | | |
| *Extra Helping* | 21¼-oz. dinner | 4,778 | 27.0 | | | |
| (Morton) | 11-oz. dinner | 1,242 | 8.0 | | | |
| (Swanson): | | | | | | |
| 4-compartment meal | 16-oz. dinner | 1,780 | 26.0 | | | |
| *Hungry-Man* | 22-oz. dinner | 2,430 | 46.0 | | | |
| (Van de Kamp's) | 11½-oz. dinner | 1,040 | 20.0 | | | |
| **MILK, CONDENSED,** | | | | | | |
| sweetened, canned: | | | | | | |
| (USDA) | 1 cup (10.8 oz.) | 343 | 26.6 | 13. | 13. | 105 |
| (Carnation) | 1 fl. oz. | 49 | 3.3 | | | 9 |
| *Dairy Sweet* (Milnot) | ⅓ cup | 125 | 9.0 | | | |
| *Eagle Brand* (Borden's) | ⅓ cup | 120 | | | | |

(USDA): United States Department of Agriculture
*Prepared as Package Directs

| Food and Description | Measure or Quantity | Sodium (mg.) | Fats in grams — Total | Satu- rated | Unsatu- rated | Choles- terol (mg.) |
|---|---|---|---|---|---|---|
| **MILK, DRY:** | | | | | | |
| Whole: | | | | | | |
| (USDA) packed | 1 cup (5.1 oz.) | 587 | 39.9 | 22. | 18. | 158 |
| (USDA) spooned | 1 cup (4.3 oz.) | 490 | 33.3 | 18. | 15. | 132 |
| Nonfat, instant: | | | | | | |
| 7/8 cup makes 1 qt. (USDA) | 7/8 cup (3.2 oz.) | 484 | .7 | | | 20 |
| 1 1/3 cups make 1 qt. | | | | | | |
| (USDA) | 1 1/3 cups (3.2 oz.) | 479 | .7 | | | 20 |
| *(Carnation) | 1 cup (8.6 oz.) | 125 | .2 | Tr. | Tr. | 4 |
| **MILK, EVAPORATED,** canned: | | | | | | |
| Regular: | | | | | | |
| Unsweetened (USDA) | 1 cup (8.9 oz.) | 297 | 19.9 | 10. | 10. | 79 |
| (Carnation) | 1 cup (8.9 oz.) | 268 | 19 | | | 74 |
| (Pet) | 1 cup | 280 | 20.0 | | | 72 |
| Skimmed: | | | | | | |
| (Carnation) | 1 cup (9 oz.) | 280 | .5 | | | 10 |
| *Pet 99* | 1 cup | 300 | 0.0 | | | 2 |
| **MILK, FRESH:** | | | | | | |
| Whole: | | | | | | |
| 3.5% fat (USDA) | 1 cup (8.6 oz.) | 122 | 8.5 | 5. | 4. | 34 |
| 3.7% fat (USDA) | 1 cup (8.5 oz.) | 121 | 8.9 | 5. | 4. | |
| (Borden's) regular or hi-calcium | 1 cup | 130 | 8.0 | | | |
| (Johanna) | 1 cup | 125 | 8.0 | | | 33 |
| Skim: | | | | | | |
| (USDA) | 1 cup (8.6 oz.) | 127 | .2 | | | 5 |
| 1% fat with 1-2% nonfat milk solids added (USDA) | 1 cup (8.7 oz.) | | 2.5 | | | 15 |
| 2% fat with 1-2% nonfat milk solids added (USDA) | 1 cup (8.7 oz.) | 150 | 4.9 | 2. | 2. | 22 |
| (Borden's): | | | | | | |
| Regular | 1 cup | 130 | 1.0 | | | |
| *Skim-line* | 1 cup | 150 | 1.0 | | | |
| Buttermilk, cultured, fresh: | | | | | | |
| (USDA) | 1 cup (8.6 oz.) | 318 | .2 | | | 5 |
| (Borden's) *Golden Churn Brand* | 1 cup | 250 | 4.0 | | | |
| (Friendship) no salt added | 1 cup | 125 | 4.0 | | | |
| Buttermilk, cultured, dried | | | | | | |
| (USDA) | 1 cup (4.2 oz.) | 608 | 6.4 | 4. | 3. | |

(USDA): United States Department of Agriculture
*Prepared as Package Directs

| Food and Description | Measure or Quantity | Sodium (mg.) | — Fats in grams — | | | Choles- terol (mg.) |
|---|---|---|---|---|---|---|
| | | | Total | Satu- rated | Unsatu- rated | |
| Chocolate milk drink, fresh: (USDA): | | | | | | |
| With whole milk | 1 cup (8.8 oz.) | 118 | 8.5 | 4. | 5. | 32 |
| With skim milk & 2% added butterfat | 1 cup (8.8 oz.) | 115 | 5.8 | 2. | 3. | 20 |
| (Borden's) *Dutch Brand* | 8 fl. oz. | 180 | 5.0 | | | |
| (Hershey's) 2% low fat | 1 cup (8 fl. oz.) | 130 | 5.0 | | | |
| (Johanna): | | | | | | |
| Regular | 1 cup | 200 | 8.0 | | | 30 |
| Low fat | 1 cup | 210 | 2.0 | | | 6 |
| **MILK, GOAT,** whole (USDA) | 1 cup (8.6 oz.) | 83 | 9.8 | 5. | 5. | |
| **MILK, HUMAN** (USDA) | 1 oz. (by wt.) | 5 | 1.1 | <1. | <1. | |
| *MILK MAKERS* (Swiss Miss): | | | | | | |
| Chocolate | 8 fl. oz. | 230 | Tr. | | | |
| Malted | 8 fl. oz. | 220 | Tr. | | | |
| Strawberry | 8 fl. oz. | 170 | Tr. | | | |
| **MILK, REINDEER** (USDA) | 1 oz. (by wt.) | 45 | 5.6 | | | |
| **MILLET,** whole-grain (USDA) | 1 lb. | | 13.2 | 4. | 9. | 0 |
| **MINCEMEAT** (See **PIE FILLING,** Mincemeat) | | | | | | |
| **MINCE PIE** (See **PIE, Mince**) | | | | | | |
| **MINERAL WATER:** | | | | | | |
| *La Croix* | 6 fl. oz. | 1 | 0.0 | | | 0 |
| (Schweppes) | 6 fl. oz. | 3 | 0.0 | | | 0 |
| *MINI-WHEATS,* cereal (Kellogg's) frosted | .25-oz. biscuit | <10 | 0.0 | | | |
| **MISO,** cereal & soybeans (USDA) | 4 oz. | 3345 | 5.2 | 1. | 4. | 0 |
| **MOLASSES:** | | | | | | |
| Blackstrap (USDA) | ½ cup (5.4 oz.) | 148 | | | | 0 |
| Blackstrap (USDA) | 1 T. (.7 oz.) | 18 | | | | 0 |
| Light (USDA) | ½ cup (5.4 oz.) | 23 | | | | 0 |

(USDA): United States Department of Agriculture
*Prepared as Package Directs

| Food and Description | Measure or Quantity | Sodium (mg.) | Total | Satu-rated | Unsatu-rated | Choles-terol (mg.) |
|---|---|---|---|---|---|---|
| | | | | —Fats in grams— | | |
| Light (USDA) | 1 T. (.7 oz.) | 3 | | | | 0 |
| Medium (USDA) | ½ cup (5.4 oz.) | 57 | | | | 0 |
| Medium (USDA) | 1 T. (.7 oz.) | 7 | | | | 0 |
| Unsulphured (Grandma's) | 1 T. (.7 oz.) | 21 | | | | (0) |
| **MORTADELLA,** sausage (See also **SAUSAGE**) (USDA) | 1 oz. | | 7.1 | | | |
| *MOST,* cereal (Kellogg's) | ½ cup (1 oz.) | 30 | 0.0 | | | |
| **MOSTACCIOLI,** frozen (Banquet) *Buffet Supper,* & sauce | 32-oz. pkg. | 5,684 | 32.0 | | | |
| **MOUSSE,** canned, dietetic (Featherweight) chocolate | ½ cup (4 oz.) | | 3.0 | | | |
| **MUFFIN:** | | | | | | |
| Apple (Pepperidge Farm) with spice | 1 muffin | 230 | 8.0 | | | |
| Blueberry: | | | | | | |
| (USDA) home recipe [1] | 3″ muffin (1.4 oz.) | 253 | 3.7 | 1. | 3. | |
| (Hostess) | 1¾-oz. muffin | 149 | 3.5 | | | 15 |
| (Morton) frozen: | | | | | | |
| Regular | 1.6-oz. muffin | 130 | 3.0 | | | 9 |
| Rounds | 1.5-oz. muffin | 180 | 3.0 | | | 14 |
| (Pepperidge Farm) regular or frozen | 1.9-oz. muffin | 250 | 7.0 | | | |
| Bran: | | | | | | |
| (USDA) home recipe [2] | 3″ muffin (1.4 oz.) | 179 | 3.9 | 2. | 1.9 | |
| (Pepperidge Farm) with raisins, regular or frozen | 1 muffin | 300 | 7.0 | | | |
| Carrot walnut (Pepperidge Farm) | 1 muffin | 220 | 4.0 | | | |
| Chocolate chip (Pepperidge Farm) | 1 muffin | 170 | 8.0 | | | |
| Cinnamon swirl (Pepperidge Farm) | 1 muffin | 170 | 6.0 | | | |

(USDA): United States Department of Agriculture
*Prepared as Package Directs
[1]Principal sources of fat: vegetable shortening, egg & milk.
[2]Principal sources of fat: butter, egg & milk.

| Food and Description | Measure or Quantity | Sodium (mg.) | Total | Satu- rated | Unsatu- rated | Choles- terol (mg.) |
|---|---|---|---|---|---|---|
| Corn: | | | | | | |
| (USDA) home recipe, prepared with whole ground cornmeal [1] | 2⅜-oz. muffin | 198 | 4.1 | 2. | 3. | |
| (Morton) frozen | 1.7-oz. muffin | 280 | 4.0 | | | 14 |
| (Pepperidge Farm) | 1.9-oz. muffin | 260 | 7.0 | | | |
| English: | | | | | | |
| (Pepperidge Farm): | | | | | | |
| Plain | 2-oz. muffin | 180 | 4.0 | | | |
| Cinnamon raisin | 2-oz. muffin | 180 | 2.0 | | | |
| *Roman Meal* | 2½-oz. muffin | | .9 | | | Tr. |
| (Thomas'): | | | | | | |
| Regular | 2-oz. muffin | 207 | 1.1 | | | 0 |
| Honey wheat | 2-oz. muffin | 227 | 1.1 | | | 0 |
| Raisin | 2.1-oz. muffin | 187 | 1.5 | | | 0 |
| Sourdough | 2-oz. muffin | 208 | 1.8 | | | 0 |
| (Wonder) | 2-oz. muffin | 284 | 1.1 | | | 0 |
| **MUFFIN MIX:** | | | | | | |
| *Apple (Betty Crocker) Spiced | ¹⁄₁₂ of pkg. | 135 | 4.0 | | | |
| Bran: | | | | | | |
| (Duncan Hines) | ¹⁄₁₂ of pkg. | 161 | 2.8 | | | 0 |
| (Elam's) natural | 1 T. (.25 oz. dry mix) | 43 | Tr. | | | |
| *Cherry (Betty Crocker) | ¹⁄₁₂ of pkg. | | | 120 | 4. | |
| Corn: | | | | | | |
| With enriched flour (USDA) [2] | 1 oz. | 187 | 3.3 | <1. | 2. | |
| Prepared with egg & milk (USDA) [3] | 2⅜″ muffin (1.4 oz.) | 136 | 3.1 | <1. | 2. | |
| With cake flour & nonfat dry milk (USDA) [2] | 1 oz. | 230 | 3.0 | <1. | 2. | |
| Prepared with egg & water (USDA) [4] | 2⅜″ muffin (1.4 oz.) | 138 | 3.1 | <1. | 2. | |
| *(Betty Crocker) | 2¾″ muffin | 315 | 4.8 | | | |
| *(Dromedary) | 2½″ muffin (1.4 oz.) | 270 | 4.0 | | | |
| *(Flako) | 1.5-oz. muffin (¹⁄₁₂ of pkg.) | 370 | 4.0 | | | |

(USDA): United States Department of Agriculture
*Prepared as Package Directs
[1]Principal sources of fat: lard, milk & egg.
[2]Principal source of fat: vegetable shortening.
[3]Principal sources of fat: vegetable shortening, milk & egg.
[4]Principal sources of fat: vegetable shortening & egg.

| Food and Description | Measure or Quantity | Sodium (mg.) | Total | Fats in grams — Satu-rated | Unsatu-rated | Choles-terol (mg.) |
|---|---|---|---|---|---|---|
| **MULLET,** raw (USDA): | | | | | | |
| Whole | 1 lb. (weighed whole) | 195 | 16.6 | | | |
| Meat only | 4 oz. | 92 | 7.8 | | | |
| **MUNG BEANSPROUT** (See **BEAN SPROUT**) | | | | | | |
| **MUSCATEL WINE** (Gold Seal) | | | | | | |
| 19% alcohol | 3 fl. oz. (3.3 oz.) | 3 | 0.0 | | | (0) |
| **MUSHROOM:** | | | | | | |
| Raw (USDA): | | | | | | |
| Whole | ½ lb. (weighed untrimmed) | 33 | .6 | | | 0 |
| Trimmed, slices | ½ cup (1.2 oz.) | 5 | .1 | | | 0 |
| Powdered (Spice Islands) | 1 tsp. | <1 | | | | (0) |
| Canned, solids & liq.: | | | | | | |
| (USDA) | ½ cup (4.3 oz.) | 488 | .1 | | | 0 |
| Sliced, chopped or whole, broiled in butter (B in B) | 6-oz. can | 710 | 2.5 | | | |
| Whole or sliced (Green Giant): | | | | | | |
| Plain | 2 oz. | 260 | Tr. | | | |
| Broiled in butter | ½ of 3-oz. can | 394 | Tr. | | | |
| Frozen, whole, in butter sauce (Green Giant) | ½ cup | 240 | 4.0 | | | |
| **MUSKELLUNGE,** raw (USDA): | | | | | | |
| Whole | 1 lb. (weighed whole) | | 5.6 | | | |
| Meat only | 4 oz. | | 2.8 | | | |
| **MUSKMELON** (See **CANTALOUPE, CASABA** or **HONEYDEW**) | | | | | | |
| **MUSKRAT,** roasted (USDA) | 4 oz. | | 4.6 | | | |
| **MUSSEL** (USDA): | | | | | | |
| Raw, Atlantic & Pacific, with liq., in shell | 1 lb. (weighed in shell) | | 3.2 | | | |

(USDA): United States Department of Agriculture
*Prepared as Package Directs

236

| Food and Description | Measure or Quantity | Sodium (mg.) | — Fats in grams — | | | Choles- terol (mg.) |
|---|---|---|---|---|---|---|
| | | | Total | Satu- rated | Unsatu- rated | |
| Raw, Atlantic & Pacific, meat only | 4 oz. | 328 | 2.5 | | | |
| Canned, Pacific, drained | 4 oz. | | 3.7 | | | |
| **MUSTARD,** prepared: | | | | | | |
| Brown: | | | | | | |
| (USDA) | 1 tsp. (9 grams) | 118 | .6 | | | 0 |
| (French's) spicy | 1 tsp. | 50 | .3 | | | (0) |
| Chinese: | | | | | | |
| (Chun King) | 1 tsp. | 74 | .4 | | | 0 |
| (La Choy) hot | 1 tsp. | 130 | <1.0 | | | (0) |
| Cream salad (French's) | 1 tsp. | 60 | .3 | | | (0) |
| Dijon (French's) | 1 tsp. | 153 | .7 | | | (0) |
| *Grey Poupon* | 1 tsp. (6 grams) | 179 | .3 | | | (0) |
| Horseradish (French's) | 1 tsp. | 93 | .3 | | | (0) |
| Medford (French's) | 1 tsp. | 83 | .3 | | | (0) |
| Onion (French's) | 1 tsp. | 67 | .3 | | | (0) |
| Yellow: | | | | | | |
| (USDA) | 1 tsp. (9 grams) | 113 | .4 | | | (0) |
| (French's) | 1 tsp. | 60 | .3 | | | (0) |
| **MUSTARD GREENS:** | | | | | | |
| Raw, whole (USDA) | 1 lb. (weighed untrimmed) | 102 | 1.6 | | | 0 |
| Boiled without salt, drained (USDA) | 1 cup (7.8 oz.) | 40 | .9 | | | 0 |
| Canned, solids & liq.: | | | | | | |
| (Allen) | ½ cup | 35 | <1.0 | | | |
| (Sunshine) | ½ cup | 371 | .3 | | | |
| Frozen: | | | | | | |
| Not thawed (USDA) | 4 oz. | 14 | .5 | | | 0 |
| Boiled, drained (USDA) | ½ cup (3.8 oz.) | 11 | .4 | | | 0 |
| (Birds Eye) chopped | ⅓ of 10-oz. pkg. | 27 | .2 | | | 0 |
| (Frosty Acres) | 3.3 oz. | 20 | 0.0 | | | (0) |
| (McKenzie) chopped | 3.3 oz. | 37 | 0.0 | | | (0) |
| (Southland) | ⅕ of 16-oz. pkg. | 20 | 0.0 | | | (0) |
| **MUSTARD SEED** (Spice Islands) | 1 tsp. | <1 | | | | (0) |
| **MUSTARD SPINACH** (USDA): | | | | | | |
| Raw | 1 lb. | | 1.4 | | | 0 |
| Boiled without salt, drained | 4 oz. | | .2 | | | 0 |

(USDA): United States Department of Agriculture
*Prepared as Package Directs

| Food and Description | Measure or Quantity | Sodium (mg.) | — Fats in grams — Total | Satu- rated | Unsatu- rated | Choles- terol (mg.) |
|---|---|---|---|---|---|---|

# N

**NATHAN'S:**

| | | | | | | |
|---|---|---|---|---|---|---|
| French fries | 1 regular order | 151 | 31.0 | | | |
| Hamburger & roll | 4½-oz. serving | 203 | 23.0 | | | |
| Hot dog & roll | ¾-oz. serving | 675 | 19.0 | | | |

**NATTO,** fermented soybean

| | | | | | | |
|---|---|---|---|---|---|---|
| (USDA) | 4 oz. | | 8.4 | 1. | 7. | |

**NATURAL CEREAL:**

*Familia:*

| | | | | | | |
|---|---|---|---|---|---|---|
| Regular | ½ cup | 8 | 2.9 | | | |
| Bran | ½ cup | 90 | 3.4 | | | |
| Granola | ½ cup | 67 | 9.5 | | | |
| No added salt | ½ cup | 2 | 3.2 | | | |

*Heartland* (Pet):

| | | | | | | |
|---|---|---|---|---|---|---|
| Regular, raisin or trail mix | ¼ cup (1 oz.) | 80 | 4.0 | | | |
| Coconut | ¼ cup (1 oz.) | 80 | 5.0 | | | |

**NATURE SNACKS** (Sun-Maid):

| | | | | | | |
|---|---|---|---|---|---|---|
| Carob crunch | 1 oz. | 13 | 7.1 | | | |
| Carob peanut | 1¼ oz. | 16 | 11.0 | | | |
| Carob raisin | 1¼ oz. | 21 | 5.0 | | | |
| Nuts galore | 1 oz. | | 15.0 | | | |
| Raisin crunch | 1 oz. | 41 | 4.3 | | | |
| Rocky road | 1 oz. | 4 | 4.9 | | | |
| Sesame nut crunch | 1 oz. | 159 | 8.9 | | | |
| Yogurt crunch | 1 oz. | 28 | 4.3 | | | |
| Yogurt raisin | 1 oz. | 20 | 6.0 | | | |

**NEAR BEER** (See **BEER, NEAR**)

**NECTARINE,** fresh (USDA):

| | | | | | | |
|---|---|---|---|---|---|---|
| Whole | 1 lb. (weighed with pits) | 25 | Tr. | | | 0 |
| Flesh only | 4 oz. | 7 | Tr. | | | 0 |

**NEW ZEALAND SPINACH** (USDA):

| | | | | | | |
|---|---|---|---|---|---|---|
| Raw | 1 lb. | 721 | 1.4 | | | |
| Boiled without salt, drained | 4 oz. | 104 | .2 | | | |

(USDA): United States Department of Agriculture
*Prepared as Package Directs

| Food and Description | Measure or Quantity | Sodium (mg.) | Total | — Fats in grams — Satu- rated | Unsatu- rated | Choles- terol (mg.) |
|---|---|---|---|---|---|---|
| **NIAGARA WINE,** white | | | | | | |
| (Pleasant Valley) | 12.5% alcohol | 24 | 0.0 | | | 0 |
| **NOODLE** (USDA): | | | | | | |
| Dry, 1½″ strips[1] | 1 cup (2.6 oz.) | 4 | 3.4 | <1. | 3. | 67 |
| Dry, 1½″ strips[1] | 1 oz. | 1 | 1.3 | Tr. | 1. | 27 |
| Cooked[1] | 1 cup (5.6 oz.) | 3 | 2.4 | <1. | 2. | 50 |
| Cooked[1] | 1 oz. | <1 | .4 | Tr. | Tr. | 9 |
| **NOODLE & BEEF:** | | | | | | |
| Canned (Hormel) *Short Orders* | 7½-oz. can | 974 | 14.0 | | | |
| Frozen (Banquet) *Buffet Supper* | 2-lb. pkg. | 5,581 | 26.4 | | | |
| **NOODLE & CHICKEN:** | | | | | | |
| Canned (Hormel) *Dinty Moore, Short Orders* | 7½-oz. can | 1,144 | 12.0 | | | |
| Frozen (Swanson) 3-compartment dinner | 10½-oz. dinner | 820 | 9.0 | | | |
| **NOODLE, CHOW MEIN,** canned: | | | | | | |
| (USDA) | 1 cup (1.6 oz.) | | 10.6 | | | 5 |
| (Chun King) | 1 oz. | | 6.7 | | | 0 |
| (La Choy) | ½ cup (1 oz.) | 230 | 8.0 | | | |
| **NOODLE MIX:** | | | | | | |
| *(Betty Crocker): | | | | | | |
| Fettucini alfredo | ¼ of pkg. | 490 | 11.0 | | | |
| Parisienne | ¼ of pkg. | 540 | 4.0 | | | |
| Romanoff | ¼ of pkg. | 705 | 12.0 | | | |
| Stroganoff | ¼ of pkg. | 605 | 12.0 | | | |
| *(Lipton) & sauce: Regular: | | | | | | |
| Beef | ½ cup | 595 | 7.0 | | | |
| Butter | ½ cup | 565 | 9.0 | | | |
| Cheese | ½ cup | 540 | 9.0 | | | |
| Sour cream & chive | ½ cup | 455 | 9.0 | | | |
| Deluxe: | | | | | | |
| Alfredo | ½ cup | 560 | 11.0 | | | |
| *Parmesano* | ½ cup | 445 | 11.0 | | | |
| Stroganoff | ½ cup | 510 | 10.0 | | | |
| *Noodle-Roni,* parmesan | ⅕ of 6-oz. pkg. | 370 | 3.0 | | | |

(USDA): United States Department of Agriculture
*Prepared as Package Directs
[1]Principal source of fat: egg.

239

| Food and Description | Measure or Quantity | Sodium (mg.) | Total | Satu-rated | Unsatu-rated | Choles-terol (mg.) |
|---|---|---|---|---|---|---|
| | | | | — Fats in grams — | | |
| **\*NOODLE, RAMEN,** canned (La Choy): | | | | | | |
| Beef | ½ of 3-oz. pkg. | 1,040 | 6.7 | | | |
| Chicken | ½ of 3-oz. pkg. | 1,159 | 6.6 | | | |
| Oriental | ½ of 3-oz. pkg. | 742 | 6.6 | | | |
| **NOODLE, RICE,** canned (La Choy) | ½ cup (1 oz.) | 420 | 5.0 | | | |
| **NUT,** mixed (See also individual kinds): | | | | | | |
| Dry roasted, salted: | | | | | | |
| (Flavor House) | 1 oz. | 81 | 14.9 | | | (0) |
| (Planters) | 1 oz. | 340 | 14.2 | 2. | 12. | 0 |
| (Skippy) | 1 oz. | 147 | 15.1 | 2. | 13. | 0 |
| Oil roasted: | | | | | | |
| With peanuts (Planters) | 1 oz. | 220 | 14.3 | | | 0 |
| Without peanuts (Planters) | 1 oz. | 220 | 15.0 | | | 0 |
| **NUT LOAF** (See **BREAD, CANNED**) | | | | | | |
| **NUTMEG:** | | | | | | |
| Whole (Spice Islands) | 1 nut | <1 | | | | (0) |
| Ground (Spice Islands) | 1 tsp. | <1 | | | | (0) |
| **NUTRI-GRAIN,** cereal (Kellogg's): | | | | | | |
| Corn | ½ cup (1 oz.) | 185 | 1.0 | | | |
| Wheat | ⅔ cup (1 oz.) | 195 | 0.0 | | | |
| Wheat & raisins | ⅔ cup | 165 | 0.0 | | | |
| **NUTRIMATO** (Mott's) | 4 oz. | | .3 | | | |

# O

| Food and Description | Measure or Quantity | Sodium (mg.) | Total | Satu-rated | Unsatu-rated | Choles-terol (mg.) |
|---|---|---|---|---|---|---|
| **OAT FLAKES,** cereal (Post) | ⅔ cup (1 oz.) | 254 | .4 | | | 0 |
| **OATMEAL:** | | | | | | |
| Instant: | | | | | | |
| (H-O) | 1 cup (2.4 oz.) | 1 | 3.9 | 1. | 3. | 0 |
| (H-O) | 1 T. (4 grams) | Tr. | .2 | Tr. | Tr. | 0 |

(USDA): United States Department of Agriculture
\*Prepared as Package Directs

| Food and Description | Measure or Quantity | Sodium (mg.) | Fats in grams — Total | Satu-rated | Unsatu-rated | Choles-terol (mg.) |
|---|---|---|---|---|---|---|
| *(Quaker) | 1-oz. packet (¾ cup cooked) | 255 | 1.7 | | | |
| Sweet and Mellow (H-O) | 1 packet (1.4 oz.) | 272 | 1.7 | Tr. | 1. | 0 |
| With apple & cinnamon (Quaker) | 1⅛-oz. packet (¾ cup cooked) | 202 | 1.3 | | | |
| With chocolate flavor (Quaker) | 1¾-oz. packet (¾ cup cooked) | 276 | 2.0 | | | |
| With dates & brown sugar (Quaker) | 1⅜-oz. packet (¾ cup cooked) | 228 | 1.2 | | | |
| With dates & caramel (H-O) | 1 packet (1.4 oz.) | 232 | 1.4 | Tr. | 1. | 0 |
| With maple & brown sugar (Quaker) | 1⅝-oz. packet (¾ cup cooked) | 275 | 1.8 | | | |
| With raisins & spice (H-O) | 1 packet (1.6 oz.) | 252 | 1.6 | Tr. | 1. | 0 |
| With raisins & spice (Quaker) | 1½-oz. packet (¾ cup cooked) | 253 | 1.3 | | | |
| Quick: | | | | | | |
| Dry: | | | | | | |
| (H-O) | 1 cup (2.5 oz.) | 2 | 4.1 | 1. | 3. | 0 |
| (H-O) | 1 T. (4 grams) | Tr. | .3 | Tr. | Tr. | 0 |
| Cooked: | | | | | | |
| *(Albers) | 1 cup | | 2.8 | | | |
| *(Quaker) | ⅔ cup (1 oz. dry) | 1 | 1.7 | | | |
| Regular: | | | | | | |
| Dry: | | | | | | |
| (USDA) | 1 cup (2.5 oz.) | 1 | 5.3 | 1. | 4. | 0 |
| (USDA) | 1 T. (4 grams) | <1 | .3 | Tr. | Tr. | 0 |
| (H-O) old fashioned | 1 cup (2.6 oz.) | 1 | .4 | | | 0 |
| (H-O) old fashioned | 1 T. (5 grams) | Tr. | .3 | Tr. | Tr. | 0 |
| Cooked: | | | | | | |
| *(USDA) | 1 cup (8.5 oz.) | 523 | 2.4 | | | 0 |
| *(Quaker) old fashioned | ⅔ cup (1 oz. dry) | 1 | 1.7 | | | (0) |

**OCEAN PERCH:**
Atlantic:

| Food and Description | Measure or Quantity | Sodium (mg.) | Total | | | |
|---|---|---|---|---|---|---|
| Raw, whole (USDA) | 1 lb. (weighed whole) | 111 | 1.7 | | | |

(USDA): United States Department of Agriculture
*Prepared as Package Directs

| Food and Description | Measure or Quantity | Sodium (mg.) | Total | Fats in grams — Saturated | Unsaturated | Cholesterol (mg.) |
|---|---|---|---|---|---|---|
| Fried, dipped in egg, milk & bread crumbs (USDA) | 4 oz. | 174 | 15.1 | | | |
| Frozen, breaded, fried, reheated (USDA) | 4 oz. | | 21.4 | | | |
| Pacific, raw: | | | | | | |
| Whole (USDA) | 1 lb. (weighed whole) | 77 | 1.8 | | | |
| Meat only (USDA) | 4 oz. | 71 | 1.7 | | | |
| Frozen (Gorton's) | ⅓ of 1-lb. pkg. | 120 | 1.8 | | | |
| **OCEAN PERCH MEALS,** frozen: (Banquet): | | | | | | |
| Fish compartment | 5 oz. | | 8.7 | | | |
| Potato compartment | 1.6 oz. | | 7.6 | | | |
| Corn compartment | 2.2 oz. | | .9 | | | |
| Complete dinner | 8.8-oz. dinner | | 17.1 | | | |
| (Weight Watchers) | 18-oz. dinner | | 6.1 | | | |
| & broccoli (Weight Watchers) | 9½-oz. luncheon | | 7.9 | | | |
| **OCTOPUS,** raw, meat only (USDA) | 4 oz. | | .9 | | | |
| **OIL,** salad or cooking: Corn: | | | | | | |
| (USDA) | ½ cup (3.9 oz.) | 0 | 110.0 | 11. | 99. | 0 |
| (USDA) | 1 T. (.5 oz.) | 0 | 14.0 | 1. | 13. | 0 |
| (Kraft) | 1 oz. | 0 | 28.4 | 4. | 24. | 0 |
| (Mazola) | 1 cup (7.7 oz.) | 0 | 221.0 | 29. | 192. | 0 |
| (Mazola) | 1 T. (.5 oz.) | 0 | 14.0 | 2. | 12. | 0 |
| Cottonseed (USDA) | ½ cup (3.9 oz.) | 0 | 110.0 | 28. | 82. | 0 |
| Cottonseed (USDA) | 1 T. (.5 oz.) | 0 | 14.0 | 4. | 10. | 0 |
| Crisco | 1 T. | 0 | 14.0 | 2. | 12. | |
| Olive (USDA) | ½ cup (3.9 oz.) | 0 | 110.0 | 12. | 98. | 0 |
| Olive (USDA) | 1 T. (.5 oz.) | 0 | 14.0 | 2. | 12. | 0 |
| Peanut: | | | | | | |
| (USDA) | ½ cup (3.9 oz.) | 0 | 110.0 | 20. | 90. | 0 |
| (USDA) | 1 T. (.5 oz.) | 0 | 14.0 | 3. | 11. | 0 |
| (Planters) | 1 T. (.5 oz.) | Tr. | 14.0 | 3. | 11. | 0 |
| Safflower: | | | | | | |
| (USDA) | ½ cup (3.9 oz.) | 0 | 110.0 | 9. | 101. | 0 |
| (USDA) | 1 T. (.5 oz.) | 0 | 14.0 | 1. | 13. | 0 |
| (Kraft) | 1 oz. | | 28.4 | 3. | 26. | 0 |
| (Saff-o-life) | 1 T. | Tr. | 14.0 | | | (0) |

(USDA): United States Department of Agriculture
*Prepared as Package Directs

| Food and Description | Measure or Quantity | Sodium (mg.) | — Fats in grams — | | | Cholesterol (mg.) |
|---|---|---|---|---|---|---|
| | | | Total | Saturated | Unsaturated | |
| *Saffola* | ½ cup (3.9 oz.) | 0 | 110.0 | 9. | 101. | 0 |
| *Saffola* | 1 T. (.5 oz.) | 0 | 14.0 | 1. | 13. | 0 |
| Sesame (USDA) | ½ cup (3.9 oz.) | 0 | 110.0 | 15. | 95. | 0 |
| Sesame (USDA) | 1 T. (.5 oz.) | 0 | 14.0 | 2. | 12. | 0 |
| Soybean (USDA) | ½ cup (3.9 oz.) | 0 | 110.0 | 16. | 94. | 0 |
| Soybean (USDA) | 1 T. (.5 oz.) | 0 | 14.0 | 2. | 12. | 0 |
| Vegetable (Kraft) | 1 oz. | 0 | 28.4 | 5. | 24. | 0 |
| *Wesson* | 1 T. (.5 oz.) | 0 | 14.0 | 3. | 11. | 0 |

## OKRA:

| Food and Description | Measure or Quantity | Sodium (mg.) | Total | Satu-rated | Unsatu-rated | Choles-terol (mg.) |
|---|---|---|---|---|---|---|
| Raw, whole (USDA) | 1 lb. (weighed untrimmed) | 12 | 1.2 | | | 0 |
| Boiled without salt, drained (USDA): | | | | | | |
| Whole | ½ cup (3.1 oz.) | 2 | .3 | | | 0 |
| Pods | 8 pods (3″ × ⅝″, 3 oz.) | 2 | .3 | | | 0 |
| Slices | ½ cup (2.8 oz.) | 2 | .2 | | | 0 |
| Frozen: | | | | | | |
| Cut & pods, not thawed (USDA) | 4 oz. | 2 | .1 | | | 0 |
| Cut, boiled, drained (USDA) | ½ cup (3.2 oz.) | 2 | <.1 | | | 0 |
| Whole, boiled, drained (USDA) | ½ cup (2.4 oz.) | 1 | <.1 | | | 0 |
| Cut (Birds Eye) | ⅓ of 10-oz. pkg. | 2 | Tr. | | | 0 |
| (Frosty Acres) | 3.3 oz. | 0 | 0 | | | (0) |
| (Larsen) | 3.3 oz. | 5 | 0 | | | (0) |
| (McKenzie) | 3.3 oz. | 19 | 0 | | | (0) |

## OLEOMARGARINE (See MARGARINE)

## OLIVE:

| Food and Description | Measure or Quantity | Sodium (mg.) | Total | Satu-rated | Unsatu-rated | Choles-terol (mg.) |
|---|---|---|---|---|---|---|
| Greek style, salt-cured, oil-coated: | | | | | | |
| Pitted (USDA) | 1 oz. | 932 | 10.1 | 1. | 9. | 0 |
| With pits, drained (USDA) | 4 oz. | 2,992 | 32.6 | 4. | 29. | 0 |
| Green, pitted & drained: | | | | | | |
| (USDA) | 1 oz. | 680 | 3.6 | | | 0 |
| (USDA) | 4 med. or 3 extra large or 2 giant (.6 oz.) | 384 | 2.0 | | | 0 |
| (USDA) | 1 olive (13⁄16″ × 1 1⁄16″, 6 grams) | 132 | .7 | | | 0 |

(USDA): United States Department of Agriculture
*Prepared as Package Directs

| Food and Description | Measure or Quantity | Sodium (mg.) | Total | Satu- rated | Unsatu- rated | Choles- terol (mg.) |
|---|---|---|---|---|---|---|
| | | | | —Fats in grams— | | |

Ripe, by variety, pitted & drained:

| Food and Description | Measure or Quantity | Sodium (mg.) | Total | Satu-rated | Unsatu-rated | Choles-terol (mg.) |
|---|---|---|---|---|---|---|
| Ascalano, any size (USDA) | 1 oz. | 230 | 3.9 | <1. | 3. | 0 |
| Manzanilla, any size (USDA) | 1 oz. | 230 | 3.9 | <1. | 3. | 0 |
| Mission, any size (USDA) | 1 oz. | 213 | 5.7 | <1. | 5. | 0 |
| Mission (USDA) | 3 small or 2 large (.4 oz.) | 75 | 2.0 | Tr. | 2. | 0 |
| Mission, slices (USDA) | ½ cup (2.2 oz.) | 465 | 12.5 | 1. | 11. | 0 |
| Sevillano, any size (USDA) | 1 oz. | 235 | 2.7 | Tr. | 2. | 0 |

**ONION:**

Raw (USDA):

| Food and Description | Measure or Quantity | Sodium (mg.) | Total | Satu-rated | Unsatu-rated | Choles-terol (mg.) |
|---|---|---|---|---|---|---|
| Whole | 1 lb. (weighed untrimmed) | 41 | .4 | | | 0 |
| Whole | 2½" onion (3.9 oz.) | 10 | .1 | | | 0 |
| Chopped | ½ cup (3 oz.) | 9 | <.1 | | | 0 |
| Chopped | 1 T. (.4 oz.) | 1 | <.1 | | | 0 |
| Grated | 1 T. (.5 oz.) | 1 | <.1 | | | 0 |
| Ground | 1 T. (.5 oz.) | 2 | <.1 | | | 0 |
| Slices | ½ cup (2 oz.) | 6 | <.1 | | | 0 |
| Boiled without salt (USDA): | | | | | | |
| Whole | ½ cup (3.7 oz.) | 7 | .1 | | | 0 |
| Halves or pieces | ½ cup (3.2 oz.) | 6 | <.1 | | | 0 |
| Pearl onions | ½ cup (3.2 oz.) | 6 | <.1 | | | 0 |
| Canned, boiled, solids & liq. (Comstock-Greenwood) | 4 oz. | 176 | .1 | | | (0) |
| Dehydrated: | | | | | | |
| Flakes (USDA) | 1 cup (2.3 oz.) | 56 | .8 | | | 0 |
| Flakes (USDA) | 1 tsp. (1 gram) | 1 | Tr. | | | 0 |
| Instant, minced or powder (Spice Islands) | 1 tsp. | 2 | | | | (0) |
| Frozen: | | | | | | |
| (Birds Eye): | | | | | | |
| Chopped | 1 oz. | 2 | Tr. | | | 0 |
| Pearl, deluxe | ⅓ of 10-oz. pkg. | 9 | .1 | | | 0 |
| Small, with cream sauce | 3 oz. | 333 | 6.1 | | | Tr. |
| Small, whole | 4 oz. | 10 | .1 | | | (0) |
| (Frosty Acres) chopped | 1 oz. | 5 | 0.0 | | | (0) |
| (Green Giant) small, in cheese flavored sauce | ½ cup | 400 | 5.0 | | | |
| (Larsen) diced | 1 oz. | Tr. | 0.0 | | | (0) |
| (Mrs. Paul's) rings, breaded & fried | ½ of 5-oz. pkg. | 305 | 6.7 | | | |

(USDA): United States Department of Agriculture
*Prepared as Package Directs

| Food and Description | Measure or Quantity | Sodium (mg.) | —Fats in grams— | | | Cholesterol (mg.) |
|---|---|---|---|---|---|---|
| | | | Total | Saturated | Unsaturated | |

**ONION BOUILLON:**

| | | | | | | |
|---|---|---|---|---|---|---|
| (Herb-Ox) | 1 cube (4 grams) | 560 | .1 | | | |
| (Herb-Ox) instant | 1 packet (5 grams) | 800 | .2 | | | |
| (Wyler's) | 1 tsp. | 670 | <.1 | | | |

**ONION, COCKTAIL** (Vlasic)

| | | | | | | |
|---|---|---|---|---|---|---|
| lightly spiced | 1 oz. | 371 | 0.0 | | | |

**ONION, GREEN** (USDA):
Raw:

| | | | | | | |
|---|---|---|---|---|---|---|
| Whole | 1 lb. (weighed untrimmed) | 22 | .9 | | | 0 |
| Bulb & entire top | 1 oz. | 1 | <.1 | | | 0 |
| Bulb & white portion of top | 3 small onions (.9 oz.) | 1 | <.1 | | | 0 |
| Slices, bulb & white portion of top | ½ cup (1.8 oz.) | 2 | .1 | | | 0 |
| Tops only | 1 oz. | 1 | .1 | | | 0 |
| Dry, shredded (Spice Islands) | 1 tsp. | 11 | | | | (0) |

**ONION SOUP** (See **SOUP,** Onion)

**ONION, WELSH,** raw (USDA):

| | | | | | | |
|---|---|---|---|---|---|---|
| Whole | 1 lb. (weighed untrimmed) | | 1.2 | | | 0 |
| Trimmed | 4 oz. | | .5 | | | 0 |

**OPOSSUM,** roasted, meat only (USDA)

| | | | | | | |
|---|---|---|---|---|---|---|
| (USDA) | 4 oz. | | 11.6 | | | |

**ORANGE,** fresh:
All varieties (USDA):

| | | | | | | |
|---|---|---|---|---|---|---|
| Whole | 1 lb. (weighed with rind & seeds) | 3 | .7 | | | 0 |
| Whole | small orange (2½" dia., 5.3 oz.) | 1 | .2 | | | 0 |
| Whole | med. orange (3" dia., 5.5 oz.) | 2 | .3 | | | 0 |
| Whole | large orange (3⅜" dia., 8.4 oz.) | 2 | .5 | | | 0 |

(USDA): United States Department of Agriculture
*Prepared as Package Directs

| Food and Description | Measure or Quantity | Sodium (mg.) | —Fats in grams— | | | Choles- terol (mg.) |
|---|---|---|---|---|---|---|
| | | | Total | Satu- rated | Unsatu- rated | |
| Diced or sliced, drained | 1 cup (7.7 oz.) | 2 | .4 | | | 0 |
| Sections | 1 cup (8.5 oz.) | 2 | .5 | | | 0 |
| California Navel (USDA): | | | | | | |
| Whole | 1 lb. (weighed with rind & seeds) | 3 | .3 | | | 0 |
| Whole | 2⅘" orange (6.3 oz.) | 1 | .1 | | | 0 |
| Sections | 1 cup (8.5 oz.) | 2 | .2 | | | 0 |
| California Valencia (USDA): | | | | | | |
| Whole | 1 lb. (weighed with rind & seeds) | 3 | 1.0 | | | 0 |
| Fruit, including peel | 2⅝" orange (6.3 oz.) | 4 | .5 | | | 0 |
| Sections | 1 cup (8.5 oz.) | 2 | .7 | | | 0 |
| Florida, all varieties (USDA): | | | | | | |
| Whole | 1 lb. (weighed with rind & seeds) | 3 | .7 | | | 0 |
| Whole | 3" orange (5.5 oz.) | 2 | .3 | | | 0 |
| Sections | 1 cup (8.5 oz.) | 2 | .5 | | | 0 |
| **ORANGE-APRICOT JUICE DRINK,** canned (USDA) 40% fruit juices | 1 cup (8.8 oz.) | Tr. | .2 | | | 0 |
| **ORANGE CREAM BAR** (Sealtest) | 2½-fl.-oz. bar | 27 | 3.1 | | | |
| **ORANGE DRINK:** | | | | | | |
| Canned: | | | | | | |
| *Bama* (Borden's) | 8.45 fl. oz. | 60 | 0.0 | | | (0) |
| *Capri Sun* | 6¾-oz. serving | 2 | 0.0 | | | (0) |
| (Lincoln) | 6 fl. oz. | 20 | 0.0 | | | (0) |
| *Ssips* (Johanna Farms) | 8.45 fl. oz. | <10 | 0.0 | | | (0) |
| *Mix: | | | | | | |
| Regular (Hi-C) | 6 fl. oz. | Tr. | 1.0 | | | (0) |
| Dietetic: | | | | | | |
| *Crystal Light* | 6 fl. oz. | <1 | Tr. | | | (0) |
| (Sunkist) | 8 fl. oz. | 70 | 0.0 | | | (0) |

(USDA): United States Department of Agriculture
*Prepared as Package Directs

| Food and Description | Measure or Quantity | Sodium (mg.) | Total | Satu- rated | Unsatu- rated | Choles- terol (mg.) |
|---|---|---|---|---|---|---|
| | | | | — Fats in grams — | | |

**ORANGE-GRAPEFRUIT JUICE:**

| Food and Description | Measure or Quantity | Sodium (mg.) | Total | Satu-rated | Unsatu-rated | Choles-terol (mg.) |
|---|---|---|---|---|---|---|
| Bottled, chilled (Kraft) | ½ cup (4.5 oz.) | 1 | .1 | | | (0) |
| Canned: | | | | | | |
| Sweetened (USDA) | ½ cup (4.4 oz.) | 1 | .1 | | | 0 |
| Sweetened (Del Monte) | 6 fl. oz. | 2 | .1 | | | 0 |
| Sweetened (Stokely-Van Camp's) | ½ cup (4.4 oz.) | | .1 | | | (0) |
| Unsweetened (USDA) | ½ cup (4.3 oz.) | 1 | .2 | | | 0 |
| Unsweetened (Libby's) | 6 fl. oz. | 5 | 0.0 | | | (0) |
| Frozen, concentrate, unsweetened: | | | | | | |
| (USDA) | 6-fl.-oz. can (7.4 oz.) | 4 | .1 | | | 0 |
| *Diluted with 3 parts water (USDA) | ½ cup (4.4 oz.) | Tr. | .1 | | | 0 |
| *(Minute Maid) | ½ cup (4.2 oz.) | <1 | <.1 | | | 0 |
| *(Snow Crop) | ½ cup (4.2 oz.) | <1 | <.1 | | | 0 |

**ORANGE JUICE:**

| Food and Description | Measure or Quantity | Sodium (mg.) | Total | Satu-rated | Unsatu-rated | Choles-terol (mg.) |
|---|---|---|---|---|---|---|
| Fresh: | | | | | | |
| All varieties (USDA) | ½ cup (4.4 oz.) | 1 | .2 | | | 0 |
| California Navel (USDA) | ½ cup (4.4 oz.) | 1 | .1 | | | 0 |
| California Valencia (USDA) | ½ cup (4.4 oz.) | 1 | .4 | | | 0 |
| California Navel or Valencia (Sunkist) | ½ cup (4.4 oz.) | <1 | Tr. | | | 0 |
| Florida, early or mid-season (USDA) | ½ cup (4.4 oz.) | 1 | .2 | | | 0 |
| Florida Temple (USDA) | ½ cup (4.4 oz.) | 1 | .2 | | | 0 |
| Florida Valencia (USDA) | ½ cup (4.4 oz.) | 1 | .2 | | | 0 |
| Chilled, fresh (Citrus Hill) | 6 fl. oz. | 10 | .2 | | | (0) |
| Canned or bottled, sweetened: | | | | | | |
| (USDA) | ½ cup (4.4 oz.) | 1 | .3 | | | 0 |
| (Borden's) *Sippin' Pak* | 8.45 fl. oz. | 25 | 0.0 | | | (0) |
| (Libby's) | 6 fl. oz. | 5 | 0.0 | | | (0) |
| (Johanna Farms) *Tree Ripe* | 8.45 fl. oz. | 2 | .4 | | | (0) |
| Canned or bottled, unsweetened: | | | | | | |
| (USDA) | ½ cup (4.4 oz.) | 1 | .2 | | | 0 |
| (Del Monte) | ½ cup (4.3 oz.) | 1 | .1 | | | 0 |
| Canned, concentrate, unsweetened: | | | | | | |
| (USDA) | 4 oz. | 1 | .3 | | | 0 |

(USDA): United States Department of Agriculture
*Prepared as Package Directs

| Food and Description | Measure or Quantity | Sodium (mg.) | —Fats in grams— | | | Cholesterol (mg.) |
|---|---|---|---|---|---|---|
| | | | Total | Saturated | Unsaturated | |
| *Diluted with 5 parts water (USDA) | ½ cup (4.4 oz.) | 1 | .4 | | | 0 |
| Dehydrated, crystals: | | | | | | |
| (USDA) | 4-oz. can | 9 | 1.9 | | | 0 |
| *Reconstituted (USDA) | ½ cup (4.4 oz.) | 1 | .2 | | | 0 |
| Frozen, concentrate: | | | | | | |
| (USDA) | 6-fl.-oz. can (7.5 oz.) | 4 | .4 | | | 0 |
| *Diluted with 3 parts water (USDA) | ½ cup (4.4 oz.) | 1 | .1 | | | 0 |
| *(Birds Eye) *Orange Plus* | 6 fl. oz. | 9 | .4 | | | 0 |
| *(Citrus Hill) | 6 fl. oz. | 10 | <1.0 | | | (0) |
| *(Sunkist) | 6 fl. oz. | Tr. | 0.0 | | | (0) |
| **ORANGE JUICE BAR** (Sunkist) | 3-fl.-oz. bar | 5 | 0.0 | | | |
| **ORANGE, MANDARIN** (See **TANGERINE**) | | | | | | |
| **ORANGE PEEL:** | | | | | | |
| Raw (USDA) | 1 oz. | 1 | .1 | | | 0 |
| Dry (Spice Islands) | 1 tsp. | <1 | | | | (0) |
| Candied (USDA) | 1 oz. | | .1 | | | 0 |
| **ORANGE-PINEAPPLE DRINK,** canned (Lincoln) | 6 fl. oz. (6.3 oz.) | 30 | 0.0 | | | (0) |
| **ORANGE SHERBET** (See **SHERBET**) | | | | | | |
| **ORCHARD BLEND JUICE,** canned (Welch's): | | | | | | |
| Apple grape | 6 fl. oz. | 15 | 0.0 | | | |
| Harvest or north country | 6 fl. oz. | 20 | 0.0 | | | |
| Vineyard | 6 fl. oz. | 5 | 0.0 | | | |
| **OREGANO** (Spice Islands) | 1 tsp. | <1 | | | | (0) |
| **OVALTINE,** dry: | | | | | | |
| Chocolate | ¾ oz. | 146 | <1.0 | | | |
| Malt | ¾ oz. | 92 | <1.0 | | | |

(USDA): United States Department of Agriculture
*Prepared as Package Directs

| Food and Description | Measure or Quantity | Sodium (mg.) | —Fats in grams— | | | Choles- terol (mg.) |
|---|---|---|---|---|---|---|
| | | | Total | Satu- rated | Unsatu- rated | |

**OYSTER:**
  Raw:
    Eastern, meat only:

| Food and Description | Measure or Quantity | Sodium (mg.) | Total | Satu- rated | Unsatu- rated | Choles- terol (mg.) |
|---|---|---|---|---|---|---|
| (USDA) | 1 lb. (weighed with shell & liq.) | 33 | .8 | | | 23 |
| (USDA) | 12 oysters (weighed in shell, 4 lb.) | 132 | 3.2 | | | 92 |
| (USDA) | 4 oz. | 83 | 2.0 | | | 57 |
| (USDA) | 19-31 small or 13-19 med. oysters (1 cup, 8.5 oz.) | 175 | 4.3 | | | 120 |
| Pacific & Western, meat only: | | | | | | |
| (USDA) | 4 oz. | | 2.5 | | | 57 |
| (USDA) | 6-9 small or 4-6 med. oysters (1 cup, 8.5 oz.) | | 5.3 | | | 120 |
| Canned, solids & liq. (USDA) | 4 oz. | | 2.5 | | | 51 |
| Fried, dipped in egg, milk & bread crumbs (USDA) | 4 oz. | 234 | 15.8 | | | |
| Frozen, solids & liq. (USDA) | 4 oz. | 431 | 6.9 | | | |

**OYSTER CRACKER** (See **CRACKER**)

**OYSTER STEW:**
  Home recipe (USDA):

| Food and Description | Measure or Quantity | Sodium (mg.) | Total | Satu- rated | Unsatu- rated | Choles- terol (mg.) |
|---|---|---|---|---|---|---|
| 1 part oysters to 1 part milk by volume | 1 cup (6-8 oysters, 8.5 oz.) | | 13.2 | | | |
| 1 part oysters to 2 parts milk by volume [1] | 1 cup (8.5 oz.) | 814 | 15.4 | | | 62 |
| 1 part oysters to 3 parts milk by volume [1] | 1 cup (8.5 oz.) | 487 | 12.7 | | | 58 |
| *Canned (Campbell's) | 1 cup | 824 | 8.0 | 2. | 6. | |
| Frozen (USDA): | | | | | | |
| Condensed | 8 oz. (by wt.) | 1542 | 14.3 | | | |
| *Prepared with equal volume water | 1 cup (8.5 oz.) | 816 | 7.7 | | | |
| *Prepared with equal volume milk | 1 cup (8.5 oz.) | 878 | 11.8 | | | |

(USDA): United States Department of Agriculture
*Prepared as Package Directs
[1]Prepared with added salt & butter.

| Food and Description | Measure or Quantity | Sodium (mg.) | — Fats in grams — | | | Cholesterol (mg.) |
|---|---|---|---|---|---|---|
| | | | Total | Satu-rated | Unsatu-rated | |

# P

**PAC-MAN,** cereal (General Mills)

| Food and Description | Measure or Quantity | Sodium (mg.) | Total | Satu-rated | Unsatu-rated | Cholesterol (mg.) |
|---|---|---|---|---|---|---|
| **PAC-MAN,** cereal (General Mills) | 1 cup (1 oz.) | 195 | 1.0 | | | |
| **PANCAKE:** | | | | | | |
| Home recipe, wheat (USDA) | 4″ pancake (1 oz.) | 115 | 1.9 | <1. | 1. | |
| Frozen, breakfast, with link sausage (Swanson) | 6-oz. breakfast | 972 | 24.0 | | | |
| **PANCAKE BATTER,** frozen (Aunt Jemima): | | | | | | |
| Regular | 4″ pancake (1.3 oz.) | 286 | .5 | | | |
| Blueberry | 4″ pancake (1.3 oz.) | 233 | .5 | | | |
| Buttermilk | 4″ pancake (1.3 oz.) | 244 | .5 | | | |
| **PANCAKE DINNER OR ENTREE,** frozen (Swanson): | | | | | | |
| & blueberry sauce | 7-oz. meal | 800 | 9.0 | | | |
| & sausage | 6-oz. meal | 940 | 22.0 | | | |
| & strawberries | 7-oz. meal | 820 | 8.0 | | | |
| **PANCAKE & WAFFLE MIX** (See also **PANCAKE & WAFFLE MIX, DIETETIC**): | | | | | | |
| Buckwheat: | | | | | | |
| (USDA) | 1 oz. | 378 | .5 | | | |
| (USDA) | 1 cup (4.8 oz.) | 1,801 | 2.6 | | | |
| *Prepared with egg & milk (USDA) | 4″ pancake (1 oz.) | 125 | 2.5 | | | |
| *(Aunt Jemima) | 4″ pancake (1.2 oz.) | 173 | 2.7 | | | |
| Buttermilk: | | | | | | |
| (USDA) | 1 oz. | 406 | .5 | | | |
| (USDA) | 1 cup (4.8 oz.) | 1,935 | 2.4 | | | |

(USDA): United States Department of Agriculture
*Prepared as Package Directs

| Food and Description | Measure or Quantity | Sodium (mg.) | —Fats in grams— | | | Cholesterol (mg.) |
|---|---|---|---|---|---|---|
| | | | Total | Saturated | Unsaturated | |
| *Prepared with milk (USDA)[1] | 4″ pancake (1 oz.) | 122 | 1.5 | <1. | 1. | |
| *Prepared with milk & egg (USDA)[2] | 4″ pancake (1 oz.) | 182 | 2.0 | <1. | 1. | |
| *(Aunt Jemima) complete | 4″ pancake (1 oz.) | 290 | 1.0 | | | |
| *(Pillsbury) | 4″ pancake (2 oz.) | 190 | 3.7 | | | |
| Plain: | | | | | | |
| (USDA) | 1 oz. | 406 | .5 | | | |
| (USDA) | 1 cup (4.8 oz.) | 1,935 | 2.4 | | | |
| *Prepared with milk (USDA)[1] | 4″ pancake (1 oz.) | 122 | 1.5 | <1. | 1. | |
| *Prepared with milk & egg (USDA)[2] | 4″ pancake (1 oz.) | 152 | 2.0 | <1. | 1. | 20 |
| *Prepared with milk & egg (USDA)[2] | 6″ × ½″ pancake (7 T. batter) | 412 | 5.3 | 2. | 3. | 54 |
| *(Aunt Jemima) complete | 4″ pancake (1.2 oz.) | 290 | 1.0 | | | |
| *(Aunt Jemima) original | 4″ pancake (1 oz.) | 183 | 2.7 | | | |
| *PANCAKE & WAFFLE MIX, DIETETIC, buttermilk or plain (Featherweight) | 4″ pancake (1.2 oz.) | 23 | .2 | | | |
| PANCAKE & WAFFLE SYRUP (See SYRUP, Pancake & Waffle) | | | | | | |
| PANCREAS, raw (USDA): | | | | | | |
| Beef, lean only | 4 oz. | 76 | 8.3 | | | |
| Beef, medium-fat | 4 oz. | | 28.4 | | | |

(USDA): United States Department of Agriculture
*Prepared as Package Directs
[1]Principal sources of fat: vegetable shortening & milk.
[2]Principal sources of fat: vegetable shortening, milk & egg.

| Food and Description | Measure or Quantity | Sodium (mg.) | — Fats in grams — | | | Choles- terol (mg.) |
|---|---|---|---|---|---|---|
| | | | Total | Satu- rated | Unsatu- rated | |
| Calf | 4 oz. | | 10.0 | | | |
| Hog or hog sweetbread | 4 oz. | 50 | 22.6 | | | |
| **PAPAW,** fresh (USDA): | | | | | | |
| Whole | 1 lb. (weighed with rind & seeds) | | 3.1 | | | 0 |
| Flesh only | 4 oz. | | 1.0 | | | 0 |
| **PAPAYA,** fresh (USDA): | | | | | | |
| Whole | 1 lb. (weighed with skin & seeds) | 9 | .3 | | | 0 |
| Flesh only | 4 oz. | 3 | .1 | | | 0 |
| Cubed | 1 cup (6.4 oz.) | 5 | .2 | | | 0 |
| **PAPRIKA** (Spice Islands) | 1 tsp. | < 2 | | | | (0) |
| **PARSLEY:** | | | | | | |
| Fresh (USDA): | | | | | | |
| Whole | ½ lb. | 102 | 1.4 | | | 0 |
| Chopped | 1 T. (4 grams) | 2 | < .1 | | | 0 |
| Dry (Spice Islands) | 1 tsp. | 5 | | | | |
| **PARSNIP** (USDA): | | | | | | |
| Raw, whole | 1 lb. (weighed unpared) | 46 | 1.9 | | | 0 |
| Boiled without salt, drained, cut in pieces | ½ cup (3.7 oz.) | 8 | .5 | | | 0 |
| **PASSION FRUIT,** fresh (USDA): | | | | | | |
| Whole | 1 lb. (weighed with shell) | 66 | 1.7 | | | 0 |
| Pulp & seeds | 4 oz. | 32 | .8 | | | 0 |
| **PASTINAS,** dry (USDA): | | | | | | |
| Carrot | 1 oz. | | .5 | | | |
| Egg [1] | 1 oz. | 1 | 1.2 | Tr. | < 1. | |
| Spinach | 1 oz. | | .5 | | | |

(USDA): United States Department of Agriculture
*Prepared as Package Directs
[1]Principal source of fat: egg.

| Food and Description | Measure or Quantity | Sodium (mg.) | Total | —Fats in grams— Satu- rated | Unsatu- rated | Choles- terol (mg.) |
|---|---|---|---|---|---|---|
| **PASTRAMI,** packaged: | | | | | | |
| (Carl Buddig) | 1 oz. | 320 | 2.0 | .9 | 1. | 16 |
| (Eckrich) | 1 oz. | 360 | 2.0 | | | |
| | | | | | | |
| ***PASTRY POCKETS,*** (Pillsbury) | 1 pocket | 550 | 13.0 | | | |
| | | | | | | |
| **PASTRY SHEET, PUFF,** frozen | | | | | | |
| (Pepperidge Farm) | 1 sheet | 1,160 | 68.0 | | | |
| | | | | | | |
| **PASTRY SHELL** (See also **PIE CRUST**): | | | | | | |
| Home recipe, made with lard, baked (USDA)[1] | 1 shell (1.5 oz.) | 260 | 14.2 | 6. | 9. | |
| Home recipe, made with vegetable shortening, baked (USDA)[2] | 1 shell (1.5 oz.) | 260 | 14.2 | 3. | 11. | 0 |
| | | | | | | |
| **PÂTÉ,** canned: | | | | | | |
| De foie gras (USDA) | 1 oz. | | 12.4 | | | |
| De foie gras (USDA) | 1 T. (.5 oz.) | | 6.6 | | | |
| Liver (Hormel) | 1 T. | | 3.0 | | | |
| Liver (Sells) | 1 T. (.5 oz.) | 119 | 4.0 | | | |
| | | | | | | |
| ***P.D.Q.:*** | | | | | | |
| Chocolate | 1 T. (.6 oz.) | | .5 | | | 0 |
| Eggnog | 2 heaping tsps. (1 oz.) | | .1 | | | Tr. |
| Strawberry | 1 T. (.5 oz.) | | Tr. | | | 0 |
| | | | | | | |
| **PEA, GREEN:** | | | | | | |
| Raw (USDA): | | | | | | |
| In pod | 1 lb. (weighed in pod) | 3 | .7 | | | 0 |
| Shelled | 1 lb. | 9 | 1.8 | | | 0 |
| Shelled | ½ cup (2.4 oz.) | 1 | .3 | | | 0 |
| Boiled without salt, drained (USDA) | ½ cup (2.9 oz.) | <1 | .3 | | | 0 |
| Canned, regular pack: | | | | | | |
| Drained solids (Del Monte) | ½ cup (3 oz.) | 198 | .4 | | | 0 |
| Seasoned, drained solids (Del Monte) | ½ cup (3 oz.) | 204 | .4 | | | 0 |

(USDA): United States Department of Agriculture
*Prepared as Package Directs
[1]Principal source of fat: lard.
[2]Principal source of fat: vegetable shortening.

253

| Food and Description | Measure or Quantity | Sodium (mg.) | — Fats in grams — | | | Choles-terol (mg.) |
|---|---|---|---|---|---|---|
| | | | Total | Satu-rated | Unsatu-rated | |
| Alaska, Early or June, solids & liq. (USDA) | 1/2 cup (4.4 oz.) | 293 | .4 | | | 0 |
| Alaska, Early or June, drained solids (USDA) | 1/2 cup (3 oz.) | 203 | .3 | | | 0 |
| Alaska, Early or June, drained liq. (USDA) | 4 oz. | 268 | Tr. | | | 0 |
| Early, solids & liq. (Le Sueur) | 1/2 of 8.5-oz. can | 374 | .2 | | | |
| Early, solids & liq. (Stokely-Van Camp's) | 1/2 cup (4.1 oz.) | | .4 | | | (0) |
| Early June, with onions (Green Giant) | 1/4 of 17-oz. can | 518 | .2 | | | (0) |
| Sweet, solids & liq. (USDA) | 1/2 cup (4.4 oz.) | 293 | .4 | | | 0 |
| Sweet, drained solids (USDA) | 1/2 cup (3 oz.) | 203 | .3 | | | 0 |
| Sweet, drained liq. (USDA) | 4 oz. | 268 | Tr. | | | 0 |
| Sweet, solids & liq. (Green Giant) | 1/2 of 8.5-oz. can | 337 | .4 | | | (0) |
| Sweet, honey pod, solids & liq. (Stokely-Van Camp's) | 1/2 cup (4 oz.) | | .4 | | | (0) |
| Canned, dietetic pack: | | | | | | |
| Alaska, Early or June, solids & liq. (USDA) | 4 oz. | 3 | .3 | | | 0 |
| Alaska, Early or June, drained solids (USDA) | 4 oz. | 3 | .5 | | | 0 |
| Alaska, Early or June, drained liq. (USDA) | 4 oz. | 3 | Tr. | | | 0 |
| Sweet, solids & liq. (USDA) | 4 oz. | 3 | .3 | | | 0 |
| Sweet, drained solids (USDA) | 4 oz. | 3 | .5 | | | 0 |
| Sweet, drained liq. (USDA) | 4 oz. | 3 | Tr. | | | 0 |
| Solids & liq. (Diet Delight) | 1/2 cup (4.4 oz.) | 10 | .2 | | | (0) |
| (S & W) Nutradiet, unseasoned | 4 oz. | 11 | .1 | | | (0) |
| Frozen: | | | | | | |
| Not thawed (USDA) | 1 cup (2.5 oz.) | 93 | .2 | | | 0 |
| Boiled, drained (USDA) | 1/2 cup (3 oz.) | 97 | .3 | | | 0 |
| Sweet (Birds Eye) | 1/2 cup (3.3 oz.) | 131 | .5 | | | 0 |
| Tender tiny (Birds Eye) | 1/2 cup (3.3 oz.) | 121 | .3 | | | 0 |
| In butter sauce, sweet (Green Giant) | 1/2 cup | 490 | 1.0 | | | |
| With cream sauce (Birds Eye) | 1/3 of pkg. (2.7 oz.) | 446 | 7.0 | | | Tr. |

(USDA): United States Department of Agriculture
*Prepared as Package Directs

| Food and Description | Measure or Quantity | Sodium (mg.) | Total | —Fats in grams— Satu- rated | Unsatu- rated | Choles- terol (mg.) |
|---|---|---|---|---|---|---|
| With cream sauce (Green Giant) | ½ cup | 320 | 4.0 | | | |
| **PEA, MATURE SEED,** dry: | | | | | | |
| Raw: | | | | | | |
| Whole (USDA) | 1 lb. | 159 | 5.9 | | | 0 |
| Whole (USDA) | 1 cup (7.1 oz.) | 70 | 2.6 | | | 0 |
| Split, without seed coat (USDA) | 1 lb. | 181 | 4.5 | | | 0 |
| Split, without seed coat (USDA) | 1 cup (7.2 oz.) | 81 | 2.0 | | | 0 |
| Cooked without salt, split, without seed coat, drained (USDA) | ½ cup (3.4 oz.) | 13 | .3 | | | 0 |
| **PEA & CARROT:** | | | | | | |
| Canned, regular pack, solids & liq.: | | | | | | |
| (Comstock) | ½ cup (4.4 oz.) | 430 | 0.0 | | | (0) |
| (Del Monte) | ½ cup | 355 | Tr. | | | (0) |
| (Larsen) *Freshlike* | ½ cup (4.6 oz.) | 340 | 0.0 | | | (0) |
| (Veg-All) | ½ cup | 340 | 0.0 | | | (0) |
| Canned, dietetic pack, solids & liq.: | | | | | | |
| (Diet Delight) | ½ cup (4.2 oz.) | 5 | 0.0 | | | (0) |
| (S & W) *Nutradiet* | 4 oz. | < 10 | 0.0 | | | (0) |
| Frozen: | | | | | | |
| Not thawed (USDA) | 4 oz. | 104 | .3 | | | 0 |
| Boiled, drained (USDA) | ½ cup (3.1 oz.) | 73 | .3 | | | 0 |
| (Birds Eye) | ½ cup (3.3 oz.) | 92 | .4 | | | 0 |
| (Frosty Acres) | 3.3 oz. | 75 | 0.0 | | | (0) |
| **PEA & ONION,** frozen: | | | | | | |
| (Frosty Acres) | 3.3 oz. | 80 | 0.0 | | | (0) |
| (Larsen) | 3.3 oz. | 100 | 0.0 | | | (0) |
| **PEA POD,** edible-podded or Chinese (USDA): | | | | | | |
| Raw | 1 lb. (weighed untrimmed) | | .9 | | | 0 |
| Boiled, drained | 4 oz. | | .2 | | | 0 |

**PEA SOUP, GREEN** (See **SOUP, Pea**)

(USDA): United States Department of Agriculture
*Prepared as Package Directs

| Food and Description | Measure or Quantity | Sodium (mg.) | — Fats in grams — | | | Cholesterol (mg.) |
|---|---|---|---|---|---|---|
| | | | Total | Saturated | Unsaturated | |

**PEACH:**

Fresh, without skin (USDA):

| Food and Description | Measure or Quantity | Sodium (mg.) | Total | Cholesterol (mg.) |
|---|---|---|---|---|
| Whole | 1 lb. (weighed unpeeled) | 4 | .4 | 0 |
| Whole | 4-oz. peach (2½″ dia.) | 1 | .1 | 0 |
| Diced | ½ cup (4.7 oz.) | 1 | .1 | 0 |
| Slices | ½ cup (3 oz.) | 1 | .1 | 0 |

Canned, regular pack, solids & liq.:

| Food and Description | Measure or Quantity | Sodium (mg.) | Total | Cholesterol (mg.) |
|---|---|---|---|---|
| Juice pack (USDA) | 4 oz. | 2 | .1 | 0 |
| Light syrup (USDA) | 4 oz. | 2 | .1 | 0 |
| Heavy syrup (USDA) | 2 med. halves & 2 T. syrup (4.1 oz.) | 2 | .1 | 0 |
| Heavy syrup, halves (USDA) | ½ cup (4.5 oz.) | 3 | .1 | 0 |
| Heavy syrup, slices (USDA) | ½ cup (4.4 oz.) | 3 | .1 | 0 |
| Heavy syrup (Del Monte) cling | ½ cup (4.6 oz.) | <10 | 0.0 | 0 |
| Heavy syrup (Del Monte) freestone | ½ cup (4.6 oz.) | <10 | .2 | 0 |
| Heavy syrup (Hunt's) diced | 5 oz. | 5 | <1 | |
| Extra heavy syrup (USDA) | 4 oz. | 2 | .1 | 0 |
| Spiced, heavy syrup (Del Monte) | ½ cup (4.5 oz.) | <10 | 0.0 | 0 |

Canned, dietetic or unsweetened pack:

| Food and Description | Measure or Quantity | Sodium (mg.) | Total | Cholesterol (mg.) |
|---|---|---|---|---|
| Water pack, solids & liq. (USDA) | ½ cup (4.3 oz.) | 2 | .1 | 0 |
| (Del Monte) lite, cling, solids, liq. | ½ cup (4 oz.) | 40 | 0.0 | 0 |

Dehydrated, sulfured, nugget or pieces:

| Food and Description | Measure or Quantity | Sodium (mg.) | Total | Cholesterol (mg.) |
|---|---|---|---|---|
| Uncooked (USDA) | 1 oz. | 6 | .3 | 0 |
| Cooked with added sugar, solids & liq. (USDA) | ½ cup (5-6 halves & 3 T. liq., 5.4 oz.) | 8 | .3 | 0 |

Dried:

| Food and Description | Measure or Quantity | Sodium (mg.) | Total | Cholesterol (mg.) |
|---|---|---|---|---|
| Uncooked (USDA) | 1 lb. | 73 | 3.2 | 0 |
| Uncooked (USDA) | ½ cup (3.1 oz.) | 14 | .6 | 0 |

(USDA): United States Department of Agriculture
*Prepared as Package Directs

| Food and Description | Measure or Quantity | Sodium (mg.) | Total | Satu- rated | Unsatu- rated | Choles- terol (mg.) |
|---|---|---|---|---|---|---|
| Cooked, unsweetened (USDA) | ½ cup (5-6 halves & 3 T. liq., 4.8 oz.) | 7 | .3 | | | 0 |
| Cooked, with added sugar (USDA) | ½ cup (5-6 halves & 3 T. liq., 5.4 oz.) | 6 | .3 | | | 0 |
| Uncooked (Del Monte) | 2 oz. | <10 | 0.0 | | | 0 |
| Frozen: | | | | | | |
| Not thawed, slices, sweetened: | | | | | | |
| (USDA) | 12-oz. pkg. | 7 | .3 | | | 0 |
| (USDA) | 16-oz. can | 9 | .5 | | | 0 |
| (USDA) | ½ cup (4.2 oz.) | 2 | .1 | | | 0 |
| Quick thaw (Birds Eye) | ½ cup (5 oz.) | 9 | .2 | | | 0 |
| **PEACH BUTTER** (Smucker's) | 1 T. (.6 oz.) | 0 | Tr. | | | (0) |
| **PEACH NECTAR,** canned: | | | | | | |
| (USDA) | 1 cup (8.8 oz.) | 2 | Tr. | | | 0 |
| (Libby's) | 1 cup (8.7 oz.) | 15 | Tr. | | | 0 |
| **PEACH PRESERVE:** | | | | | | |
| Sweetened (Bama) | 1 T. (.7 oz.) | 7 | 0.0 | | | (0) |
| Low calorie or dietetic (Featherweight) | 1 T. | 40-50 | 0.0 | | | (0) |
| **PEANUT:** | | | | | | |
| Raw (USDA): | | | | | | |
| In shell | 1 lb. (weighed in shell) | 17 | 157.3 | 35. | 122. | 0 |
| With skins | 1 oz. | 1 | 13.5 | 3. | 11. | 0 |
| Without skins, whole, unsalted | 1 oz. | 1 | 13.7 | 3. | 11. | 0 |
| Boiled (USDA) | 1 oz. | 1 | 8.9 | 2. | 7. | 0 |
| Roasted: | | | | | | |
| (USDA): | | | | | | |
| Whole, unsalted | 1 lb. (weighed in shell) | 17 | 157.3 | 35. | 122. | 0 |
| With skins, unsalted | 1 oz. | 1 | 13.5 | 3. | 11. | 0 |
| Without skins, salted | 1 oz. | 119 | 14.1 | 3. | 11. | 0 |
| Halves, salted | ½ cup (2.5 oz.) | 301 | 35.9 | 8. | 38. | 0 |

(USDA): United States Department of Agriculture
*Prepared as Package Directs

PEANUT (Continued)

| Food and Description | Measure or Quantity | Sodium (mg.) | Total | — Fats in grams — Satu- rated | Unsatu- rated | Choles- terol (mg.) |
|---|---|---|---|---|---|---|
| Chopped, salted | ½ cup (2.4 oz.) | 288 | 34.4 | 8. | 27. | 0 |
| Chopped, salted | 1 T. (9 grams) | 38 | 4.5 | 1. | 3. | 0 |
| *All American Nut* (Adams): | | | | | | |
| Regular | 1 oz. | 85 | 15.0 | | | 0 |
| Butter toffee | 1 oz. | 85 | 5.0 | | | |
| (Eagle) honey roast | 1 oz. | 170 | 13.0 | | | 0 |
| (Fisher): | | | | | | |
| Dry roasted: | | | | | | |
| Lightly salted | 1 oz. | 85 | 14.0 | | | 0 |
| Salted | 1 oz. | 220 | 14.0 | | | 0 |
| Unsalted | 1 oz. | 0 | 13.0 | | | 0 |
| Honey roasted | 1 oz. | 100 | 13.0 | | | 0 |
| Oil roasted: | | | | | | |
| Salted, party | 1 oz. | 140 | 14.0 | | | 0 |
| Lightly salted | 1 oz. | 35 | 14.0 | | | 0 |
| (Planters): | | | | | | |
| In shell: | | | | | | |
| Salted | 1 oz. | 160 | 14.0 | | | 0 |
| Unsalted | 1 oz. | 0 | 14.0 | | | 0 |
| Dry roasted: | | | | | | |
| Salted | 1 oz. | 250 | 14.0 | | | 0 |
| Unsalted | 1 oz. | 0 | 15.0 | | | 0 |
| Oil roasted: | | | | | | |
| Salted | 1 oz. | 160 | 15.0 | | | 0 |
| Sweet & crunchy | 1 oz. | 20 | 8.0 | | | 0 |
| Tavern nuts | 1 oz. | 65 | 15.0 | | | 0 |
| Unsalted | 1 oz. | 0 | 15.0 | | | 0 |
| **PEANUT BUTTER:** | | | | | | |
| (USDA): | | | | | | |
| Small amounts of fat & salt added | ½ cup (4.4 oz.) | 765 | 62.2 | 11. | 51. | 0 |
| Small amounts of fat & salt added | 1 T. (.6 oz.) | 97 | 7.9 | 1. | 6. | 0 |
| Small amounts of fat, sweetener & salt added | ½ cup (4.4 oz.) | 764 | 62.4 | 11. | 51. | 0 |
| Small amounts of fat, sweetener & salt added | 1 T. (.6 oz.) | 97 | 7.9 | 1. | 6. | 0 |
| Moderate amounts of fat, sweetener & salt added | ½ cup (4.4 oz.) | 762 | 63.8 | 11. | 52. | 0 |
| Moderate amounts of fat, sweetener & salt added | 1 T. (.6 oz.) | 97 | 8.1 | 1. | 7. | 0 |
| (Adams) low sodium | 1 T. (.6 oz.) | <3 | 8.0 | | | 0 |

(USDA): United States Department of Agriculture
*Prepared as Package Directs

| Food and Description | Measure or Quantity | Sodium (mg.) | Total | Satu- rated | Unsatu- rated | Choles- terol (mg.) |
|---|---|---|---|---|---|---|
| | | | | —Fats in grams— | | |
| (Bama) crunchy | 1 T. (.6 oz.) | 57 | 8.5 | | | (0) |
| (Bama) smooth | 1 T. (.6 oz.) | 70 | 8.4 | 1. | 7. | (0) |
| (Home Brand): | | | | | | |
|   Lightly salted | 1 T. | 62 | 8.5 | | | |
|   No sugar added | 1 T. | 62 | 8.0 | | | |
|   Unsalted | 1 T. | <4 | 8.0 | | | |
| (Peter Pan) creamy | 1 T. (.6 oz.) | 75 | 4.0 | | | 0 |
| (Planters) | 1 T. (.5 oz.) | 95 | 8.1 | 3. | 6. | 0 |
| (Skippy) creamy [1] | 1 T. (.6 oz.) | 80 | 8.2 | | | 0 |
| (Skippy) chunk [1] | 1 T. (.6 oz.) | 75 | 8.5 | | | 0 |
| With crackers (See **CRACKERS**) | | | | | | |

**PEANUT BUTTER MORSELS:**

| Food and Description | Measure or Quantity | Sodium (mg.) | Total | Satu- rated | Unsatu- rated | Choles- terol (mg.) |
|---|---|---|---|---|---|---|
| (Nestle's) | 1 oz. | 60 | 10.0 | | | |
| (Reese's) | 1 oz. | 60 | 12.0 | | | Tr. |

**PEAR:**

| Food and Description | Measure or Quantity | Sodium (mg.) | Total | Satu- rated | Unsatu- rated | Choles- terol (mg.) |
|---|---|---|---|---|---|---|
| Fresh: | | | | | | |
|   Whole (USDA) | 1 lb. (weighed with stems & core) | 8 | 1.7 | | | 0 |
|   Whole (USDA) | 6.4-oz. pear (3″ × 2½″) | 3 | .6 | | | 0 |
|   Quartered (USDA) | ½ cup (3.4 oz.) | 2 | .4 | | | 0 |
|   Slices, including skin (USDA) | ½ cup (2.9 oz.) | 2 | .3 | | | 0 |
| Canned, regular pack, solids & liq.: | | | | | | |
|   Juice pack (USDA) | 4 oz. | 1 | .3 | | | 0 |
|   Light syrup (USDA) | 4 oz. | 1 | .2 | | | 0 |
|   Heavy syrup, halves (USDA) | ½ cup (4 oz.) | 1 | .2 | | | 0 |
|   Heavy syrup, halves (USDA) | 2 med. halves & 2 T. syrup (4.1 oz.) | 1 | .2 | | | 0 |
|   Heavy syrup (Del Monte) | ½ cup (4 oz.) | 7 | .6 | | | 0 |
|   Extra heavy syrup: | | | | | | |
|     (USDA) | 4 oz. | 1 | .2 | | | 0 |
|     (Stokely-Van Camp's) | ½ cup (4 oz.) | | .2 | | | (0) |

(USDA): United States Department of Agriculture
*Prepared as Package Directs
[1]Principal sources of fat: peanuts & vegetable oil.

| Food and Description | Measure or Quantity | Sodium (mg.) | Total | Fats in grams — Saturated | Fats in grams — Unsaturated | Cholesterol (mg.) |
|---|---|---|---|---|---|---|
| Canned, unsweetened or low calorie: | | | | | | |
| Water pack, solids & liq. (USDA) | ½ cup (4.3 oz.) | 1 | .2 | | | 0 |
| Solids & liq. (Blue Boy) Bartlett | 4 oz. | 1 | .1 | | | (0) |
| Solids & liq. (Diet Delight) halves or quarters | ½ cup (4.4 oz.) | 4 | <.1 | | | (0) |
| (S & W) *Nutradiet* | 4 halves (3.5 oz.) | 3 | .1 | | | (0) |
| Dried: | | | | | | |
| (USDA) | 1 lb. | 32 | 8.2 | | | 0 |
| Uncooked (Del Monte) | ½ cup (2.8 oz.) | 3 | .6 | | | 0 |
| Cooked without added sugar, solids & liq. (USDA) | 4 oz. | 3 | .9 | | | 0 |
| Cooked with added sugar, solids & liq. (USDA) | 4 oz. | 3 | .9 | | | 0 |
| **PEAR, CANDIED** (USDA) | 1 oz. | | .2 | | | (0) |
| **PEAR NECTAR:** | | | | | | |
| Sweetened (USDA) | 1 cup (8.5 oz.) | 2 | .5 | | | 0 |
| Sweetened (Del Monte) | 6 fl. oz. | 6 | 0.0 | | | 0 |
| *PEBBLES,* cereal (Post): | | | | | | |
| Cocoa | ⅞ cup (1 oz.) | 136 | 1.5 | | | |
| Fruity | ⅞ cup (1 oz.) | 158 | 1.5 | | | 0 |
| **PECAN:** | | | | | | |
| In shell (USDA) | 1 lb. (weighed in shell) | Tr. | 171.2 | 12. | 159. | 0 |
| Shelled, unsalted (USDA): | | | | | | |
| Whole | 1 lb. | Tr. | 323.0 | 23. | 300. | 0 |
| Halves | ½ cup (1.9 oz.) | Tr. | 38.4 | 3. | 36. | 0 |
| Halves | 12-14 halves (.5 oz.) | Tr. | 10.0 | <1. | 9. | 0 |
| Chopped | ½ cup (1.8 oz.) | Tr. | 37.0 | 3. | 34. | 0 |
| Chopped | 1 T. (7 grams) | Tr. | 5.0 | Tr. | 5. | 0 |
| Dry, roasted, salted (Fisher) | 1 oz. | 75 | 18.0 | | | (0) |

(USDA): United States Department of Agriculture
*Prepared as Package Directs

| Food and Description | Measure or Quantity | Sodium (mg.) | Fats in grams — Total | Satu- rated | Unsatu- rated | Choles- terol (mg.) |
|---|---|---|---|---|---|---|
| **PECTIN, FRUIT:** | | | | | | |
| *Certo* | 1 T. (.5 oz.) | < 1 | 0 | | | 0 |
| *Certo* | 6 oz. pkg. | 5 | 0 | | | 0 |
| *Sure-Jell:* | | | | | | |
| Regular | 1¾-oz. pkg. | 12 | 0 | | | 0 |
| Light | 1¾-oz. pkg. | 5 | 0 | | | 0 |
| **PEP,** cereal (Kellogg's) | ¾ cup (1 oz.) | 200 | 0.0 | | | (0) |
| **PEPPER:** | | | | | | |
| Black: | | | | | | |
| (USDA) | 1 cup (3.9 oz.) | 13 | 7.5 | | | 0 |
| (USDA) | 1 tsp. (2 grams) | < 1 | .2 | | | 0 |
| Seasoned (French's) | 1 tsp. (3 grams) | 4 | .2 | | | (0) |
| Seasoned (Lawry's) | 1 pkg. (1.6 oz.) | | 2.4 | | | (0) |
| Seasoned (Lawry's) | 1 tsp. (2 grams) | | .1 | | | (0) |
| Whole or ground (Spice Islands) | 1 tsp. | < 1 | | | | (0) |
| Cayenne (Spice Islands) | 1 tsp. | < 1 | | | | (0) |
| Lemon (Durkee) | 1 tsp. (3 grams) | 698 | Tr. | | | (0) |
| & lemon seasoning (French's) | 1 tsp. (3 grams) | 800 | Tr. | | | (0) |
| White, whole or ground (Spice Islands) | 1 tsp. | < 1 | | | | (0) |
| **PEPPER, BANANA** (Vlasic) hot rings | 1 oz. | 465 | 0.0 | | | |
| **PEPPER, CHERRY** (Vlasic) mild | 1 oz. | 410 | 0.0 | | | |
| **PEPPER, HOT CHILI:** | | | | | | |
| Green (USDA): | | | | | | |
| Raw, whole | 4 oz. | | .2 | | | 0 |
| Raw, without seeds | 4 oz. | | .2 | | | 0 |
| Canned, chili sauce | 1 oz. | | < .1 | | | 0 |
| Canned, pods, without seeds, solids & liq. | 4 oz. | | 1.1 | | | 0 |
| Red: | | | | | | |
| Raw, whole (USDA) | 4 oz. (weighed with seeds) | | 2.6 | | | 0 |

(USDA): United States Department of Agriculture
*Prepared as Package Directs

| Food and Description | Measure or Quantity | Sodium (mg.) | Fats in grams — Total | Satu- rated | Unsatu- rated | Choles- terol (mg.) |
|---|---|---|---|---|---|---|
| Raw, trimmed, pods only (USDA) | 4 oz. | 21 | 3.2 | | | 0 |
| Canned, chili sauce (USDA) | 1 oz. | | .2 | | | 0 |
| Canned, solids & liq. (Del Monte) | ¼ cup | 554 | .3 | | | 0 |
| Canned, drained (Ortega) | ¼ cup (1.8 oz.) | 42 | .1 | | | (0) |
| Dried: | | | | | | |
| Pods (USDA) | 1 oz. | 106 | 2.6 | | | 0 |
| Pods (Chili Products) | 1 oz. | | 2.5 | | | (0) |
| Powder with added seasoning (USDA) | 1 T. (.5 oz.) | 236 | 1.9 | | | 0 |

**PEPPER, STUFFED:**

| Food and Description | Measure or Quantity | Sodium (mg.) | Total | Satu- rated | Unsatu- rated | Choles- terol (mg.) |
|---|---|---|---|---|---|---|
| Home recipe, with beef & crumbs (USDA)[1] | 2¾" × 2½" pepper with 1⅛ cups stuffing (6.5 oz.) | 5,881 | 10.2 | 6. | 5. | 56 |
| Frozen: | | | | | | |
| (Armour) *Dinner Classics,* green | 12-oz. meal | 1,750 | 18.0 | | | 70 |
| (Celentano) with beef, red, in sauce | 12½-oz. pkg. | 530 | 13.0 | | | 55 |
| (Weight Watchers) with veal stuffing | 11¾-oz. pkg. | 1,180 | 6.0 | | | |

**PEPPER, SWEET:**

| Food and Description | Measure or Quantity | Sodium (mg.) | Total | Satu- rated | Unsatu- rated | Choles- terol (mg.) |
|---|---|---|---|---|---|---|
| Green: | | | | | | |
| Raw, whole (USDA) | 1 lb. (weighed untrimmed) | 48 | .7 | | | 0 |
| Raw, without stem & seeds: | | | | | | |
| (USDA) | 1 med. pepper (2.6 oz.) | 8 | .1 | | | 0 |
| Chopped (USDA) | ½ cup (2.6 oz.) | 10 | .2 | | | 0 |
| Slices (USDA) | ½ cup (1.4 oz.) | 5 | .1 | | | 0 |
| Strips (USDA) | ½ cup (1.7 oz.) | 6 | .1 | | | 0 |
| Boiled without salt, drained, (USDA) | 1 med. pepper (2.6 oz.) | 7 | .1 | | | 0 |
| Boiled without salt, strips, drained (USDA) | ½ cup (2.4 oz.) | 6 | .1 | | | 0 |

(USDA): United States Department of Agriculture
*Prepared as Package Directs
[1]Principal sources of fat: beef, butter, bread & milk.

| Food and Description | Measure or Quantity | Sodium (mg.) | — Fats in grams — | | | Choles-terol (mg.) |
|---|---|---|---|---|---|---|
| | | | Total | Satu-rated | Unsatu-rated | |
| Frozen: | | | | | | |
| (Frosty Acres) dried | 1 oz. | 1 | 0.0 | | | (0) |
| (Larsen) | 1 oz. | 0 | 0.0 | | | (0) |
| Red (USDA): | | | | | | |
| Raw, whole | 1 lb. (weighed with stems & seeds) | | 1.1 | | | 0 |
| Raw, without stem & seeds | 1 med. pepper (2.2 oz.) | | .2 | | | 0 |
| Frozen (Larsen) | 1 oz. | 0 | 0.0 | | | (0) |
| **PEPPERMINT,** dry (Spice Islands) | 1 tsp. | 3 | | | | (0) |
| **PEPPERONCINI** (Vlasic) Greek, mild | 1 oz. | 450 | 0.0 | | | |
| **PEPPERONI:** | | | | | | |
| (Eckrich) | 1 oz. | | 12.0 | | | |
| (Hormel): | | | | | | |
| Regular | 1 oz. | 462 | 13.0 | | | |
| Canned, bits | 1 T. | | 3.0 | | | |
| *Leoni Brand* | 1 oz. | 508 | 12.0 | | | |
| Packaged, sliced | 1 slice | 140 | 3.5 | | | |
| *Rosa* | 1 oz. | 626 | 13.0 | | | |
| *Rosa Grande* | 1 oz. | 512 | 13.0 | | | |
| **PEPPER STEAK:** | | | | | | |
| Canned: | | | | | | |
| *(Chun King) stir fry | 6-oz. serving | 1,003 | 16.6 | | | 51 |
| *(La Choy) | ¾ cup | 960 | 9.0 | | | |
| Frozen: | | | | | | |
| (Armour) *Classic Lite,* beef | 10-oz. meal | 1,020 | 7.0 | | | 60 |
| (Blue Star) *Dining Lite,* with rice | 9¼-oz. meal | 1,400 | 6.4 | | | |
| (Le Menu) | 11½-oz. meal | 1,110 | 14.0 | | | |
| **PERCH:** | | | | | | |
| Raw (USDA): | | | | | | |
| White, whole | 1 lb. (weighed whole) | | 6.5 | | | |
| White, meat only | 4 oz. | | 4.5 | | | |

(USDA): United States Department of Agriculture
*Prepared as Package Directs

| Food and Description | Measure or Quantity | Sodium (mg.) | —Fats in grams— | | | Cholesterol (mg.) |
|---|---|---|---|---|---|---|
| | | | Total | Satu-rated | Unsatu-rated | |
| Yellow, whole | 1 lb. (weighed whole) | 120 | 1.6 | | | |
| Yellow, meat only | 4 oz. | 77 | 1.0 | | | |
| Frozen: | | | | | | |
| (Frionor) *Norway Gourmet* | 4-oz. fillet | 85 | 4.0 | | | 74 |
| (Gorton's) *Fishmarket Fresh* | 4-oz. fillet | 100 | 2.0 | | | |
| (Mrs. Paul's) breaded & fried, fillet | 2-oz. fillet | 240 | 8.5 | | | |
| (Van de Kamp's): | | | | | | |
| Regular, batter dipped | 2-oz. piece | 355 | 7.5 | | | |
| *Light & Crispy* | 2-oz. piece | 115 | 10.0 | | | |
| *Today's Catch* | 4 oz. | 180 | 0.0 | | | |
| **PERSIMMON** (USDA): | | | | | | |
| Japanese or Kaki, fresh: | | | | | | |
| With seeds | 1 lb. (weighed with skin, calyx & seeds) | 22 | 1.5 | | | 0 |
| With seeds | 4.4-oz. persimmon | 6 | .4 | | | 0 |
| Seedless | 1 lb. (weighed with skin & calyx) | 23 | 1.5 | | | 0 |
| Seedless | 4.4-oz. persimmon | 6 | .4 | | | 0 |
| Native, fresh, whole | 1 lb. (weighed with seeds & calyx) | 4 | 1.5 | | | 0 |
| Native, fresh, flesh only | 4 oz. | 1 | .5 | | | 0 |
| **PHEASANT,** raw (USDA): | | | | | | |
| Ready-to-cook | 1 lb. (weighed with bones) | | 20.5 | | | |
| Meat & skin | 4 oz. | | 5.9 | | | |
| Meat only | 4 oz. | | 7.7 | | | |
| Giblets | 2 oz. | | 2.8 | | | |
| **PICKEREL,** chain, raw (USDA): | | | | | | |
| Whole | 1 lb. (weighed whole) | | 1.2 | | | |
| Meat only | 4 oz. | | .6 | | | |
| **PICKLE:** | | | | | | |
| Chow chow (See **CHOW CHOW**) | | | | | | |

(USDA): United States Department of Agriculture
*Prepared as Package Directs

| Food and Description | Measure or Quantity | Sodium (mg.) | — Fats in grams — | | | Cholesterol (mg.) |
|---|---|---|---|---|---|---|
| | | | Total | Saturated | Unsaturated | |
| Cucumber, fresh or bread & butter: | | | | | | |
| (USDA) | ½ cup (3 oz.) | 572 | .2 | | | 0 |
| (USDA) | 3 slices (¼″ × 1½″, .7 oz.) | 141 | <.1 | | | 0 |
| (Fanning's) | 1 fl.-oz. | 189 | Tr. | | | 0 |
| (Featherweight) no added salt | 1 med. pickle (1 oz.) | 3 | 0.0 | | | (0) |
| (Vlasic): | | | | | | |
|   Chips | 1 oz. | 160 | 0.0 | | | (0) |
|   Chunks | 1 oz. | 120 | 0.0 | | | (0) |
|   Stix | 1 oz. | 110 | 0.0 | | | (0) |
| Dill: | | | | | | |
| (USDA) | 4″ × 1¾″ pickle (4.8 oz.) | 1,928 | .3 | | | 0 |
| (USDA) | 3¾″ × 1¼″ pickle (2.3 oz.) | 928 | .1 | | | 0 |
| (Featherweight) whole, low sodium | 1 med. pickle (1 oz.) | <5 | 0.0 | | | (0) |
| (Vlasic): | | | | | | |
|   No garlic | 1 oz. | 210 | 0.0 | | | (0) |
|   Original | 1 oz. | 375 | 0.0 | | | (0) |
| (Heinz) | 4″ pickle | 1207 | .1 | | | (0) |
| Processed (Heinz) | 3″ pickle | 511 | .1 | | | (0) |
| (Smucker's) baby, fresh pack | 2¾″ pickle (.8 oz.) | 283 | Tr. | | | (0) |
| Hamburger (Vlasic) dill, chips | 1 oz. | 175 | 0.0 | | | (0) |
| Hot & spicy (Vlasic) garden mix | 1 oz. | 380 | 0.0 | | | (0) |
| Kosher dill: | | | | | | |
| (Claussen) whole | 1.9-oz. pickle | 581 | .1 | | | (0) |
| (Featherweight) low sodium | 1 oz. | <5 | 0.0 | | | (0) |
| (Vlasic): | | | | | | |
|   Baby, crunchy or gherkins | 1 oz. | 210 | 0.0 | | | (0) |
|   Crunchy, half the salt | 1 oz. | 125 | 0.0 | | | (0) |
|   Deli | 1 oz. | 290 | 0.0 | | | (0) |
|   Spear: | | | | | | |
|     Regular | 1 oz. | 175 | 0.0 | | | (0) |
|     Half the salt | 1 oz. | 120 | 0.0 | | | (0) |
| Sour, cucumber (USDA) | 1¾″ × 4″ pickle (4.8 oz.) | 1,827 | .3 | | | 0 |

(USDA): United States Department of Agriculture
*Prepared as Package Directs

| Food and Description | Measure or Quantity | Sodium (mg.) | — Fats in grams — | | | Choles- terol (mg.) |
|---|---|---|---|---|---|---|
| | | | Total | Satu- rated | Unsatu- rated | |
| Sweet, cucumber (USDA): | | | | | | |
| Whole | 1 oz. | | .1 | | | 0 |
| Whole, gherkin | 2½″ × ¾″ pickle (.5 oz.) | | <.1 | | | 0 |
| Chopped | ½ cup (2.6 oz.) | | .3 | | | 0 |
| **PICKLING SPICE** (Spice Islands) | 1 tsp. | 1 | | | | (0) |
| **PIE:** | | | | | | |
| Regular, nonfrozen: | | | | | | |
| Apple: | | | | | | |
| Home recipe, two crust (USDA) | ⅙ of 9″ pie | 476 | 17.5 | 6.3 | 11.2 | |
| (Hostess) | 4½-oz. pie | 563 | 20.4 | | | 19 |
| Banana, home recipe, cream or custard (USDA) | ⅙ of 9″ pie | 295 | 14.1 | | | |
| Berry (Hostess) | 4½-oz. pie | 415 | 20.5 | | | 19 |
| Blackberry: | | | | | | |
| Home recipe, 2-crust, made with lard (USDA)[1] | ⅙ of 9″ pie (5.6 oz.) | 423 | 17.4 | 6. | 11. | |
| Home recipe, 2-crust, made with vegetable shortening (USDA)[2] | ⅙ of 9″ pie (5.6 oz.) | 423 | 17.4 | 5. | 13. | |
| Frozen (Banquet) | 5-oz. serving | | 15.3 | | | |
| Blueberry: | | | | | | |
| Home recipe, two-crust (USDA) | ⅙ of 9″ pie | 423 | 17.1 | 6.3 | 10.7 | |
| (Hostess) | 4½-oz. pie | 415 | 20.5 | | | 19 |
| Boston cream, home recipe (USDA)[3] | ¹⁄₁₂ of 8″ pie | 128 | 6.5 | | | |
| Butterscotch, home recipe, one-crust (USDA) | ⅙ of 9″ pie | 325 | 16.7 | 6.1 | 10.6 | |
| Cherry: | | | | | | |
| Home recipe, two-crust (USDA) | ⅙ of 9″ pie | 480 | 17.9 | 6.3 | 11.5 | |
| (Hostess) | 4½-oz. pie | 537 | 20.5 | | | 19 |

(USDA): United States Department of Agriculture
*Prepared as Package Directs
[1]Principal sources of fat: lard, butter.
[2]Principal sources of fat: vegetable shortening, butter.
[3]Made with sodium aluminum sulfate-type baking powder.

| Food and Description | Measure or Quantity | Sodium (mg.) | — Fats in grams — | | | Choles- terol (mg.) |
|---|---|---|---|---|---|---|
| | | | Total | Satu- rated | Unsatu- rated | |
| Chocolate chiffon, home recipe, (USDA) | ⅙ of 9″ pie | 353 | 21.4 | 8.4 | 13. | |
| Chocolate meringue, home recipe (USDA) | ⅙ of 9″ pie | 358 | 16.8 | 5.6 | 11.2 | |
| Coconut custard, home recipe (USDA) | ⅙ of 9″ pie | 375 | 19.0 | | | |
| Lemon (Hostess) | 4½-oz. pie | 422 | 21.7 | | | 32 |
| Lemon meringue, home recipe, one-crust (USDA) | ⅙ of 9″ pie | 395 | 14.3 | 5.2 | 9.1 | 130 |
| Mince, home recipe, two-crust (USDA) | ⅙ of 9″ pie | 708 | 18.2 | | | |
| Peach (Hostess) | 4½-oz. pie | 447 | 20.4 | | | 19 |
| Pumpkin, home recipe, one-crust (USDA) | ⅙ of 9″ pie | 325 | 17.0 | 6.1 | 10.9 | 93 |
| Raisin, home recipe, two-crust (USDA) | ⅙ of 9″ pie | 450 | 16.9 | 6.3 | 10.6 | |
| Strawberry (Hostess) | 4½-oz. pie | 396 | 14.1 | | | 13 |
| Frozen: | | | | | | |
| Apple: | | | | | | |
| (Banquet) family size | ⅙ of 20-oz. pie | 282 | 11.0 | | | |
| (Morton): | | | | | | |
| Regular | ⅙ of 24-oz. pie | 240 | 13.0 | | | 12 |
| Great Little Desserts, regular | 8-oz. pie | 510 | 25.0 | | | 13 |
| (Weight Watchers) | 3 oz. | 290 | 4.0 | | | |
| Banana cream: | | | | | | |
| (Banquet) | ⅙ of 14-oz. pie | 146 | 10.0 | | | |
| (Morton) regular | ⅙ of 14-oz. pie | 130 | 10.0 | | | 9 |
| Blackberry (Banquet) | ⅙ of 20-oz. pie | 342 | 11.0 | | | |
| Blueberry: | | | | | | |
| (Banquet) | ⅙ of 20-oz. pie | 342 | 11.0 | | | |
| (Morton) Great Little Desserts | 8-oz. pie | 525 | 25.0 | | | 23 |
| Cherry: | | | | | | |
| (Banquet) | ⅙ of 20-oz. pie | 258 | 11.0 | | | |
| (Morton) regular | ⅙ of 24-oz. pie | 240 | 14.0 | | | 23 |
| (Weight Watchers) | 3 oz. | 190 | 5.0 | | | |
| Chocolate (Morton) | ⅙ of 14-oz. pie | 140 | 11.0 | | | 9 |
| Chocolate cream: | | | | | | |
| (Banquet) | ⅙ of 14-oz. pie | 106 | 10.0 | | | |
| (Morton) Great Little Desserts | 3½-oz. pie | 200 | 17.0 | | | 15 |
| Coconut cream (Banquet) | ⅙ of 14-oz. pie | 113 | 11.0 | | | |

(USDA): United States Department of Agriculture
*Prepared as Package Directs

| Food and Description | Measure or Quantity | Sodium (mg.) | —Fats in grams— | | | Choles- terol (mg.) |
|---|---|---|---|---|---|---|
| | | | Total | Satu- rated | Unsatu- rated | |
| Coconut custard (Morton) | | | | | | |
| *Great Little Desserts* | 6½-oz. pie | 495 | 15.0 | | | 110 |
| Lemon cream: | | | | | | |
| (Banquet) | ⅙ of 14-oz. pie | 111 | 9.0 | | | |
| (Morton) *Great Little* | | | | | | |
| *Desserts* | 3½-oz. pie | 200 | 15.0 | | | 200 |
| Mince: | | | | | | |
| (Banquet) | ⅙ of 20-oz. pie | 364 | 11.0 | | | |
| (Morton) | ⅙ of 24-oz. pie | 355 | 14.0 | | | 12 |
| Peach (Banquet) | ⅙ of 20-oz. pie | 275 | 11.0 | | | |
| Pumpkin: | | | | | | |
| (Banquet) | ⅙ of 20-oz. pie | 341 | 8.0 | | | |
| (Morton) | ⅙ of 24-oz. pie | 310 | 8.0 | | | 44 |
| Strawberry cream (Banquet) | ⅙ of 14-oz. pie | 112 | 9.0 | | | |
| **PIECRUST** (See also **PASTRY SHELL**): | | | | | | |
| Home recipe, baked, 9″ (USDA): | | | | | | |
| Made with lard[1] | 1 crust (6.3 oz.) | 1,100 | 60.1 | 23. | 37. | |
| Made with vegetable shortening[2] | 1 crust (6.3 oz.) | 1,100 | 60.1 | 14. | 46. | |
| Refrigerated (Pillsbury) | ⅛ of 2 crust pie shell | 210 | 15.0 | | | |
| **PIECRUST MIX:** | | | | | | |
| USDA: | | | | | | |
| Dry pkg. or stick[2] | 10-oz. pkg. (2 crusts) | 1,968 | 92.9 | 20. | 73. | |
| *Prepared with water, baked[2] | 4 oz. | 922 | 33.0 | 8. | 25. | |
| (Betty Crocker) | ⅙ of pkg. or ⅛ of stick | 140 | 8.0 | | | |
| *(Flako) | ⅙ of 9″ piecrust | 314 | 14.5 | | | |
| *(Pillsbury) mix or stick | ⅙ of 2 crust pie shell | 420 | 17.0 | | | |
| **PIE FILLING** (See also **PUDDING OR PIE FILLING**): | | | | | | |
| Apple: | | | | | | |
| (Comstock) | ⅙ of 21-oz. can | 150 | 1.0 | | | |
| (Thank You Brand) | 3½ oz. | 94 | 0.0 | | | 0 |

(USDA): United States Department of Agriculture
*Prepared as Package Directs
[1]Principal source of fat: lard.
[2]Principal source of fat: vegetable shortening.

| Food and Description | Measure or Quantity | Sodium (mg.) | Total | Satu-rated | Unsatu-rated | Choles-terol (mg.) |
|---|---|---|---|---|---|---|
| Apple rings or slices (See **APPLE,** canned) | | | | | | |
| Apricot (Comstock) | ⅙ of 21-oz. can | 250 | 1.0 | | | |
| Banana cream (Comstock) | ⅙ of 21-oz. can | 700 | 4.0 | | | |
| Blackberry: | | | | | | |
| (Comstock) | 1 cup (10¾ oz.) | 320 | <.1 | | | |
| (Lucky Leaf) | 8 oz. | 276 | .4 | | | |
| Blueberry (Comstock) | ⅙ of 21-oz. can | 350 | 2.0 | | | |
| Cherry (Thank You Brand) regular | 3½ oz. | 15 | 0.0 | | | 0 |
| Coconut cream (Comstock) | ⅙ of 21-oz. can | 650 | 4.0 | | | |
| Lemon (Comstock) | ⅙ of 21-oz. can | 300 | 4.0 | | | |
| Mincemeat (Comstock) | ½ of 21-oz. can | | 4.0 | | | |
| Pumpkin (Libby's) (See also **PUMPKIN,** canned) | 1 cup | 420 | 0.0 | | | |
| Raisin (Comstock)[1] | ⅙ of 21-oz. can | 200 | 2.0 | | | |
| **\*PIE MIX:** | | | | | | |
| Boston Cream (Betty Crocker) | ⅛ of pie | 405 | 6.0 | | | |
| Chocolate (Royal) No Bake | ⅛ of pie | 280 | 15.0 | | | |
| **PIEROGIE,** frozen: | | | | | | |
| (Empire Kosher): | | | | | | |
| Cheese | 1½ oz. | 120 | 5.0 | | | 5 |
| Onion | 1½ oz. | 138 | 4.0 | | | 4 |
| (Mrs. Paul's) potato & cheese | 1.7-oz. piece | 260 | 2.0 | | | |
| **PIGEON** (See **SQUAB**) | | | | | | |
| **PIGEONPEA** (USDA): | | | | | | |
| Raw, immature seeds in pods | 1 lb. | 9 | 1.1 | | | 0 |
| Dry seeds | 1 lb. | 118 | 6.4 | | | 0 |
| **PIGNOLIA** (See **PINE NUT**) | | | | | | |
| **PIGS FEET,** pickled: | | | | | | |
| (USDA) | 4 oz. | | 16.8 | 6. | 11. | |
| (Hormel) | 1-pt. can (8.6 oz.) | | 37.3 | | | |
| **PIKE,** raw (USDA): | | | | | | |
| Blue, whole | 1 lb. (weighed whole) | | 1.8 | | | |
| Blue, meat only | 4 oz. | | 1.0 | | | |

(USDA): United States Department of Agriculture
\*Prepared as Package Directs
[1]Principal sources of fat: vegetable shortening & butter.

| Food and Description | Measure or Quantity | Sodium (mg.) | Total | Fats in grams — Satu- rated | Unsatu- rated | Choles- terol (mg.) |
|---|---|---|---|---|---|---|
| Northern, whole | 1 lb. (weighed whole) | | 1.3 | | | |
| Northern, meat only | 4 oz. | | 1.2 | | | |
| Walleye, whole | 1 lb. (weighed whole) | 132 | 3.1 | | | |
| Walleye, meat only | 4 oz. | 58 | 1.4 | | | |
| **PILI NUT** (USDA): | | | | | | |
| In shell | 1 lb. (weighed in shell) | 2 | 58.0 | | | 0 |
| Shelled | 4 oz. | 3 | 80.6 | | | 0 |
| **PIMIENTO,** canned: | | | | | | |
| Solids & liq. (USDA) | 1 med. pod (1.3 oz.) | | .2 | | | 0 |
| (Dromedary) whole pods, slices, pieces | 1 oz. | 5 | 0.0 | | | 0 |
| (Sunshine) Diced or sliced, solids & liq. | 1 T. (.6 oz.) | 3 | Tr. | | | |
| *PINA COLADA:* | | | | | | |
| Cocktail (Mr. Boston) 12½% alcohol | 3 fl. oz. | 29 | | | | |
| Mix: | | | | | | |
| *(Bar-Tender's) | 5 fl. oz. | 45 | 3.0 | | | 12 |
| (Holland House): | | | | | | |
| Liquid | 1 oz. | 4 | 0.0 | | | |
| Instant | .56 oz. | <1 | 3.0 | | | |
| **PINEAPPLE:** | | | | | | |
| Fresh: | | | | | | |
| Whole (USDA) | 1 lb. (weighed untrimmed) | 2 | .5 | | | 0 |
| Diced (USDA) | ½ cup (2.8 oz.) | <1 | .2 | | | 0 |
| Slices (USDA) | ¾" × 3½" slice (3 oz.) | <1 | .2 | | | 0 |
| (Del Monte) | ½ cup (2.5 oz.) | <1 | .4 | | | (0) |
| Canned, regular pack, solids & liq.: | | | | | | |
| Juice pack: | | | | | | |
| (USDA) | 4 oz. | 1 | .1 | | | 0 |
| (Del Monte) | ½ cup (4.9 oz.) | 26 | .3 | | | 0 |

(USDA): United States Department of Agriculture
*Prepared as Package Directs

| Food and Description | Measure or Quantity | Sodium (mg.) | — Fats in grams — | | | Cholesterol (mg.) |
|---|---|---|---|---|---|---|
| | | | Total | Satu- rated | Unsatu- rated | |
| Chunks or crushed (Dole) | ½ cup (includes 2½ T. juice, 3.7 oz.) | 1 | .1 | | | 0 |
| Slices (Dole) | 2 med. slices & 2½ T. juice (3.7 oz.) | 1 | .1 | | | 0 |
| Light syrup (USDA) | 4 oz. | 1 | .1 | | | 0 |
| Heavy syrup: | | | | | | |
| Crushed (USDA) | ½ cup (4.6 oz.) | 1 | .1 | | | 0 |
| Slices (USDA) | ½ cup (4.9 oz.) | 1 | .1 | | | 0 |
| Slices (USDA) | 2 small or 1 large slice & 2 T. syrup (4.3 oz.) | 1 | .1 | | | 0 |
| Tidbits (USDA) | ½ cup (4.6 oz.) | 1 | .1 | | | 0 |
| (Del Monte) | ½ cup (5 oz.) | < 10 | 0.0 | | | 0 |
| Chunks (Dole) | 10 pieces & 2½ T. syrup (4 oz.) | 1 | .1 | | | 0 |
| Crushed or tidbits (Dole) | ½ cup (includes 2½ T. syrup, 4 oz.) | 2 | .1 | | | 0 |
| Slices (Dole) | 2 med. slices & 2½ T. syrup (4 oz.) | 1 | .1 | | | 0 |
| Extra heavy syrup (USDA) | 4 oz. | 1 | .1 | | | 0 |
| Canned, unsweetened, low calorie or dietetic, solids & liq.: | | | | | | |
| Water pack, except crushed: | | | | | | |
| (USDA) | 4 oz. | 1 | .1 | | | 0 |
| (Diet Delight) | ½ cup (4.4 oz.) | 5 | Tr. | | | (0) |
| (S&W) *Nutradiet* | 4 oz. | 3 | Tr. | | | (0) |
| Frozen: | | | | | | |
| Chunks, sweetened, not thawed (USDA) | ½ cup (4.3 oz.) | 2 | .1 | | | 0 |
| Chunks in heavy syrup (Dole) | 11 chunks & 2½ T. syrup (4 oz.) | 2 | .1 | | | 0 |
| **PINEAPPLE, CANDIED** | | | | | | |
| (USDA) | 1 oz. | | .1 | | | 0 |
| **PINEAPPLE & GRAPEFRUIT JUICE DRINK,** canned: | | | | | | |
| (USDA) 40% fruit juices | ½ cup (4.4 oz.) | Tr. | Tr. | | | 0 |

(USDA): United States Department of Agriculture
*Prepared as Package Directs

PINEAPPLE & GRAPEFRUIT JUICE DRINK (Continued)

| Food and Description | Measure or Quantity | Sodium (mg.) | Total | Satu- rated | Unsatu- rated | Choles- terol (mg.) |
|---|---|---|---|---|---|---|
| (Del Monte) | ½ cup (4.3 oz.) | 50 | 0.0 | | | 0 |
| (Dole) regular or pink | 6 fl. oz. can | Tr. | Tr. | | | 0 |
| (Hi-C) | ½ cup (4.2 oz.) | 40 | Tr. | | | 0 |
| **PINEAPPLE JUICE:** | | | | | | |
| Canned, unsweetened: | | | | | | |
| (USDA) | ½ cup (4.4 oz.) | 1 | .1 | | | 0 |
| (Del Monte) | ½ cup (4.3 oz.) | < 10 | 0.0 | | | 0 |
| (Dole) | 6 fl. oz. can | 2 | .2 | | | 0 |
| Frozen, concentrate: | | | | | | |
| Unsweetened, undiluted (USDA) | 6 fl. oz. can (7.6 oz.) | 6 | .2 | | | 0 |
| *Unsweetened, diluted with 3 parts water (USDA) | ½ cup (4.4 oz.) | 1 | Tr. | | | 0 |
| *Unsweetened (Minute Maid) | 6 fl. oz. | 2 | .2 | | | 0 |
| **PINEAPPLE & ORANGE JUICE DRINK,** canned: | | | | | | |
| (USDA) 40% fruit juices | ½ cup (4.4 oz.) | Tr. | .1 | | | 0 |
| (Del Monte) | 6 fl. oz. | 20 | 0.0 | | | (0) |
| (Hi-C) | 6 fl. oz. | Tr. | Tr. | | | (0) |
| (Johanna Farms) *Tree-Ripe* | 8.45-fl.-oz. container | 3 | .1 | | | (0) |
| **PINEAPPLE PRESERVE:** | | | | | | |
| Sweetened (Home Brand) | 1 T. (.7 oz.) | 7 | 0.0 | | | (0) |
| Low calorie (Tillie Lewis) | 1 T. (.5 oz.) | 3 | Tr. | | | 0 |
| **PINE NUT** (USDA): | | | | | | |
| Pignolias, shelled | 4 oz. | | 53.8 | | | 0 |
| Piñon, whole | 4 oz. (weighed in shell) | | 39.8 | | | 0 |
| Piñon, shelled | 4 oz. | | 68.6 | | | 0 |
| **PISTACHIO NUT:** | | | | | | |
| In shell (USDA) | 4 oz. (weighed in shell) | | 30.4 | 3. | 27. | 0 |
| In shell (USDA) | ½ cup (2.3 oz.) | | 17.8 | 2. | 16. | 0 |
| Shelled (USDA) | ½ cup (2.2 oz.) | | 33.3 | 3. | 30. | 0 |
| Shelled (USDA) | 1 T. (8 grams) | | 4.2 | Tr. | 4. | 0 |
| (Planters) | 1 oz. | 250 | 15.0 | | | 0 |
| In shell, salted, red or natural (Planters) | 1 oz. | 250 | 15.0 | | | 0 |

(USDA): United States Department of Agriculture
*Prepared as Package Directs

272

| Food and Description | Measure or Quantity | Sodium (mg.) | —Fats in grams— | | | Choles- terol (mg.) |
|---|---|---|---|---|---|---|
| | | | Total | Satu- rated | Unsatu- rated | |
| Dry roasted, salted, shelled: (Flavor House) | 1 oz. | 32 | 15.2 | | | (0) |
| **PITANGA,** fresh (USDA): | | | | | | |
| Whole | 1 lb. (weighed whole) | | 1.5 | | | 0 |
| Flesh only | 4 oz. | | .5 | | | 0 |
| **PIZZA PIE** (See also **SHAKEY'S**): | | | | | | |
| Home recipe, with cheese topping: | | | | | | |
| (USDA)[1] | 4 oz. | 796 | 9.4 | 3. | 6. | |
| (USDA)[1] | 5½" sector (⅛ of 14" pie, 2.6 oz.) | 527 | 6.2 | 2. | 4. | |
| Home recipe, with sausage topping: | | | | | | |
| (USDA)[2] | 4 oz. | 827 | 10.5 | 3. | 7. | |
| (USDA)[2] | 5½" sector (⅛ of 14" pie, 2.6 oz.) | 547 | 7.0 | 2. | 5. | |
| Chilled, partially baked (USDA)[1] | 4 oz. | 610 | 6.6 | 2. | 4. | |
| Chilled, baked (USDA)[1] | 4 oz. | 718 | 7.7 | 2. | 5. | |
| Regular, nonfrozen, *(Domino's):* | | | | | | |
| Beef, ground: | | | | | | |
| Plain: | | | | | | |
| 12" pizza (small) | 1 slice | 390 | 6.1 | | | 15 |
| 16" pizza (large) | 1 slice | 399 | 17.0 | | | 17 |
| With pepperoni: | | | | | | |
| 12" pizza (small) | 1 slice | 410 | 8.2 | | | 23 |
| 16" pizza (large) | 1 slice | 979 | 11.0 | | | 26 |
| Cheese: | | | | | | |
| Plain: | | | | | | |
| 12" pizza (small) | 1 slice | 255 | 4.2 | | | 9 |
| 16" pizza (large) | 1 slice | 335 | 5.1 | | | 10 |
| Double cheese: | | | | | | |
| 12" pizza (small) | 1 slice | 318 | 7.8 | | | 17 |
| 16" pizza (large) | 1 slice | 421 | 9.4 | | | 21 |

(USDA): United States Department of Agriculture
*Prepared as Package Directs
[1]Principal sources of fat: cheese, vegetable shortening & olive oil.
[2]Principal sources of fat: sausage, vegetable shortening & olive oil.

273

| Food and Description | Measure or Quantity | Sodium (mg.) | Fats in grams — Total | Satu- rated | Unsatu- rated | Choles- terol (mg.) |
|---|---|---|---|---|---|---|
| Double, with pepperoni: | | | | | | |
| 12" pizza (small) | 1 slice | 429 | 11.1 | | | 23 |
| 16" pizza (large) | 1 slice | 561 | 13.0 | | | 30 |
| Mushroom & sausage: | | | | | | |
| 12" pizza (small) | 1 slice | 301 | 6.3 | | | 14 |
| 16" pizza (large) | 1 slice | 396 | 7.3 | | | 16 |
| Pepperoni: | | | | | | |
| Plain: | | | | | | |
| 12" pizza (small) | 1 slice | 365 | 7.5 | | | 17 |
| 16" pizza (large) | 1 slice | 474 | 8.7 | | | 20 |
| With mushrooms: | | | | | | |
| 12" pizza (small) | 1 slice | 366 | 7.5 | | | 17 |
| 16" pizza (large) | 1 slice | 475 | 8.5 | | | 19 |
| With sausage: | | | | | | |
| 12" pizza (small) | 1 slice | 411 | 9.5 | | | 22 |
| 16" pizza (large) | 1 slice | 534 | 10.0 | | | 25 |
| Sausage: | | | | | | |
| 12" pizza (small) | 1 slice | 300 | 6.3 | | | 14 |
| 16" pizza (large) | 1 slice | 395 | 7.3 | | | 16 |
| Frozen: | | | | | | |
| Canadian style bacon (Celeste) | 8-oz. pie | | 11.5 | | | |
| Cheese: | | | | | | |
| (Celentano): | | | | | | |
| Mini slice | 1 slice | 166 | 5.0 | | | |
| Thick crust | 1/3 of 13-oz. pie | 252 | 7.0 | | | |
| (Stouffer's) French bread | 1/2 of 10 3/8-oz. pkg. | 850 | 13.0 | | | |
| (Weight Watchers) | 6-oz. pie | 670 | 14.0 | | | |
| Combination: | | | | | | |
| (Celeste) Chicago style | 1/4 of 24-oz. pie | 1,156 | 16.3 | | | |
| (La Pizzeria) | 1/2 of 13 1/2-oz. pie | 959 | 22.0 | | | |
| (Weight Watchers) | 7 1/4-oz. pie | 944 | 12.0 | | | |
| Deluxe: | | | | | | |
| (Celeste) | 1/2 of 9-oz. pie | 794 | 11.8 | | | |
| (Stouffer's) French bread | 1/2 of 12 3/8 oz. pkg. | 1,150 | 18.0 | | | |
| Mushroom (Stouffer's) French bread | 1/2 of 12-oz. pkg. | 1,755 | 13.0 | | | |
| Pepperoni: | | | | | | |
| (Stouffer's) French bread | 1/2 of 11 1/4-oz. pkg. | 1,190 | 20.0 | | | |
| (Weight Watchers) | 6 1/4-oz. pie | 802 | 15.0 | | | |

(USDA): United States Department of Agriculture
*Prepared as Package Directs

| Food and Description | Measure or Quantity | Sodium (mg.) | Total | Saturated | Unsaturated | Cholesterol (mg.) |
|---|---|---|---|---|---|---|
| Sausage: | | | | | | |
| (Celeste) | ½ of 8-oz. pie | 764 | 10.6 | | | |
| (Stouffer's) French bread | ½ of 12-oz. pkg. | 1,320 | 20.0 | | | |
| (Weight Watchers) veal | 6¾-oz. pie | 936 | 12.0 | | | |
| Sausage & mushroom: | | | | | | |
| (Celeste) | ¼ of 24-oz. pie | 1,195 | 17.0 | | | |
| (Stouffer's) French bread | ½ of 12½-oz. pkg. | 1,120 | 18.0 | | | |
| Sicilian style (Celeste) deluxe | ¼ of 26-oz. pie | 1,190 | 17.1 | | | |
| Supreme (Celeste) without meat | ½ of 8-oz. pie | | 8.3 | | | |
| *Mix (Ragú) Pizza Quick | ¼ of pie | 810 | 11.0 | | | 25 |
| **PIZZA PIE CRUST,** refrigerated | | | | | | |
| (Pillsbury) | ⅛ of crust | 170 | 1.0 | | | |
| **PIZZA SAUCE,** canned: | | | | | | |
| (Contadina): | | | | | | |
| Regular | ½ cup | 790 | 4.0 | | | 0 |
| With cheese | ½ cup | 760 | 4.0 | | | Tr. |
| With pepperoni | ½ cup | 720 | 4.0 | | | 4 |
| With tomato chunks | ½ cup | 600 | 0.0 | | | 0 |
| (Ragú) Pizza Quick: | | | | | | |
| Chunky | 4 oz. | 672 | 4.1 | | | 0 |
| Mushroom | 4 oz. | 706 | 4.7 | | | 0 |
| Pepperoni | 4 oz. | 777 | 7.1 | | | 0 |
| **PLANTAIN,** raw (USDA): | | | | | | |
| Whole | 1 lb. (weighed with skin) | 16 | 1.3 | | | 0 |
| Flesh only | 4 oz. | 6 | .5 | | | 0 |
| **PLUM:** | | | | | | |
| Damson, fresh (USDA): | | | | | | |
| Whole | 1 lb. (weighed with pits) | 8 | Tr. | | | 0 |
| Flesh only | 4 oz. | 2 | Tr. | | | 0 |
| Japanese & hybrid, fresh (USDA): | | | | | | |
| Whole | 1 lb. (weighed with pits) | 4 | .9 | | | 0 |
| Whole | 2" plum (2.1 oz.) | <1 | .1 | | | 0 |
| Diced | ½ cup (2.3 oz.) | <1 | .2 | | | 0 |

(USDA): United States Department of Agriculture
*Prepared as Package Directs

| Food and Description | Measure or Quantity | Sodium (mg.) | Total | Fats in grams — Satu- rated | Unsatu- rated | Choles- terol (mg.) |
|---|---|---|---|---|---|---|
| Halves | ½ cup (3.1 oz.) | <1 | .2 | | | 0 |
| Slices | ½ cup (3 oz.) | <1 | .2 | | | 0 |
| Prune-type, fresh (USDA): | | | | | | |
| Whole | 1 lb. (weighed with pits) | 4 | .9 | | | 0 |
| Halves | ½ cup (2.8 oz.) | <1 | .2 | | | 0 |
| Canned, purple, regular pack, solids & liq.: | | | | | | |
| Light syrup (USDA) | 4 oz. | 1 | .1 | | | 0 |
| Heavy syrup (USDA) | ½ cup (with pits, 4.5 oz.) | 1 | .1 | | | 0 |
| Heavy syrup (USDA) | ½ cup (without pits, 4.2 oz.) | 1 | .1 | | | 0 |
| Heavy syrup (USDA) | 3 plums without pits & 2 T. syrup (4.3 oz.) | 1 | .1 | | | 0 |
| Heavy syrup (Del Monte) | ½ cup (4.1 oz.) | 6 | .1 | | | 0 |
| Extra heavy syrup (USDA) | 4 oz. | 1 | .1 | | | 0 |
| (Stokely-Van Camp) | ½ cup (4.2 oz.) | | .1 | | | (0) |
| Canned, unsweetened or low calorie, solids & liq.: | | | | | | |
| Greengage, water pack (USDA) | 4 oz. | 1 | .1 | | | 0 |
| Purple: | | | | | | |
| Water pack (USDA) | 4 oz. | 2 | .2 | | | 0 |
| (Diet Delight) | ½ cup (4.4 oz.) | 4 | <.1 | | | (0) |
| (S&W) *Nutradiet* | 4 oz. | 2 | .1 | | | (0) |
| **PLUM PRESERVE OR JAM,** sweetened, Damson or red (Bama) | 1 T. (.7 oz.) | 7 | 0.0 | | | (0) |
| **PLUM PUDDING** (Richardson & Robbins) | 2″ piece (3.6 oz.) | 150 | 1.0 | | | |
| ***P.M.,*** fruit juice drink (Mott's) | ½ cup | | .1 | | | (0) |
| **POHA** (See **GROUND-CHERRY**) | | | | | | |
| **POKE SHOOTS** (USDA) | | | | | | |
| Raw | 1 lb. | | 1.8 | | | 0 |
| Boiled, drained | 4 oz. | | .5 | | | 0 |

(USDA): United States Department of Agriculture
*Prepared as Package Directs

| Food and Description | Measure or Quantity | Sodium (mg.) | — Fats in grams — | | Choles- terol (mg.) |
|---|---|---|---|---|---|
| | | | Total | Satu- rated | Unsatu- rated |

**POLISH-STYLE SAUSAGE**
(See **SAUSAGE**)

**POLLOCK** (USDA):

| | | | | | |
|---|---|---|---|---|---|
| Raw, drawn | 1 lb. (weighed with head, tail, fins & bones) | 98 | 1.8 | | |
| Raw, meat only | 4 oz. | 5.4 | 1.0 | | |
| Creamed [1] | 4 oz. | 126 | 6.7 | | |

**POLYNESIAN-STYLE**

| | | | | | |
|---|---|---|---|---|---|
| **DINNER,** frozen (Swanson) | 12 oz. dinner | 1,430 | 8.0 | | |

**POMEGRANATE,** raw (USDA):

| | | | | | |
|---|---|---|---|---|---|
| Whole | 1 lb. (weighed whole) | 8 | .8 | | 0 |
| Pulp only | 4 oz. | 3 | .3 | | 0 |

**POMPANO,** raw (USDA):

| | | | | | |
|---|---|---|---|---|---|
| Whole | 1 lb. (weighed whole) | 119 | 24.1 | | |
| Meat only | 4 oz. | 53 | 10.8 | | |

***PONDEROSA STEAKHOUSE:***

| | | | | | |
|---|---|---|---|---|---|
| *A-1* | 1 tsp. | 82 | | | |
| Beef, chopped, patty only: | | | | | |
| Regular | 3½ oz. | 58 | 10.8 | | 67 (raw) |
| Double Deluxe | 5.9 oz. | 99 | 18.8 | | 116 |
| Junior *(Square Shooters)* | 1.6 oz. | 27 | 5.1 | | 31 (raw) |
| Steakhouse Deluxe | 2.96 oz. | 50 | 9.4 | | 58 |
| Beverages: | | | | | |
| *Coca-Cola* | 8 fl. oz. | 1 | 0.0 | | |
| Coffee | 6 fl. oz. | 26 | | | |
| *Dr Pepper* | 8 fl. oz. | 18 | 0.0 | | |
| Milk, chocolate | 8 fl. oz. | 149 | 8.5 | | 33 |
| Orange drink | 8 fl. oz. | 12 | Tr. | | |
| Root beer | 8 fl. oz. | 18 | 0.0 | | |
| *Sprite* | 8 fl. oz. | 18 | 0.0 | | |
| *Tab* | 8 fl. oz. | 18 | 0.0 | | |

(USDA): United States Department of Agriculture
*Prepared as Package Directs
[1]Prepared with flour, butter & milk.

| Food and Description | Measure or Quantity | Sodium (mg.) | —Fats in grams— | | | Choles- terol (mg.) |
|---|---|---|---|---|---|---|
| | | | Total | Satu- rated | Unsatu- rated | |
| Bun: | | | | | | |
| Regular | 2.4-oz. bun | 334 | 3.0 | | | |
| Hot dog | 1 bun | 263 | 1.8 | | | 15 |
| Junior | 1.4-oz. bun | | | | | |
| Steakhouse deluxe | 2.4-oz. bun | 334 | 3.0 | | | |
| Cocktail sauce | 1½ oz. | 143 | .3 | | | |
| Filet mignon | 3.8 oz. (edible portion) | 82 | 8.3 | | | 70 (raw) |
| Filet of sole, fish only (See also Bun) | 3-oz. piece | 46 | 4.9 | | | 59 |
| Fish, baked | 4.9-oz. serving | 363 | 13.5 | | | 98 (raw) |
| Gelatin dessert | ½ cup | 55 | Tr. | | | |
| Gravy, au jus | 1 oz. | 125 | .2 | | | |
| Hot dog, child's, meat only (See also Bun) | 1.6-oz. hot dog | 542 | 13.0 | | | 35 |
| Margarine: | | | | | | |
| Pat | 1 tsp. | 49 | 4.1 | | | 12 |
| On potato, as served | ½ oz. | 138 | 11.3 | | | |
| Mustard sauce, sweet & sour | 1 oz. | | 1.1 | | | |
| New York strip steak | 6.1 oz. (edible portion) | 79 | 19.2 | | | 122 |
| Onion, chopped | 1 T. | 1 | Tr. | | | |
| Pickle, dill | 3 slices (.7 oz.) | 279 | Tr. | | | |
| Potato: | | | | | | |
| Baked | 7.2-oz. potato | 6 | .2 | | | |
| French fries | 3-oz. serving | 5 | 11.1 | | | |
| Pudding, chocolate | 4½ oz. | 177 | 10.6 | | | 15 |
| Ribeye | 3.2 oz. (edible portion) | 271 | 10.9 | | | 56 (raw) |
| Ribeye & shrimp: | | | | | | |
| Ribeye | 3.2 oz. | 271 | 10.9 | | | 56 (raw) |
| Shrimp | 2.2 oz. | 114 | 6.7 | | | 77 (raw) |
| Roll, kaiser | 2.2-oz. roll | 311 | 3.4 | | | |
| Salad bar: | | | | | | |
| Bean sprouts | 1 oz. | 3 | .4 | | | |
| Broccoli | 1 oz. | 4 | .1 | | | |
| Cabbage, red | 1 oz. | 7 | .1 | | | |
| Carrots | 1 oz. | 13 | .1 | | | |

(USDA): United States Department of Agriculture
*Prepared as Package Directs

| Food and Description | Measure or Quantity | Sodium (mg.) | Fats in grams Total | Satu- rated | Unsatu- rated | Choles- terol (mg.) |
|---|---|---|---|---|---|---|
| Cauliflower | 1 oz. | 4 | .1 | | | |
| Celery | 1 oz. | 35 | Tr. | | | |
| Chickpeas (Garbanzos) | 1 oz. | 7 | | | | |
| Mushrooms | 1 oz. | 4 | .1 | | | |
| Pepper, green | 1 oz. | 4 | .1 | | | |
| Radish | 1 oz. | 5 | Tr. | | | |
| Tomato | 1 oz. | <1 | .1 | | | |
| Salad dressing: | | | | | | |
| Blue cheese | 1 oz. | 264 | 12.9 | | | |
| Italian, creamy | 1 oz. | 418 | 12.9 | | | |
| Low calorie | 1 oz. | 220 | Tr. | | | |
| Oil & vinegar | 1 oz. | Tr. | 13.8 | | | |
| Thousand island | 1 oz. | 170 | 10.6 | | | |
| Shrimp dinner, shrimp only | 7 pieces (3½ oz.) | 182 | 10.6 | | | 122 (raw) |
| Steak sauce | 1 oz. | 329 | .5 | | | |
| Tartar sauce | 1.5 oz. | 300 | 3.0 | | | |
| T-Bone | 4.3 oz. (edible portion) | 545 | 8.8 | | | 84 (raw) |
| Tomato (See also Salad bar): | | | | | | |
| Slices | 2 slices (.9 oz.) | <1 | Tr. | | | |
| Whole, small | 3.5 oz. | 3 | .2 | | | |
| Topping, whipped | ¼ oz. | 4 | 1.6 | | | 5 |
| Worcestershire sauce | 1 tsp. | | Tr. | | | |
| **POPCORN:** | | | | | | |
| Unpopped (USDA) | 1 oz. | <1 | 1.3 | Tr. | 1. | 0 |
| Popped, fresh: | | | | | | |
| (USDA): | | | | | | |
| Plain, large kernel | 1 oz. | Tr. | 1.4 | Tr. | 1. | 0 |
| Butter & salt added[1] | 1 oz. | 550 | 6.2 | 4. | 4. | |
| Coconut oil & salt added[2] | 1 oz. | 550 | 6.2 | 4. | 2. | |
| Sugar coated, without salt[2] | 1 oz. | Tr. | 1.0 | Tr. | Tr. | |
| (Jolly Time) no added butter or salt: | | | | | | |
| Regular | 1 cup | Tr. | .2 | | | |
| Microwave: | | | | | | |
| Natural | 1 cup | 60 | 3.5 | | | |
| Butter flavor | 1 cup | 68 | 3.5 | | | |

(USDA): United States Department of Agriculture
*Prepared as Package Directs
[1]Principal source of fat: butter.
[2]Principal source of fat: coconut oil.

| Food and Description | Measure or Quantity | Sodium (mg.) | — Fats in grams — | | | Cholesterol (mg.) |
|---|---|---|---|---|---|---|
| | | | Total | Saturated | Unsaturated | |
| (Orville Redenbacher's): | | | | | | |
| Caramel crunch | 1 oz. | 100 | 7.0 | | | |
| Hot air corn | 1 cup | 0 | .3 | | | |
| Microwave: | | | | | | |
| Regular, butter flavor, salted | 1 cup | 50 | 1.5 | | | |
| Natural, without salt | 1 cup | 0 | 2.0 | | | |
| Original, plain | 1 cup | 0 | .3 | | | |
| (Pillsbury) microwave: | | | | | | |
| Regular | 1 cup | 129 | 4.5 | | | |
| Butter flavor | 1 cup | 176 | 4.0 | | | |
| Packaged: | | | | | | |
| Plain (Tom's) | 1 oz. | 300 | 8.0 | | | |
| Butter flavored (Wise) | 1 oz. | 110 | | | | |
| Caramel coated: | | | | | | |
| (Bachman) | 1 oz. | | 1.0 | | | |
| *Cracker Jack* | 1 oz. | 85 | 3.0 | | | |
| Cheese flavored: | | | | | | |
| (Snyder's) | 1 oz. | 250 | 10.0 | | | |
| (Tom's) | 1 oz. | 460 | 8.0 | | | |

**POPCORN POPPING OIL**

| Food and Description | Measure or Quantity | Sodium (mg.) | Total | Saturated | Unsaturated | Cholesterol (mg.) |
|---|---|---|---|---|---|---|
| (Orville Redenbacher's) buttery flavor | 1 T. (.5 oz.) | 0 | 14.0 | | | 0 |

**POPOVER:**

| Food and Description | Measure or Quantity | Sodium (mg.) | Total | Saturated | Unsaturated | Cholesterol (mg.) |
|---|---|---|---|---|---|---|
| Home recipe (USDA)[1] | 1.4 oz. popover (2¾" dia. at top, ¼ cup batter) | 88 | 3.7 | 1. | 2. | 59 |
| *Mix (Flako) | 2.3 oz. popover (⅙ of pkg.) | 355 | 4.8 | | | |

**POPPY SEED** (Spice Islands)

| Food and Description | Measure or Quantity | Sodium (mg.) | Total | Saturated | Unsaturated | Cholesterol (mg.) |
|---|---|---|---|---|---|---|
| POPPY SEED (Spice Islands) | 1 tsp. | <1 | | | | 0 |

**POP-UP** (See **TOASTER CAKE**)

**PORGY,** raw (USDA):

| Food and Description | Measure or Quantity | Sodium (mg.) | Total | Saturated | Unsaturated | Cholesterol (mg.) |
|---|---|---|---|---|---|---|
| Whole | 1 lb. (weighed whole) | 117 | 6.3 | | | |
| Meat only | 4 oz. | 71 | 3.9 | | | |

(USDA): United States Department of Agriculture
*Prepared as Package Directs
[1]Principal sources of fat: vegetable shortening, egg & milk.

| Food and Description | Measure or Quantity | Sodium (mg.) | — Fats in grams — | | | Choles- terol (mg.) |
|---|---|---|---|---|---|---|
| | | | Total | Satu- rated | Unsatu- rated | |
| **PORK,** medium-fat: | | | | | | |
| Fresh (USDA): | | | | | | |
| All lean cuts: | | | | | | |
| Lean only: | | | | | | |
| Raw, diced | 1 cup (8.2 oz.) | 667 | 26.4 | 10. | 17. | 140 |
| Raw, strips | 1 cup (8.2 oz.) | 664 | 26.3 | 10. | 17. | 140 |
| Roasted, chopped | 1 cup (5 oz.) | 554 | 20.0 | 7. | 13. | 125 |
| Boston butt: | | | | | | |
| Raw | 1 lb. (weighed with bone & skin) | 260 | 104.1 | 37. | 67. | 264 |
| Roasted, lean & fat | 4 oz. | 74 | 32.3 | 11. | 21. | 101 |
| Roasted, lean only | 4 oz. | 74 | 16.2 | 6. | 10. | 100 |
| Chop: | | | | | | |
| Broiled, lean & fat | 4-oz. chop (weighed with bone) | 49 | 23.9 | 8. | 16. | 67 |
| Broiled, lean & fat | 3-oz. chop (weighed without bone) | 55 | 26.9 | 9. | 18. | 76 |
| Broiled, lean only | 3-oz. chop (weighed without bone) | 55 | 13.1 | 5. | 8. | 75 |
| Fat, separable, cooked | 1 oz. | | 23.6 | 9. | 15. | |
| Ham (See also **HAM**): | | | | | | |
| Raw | 1 lb. (weighed with bone & skin) | 320 | 102.6 | 37. | 66. | 239 |
| Roasted, lean & fat | 4 oz. | 74 | 34.7 | 12. | 22. | 101 |
| Roasted, lean only | 4 oz. | 74 | 11.3 | 5. | 7. | 100 |
| Loin: | | | | | | |
| Raw | 1 lb. (weighed with bone) | 260 | 89.0 | 32. | 57. | 221 |
| Broiled, lean & fat | 4 oz. | 74 | 35.9 | 12. | 24. | 101 |
| Broiled, lean only | 4 oz. | 74 | 17.5 | 7. | 11. | 100 |
| Roasted, lean & fat | 4 oz. | 74 | 32.3 | 11. | 21. | 101 |
| Roasted, lean only | 4 oz. | 74 | 16.1 | 6. | 10. | 100 |
| Picnic: | | | | | | |
| Raw | 1 lb. (weighed with bone & skin) | 260 | 92.2 | 33. | 59. | 231 |
| Simmered, lean & fat | 4 oz. | 74 | 34.6 | 12. | 22. | 101 |
| Simmered, lean only | 4 oz. | 74 | 11.1 | 5. | 7. | 100 |
| Spareribs: | | | | | | |
| Raw, with bone | 1 lb. (weighed with bone) | 775 | 89.7 | 32. | 58. | 169 |

(USDA): United States Department of Agriculture
*Prepared as Package Directs

281

| Food and Description | Measure or Quantity | Sodium (mg.) | Fats in grams — Total | Satu- rated | Unsatu- rated | Choles- terol (mg.) |
|---|---|---|---|---|---|---|
| Raw, without bone | 1 lb. (weighed without bone) | 1,295 | 150.6 | 54. | 97. | 281 |
| Braised, lean & fat | 4 oz. | 74 | 44.1 | 16. | 28. | 101 |
| Cured, light commercial cure: | | | | | | |
| Bacon (see **BACON**) | | | | | | |
| Boston butt (USDA): | | | | | | |
| Raw | 1 lb. (weighed with bone & skin) | | 101.7 | 37. | 65. | |
| Roasted, lean & fat | 4 oz. | | 29.1 | 10. | 19. | |
| Roasted, lean only | 4 oz. | 1,055 | 15.6 | 7. | 9. | |
| Ham (See also **HAM**) (USDA): | | | | | | |
| Raw | 1 lb. (weighed with bone & skin) | | 89.7 | 32. | 58. | |
| Raw, lean only, ground | 1 cup (6 oz.) | 1,870 | 14.4 | 5. | 9. | |
| Roasted, lean & fat | 4 oz. | | 25.1 | 9. | 16. | |
| Roasted, lean only: | 4 oz. | 1,055 | 10.0 | 3. | 7. | |
| Chopped | 1 cup (4.9 oz.) | 1,283 | 12.1 | 4. | 8. | |
| Diced | 1 cup (5.2 oz.) | 1,367 | 12.9 | 4. | 9. | |
| Ground | 1 cup (3.8 oz.) | 1,014 | 9.6 | 3. | 6. | |
| Picnic (USDA): | | | | | | |
| Raw | 1 lb. (weighed with bone & skin) | | 87.8 | 32. | 56. | |
| Roasted, lean & fat | 4 oz. | | 28.6 | 10. | 18. | |
| Roasted, lean only | 4 oz. | 1,055 | 11.2 | 5. | 7. | |
| **PORK, CANNED,** chopped luncheon meat (USDA)[1]: | 1 oz. | 350 | 7.1 | 3. | 5. | |
| Chopped | 1 cup (4.8 oz.) | 1,678 | 33.9 | 12. | 22. | |
| Diced | 1 cup (5 oz.) | 1,740 | 35.1 | 13. | 22. | |
| **PORK DINNER OR ENTREE:** | | | | | | |
| Canned (Hunt's) *Minute Gourmet* Microwave Entree Maker, cajun: | | | | | | |
| Without pork | 3.9 oz. | 1,220 | 1. | | | |
| *With pork | 6.6 oz. | 1,270 | 23. | | | |
| Frozen (Swanson) loin of | 11¼-oz. dinner | 710 | 11. | | | |
| **PORK & GRAVY,** 90% pork, canned (USDA) | 4 oz. | | 20.2 | 7. | 13. | |

(USDA): United States Department of Agriculture
*Prepared as Package Directs
[1]Principal source of fat: pork.

| Food and Description | Measure or Quantity | Sodium (mg.) | Total | Satu-rated | Unsatu-rated | Choles-terol (mg.) |
|---|---|---|---|---|---|---|
| **PORK RINDS,** fried, *Baken-ets* (See also other brand names) | 1 oz. | 490 | 7.4 | 3. | 5. | 6 |
| **PORK SAUSAGE** (See **SAUSAGE, Pork**) | | | | | | |
| **PORT WINE:** | | | | | | |
| (Gold Seal) 19% alcohol | 3 fl. oz. (3.3 oz.) | 3 | 0.0 | | | (0) |
| (Great Western) Solera, 18% alcohol | 3 fl. oz. | 34 | 0.0 | | | 0 |
| (Great Western) Solera, tawny, 18% alcohol | 3 fl. oz. | 34 | 0.0 | | | 0 |
| *POSTUM,* instant | 1 cup (6 oz.) | 3 | Tr. | | | 0 |
| **POTATO:** | | | | | | |
| Raw, whole (USDA) | 1 lb. (weighed unpared) | 11 | .4 | | | 0 |
| Raw, pared (USDA): | | | | | | |
| Chopped | 1 cup (5.2 oz.) | 4 | .1 | | | 0 |
| Diced | 1 cup (5.5 oz.) | 5 | .2 | | | 0 |
| Slices | 1 cup (5.2 oz.) | 4 | .1 | | | 0 |
| Cooked: | | | | | | |
| Au gratin or scalloped, without cheese (USDA)[1] | ½ cup (4.3 oz.) | 433 | 4.8 | 2. | 2. | 7 |
| Au gratin, with cheese (USDA)[2] | ½ cup (4.3 oz.) | 545 | 9.6 | 5. | 5. | 18 |
| Baked, peeled after baking, no salt added (USDA) | 2½" dia. potato (3.5 oz., 3 raw per lb.) | 4 | .1 | | | 0 |
| Baked, peeled after baking, salt added (USDA) | 2½" dia. potato (3.5 oz., 3 raw per lb.) | 234 | .1 | | | 0 |
| Boiled, peeled after boiling, no salt added (USDA) | 4.8-oz. potato (3 raw per lb.) | 4 | .1 | | | 0 |
| Boiled, peeled after boiling, salt added (USDA) | 4.8-oz. potato (3 raw per lb.) | 321 | .1 | | | 0 |

(USDA): United States Department of Agriculture
*Prepared as Package Directs
[1]Principal sources of fat: butter & milk.
[2]Principal sources of fat: cheese, butter & milk.

| Food and Description | Measure or Quantity | Sodium (mg.) | — Fats in grams — | | | Cholesterol (mg.) |
|---|---|---|---|---|---|---|
| | | | Total | Saturated | Unsaturated | |
| Boiled, peeled before boiling, no salt added (USDA): | | | | | | |
| Whole | 4.3-oz. potato (3 raw per lb.) | 2 | .1 | | | 0 |
| Diced | ½ cup (2.8 oz.) | 2 | <.1 | | | 0 |
| Mashed | ½ cup (3.7 oz.) | 2 | .1 | | | 0 |
| Riced | ½ cup (4 oz.) | 2 | .1 | | | 0 |
| Slices | ½ cup (2.8 oz.) | 2 | <.1 | | | 0 |
| Boiled, peeled before boiling, salt added (USDA): | | | | | | |
| Whole | 4.3-oz. potato (3 raw per lb.) | 288 | .1 | | | 0 |
| Diced | ½ cup (2.8 oz.) | 184 | <.1 | | | 0 |
| Mashed | ½ cup (3.7 oz.) | 245 | .1 | | | 0 |
| Riced | ½ cup (4 oz.) | 269 | .1 | | | 0 |
| Slices | ½ cup (2.8 oz.) | 189 | <.1 | | | 0 |
| French-fried in deep fat, no salt added (USDA)[1] | 10 pieces (2" × ½" × ½", 2 oz.) | 3 | 7.5 | 2. | 6. | |
| French-fried in deep fat, salt added (USDA)[1] | 10 pieces (2" × ½" × ½", 2 oz.) | 135 | 7.5 | 2. | 6. | |
| French-fried (McDonald's) | 1 serving (2.4 oz.) | 117 | 10.4 | | | |
| Hash-browned (USDA)[2] | ½ cup (3.4 oz.) | 281 | 11.4 | 3. | 8. | |
| Mashed, milk added (USDA) | ½ cup (3.5 oz.) | 295 | .7 | | | |
| Mashed, milk & butter added (USDA)[3] | ½ cup (3.5 oz.) | 324 | 4.2 | 2. | 2. | |
| Pan-fried from raw (USDA) | ½ cup (3 oz.) | 190 | 12.1 | 3. | 10. | |
| Scalloped (See Au gratin) | | | | | | |
| Canned: | | | | | | |
| Solids & liq., no added salt (USDA) | 1 cup (8.8 oz.) | 2 | .5 | | | 0 |
| Solids & liq., added salt (USDA) | 1 cup (8.8 oz.) | 590 | .5 | | | 0 |
| (Allen) *Butterfield* | ½ cup (4 oz.) | 360 | <1.0 | | | |
| (Del Monte) sliced or whole, solids & liq. | ½ cup (4 oz.) | 355 | 0.0 | | | |

(USDA): United States Department of Agriculture
*Prepared as Package Directs
[1]Principal source of fat: cottonseed oil.
[2]Principal source of fat: vegetable shortening.
[3]Principal sources of fat: butter & milk.

| Food and Description | Measure or Quantity | Sodium (mg.) | — Fats in grams — | | Choles- terol (mg.) |
|---|---|---|---|---|---|
| | | | Total | Satu- rated | Unsatu- rated | |

| Food and Description | Measure or Quantity | Sodium (mg.) | Total | Saturated | Unsaturated | Cholesterol (mg.) |
|---|---|---|---|---|---|---|
| (Larsen) *Freshlike* solids & liq. | ½ cup (4.5 oz.) | 260 | 0.0 | | | |
| Dehydrated, mashed: | | | | | | |
| Flakes, without milk (USDA): | | | | | | |
| Dry | ½ cup (.8 oz.) | 20 | .1 | | | 0 |
| *Prepared with water, milk & fat [1] | ½ cup (3.8 oz.) | 247 | 3.4 | 2. | 1. | |
| Granules, without milk (USDA): | | | | | | |
| Dry | ½ cup (3.5 oz.) | 84 | .6 | | | 0 |
| *Prepared with water. milk & butter [1] | ½ cup (3.7 oz.) | 256 | 3.8 | 2. | 2. | |
| Granules with milk (USDA): | | | | | | |
| Dry | ½ cup (3.5 oz.) | 82 | 1.1 | | | |
| *Prepared with water & fat [2] | ½ cup (3.7 oz.) | 246 | 2.3 | 1. | 1. | |
| Frozen: | | | | | | |
| (USDA): | | | | | | |
| Diced for hash browning | 4 oz. | 9 | Tr. | | | |
| Diced, hash browned [3] | 4 oz. | 339 | 13.0 | 3. | 10. | |
| French fried: | | | | | | |
| Not thawed: | | | | | | |
| No salt added [3] | 9-oz. pkg. | 8 | 16.6 | 5. | 12. | |
| Salt added [3] | 9-oz. pkg. | 602 | 16.6 | 5. | 12. | |
| Heated, no added salt [3] | 10 pieces (2″ × 1 ½″ × ½″) .2 oz. | 2 | 4.8 | 2. | 3. | |
| Mashed, not thawed | 4 oz. | 90 | .1 | | | |
| (Birds Eye): | | | | | | |
| Cottage fries | ¼ of 14-oz. pkg. | 14 | 4.2 | | | 0 |
| Crinkle cuts, regular | 3 oz. | 36 | 3.8 | | | 0 |
| French fries: | | | | | | |
| Regular | 3 oz. | 23 | 4.0 | | | 0 |
| *Deep Gold* | 3 oz. | 280 | 6.0 | | | 0 |
| Hash browns, shredded | 3 oz. | 21 | .3 | | | 0 |
| Shoestring | 3 oz. | 45 | 5.2 | | | 0 |
| Steak fries | 3 oz. | 25 | 3.4 | | | 0 |
| Tasti-fries | 2½ oz. | 268 | 6.9 | | | 0 |
| Tasti-puffs | 2½ oz. | 401 | 11.6 | | | 32 |
| Whole, peeled | ⅒ of 32-oz. pkg. | 5 | Tr. | | | 0 |

(USDA): United States Department of Agriculture
*Prepared as Package Directs
[1]Principal sources of fat: butter & milk.
[2]Principal source of fat: butter.
[3]Principal source of fat: cottonseed oil.

285

| Food and Description | Measure or Quantity | Sodium (mg.) | Fats in grams — Total | Satu- rated | Unsatu- rated | Choles- terol (mg.) |
|---|---|---|---|---|---|---|
| (Empire Kosher) french fries | 3 oz. | 35 | 4.0 | | | |
| (Green Giant) sliced in butter sauce | 1/2 cup | 470 | 2.0 | | | |
| (Larsen) diced | 4 oz. | 40 | 0.0 | | | |
| (McKenzie) whole | 3 1/2 oz. | 20 | 0.0 | | | |
| **POTATO & BACON,** canned au gratin (Hormel), *Short Orders* | 7 1/2-oz. can | 942 | 14.0 | | | |
| **POTATO & BEEF,** canned (Hormel) *Dinty Moore, Short Orders* | 7 1/2-oz. can | | 12.0 | | | |
| **POTATO CHIP:** | | | | | | |
| (Cottage Fries) no salt added | 1 oz. | 5 | 11.0 | | | |
| *Delta Gold:* | | | | | | |
| Regular or dip style | 1 oz. | 160 | 11.0 | | | 0 |
| Mesquite flavored Barbecue | 1 oz. | 240 | 11.0 | | | 0 |
| (Featherweight) unsalted | 1 oz. | 6 | 11.0 | | | |
| (Laura Scudder's): | | | | | | |
| Barbecue | 1 oz. | 200 | 9.0 | | | 0 |
| Sour cream & onion | 1 oz. | 170 | 9.0 | | | |
| (Lay's): | | | | | | |
| Regular | 1 oz. | 200 | 10.0 | | | 0 |
| Barbecue | 1 oz. | 310 | 9.0 | | | 0 |
| Italian cheese | 1 oz. | 210 | 9.0 | | | 0 |
| Salt & vinegar | 1 oz. | 460 | 9.0 | | | 0 |
| Sour cream & onion | 1 oz. | 250 | 10.0 | | | 0 |
| Unsalted | 1 oz. | 10 | 10.0 | | | 0 |
| (New York Deli) | 1 oz. | 120 | 11.0 | | | (0) |
| (O'Grady's): | | | | | | |
| Regular | 1 oz. | 210 | 9.0 | | | 0 |
| Au gratin | 1 oz. | 330 | 8.0 | | | 0 |
| (Pringle's): | | | | | | |
| Regular | 1 oz. | 216 | 9.0 | | | 0 |
| Light | 1 oz. | 152 | 8.2 | | | 0 |
| Rippled | 1 oz. | 250 | 11.9 | | | 0 |
| (Ruffles): | | | | | | |
| Regular | 1 oz. | 190 | 10.0 | | | 0 |
| Cajun spice | 1 oz. | 240 | 10.0 | | | 0 |
| Sour cream & onion | 1 oz. | 240 | 9.0 | | | 0 |

(USDA): United States Department of Agriculture
*Prepared as Package Directs

| Food and Description | Measure or Quantity | Sodium (mg.) | —Fats in grams— | | | Choles-terol (mg.) |
|---|---|---|---|---|---|---|
| | | | Total | Satu-rated | Unsatu-rated | |
| (Snyder's): | | | | | | |
| Regular | 1 oz. | 140 | 10.0 | | | 0 |
| No salt added | 1 oz. | 10 | 10.0 | | | 0 |
| (Tom's): | | | | | | |
| Regular | 1 oz. | 200 | 11.0 | | | (0) |
| Barbecue | 1 oz. | 280 | 11.0 | | | (0) |
| Hot | 1 oz. | 310 | 10.0 | | | (0) |
| Vinegar & salt | 1 oz. | 280 | 10.0 | | | (0) |
| (Wise): | | | | | | |
| Regular: | | | | | | |
| Barbecue | 1 oz. | 240 | | | | |
| Garlic & onion | 1 oz. | 250 | | | | |
| Natural | 1 oz. | 150 | | | | |
| Cottage fries, no salt added | 1 oz. | 10 | | | | |
| *Ridgies*, natural | 1 oz. | 150 | | | | |
| **POTATO & HAM,** canned | | | | | | |
| (Hormel) scalloped | 7 1/2-oz. can | 1,189 | 16.0 | | | |
| **POTATO MIX:** | | | | | | |
| *Au gratin (Betty Crocker) | 1/2 cup | 605 | 6.0 | | | |
| *Au gratin (French's) | 1/2 cup | 460 | 5.0 | | | |
| *Buds (Betty Crocker) | 1/2 cup | 355 | 6.0 | | | |
| *Mashed, granules, salt added (French's) | 1/2 cup | 320 | 6.0 | | | |
| *Scalloped (Betty Crocker) | 1/2 cup | 570 | 6.0 | | | |
| *Scalloped (French's) real cheese | 1/2 cup | 380 | 5.0 | | | |
| **\*POTATO PANCAKE MIX** | | | | | | |
| (French's) | 3" pancake | 130 | .7 | | | |
| (French's) | 3 small pancakes (1/4 pkg.) | 375 | 1.4 | | | |
| **POTATO SALAD:** | | | | | | |
| Home recipe, with cooked salad dressing & seasonings (USDA)[1] | 4 oz. | 599 | 3.2 | 1. | 2. | |
| Home recipe, with mayonnaise & French dressing, hard-cooked eggs & seasonings (USDA)[2] | 1/2 cup (4.4 oz.) | 600 | 11.5 | 2. | 9. | 81 |

(USDA): United States Department of Agriculture
*Prepared as Package Directs
[1]Principal sources of fat: butter, milk & egg.
[2]Principal sources of fat: soybean oil, cottonseed oil, corn oil & eggs.

| Food and Description | Measure or Quantity | Sodium (mg.) | Total | Fats in grams — Satu- rated | Unsatu- rated | Choles- terol (mg.) |
|---|---|---|---|---|---|---|
| **POTATO STARCH** | | | | | | |
| (Manischewitz) pure | ½ cup (3.1 oz.) | 0 | 0.0 | | | 0 |
| **POTATO STICK:** | | | | | | |
| (USDA)[1,2] | 1 oz. | 284 | 10.3 | 3. | 8. | |
| (Durkee) O & C | 1½ oz. | 383 | 15.0 | | | |
| **POTATO, STUFFED, BAKED** | | | | | | |
| frozen (Green Giant) with sour cream & chives | 5 oz. | 580 | 10.0 | | | |
| **POUND CAKE (See CAKE, Pound)** | | | | | | |
| **PRESERVE,** sweetened (See also individual listings by flavor): | | | | | | |
| (USDA) | 1 oz. | 3 | <.1 | | | 0 |
| (USDA) | 1 T. (.7 oz.) | 2 | Tr. | | | 0 |
| **PRETZEL:** | | | | | | |
| (USDA)[3] | 1 oz. | 476 | 1.3 | | | |
| Dutch, twist (USDA)[3] | 1 pretzel (.6 oz.) | 269 | .7 | | | |
| Stick, small (USDA)[3] | 10 small sticks (2¼", 3 grams) | 50 | .1 | | | |
| Stick, regular (USDA)[3] | 5 regular sticks (3⅛", 3 grams) | 50 | .1 | | | |
| Thin, twist (USDA)[3] | 1 pretzel (6 grams) | 101 | .3 | | | |
| (Eagle Snacks) | 1 oz. | 570 | 2.0 | | | 0 |
| (Estee) unsalted | 1 piece (1.3 grams) | <1 | Tr. | | | 0 |
| *Mister Salty* (Nabisco): | | | | | | |
| Regular: | | | | | | |
| Dutch | 1 piece | 220 | .5 | | | 0 |
| Logs | 1 piece | 57 | .1 | | | 0 |
| Nuggets | 1 piece | 26 | Tr. | | | 0 |
| Rods | 1 piece | 250 | .5 | | | 0 |

(USDA): United States Department of Agriculture
\*Prepared as Package Directs
[1]Principal source of fat: cottonseed oil.
[2]Sodium content is variable & may be as high as 284 mg. per oz.
[3]Sodium content is variable. For example, *Very-Thin* pretzel sticks contain about twice the average amount listed.

| Food and Description | Measure or Quantity | Sodium (mg.) | Fats in grams — Total | Satu- rated | Unsatu- rated | Choles- terol (mg.) |
|---|---|---|---|---|---|---|
| Sticks, *Veri-Thin* | 1 piece | 17 | Tr. | | | 0 |
| Twists | 1 piece | 118 | .4 | | | 0 |
| Juniors | 1 piece | 18 | Tr. | | | 0 |
| *Rold Gold* (Frito-Lay): | | | | | | |
| Rods | 1 oz. | 550 | 2.0 | | | 0 |
| *Tiny Tim* | 1 oz. | 610 | 1.0 | | | 0 |
| Twists | 1 oz. | 470 | 1.0 | | | 0 |
| (Snyder's) hard | 1 oz. | 548 | 7.1 | | | (0) |
| (Wise) nugget | 1 oz. | 600 | | | | |

**PRICKLY PEAR,** fresh (USDA):

| | | | | | | |
|---|---|---|---|---|---|---|
| Whole | 1 lb. (weighed with rind & seeds) | 4 | .2 | | | 0 |
| Flesh only | 4 oz. | 2 | .1 | | | 0 |

**PRODUCT 19,** cereal

| | | | | | | |
|---|---|---|---|---|---|---|
| (Kellogg's) | 1 cup (1 oz.) | 290 | 0.0 | | | (0) |

**PROSCIUTTO** (Hormel)

| | | | | | | |
|---|---|---|---|---|---|---|
| boneless | 1 oz. | 502 | 7.0 | | | |

**PRUNE:**

Dried, "softenized," uncooked:

| | | | | | | |
|---|---|---|---|---|---|---|
| Small (USDA) | 1 prune (5 grams) | <1 | Tr. | | | 0 |
| Medium, whole with pits (USDA) | 1 cup (6.6 oz.) | 13 | 1.0 | | | 0 |
| Medium (USDA) | 1 prune (7 grams) | <1 | Tr. | | | 0 |
| Large (USDA) | 1 prune (9 grams) | <1 | Tr. | | | 0 |
| Pitted, chopped (USDA) | 1 cup (5.3 oz.) | 12 | .9 | | | 0 |
| Pitted, ground (USDA) | 1 cup (9.7 oz.) | 22 | 1.6 | | | 0 |
| Dried, moist-pak (Del Monte) | 1 cup (8 oz.) | 5 | .9 | | | 0 |
| Dried, ready-to-eat (Del Monte) | 1 cup (6.6 oz.) | 2 | 4.7 | | | 0 |
| Dried, "softenized," cooked, unsweetened (USDA) | 1 cup (17-18 med. with 1/3 cup liq., 9.5 oz.) | 10 | .7 | | | 0 |
| Dried, "softenized," cooked with sugar (USDA) | 1 cup (16-18 prunes & 1/3 cup liq., 11.1 oz.) | 9 | .6 | | | 0 |

(USDA): United States Department of Agriculture
*Prepared as Package Directs

PRUNE (Continued)

| Food and Description | Measure or Quantity | Sodium (mg.) | Total | Satu-rated | Unsatu-rated | Choles-terol (mg.) |
|---|---|---|---|---|---|---|
| **Dehydrated (USDA):** | | | | | | |
| Nugget-type & pieces | 8 oz. | 25 | 1.1 | | | 0 |
| Nugget-type & pieces, cooked with sugar, solids & liq. | 1 cup (8.9 oz.) | 10 | .5 | | | 0 |
| Canned: | | | | | | |
| Cooked (Sunsweet) | 1 cup | | .4 | | | (0) |
| Stewed (Del Monte) | 1 cup (9.4 oz.) | 3 | 1.1 | | | 0 |
| Stewed, pitted (Del Monte) | 1 cup (9.2 oz.) | 14 | 1.3 | | | 0 |
| **PRUNE JUICE:** | | | | | | |
| (USDA) | ½ cup (4.5 oz.) | 2 | .1 | | | 0 |
| (Del Monte) | ½ cup (4.3 oz.) | <10 | 0.0 | | | 0 |
| (Sunsweet) | 6 fl. oz. | 4 | <.1 | | | (0) |
| **PRUNE WHIP,** home recipe | | | | | | |
| (USDA) | 1 cup (4.8 oz.) | 221 | .3 | | | |
| **PUDDING OR PIE FILLING:** | | | | | | |
| Home recipe (USDA): | | | | | | |
| Chocolate | ½ cup (4.6 oz.) | 73 | 6.9 | | | |
| Rice, with raisins [1] | ½ cup (4.7 oz.) | 94 | 4.1 | 2.6 | 1.5 | 15 |
| Tapioca: | | | | | | |
| Apple | ½ cup (4.4 oz.) | 64 | .1 | | | |
| Cream | ½ cup (2.9 oz.) | 128 | 4.2 | | | 80 |
| Vanilla, blancmange | ½ cup (4.5 oz.) | 83 | 5.0 | | | 18 |
| Canned, regular pack: | | | | | | |
| Banana: | | | | | | |
| (Del Monte) | 5 oz. | 277 | 5.3 | | | |
| (Hunt's) *Snack-Pak* | 4¼ oz. | 180 | 9.0 | | | |
| (Thank You Brand) | ½ cup (4.6 oz.) | 182 | 3.9 | | | 1 |
| Butterscotch: | | | | | | |
| (Hunt's) *Snack-Pak* | 4¼ oz. | 200 | 8.0 | | | |
| (Swiss Miss) | 4 oz. | 210 | 6.0 | | | |
| (Thank You Brand) | ½ cup (4.6 oz.) | 221 | 3.9 | | | 1 |
| Chocolate: | | | | | | |
| (Hunt's) *Snack-Pak:* | | | | | | |
| Regular, German or marshmallows | 4¼ oz. | 135 | 7.0 | | | |
| Fudge | 4¼ oz. | 140 | 9.0 | | | |
| (Swiss Miss) regular | 4 oz. | 200 | 6.0 | | | |
| (Thank You Brand) fudge | ½ cup (4.6 oz.) | 130 | 3.9 | | | 1 |
| Lemon (Hunt's) *Snack-Pak* | 4¼ oz. | 70 | 3.0 | | | |

(USDA): United States Department of Agriculture
*Prepared as Package Directs
[1]Principal source of fat: milk.

290

| Food and Description | Measure or Quantity | Sodium (mg.) | —Fats in grams— | | | Choles- terol (mg.) |
|---|---|---|---|---|---|---|
| | | | Total | Satu- rated | Unsatu- rated | |
| **Rice:** | | | | | | |
| (Comstock) | 3¾ oz. | 450 | 3.0 | | | |
| (Hunt's) *Snack-Pak* | 4¼ oz. | 200 | 10.0 | | | |
| **Tapioca:** | | | | | | |
| (Hunt's) *Snack-Pak* | 4¼ oz. | 140 | 5.0 | | | |
| (Swiss Miss) | 4 oz. | 190 | 4.0 | | | |
| (Thank You Brand) | ½ cup (4.6 oz.) | 169 | 2.6 | | | 1 |
| **Vanilla:** | | | | | | |
| (Hunt's) *Snack-Pak* | 4¼ oz. | 160 | 7.0 | | | |
| (Swiss Miss) | 4 oz. | 200 | 6.0 | | | |
| **Canned, dietetic** | | | | | | |
| **(Estee):** | | | | | | |
| Butterscotch | ½ cup | 80 | <1 | | | 2 |
| Chocolate or vanilla | ½ cup | 75 | <1 | | | 2 |
| *Mix, regular: | | | | | | |
| **Banana cream:** | | | | | | |
| **(Jell-O):** | | | | | | |
| Regular | ½ cup | 257 | 4.1 | | | 18 |
| Instant | ½ cup | 445 | 4.2 | | | 16 |
| **(Royal):** | | | | | | |
| Regular | ½ cup | 210 | 4.0 | | | 14 |
| Instant | ½ cup | 390 | 5.0 | | | 15 |
| Butter pecan (Jell-O) instant | ½ cup | 442 | 4.9 | | | 16 |
| **Butterscotch:** | | | | | | |
| **(Jell-O):** | | | | | | |
| Regular | ½ cup | 247 | 4.3 | | | 16 |
| Instant | ½ cup | 483 | 4.3 | | | 16 |
| **(Royal):** | | | | | | |
| Regular | ½ cup | 210 | 4.0 | | | 14 |
| Instant | ½ cup | 390 | 5.0 | | | 15 |
| **Chocolate:** | | | | | | |
| **(Jell-O):** | | | | | | |
| Plain, regular | ½ cup | 170 | 4.4 | | | 16 |
| **Fudge:** | | | | | | |
| Regular | ½ cup | 171 | 4.4 | | | 17 |
| Instant | ½ cup | 482 | 4.4 | | | 17 |
| Milk, regular | ½ cup | 173 | 4.4 | | | 17 |
| **(Royal) plain:** | | | | | | |
| Regular | ½ cup | 150 | 4.0 | | | 15 |
| Instant | ½ cup | 390 | 4.0 | | | 15 |
| **Coconut:** | | | | | | |
| (Jell-O) cream, regular | ½ cup | 216 | 6.6 | | | 18 |
| (Royal) toasted, instant | ½ cup | 350 | 4.0 | | | 15 |

(USDA): United States Department of Agriculture
*Prepared as Package Directs

291

| Food and Description | Measure or Quantity | Sodium (mg.) | Fats in grams — Total | Satu- rated | Unsatu- rated | Choles- terol (mg.) |
|---|---|---|---|---|---|---|
| Custard: | | | | | | |
| (Jell-O) | ½ cup | 222 | 5.0 | | | 81 |
| (Royal) | ½ cup | 115 | 5.0 | | | 14 |
| Flan (Royal) regular, with caramel sauce | ½ cup | 115 | 5.0 | | | 14 |
| Lemon: | | | | | | |
| (Jell-O): | | | | | | |
| Regular | ½ cup | 94 | 1.9 | | | 93 |
| Instant | ½ cup | 397 | 4.3 | | | 16 |
| (Royal) instant | ½ cup | 350 | 5.0 | | | 15 |
| Lime (Royal) regular | ½ cup | 120 | 3.0 | | | |
| Pineapple cream (Jell-O) instant | ½ cup | 400 | 4.3 | | | 16 |
| Pistachio (Jell-O) instant | ½ cup | 445 | 4.9 | | | 17 |
| Raspberry (Salada) Danish Dessert | ½ cup | 5 | 0.0 | | | |
| Rice (Jell-O) | ½ cup | 158 | 4.1 | | | 16 |
| Tapioca: | | | | | | |
| (Jell-O) | ½ cup | 170 | 4.0 | | | 16 |
| (Royal) vanilla | ½ cup | 150 | 1.0 | | | 14 |
| Vanilla: | | | | | | |
| (Jell-O): | | | | | | |
| Regular | ½ cup | 198 | 4.0 | | | 17 |
| Instant | ½ cup | 422 | 4.0 | | | 16 |
| (Royal) regular | ½ cup | 210 | 4.0 | | | 15 |
| *Mix, dietetic: | | | | | | |
| Butterscotch: | | | | | | |
| (Dia-Mel) | ½ cup | 80 | 0.0 | | | 2 |
| (D-Zerta) | ½ cup | 115 | Tr. | | | 3 |
| (Estee) | ½ cup | 80 | <1 | | | 2 |
| (Royal) instant | ½ cup | 470 | 2.0 | | | |
| Chocolate: | | | | | | |
| (D-Zerta) | ½ cup | 116 | .4 | | | 3 |
| (Estee) instant | ½ cup | 75 | <1 | | | 2 |
| (Louis Sherry) | ½ cup | 80 | <1 | | | 2 |
| Lemon (Estee) | ½ cup | 75 | <1 | | | 2 |
| Vanilla: | | | | | | |
| (Estee) | ½ cup | 75 | <1 | | | 2 |
| (Royal) instant | ½ cup | 470 | 2.0 | | | |
| **PUDDING STIX** (Good Humor) | 1¾ fl. oz. pop | 65 | 2.0 | | | |

(USDA): United States Department of Agriculture
*Prepared as Package Directs

| Food and Description | Measure or Quantity | Sodium (mg.) | —Fats in grams— | | | Choles-terol (mg.) |
|---|---|---|---|---|---|---|
| | | | Total | Satu-rated | Unsatu-rated | |
| **PUDDING SUNDAE** (Swiss Miss): | | | | | | |
| Chocolate | 4 oz. | 180 | 7.0 | | | |
| Mint or peanut butter | 4 oz. | 180 | 11.0 | | | |
| **PUFF** (See **CRACKER** or individual kinds of hors d'oeuvres, such as **CHICKEN PUFF**) | | | | | | |
| **PUFFED OAT CEREAL** (USDA): | | | | | | |
| Added nutrients | 1 oz. | 359 | 1.6 | | | 0 |
| Sugar-coated, added nutrients | 1 oz. | 167 | 1.0 | | | 0 |
| **PUFFED RICE CEREAL:** | | | | | | |
| (USDA) added nutrients, unsalted | 1 cup (.5 oz.) | < 1 | < .1 | | | 0 |
| (USDA) honey & added nutrients | 1 oz. | 200 | .2 | | | 0 |
| (USDA) honey or cocoa fat, added nutrients | 1 oz. | 101 | 1.1 | | | 0 |
| (Malt-O-Meal) | ½ oz. | 1 | < .1 | | | (0) |
| (Quaker) | 1 cup (½ oz.) | < 1 | .1 | | | (0) |
| **PUMPKIN:** | | | | | | |
| Fresh, whole (USDA) | 1 lb. (weighed with rind & seeds) | 3 | .3 | | | 0 |
| Flesh only (USDA) | 4 oz. | 1 | .1 | | | 0 |
| Canned: | | | | | | |
| Salted (USDA) | ½ cup (4.3 oz.) | 288 | .4 | | | 0 |
| Unsalted (USDA) | ½ cup (4.3 oz.) | 2 | .4 | | | 0 |
| (Del Monte) | ½ cup (4.3 oz.) | < 10 | 0.0 | | | 0 |
| (Libby's) | ½ cup (4.1 oz.) | 5 | .5 | | | (0) |
| **PUMPKIN SEED,** dry (USDA): | | | | | | |
| Whole | 4 oz. (weighed in hull) | | 39.2 | 7. | 32. | 0 |
| Hulled | 4 oz. | | 53.0 | 9. | 44. | 0 |

(USDA): United States Department of Agriculture
*Prepared as Package Directs

| Food and Description | Measure or Quantity | Sodium (mg.) | —Fats in grams— | | | Choles-terol (mg.) |
| --- | --- | --- | --- | --- | --- | --- |
| | | | Total | Satu-rated | Unsatu-rated | |
| **PURSLANE,** including stems (USDA): | | | | | | |
| Raw | 1 lb. | | 1.8 | | | 0 |
| Boiled, drained | 4 oz. | | .3 | | | 0 |

# Q

| | | | | | | |
| --- | --- | --- | --- | --- | --- | --- |
| **QUAIL,** raw (USDA): | | | | | | |
| Ready-to-cook | 1 lb. (weighed with bones) | | 27.8 | | | |
| Meat & skin only | 4 oz. | 45 | 7.9 | | | |
| Giblets | 2 oz. | | 3.5 | | | |
| **QUIK** (Nestlé): | | | | | | |
| Chocolate | 1 tsp. | 18 | .5 | | | 0 |
| Strawberry | 1 tsp. | 0 | 0.0 | | | |
| **QUINCE,** fresh (USDA): | | | | | | |
| Untrimmed | 1 lb. (weighed with skin & seeds) | 11 | .3 | | | 0 |
| Flesh only | 4 oz. | 5 | .1 | | | 0 |
| **QUISP,** cereal (Quaker) | 1⅙ cups (1 oz.) | 189 | 2.7 | | | 0 |

# R

| | | | | | | |
| --- | --- | --- | --- | --- | --- | --- |
| **RABBIT** (USDA): | | | | | | |
| Domesticated: | | | | | | |
| Ready-to-cook | 1 lb. (weighed with bones) | 154 | 29.0 | 11. | 18. | |
| Raw meat only | 4 oz. | 49 | 9.1 | | | 74 |
| Stewed, flesh only | 4 oz. | 46 | 11.5 | | | 103 |
| Stewed, flesh only, chopped or diced | 1 cup (4.9 oz.) | 57 | 14.1 | | | 127 |
| Wild, ready-to-cook | 1 lb. (weighed with bones) | | 18.1 | | | |
| Wild, raw, meat only | 4 oz. | | 5.7 | | | |
| **RACCOON,** roasted, meat only (USDA) | 4 oz. | | 16.4 | | | |

(USDA): United States Department of Agriculture
*Prepared as Package Directs

| Food and Description | Measure or Quantity | Sodium (mg.) | — Fats in grams — | | | Cholesterol (mg.) |
|---|---|---|---|---|---|---|
| | | | Total | Saturated | Unsaturated | |

**RADISH** (USDA):
Common, raw:

| Food and Description | Measure or Quantity | Sodium (mg.) | Total | Saturated | Unsaturated | Cholesterol (mg.) |
|---|---|---|---|---|---|---|
| Untrimmed, without tops | ½ lb. (weighed untrimmed) | 36 | .2 | | | 0 |
| Trimmed, whole | 4 small radishes (1.4 oz.) | 7 | <.1 | | | 0 |
| Trimmed, whole | 1 cup (4.7 oz.) | 24 | .1 | | | 0 |
| Trimmed, sliced | ½ cup (2 oz.) | 10 | <.1 | | | 0 |
| Oriental, raw, without tops | ½ lb. (weighed unpared) | | .2 | | | 0 |
| Oriental, raw, trimmed & pared | 4 oz. | | .1 | | | 0 |

**RAISIN:**
Dried:

| Food and Description | Measure or Quantity | Sodium (mg.) | Total | Saturated | Unsaturated | Cholesterol (mg.) |
|---|---|---|---|---|---|---|
| Whole (USDA) | 4 oz. | 31 | .2 | | | 0 |
| Whole (USDA) | 1 pkg. (.5 oz.) | 4 | <.1 | | | 0 |
| Whole, pressed down (USDA) | ½ cup (2.9 oz.) | 22 | .2 | | | 0 |
| Whole, pressed down (USDA) | 1 T. (.4 oz.) | 3 | <.1 | | | 0 |
| Chopped (USDA) | ½ cup (2.9 oz.) | 22 | .2 | | | 0 |
| Ground (USDA) | ½ cup (4.7 oz.) | 36 | .3 | | | 0 |
| Seedless, California Thompson (Sun-Maid) | 1 oz. | 4 | 0.0 | | | 0 |
| Seedless, golden (Del Monte) | 3 oz. | 15 | 0.0 | | | 0 |
| Cooked, added sugar, solids & liq. (USDA) | ½ cup (4.3 oz.) | 16 | .1 | | | 0 |

**RAISINS RICE & RYE,** cereal

| Food and Description | Measure or Quantity | Sodium (mg.) | Total | Saturated | Unsaturated | Cholesterol (mg.) |
|---|---|---|---|---|---|---|
| (Kellogg's) | ¾ cup (1.3 oz.) | 235 | 0.0 | | | |

**RAJA FISH** (See **SKATE**)

**RALSTON,** cereal, regular or instant

| Food and Description | Measure or Quantity | Sodium (mg.) | Total | Saturated | Unsaturated | Cholesterol (mg.) |
|---|---|---|---|---|---|---|
| instant | ¼ cup (1 oz.) | 3 | .6 | | | |

**RASPBERRY:**
Black:
Fresh:

| Food and Description | Measure or Quantity | Sodium (mg.) | Total | Saturated | Unsaturated | Cholesterol (mg.) |
|---|---|---|---|---|---|---|
| (USDA) | ½ lb. (weighed with caps & stems) | 2 | 3.1 | | | 0 |

(USDA): United States Department of Agriculture
*Prepared as Package Directs

295

| Food and Description | Measure or Quantity | Sodium (mg.) | Total | —Fats in grams— Satu- rated | Unsatu- rated | Choles- terol (mg.) |
|---|---|---|---|---|---|---|
| (USDA) without caps & stems | ½ cup (2.4 oz.) | <1 | .9 | | | 0 |
| Canned, water pack, unsweetened, solids & liq. (USDA) | 4 oz. | 1 | 1.2 | | | 0 |
| Red: | | | | | | |
| Fresh: | | | | | | |
| (USDA) | ½ lb. (weighed with caps & stems) | 2 | 1.1 | | | 0 |
| (USDA) without caps & stems | ½ cup (2.5 oz.) | <1 | .4 | | | 0 |
| Canned, water pack, unsweetened, or low calorie: | | | | | | |
| Solids & liq. (USDA) | 4 oz. | 1 | .1 | | | 0 |
| Solids & liq. (Blue Boy) | 4 oz. | 1 | 1.0 | | | (0) |
| Frozen, sweetened: | | | | | | |
| Not thawed (USDA) | 10-oz. pkg. | 3 | .6 | | | 0 |
| Not thawed (USDA) | ½ cup (4.4 oz.) | 1 | .2 | | | 0 |
| Quick-thaw (Birds Eye) | ½ cup (5 oz.) | 1 | .2 | | | 0 |
| **RASPBERRY PRESERVE or JAM:** | | | | | | |
| Sweetened, black or red (Bama) | 1 T. (.7 oz.) | 2 | <.1 | | | (0) |
| Low calorie or dietetic (Estee) | 1 T. | <3 | 0.0 | | | 0 |
| **RATATOUILLE,** frozen | | | | | | |
| (Stouffer's) | 5 oz. | 1,320 | 3.0 | | | |
| **RAVIOLI:** | | | | | | |
| Canned: | | | | | | |
| Regular pack (Franco-American) beef: | | | | | | |
| In meat sauce | 7½-oz. can | 1,090 | 5.0 | | | |
| In meat sauce, *RavioliOs* | 7½-oz. can | 890 | 7.0 | | | |
| Dietetic: | | | | | | |
| (Dia-Mel) beef | 8 oz. | 75 | 10.0 | | | |
| (Estee) beef | 7½-oz. can | 110 | 8.0 | | | |
| (Featherweight) beef | 8 oz. | 68 | 10.0 | | | |

(USDA): United States Department of Agriculture
*Prepared as Package Directs

| Food and Description | Measure or Quantity | Sodium (mg.) | Total | Fats in grams — Saturated | Unsaturated | Cholesterol (mg.) |
|---|---|---|---|---|---|---|
| Frozen: | | | | | | |
| (Celentano) cheese: | | | | | | |
| Regular size | ½ of 13-oz. pkg. | 360 | 12.0 | | | 112 |
| Mini | ½ of 8-oz. pkg. | 180 | 6.0 | | | 50 |
| (Weight Watchers) cheese, | | | | | | |
| baked | 8 1/16-oz. pkg. | 685 | 11.0 | | | |

**REDFISH** (See **DRUM, RED & OCEAN PERCH,** Atlantic)

**RED & GRAY SNAPPER,** raw (USDA):

| | | | | | | |
|---|---|---|---|---|---|---|
| Whole | 1 lb. (weighed whole) | 158 | 2.1 | | | |
| Meat only | 4 oz. | 76 | 1.0 | | | |

**REDHORSE, SILVER,** raw (USDA):

| | | | | | | |
|---|---|---|---|---|---|---|
| Drawn | 1 lb. (weighed eviscerated) | | 4.8 | | | |
| Meat only | 4 oz. | | 2.6 | | | |

**RED LOBSTER:** (All "lunch portions" weigh 5 oz. before cooking):

| | | | | | | |
|---|---|---|---|---|---|---|
| Calamari, breaded & fried | 1 lunch portion | 1,150 | 21.0 | | | 140 |
| Catfish | 1 lunch portion | 50 | 10.0 | | | 85 |
| Chicken breast | 4-oz. serving | 60 | 3.0 | | | 65 |
| Clam, cherrystone | 1 order | 540 | 2.0 | | | 80 |
| Cod, Atlantic | 1 lunch portion | 200 | 1.0 | | | 70 |
| Crab legs: | | | | | | |
| King | 16-oz. serving | 900 | 2.0 | | | 100 |
| Snow | 16-oz. serving | 1,630 | 2.0 | | | 130 |
| Flounder | 1 lunch portion | 95 | 1.0 | | | 70 |
| Grouper | 1 lunch portion | 70 | 1.0 | | | 65 |
| Haddock | 1 lunch portion | 180 | 1.0 | | | 85 |
| Halibut | 1 lunch portion | 105 | 1.0 | | | 60 |
| Hamburger patty, no bun | 5.3-oz. serving | 70 | 23.0 | | | 105 |
| Lobster tail, rock | 1 tail | 1,090 | 3.0 | | | 200 |
| Mackerel | 1 lunch portion | 250 | 12.0 | | | 100 |
| Mussels | 3-oz. serving | 150 | 2.0 | | | 50 |
| Oysters | 6 raw oysters | 90 | 4.0 | | | 60 |
| Perch, ocean | 1 lunch portion | 190 | 4.0 | | | 75 |

(USDA): United States Department of Agriculture
*Prepared as Package Directs

| Food and Description | Measure or Quantity | Sodium (mg.) | —Fats in grams— Total | Saturated | Unsaturated | Cholesterol (mg.) |
|---|---|---|---|---|---|---|
| Pollock | 1 lunch portion | 90 | 1.0 | | | 90 |
| Rockfish, red | 1 lunch portion | 95 | 1.0 | | | 85 |
| Salmon: | | | | | | |
|   Norwegian | 1 lunch portion | 60 | 12.0 | | | 80 |
|   Sockeye | 1 lunch portion | 60 | 4.0 | | | 50 |
| Scallop: | | | | | | |
|   Calico | 1 lunch portion | 260 | 2.0 | | | 115 |
|   Deep sea | 1 lunch portion | 260 | 2.0 | | | 50 |
| Shark: | | | | | | |
|   Blacktip | 1 lunch portion | 90 | 1.0 | | | 60 |
|   Mako | 1 lunch portion | 60 | 1.0 | | | 100 |
| Shrimp | 8-12 pieces | 110 | 2.0 | | | 230 |
| Snapper, red | 1 lunch portion | 140 | 1.0 | | | 70 |
| Sole, lemon | 1 lunch portion | 90 | 1.0 | | | 65 |
| Steak: | | | | | | |
|   Porterhouse | 18-oz. steak | 150 | 131.0 | | | 290 |
|   Sirloin | 7-oz. steak | 85 | 48.0 | | | 140 |
|   Strip | 7-oz. steak | 70 | 64.0 | | | 140 |
| Swordfish | 1 lunch portion | 140 | 4.0 | | | 100 |
| Tuna, yellowfin | 1 lunch portion | 70 | 6.0 | | | 70 |
| | | | | | | |
| **REINDEER,** raw, lean only | | | | | | |
|   (USDA) | 4 oz. | | 4.3 | | | |
| | | | | | | |
| **RELISH:** | | | | | | |
|   Dill (Vlasic) | 1 oz. | 415 | 0.0 | | | (0) |
|   Hamburger (Vlasic) | 1 oz. | 255 | 0.0 | | | (0) |
|   Hot dog (Vlasic) | 1 oz. | 255 | 0.0 | | | (0) |
|   Sour (USDA) | 1 T. (.5 oz.) | | .1 | | | 0 |
|   Sweet: | | | | | | |
|     (USDA) finely chopped | 1 T. (.5 oz.) | 107 | <.1 | | | 0 |
|     (Vlasic) | 1 oz. | 220 | 0.0 | | | (0) |
| | | | | | | |
| **RENNET MIX** (Junket): | | | | | | |
|   *Powder: | | | | | | |
|     Chocolate: | | | | | | |
|       Skim milk | ½ cup | 70 | 0.0 | | | |
|       Whole milk | ½ cup | 65 | 4.0 | | | |
|     Raspberry or strawberry: | | | | | | |
|       Skim milk | ½ cup | 65 | 0.0 | | | |
|       Whole milk | ½ cup | 60 | 4.0 | | | |
|   *Tablet: | | | | | | |
|     Skim milk | ½ cup | 70 | 0.0 | | | |
|     Whole milk | ½ cup | 65 | 4.0 | | | |

(USDA): United States Department of Agriculture
*Prepared as Package Directs

| Food and Description | Measure or Quantity | Sodium (mg.) | Total | Fats in grams Satu- rated | Unsatu- rated | Choles- terol (mg.) |
|---|---|---|---|---|---|---|
| **RHINE WINE:** | | | | | | |
| (Gold Seal) 12% alcohol | 3 fl. oz. (3.1 oz.) | 3 | 0.0 | | | (0) |
| (Great Western) 12.5% alcohol, regular | 3 fl. oz. | 25 | 0.0 | | | 0 |
| (Great Western) 12.5% alcohol, Dutchess | 3 fl. oz. | 27 | 0.0 | | | 0 |
| **RHUBARB:** | | | | | | |
| Fresh (USDA): | | | | | | |
| Partly trimmed | 1 lb. (weighed with part leaves, ends & trimmings) | 7 | .3 | | | 0 |
| Trimmed | 4 oz. | 2 | .1 | | | 0 |
| Diced | ½ cup (2.2 oz.) | 1 | <.1 | | | 0 |
| Cooked, sweetened, solids & liq. (USDA) | ½ cup (4.2 oz.) | 2 | .1 | | | 0 |
| Frozen, sweetened: | | | | | | |
| Not thawed (USDA) | ½ cup (3.9 oz.) | 4 | .2 | | | 0 |
| Cooked, added sugar, solids & liq. (USDA) | ½ cup (4.4 oz.) | 4 | .2 | | | 0 |
| (Birds Eye) | ½ cup (4 oz.) | 2 | .1 | | | 0 |
| **RICE:** | | | | | | |
| Brown: | | | | | | |
| Raw (USDA) | ½ cup (3.7 oz.) | 9 | 2.0 | | | 0 |
| Raw (USDA) | 1 oz. | 3 | .5 | | | 0 |
| Cooked: | | | | | | |
| With salt added: | | | | | | |
| (USDA) | 4 oz. | 320 | .7 | | | 0 |
| (Carolina) | 4 oz. | 320 | .7 | | | (0) |
| (River Brand) | 4 oz. | 320 | .7 | | | (0) |
| (Water Maid) | 4 oz. | 320 | .7 | | | (0) |
| Parboiled (Uncle Ben's) with no added butter or salt | ⅔ cup (4.2 oz.) | 6 | 1.1 | | | 0 |
| Parboiled (Uncle Ben's) with added butter | ⅔ cup (4.3 oz.) | 32 | 3.2 | | | |
| Frozen, in beef stock (Green Giant) | ⅓ of 12-oz. pkg. | 782 | 2.8 | | | |
| White: | | | | | | |
| Instant or precooked: | | | | | | |
| Dry, long-grain (USDA) | ½ cup (1.9 oz.) | <1 | .1 | | | 0 |
| Dry, long-grain (USDA) | 1 oz. | <1 | <.1 | | | 0 |

(USDA): United States Department of Agriculture
*Prepared as Package Directs

| Food and Description | Measure or Quantity | Sodium (mg.) | Fats in grams Total | Fats in grams Saturated | Fats in grams Unsaturated | Cholesterol (mg.) |
|---|---|---|---|---|---|---|
| Cooked: | | | | | | |
| With salt added: | | | | | | |
| Long-grain (USDA) | ⅔ cup (3.3 oz.) | 254 | Tr. | | | 0 |
| (Carolina) | ⅔ cup (3.3 oz.) | 254 | Tr. | | | (0) |
| Without salt: | | | | | | |
| (Minute Rice) no added butter | ⅔ cup (4 oz.) | 1 | Tr. | | | 0 |
| Long-grain (Uncle Ben's Quick) no added butter | ⅔ cup (4 oz.) | 9 | <.1 | | | 0 |
| Long-grain (Uncle Ben's Quick) with added butter | ⅔ cup (4.1 oz.) | 37 | 2.5 | | | |
| Parboiled: | | | | | | |
| Dry, long-grain (USDA) | 1 oz. | 3 | <.1 | | | 0 |
| Cooked: | | | | | | |
| With added salt: | | | | | | |
| Long-grain (USDA) | ⅔ cup (4.1 oz.) | 419 | .1 | | | 0 |
| (Aunt Caroline) | ⅔ cup (4.1 oz.) | 419 | .1 | | | (0) |
| No added salt, long-grain (Uncle Ben's Converted), no added butter | ⅔ cup (4.3 oz.) | 3 | .2 | | | 0 |
| Regular: | | | | | | |
| Raw (USDA) | ½ cup (3.5 oz.) | 5 | .4 | | | 0 |
| Cooked with salt: | | | | | | |
| (USDA) | ⅔ cup (4.8 oz.) | 512 | .1 | | | 0 |
| Extra long-grain (Carolina) | ⅔ cup (4.8 oz.) | 512 | .1 | | | (0) |
| Long-grain (Mahatma) | ⅔ cup (4.8 oz.) | 512 | .1 | | | (0) |
| (River Brand) fluffy | ⅔ cup (4.8 oz.) | 512 | .1 | | | (0) |
| (Water Maid) | ⅔ cup (4.8 oz.) | 512 | .1 | | | (0) |
| White & wild, frozen (Green Giant) | ⅓ of 12-oz. pkg. | 522 | 1.1 | | | |
| Wild (See **WILD RICE**) | | | | | | |
| **RICE BRAN** (USDA) | 1 oz. | Tr. | 4.5 | | | 0 |
| **RICE CEREAL** (USDA): | | | | | | |
| With casein & other added nutrients | 1 oz. | 170 | <.1 | | | 0 |
| Wheat gluten & other added nutrients | 1 oz. | 227 | <.1 | | | 0 |

(USDA): United States Department of Agriculture
*Prepared as Package Directs

| Food and Description | Measure or Quantity | Sodium (mg.) | Fats in grams — Total | Satu- rated | Unsatu- rated | Choles- terol (mg.) |
|---|---|---|---|---|---|---|
| **RICE FLAKES,** cereal, added nutrients (USDA) | 1 cup (1.1 oz.) | 296 | <.1 | | | 0 |
| **RICE, FRIED** (See also **RICE MIX**): | | | | | | |
| *Canned (La Choy) | ⅓ of 11-oz. can | 965 | 2.0 | | | |
| Frozen: | | | | | | |
| (Birds Eye) | ⅓ of 11-oz. pkg. | 432 | .3 | | | Tr. |
| (La Choy) with meat | 8-oz. entree | 1,770 | 4.0 | | | |
| Seasoning mix: | | | | | | |
| *(Durkee) | 1 cup | 1,597 | .7 | | | |
| (Kikkoman) | 1-oz. pkg. | 2,000 | .2 | | | <1 |
| ***RICE KRISPIES,*** cereal (Kellogg's): | | | | | | |
| Regular | 1 cup (1 oz.) | 285 | 0.0 | | | |
| Cocoa | ¾ cup (1 oz.) | 195 | 0.0 | | | |
| Frosted | ¾ cup (1 oz.) | 200 | 0.0 | | | |
| Strawberry | ¾ cup (1 oz.) | 200 | 0.0 | | | |
| **RICE MIX:** | | | | | | |
| Beef: | | | | | | |
| *(Lipton) and sauce | ½ cup | 665 | 4.0 | | | |
| *(Minute Rice) rib roast | ½ cup | 720 | 4.1 | | | 10 |
| *Rice-A-Roni* | ⅙ of pkg. | 780 | 1.0 | | | |
| Chicken: | | | | | | |
| *(Lipton) and sauce | ½ cup | 525 | 4.0 | | | |
| *(Minute Rice) | ½ cup | 694 | 4.3 | | | 11 |
| *Rice-A-Roni* | ⅙ of pkg. | 800 | 1.0 | | | |
| *Fried (Minute Rice) | ½ cup | 549 | 4.7 | | | 0 |
| *Herb & Butter (Lipton) and sauce | ½ cup | 500 | 5.0 | | | |
| *Long grain & wild (Minute Rice) | ½ cup | 578 | 4.1 | | | 10 |
| *Medley (Lipton) & sauce | ½ cup | 400 | 3.0 | | | |
| Spanish (See also **RICE, SPANISH**): | | | | | | |
| *(Lipton) & sauce | ½ cup | 520 | 3.0 | | | |
| *(Minute Rice) | ½ cup | 839 | 4.1 | | | |
| *Rice-A-Roni* | ⅐ of pkg. | 720 | 1.0 | | | |
| **RICE, POLISH** (USDA) | 1 oz. | Tr. | 3.6 | | | 0 |

(USDA): United States Department of Agriculture
*Prepared as Package Directs

| Food and Description | Measure or Quantity | Sodium (mg.) | — Fats in grams — | | | Cholesterol (mg.) |
|---|---|---|---|---|---|---|
| | | | Total | Satu- rated | Unsatu- rated | |
| **\*RICE SEASONING** (French's) | | | | | | |
| Spice Your Rice: | | | | | | |
| Beef flavor & onion | ½ cup | 560 | 4.0 | | | |
| Buttery herb | ½ cup | 430 | 5.0 | | | |
| Cheese 'n chives | ½ cup | 400 | 4.0 | | | |
| Chicken flavor & herb or chicken flavor & parmesan | ½ cup | 440 | 4.0 | | | |
| **RICE, SPANISH:** | | | | | | |
| Home recipe (USDA) | 4 oz. | 358 | 1.9 | | | |
| Canned: | | | | | | |
| Regular pack (Menner's) | ½ of 7½-oz. can | 850 | 1.0 | | | |
| Dietetic (Featherweight) | 7½ oz. | 32 | 0.0 | | | |
| Frozen (Birds Eye) | ⅓ of 11-oz. pkg. | 495 | .5 | | | 0 |
| **RICE & VEGETABLE:** | | | | | | |
| Frozen (Birds Eye): | | | | | | |
| French style | ⅓ of 11-oz. pkg. | 637 | .4 | | | 0 |
| & peas with mushroom | ⅓ of 7-oz. pkg. | 322 | .2 | | | 0 |
| \*Mix (Lipton) with peas & sauce | ½ cup | 400 | 3.0 | | | |
| **ROCKFISH** (USDA): | | | | | | |
| Raw, meat only | 1 lb. | 272 | 8.2 | | | |
| Oven-steamed, with onion | 4 oz. | 77 | 2.8 | | | |
| **ROE** (USDA): | | | | | | |
| Raw, carp, cod, haddock, herring, pike or shad | 4 oz. | | 2.6 | | | |
| Raw, salmon, sturgeon, turbot | 4 oz. | | 11.8 | | | 401 |
| Baked or broiled,[1] cod & shad | 4 oz. | 83 | 3.2 | | | |
| Canned, cod, haddock or herring, solids & liq. | 4 oz. | | 3.2 | | | |
| **ROLL & BUN:** | | | | | | |
| Commercial-type, nonfrozen: | | | | | | |
| Biscuit (Wonder) | 1¼-oz. piece | 188 | 2.1 | | | < 2 |
| Brown & serve: | | | | | | |
| (USDA): | | | | | | |
| Unbrowned[2] | 1 oz. | 145 | 1.9 | .3 | 1.6 | |
| Browned[2] | 1 oz. | 159 | 2.2 | .3 | 2. | |

(USDA): United States Department of Agriculture
\*Prepared as Package Directs
[1]Prepared with butter or margarine & lemon juice or vinegar.
[2]Principal source of fat: vegetable shortening.

| Food and Description | Measure or Quantity | Sodium (mg.) | — Fats in grams — | | | Choles- terol (mg.) |
|---|---|---|---|---|---|---|
| | | | Total | Satu- rated | Unsatu- rated | |
| (Pepperidge Farm) | 1.3-oz. roll | 220 | 1.0 | | | |
| (Wonder): | | | | | | |
| Buttermilk | 1-oz. roll | 142 | 2.6 | | | Tr. |
| French | 1-oz. roll | 151 | 2.6 | | | Tr. |
| Home bake | 1-oz. roll | 114 | 1.4 | | | Tr. |
| Cloverleaf (USDA) home recipe[1] | 1.2-oz. roll | 98 | 3.0 | .7 | 2.3 | |
| Crescent (Pepperidge Farm) butter | 1-oz. roll | 160 | 6.0 | | | |
| Croissant (Pepperidge Farm): | | | | | | |
| Almond | 2-oz. roll | 260 | 11.0 | | | |
| Butter | 2-oz. roll | 310 | 13.0 | | | |
| Chocolate | 2.4-oz. roll | 325 | 16.0 | | | |
| Raisin | 2-oz. roll | 265 | 10.0 | | | |
| Walnut | 2-oz. roll | 275 | 12.0 | | | |
| Dinner: | | | | | | |
| Home Pride | 1-oz. roll | 170 | 2.3 | | | Tr. |
| (Wonder) | 1¼-oz. roll | 188 | 2.1 | | | <2 |
| Frankfurter: | | | | | | |
| (USDA)[2] | 1.4-oz. roll | 202 | 2.2 | .4 | 1.8 | |
| (Arnold) | 1.3-oz. roll | 290 | 1.0 | | | 0 |
| (Pepperidge Farm) | 1¾-oz. roll | 240 | 3.0 | | | |
| (Wonder) | 2-oz. roll | 153 | 2.8 | | | Tr. |
| French: | | | | | | |
| (Arnold) Francisco | 1.1-oz. roll | 160 | 1.0 | | | 1 |
| (Pepperidge Farm) regular | 1.3-oz. roll | 250 | 2.0 | | | |
| Golden twist (Pepperidge Farm) | 1-oz. roll | 160 | 6.0 | | | |
| Hamburger: | | | | | | |
| (Arnold) | 1.4 oz. bun | 285 | 1.0 | | | 0 |
| (Pepperidge Farm) | 1½-oz. bun | 260 | 3.0 | | | 0 |
| (Wonder) | 2-oz. bun | 153 | 2.8 | | | 0 |
| Hard (USDA) round or rectangular | 1.8-oz. roll | 312 | 1.6 | .5 | 1.1 | |
| Hoagie (Wonder) | 6-oz. roll | 869 | 8.5 | | | <8 |
| Honey (Hostess) glazed | 3¾-oz. piece | 522 | 21.3 | | | 23 |
| Kaiser (Wonder) | 6-oz. roll | 869 | 8.5 | | | <8 |
| Parker House (Pepperidge Farm) | .6-oz. roll | 90 | 1.0 | | | |
| Party (Pepperidge Farm) | .4-oz. roll | 50 | 4.0 | | | |
| Sandwich (Arnold) plain | 1.3-oz. roll | 260 | 2.0 | | | <5 |

(USDA): United States Department of Agriculture
*Prepared as Package Directs
[1]Principal sources of fat: vegetable shortening, milk & egg.
[2]Principal source of fat: vegetable shortening.

| Food and Description | Measure or Quantity | Sodium (mg.) | Fats in grams — Total | Saturated | Unsaturated | Cholesterol (mg.) |
|---|---|---|---|---|---|---|
| Soft (Pepperidge Farm) | 1.2-oz. roll | 235 | 3.0 | | | |
| Sourdough French (Pepperidge Farm) | 1.3-oz. roll | 255 | 2.0 | | | |
| Frozen: | | | | | | |
| Caramel sticky bun (Sara Lee) | 1-oz. bun | 110 | 5.4 | | | |
| Cinnamon (Sara Lee) | .9-oz. roll | 96 | 4.2 | | | |
| Honey (Morton): | | | | | | |
| Regular | 2.3-oz. piece | 150 | 11.0 | | | 1 |
| Mini | 1.3-oz. piece | 90 | 6.0 | | | 0 |

**ROLL OR BUN DOUGH:**
| | | | | | | |
|---|---|---|---|---|---|---|
| Frozen: | | | | | | |
| (USDA): | | | | | | |
| Unbaked | 1 oz. | 137 | 1.4 | Tr. | 1. | |
| Baked | 1 oz. | 159 | 1.5 | Tr. | 1. | |
| *(Rich's): | | | | | | |
| Cinnamon | 2¼-oz. piece | 226 | 2.5 | | | 4 |
| Frankfurter | 1.6-oz. roll | 237 | 1.9 | | | |
| Hamburger | 1.6-oz. bun | 227 | 1.7 | | | 0 |
| *Refrigerated (Pillsbury): | | | | | | |
| Apple danish | 1 piece | 260 | 11.0 | | | |
| Caramel danish with nuts | 1 piece | 245 | 8.0 | | | |
| Cinnamon & raisin danish | 1 piece | 225 | 7.0 | | | |
| Crescent | 1 piece | 230 | 5.5 | | | |

**ROLL MIX:**
| | | | | | | |
|---|---|---|---|---|---|---|
| Dry (USDA)[1] | 1 oz. | 117 | 1.7 | Tr. | 1. | |
| *Prepared with water (USDA)[1] | 1 oz. | 89 | 1.3 | Tr. | 1. | |
| (Pillsbury) hot | 1 oz. | 215 | 2.0 | | | |

**\*ROMAN MEAL CEREAL,** dry
| | | | | | | |
|---|---|---|---|---|---|---|
| *ROMAN MEAL CEREAL, dry | ⅓ cup (1 oz.) | 2 | .7 | Tr. | <1. | Tr. |

**ROSE APPLE,** raw (USDA):
| | | | | | | |
|---|---|---|---|---|---|---|
| Whole | 1 lb. (weighed with caps & seeds) | | .9 | | | 0 |
| Flesh only | 4 oz. | | .3 | | | 0 |

**ROSEMARY** (Spice Islands)
| | | | | | | |
|---|---|---|---|---|---|---|
| ROSEMARY (Spice Islands) | 1 tsp. | <1 | | | | (0) |

(USDA): United States Department of Agriculture
*Prepared as Package Directs
[1]Principal source of fat: vegetable shortening.

| Food and Description | Measure or Quantity | Sodium (mg.) | — Fats in grams — Total | Satu- rated | Unsatu- rated | Choles- terol (mg.) |
|---|---|---|---|---|---|---|
| **ROSE WINE:** | | | | | | |
| (Great Western) 12.5% alcohol | 3 fl. oz. | 38 | 0.0 | | | 0 |
| (Great Western) Isabella, 12.5% alcohol | 3 fl. oz. | <1 | 0.0 | | | 0 |
| | | | | | | |
| **ROY ROGERS:** | | | | | | |
| Bar Burger, R.R. | 1 burger | 1,826 | 39.4 | | | 115 |
| Biscuit | 1 biscuit | 575 | 12.1 | | | <5 |
| Breakfast crescent sandwich: | | | | | | |
| Regular | 4.5-oz. sandwich | 867 | 27.3 | | | 148 |
| With bacon | 4.7-oz. sandwich | 1,035 | 29.7 | | | 156 |
| With ham | 5.8-oz. sandwich | 1,192 | 41.7 | | | 189 |
| With sausage | 5.7-oz. sandwich | 1,289 | 29.4 | | | 168 |
| Brownie | 1 piece | 150 | 11.4 | | | 10 |
| Cheeseburger: | | | | | | |
| Regular | 1 burger | 1,404 | 37.3 | | | 95 |
| With bacon | 1 burger | 1,535 | 39.2 | | | 102 |
| Chicken: | | | | | | |
| Breast | 1 piece | 609 | 23.7 | | | 118 |
| Leg | 1 piece | 190 | 8.0 | | | 40 |
| Thigh | 1 piece | 406 | 19.5 | | | 85 |
| Wing | 1 piece | 285 | 12.8 | | | 47 |
| Coleslaw | 3½-oz. serving | 261 | 6.9 | | | <5 |
| Danish: | | | | | | |
| Apple | 1 piece | 255 | 11.6 | | | 15 |
| Cheese | 1 piece | 260 | 12.2 | | | 11 |
| Cherry | 1 piece | 242 | 14.4 | | | 11 |
| Drinks: | | | | | | |
| Coffee, black | 6 fl. oz. | 2 | Tr. | | | (0) |
| Coca-Cola: | | | | | | |
| Regular | 12 fl. oz. | 22 | 0.0 | | | 0 |
| Diet | 12 fl. oz. | 52 | 0.0 | | | 0 |
| Hot chocolate | 6 fl. oz. | 124 | 2.0 | | | 35 |
| Milk | 8 fl. oz. | 120 | 8.2 | | | 33 |
| Orange juice: | | | | | | |
| Regular | 7 fl. oz. | 2 | .2 | | | 0 |
| Large | 10 fl. oz. | 3 | .3 | | | 0 |
| Shake: | | | | | | |
| Chocolate | 1 shake | 290 | 10.2 | | | 37 |
| Strawberry | 1 shake | 261 | 10.2 | | | 37 |
| Vanilla | 1 shake | 282 | 10.7 | | | 40 |
| Tea, iced, plain | 8 fl. oz. | Tr. | 0.0 | | | 0 |

(USDA): United States Department of Agriculture
*Prepared as Package Directs

| Food and Description | Measure or Quantity | Sodium (mg.) | Total | Fats in grams — Saturated | Fats in grams — Unsaturated | Cholesterol (mg.) |
|---|---|---|---|---|---|---|
| Egg & biscuit platter: | | | | | | |
| Regular | 1 meal | 734 | 26.5 | | | 284 |
| With bacon | 1 meal | 957 | 29.6 | | | 294 |
| With ham | 1 meal | 1,156 | 28.6 | | | 304 |
| With sausage | 1 meal | 1,059 | 40.9 | | | 325 |
| Hamburger | 1 burger | 495 | 28.3 | | | 73 |
| Pancake platter, with syrup & butter: | | | | | | |
| Plain | 1 order | 842 | 15.2 | | | 53 |
| With bacon | 1 order | 1,065 | 18.3 | | | 63 |
| With ham | 1 order | 1,264 | 17.3 | | | 73 |
| With sausage | 1 order | 1,167 | 29.6 | | | 94 |
| Potato: | | | | | | |
| Baked, Hot Topped: | | | | | | |
| Plain | 1 potato | 10 | .2 | | | 0 |
| With bacon & cheese | 1 potato | 778 | 21.7 | | | 34 |
| With broccoli & cheese | 1 potato | 523 | 18.1 | | | <20 |
| With margarine | 1 potato | 106 | 7.3 | | | 0 |
| With sour cream & chives | 1 potato | 138 | 20.9 | | | 31 |
| With taco beef & cheese | 1 potato | 726 | 21.8 | | | 37 |
| French fries: | | | | | | |
| Regular | 3 oz. | 165 | 13.5 | | | 42 |
| Large | 4 oz. | 220 | 18.4 | | | 56 |
| Potato salad | 3½-oz. order | 696 | 6.1 | | | <5 |
| Roast beef sandwich: | | | | | | |
| Plain: | | | | | | |
| Regular | 1 sandwich | 785 | 10.2 | | | 55 |
| Large | 1 sandwich | 1,044 | 11.9 | | | 73 |
| With cheese: | | | | | | |
| Regular | 1 sandwich | 1,694 | 19.2 | | | 77 |
| Large | 1 sandwich | 1,953 | 20.9 | | | 95 |
| Salad bar: | | | | | | |
| Bacon bits | 1 T. | 210 | 1.0 | | | |
| Beets, sliced | ¼ cup | 100 | 0.0 | | | |
| Broccoli | ½ cup | 7 | 0.0 | | | |
| Carrot, shredded | ¼ cup | 7 | 0.0 | | | |
| Cheese, cheddar | ¼ cup | 195 | 9.0 | | | |
| Croutons | 1 T. | 130 | 0.0 | | | |
| Egg, chopped | 1 T. | 21 | 2.0 | | | |
| Lettuce | 1 cup | 7 | 0.0 | | | |
| Macaroni salad | 1 T. | 155 | 1.8 | | | |
| Mushrooms | ¼ cup | 3 | 0.0 | | | |
| Noodle, Chinese | ¼ cup | 100 | 2.8 | | | |

(USDA): United States Department of Agriculture
*Prepared as Package Directs

| Food and Description | Measure or Quantity | Sodium (mg.) | —Fats in grams— | | | Choles-terol (mg.) |
|---|---|---|---|---|---|---|
| | | | Total | Satu-rated | Unsatu-rated | |
| Pepper, green | 1 T. | 66 | 0.0 | | | |
| Potato salad | 1 T. | 175 | 1.5 | | | |
| Tomato | 1 slice | 1 | 0.0 | | | |
| Salad dressing: | | | | | | |
| Regular: | | | | | | |
| Bacon & tomato | 1 T. | 75 | 6.0 | | | |
| Bleu cheese | 1 T. | 76 | 8.0 | | | |
| Ranch | 1 T. | 50 | 7.0 | | | |
| Thousand island | 1 T. | 75 | 8.0 | | | |
| Low calorie, Italian | 1 T. | 50 | 3.0 | | | |
| Strawberry shortcake | 7.2-oz. serving | 674 | 19.2 | | | 28 |
| Sundae: | | | | | | |
| Caramel | 1 sundae | 193 | 8.5 | | | 23 |
| Hot fudge | 1 sundae | 230 | 12.5 | | | 186 |
| Strawberry | 1 sundae | 99 | 7.1 | | | 23 |
| **RUSK:** | | | | | | |
| (USDA)[1] | 1 piece (.5 oz.) | 35 | 1.2 | Tr. | 1. | |
| Holland (Nabisco) | 1 piece (.4 oz.) | 34 | .6 | | | |
| **RUTABAGA:** | | | | | | |
| Raw, without tops (USDA) | 1 lb. (weighed with skin) | 19 | .4 | | | 0 |
| Raw, diced (USDA) | ½ cup (2.5 oz.) | 4 | <.1 | | | 0 |
| Boiled without salt, diced, drained (USDA) | ½ cup (3 oz.) | 3 | <.1 | | | 0 |
| Boiled without salt, mashed (USDA) | ½ cup (4.3 oz.) | 5 | .1 | | | 0 |
| Canned (Sunshine) solids & liq. | ½ cup (4.2 oz.) | 393 | .1 | | | |
| Frozen (Southland) | 4 oz. | 200 | 0.0 | | | |
| Canned (King Pharr) | ½ cup | | | | | |
| **RYE,** whole grain (USDA) | 1 oz. | <1 | .5 | | | 0 |

**RYE FLOUR (See FLOUR)**

**RYE WHISKEY (See DISTILLED LIQUOR)**

**RYKRISP (See CRACKER)**

(USDA): United States Department of Agriculture
*Prepared as Package Directs
[1]Principal sources of fat: vegetable shortening, egg & milk.

| Food and Description | Measure or Quantity | Sodium (mg.) | —Fats in grams— | | | Cholesterol (mg.) |
|---|---|---|---|---|---|---|
| | | | Total | Saturated | Unsaturated | |

# S

**SABLEFISH,** raw (USDA):

| | | | | | | |
|---|---|---|---|---|---|---|
| Whole | 1 lb. (weighed whole) | 107 | 28.4 | | | |
| Meat only | 4 oz. | 64 | 16.9 | | | |

**SAFFLOWER SEED** (USDA):

| | | | | | | |
|---|---|---|---|---|---|---|
| Kernels, dry, in hull | ½ lb. (weighed in hull) | | 68.8 | 6. | 63. | |
| Kernels, dry, hulled | 1 oz. | | 16.9 | 1. | 15. | |
| Meal, partially defatted | 1 oz. | | 2.3 | Tr. | 2. | |

| | | | | | | |
|---|---|---|---|---|---|---|
| **SAFFRON** (Spice Islands) | 1 tsp. | < 1 | | | | (0) |
| **SAGE** (Spice Islands) | 1 tsp. | < 1 | | | | (0) |

**SAINT JOHN'S-BREAD FLOUR** (See **FLOUR,** Carob)

**SALAD DRESSING:**

| | | | | | | |
|---|---|---|---|---|---|---|
| Regular: | | | | | | |
| Bacon & tomato (Henri's) | 1 T. (.5 oz.) | 150 | 6.0 | | | |
| Blue or bleu cheese: | | | | | | |
| (USDA) | 1 T. (.5 oz.) | 164 | 7.8 | 1.6 | 6.2 | |
| (Henri's) | 1 T. (.5 oz.) | 220 | 5.0 | | | |
| (Wish-Bone) chunky | 1 T. | 150 | 8.0 | | | Tr. |
| Boiled, home recipe (USDA) | 1 T. (.6 oz.) | 116 | 1.6 | .8 | .8 | 12 |
| Caesar (Wish-Bone) | 1 T. (.5 oz.) | 250 | 8.0 | | | Tr. |
| Cheddar & bacon (Wish-Bone) | 1 T. (.5 oz.) | 110 | 7.0 | | | Tr. |
| Cucumber (Wish-Bone) creamy | 1 T. | 115 | 8.0 | | | Tr. |
| French: | | | | | | |
| Home recipe (USDA) | 1 T. (.6 oz.) | 105 | 11.2 | 1.1 | 10.1 | |
| (Henri's) hearty | 1 T. | 95 | 6.0 | | | |
| (Wish-Bone): | | | | | | |
| Deluxe | 1 T. (.5 oz.) | 80 | 5.0 | | | 0 |
| Garlic | 1 T. (.5 oz.) | 150 | 6.0 | | | 0 |
| Sweet & spicy | 1 T. (.5 oz.) | 150 | 6.0 | | | 0 |
| Garlic (Wish-Bone) creamy | 1 T. (.5 oz.) | 170 | 8.0 | | | 0 |

(USDA): United States Department of Agriculture
*Prepared as Package Directs

| Food and Description | Measure or Quantity | Sodium (mg.) | Total | —Fats in grams—<br>Satu-<br>rated | Unsatu-<br>rated | Choles-<br>terol<br>(mg.) |
|---|---|---|---|---|---|---|
| Italian: | | | | | | |
| (USDA) | 1 T. | 314 | 9.0 | 1.5 | 7.5 | |
| (Henri's): | | | | | | |
| Authentic | 1 T. | 260 | 9.0 | | | |
| Creamy garlic | 1 T. | 140 | 4.0 | | | |
| (Wish-Bone): | | | | | | |
| Regular | 1 T. | 240 | 7.0 | | | 0 |
| Creamy | 1 T. | 145 | 6.0 | | | 0 |
| Robusto | 1 T. | 285 | 8.0 | | | 0 |
| Mayonnaise-type: | | | | | | |
| (USDA) | 1 T. | 88 | 6.3 | 1.2 | 5.1 | 8 |
| Miracle Whip (Kraft) | 1 T. | 85 | | | | 5 |
| Ranchouse (Henri's) Chef's | | | | | | |
| Recipe | 1 T. | 135 | 7.0 | | | |
| Roquefort (USDA) | 1 T. (.5 oz.) | 164 | 7.8 | 1.6 | 6.2 | |
| Russian: | | | | | | |
| (USDA) | 1 T. (.5 oz.) | 130 | 7.6 | 1.4 | 6.3 | |
| (Henri's) | 1 T. (.5 oz.) | 90 | 5.0 | | | |
| (Wish-Bone) | 1 T. (.5 oz.) | 140 | 2.0 | | | 0 |
| Sour cream & bacon | | | | | | |
| (Wish-Bone) | 1 T. | 95 | 7.0 | | | 0 |
| Spin Blend (Hellmann's) | 1 T. (.5 oz.) | 112 | 5.1 | | | 7 |
| Tas-Tee (Henri's) | 1 T. | 95 | 4.0 | | | |
| Thousand island: | | | | | | |
| (USDA) | 1 T. (.6 oz.) | 112 | 8.0 | 1.4 | 6.6 | |
| (Henri's) | 1 T. | 130 | 5.0 | | | |
| (Wish-Bone): | | | | | | |
| Regular | 1 T. | 130 | 6.0 | | | 5 |
| Southern recipe | 1 T. | 90 | 6.0 | | | 10 |
| Low calorie: | | | | | | |
| Bacon & tomato (Estee) | 1 T. (.5 oz.) | 35 | 1.0 | | | 3 |
| Bleu cheese: | | | | | | |
| (Estee) | 1 T. (.5 oz.) | 50 | 1.0 | | | 10 |
| (Henri's) | 1 T. (.5 oz.) | 200 | 2.0 | | | |
| (Pritikin) regular or | | | | | | |
| creamy | 1 T. | 0 | 1.0 | | | 0 |
| (Walden Farms) | 1 T. | 270 | 1.9 | | | 6 |
| (Wish-Bone) | 1 T. | 190 | 4.0 | | | Tr. |
| Buttermilk: | | | | | | |
| (Estee) creamy | 1 T. | 30 | 0.0 | | | 5 |
| (Wish-Bone) | 1 T. | 150 | 5.0 | | | Tr. |
| Catalina (Kraft) | 1 T. | 125 | | | | |

(USDA): United States Department of Agriculture
*Prepared as Package Directs

| Food and Description | Measure or Quantity | Sodium (mg.) | —Fats in grams— | | | Cholesterol (mg.) |
|---|---|---|---|---|---|---|
| | | | Total | Saturated | Unsaturated | |
| *Chef's Recipe Ranchouse* | | | | | | |
| (Henri's) | 1 T. | 115 | 1.0 | | | |
| Cucumber, creamy: | | | | | | |
| (Featherweight) | 1 T. | 12 | 2.0 | | | |
| (Kraft) | 1 T. | 210 | | | | |
| (Wish-Bone) | 1 T. (.5 oz.) | 164 | 4.0 | | | 0 |
| Cucumber & onion: | | | | | | |
| (Featherweight) | 1 T. | 128 | 0.0 | | | |
| (Henri's) | 1 T. | 200 | 2.0 | | | |
| Dijon (Estee) | 1 T. | 100 | 1.0 | | | 30 |
| French: | | | | | | |
| (USDA): | | | | | | |
| Low fat, 6% fat | 1 T. (.6 oz.) | 126 | .7 | .2 | .5 | |
| Medium fat, with artificial sweetener | 1 T. | 118 | 2.5 | .4 | 2.1 | |
| (Estee) | 1 T. (.5 oz.) | 15 | 0.0 | | | 5 |
| (Henri's) | 1 T. | 130 | 2.0 | | | |
| (Pritikin) | 1 T. | 0 | 0.0 | | | 0 |
| (Walden Farms) | 1 T. | 132 | 2.4 | | | 0 |
| (Wish-Bone) Regular | 1 T. | 70 | 2.0 | | | 0 |
| Garlic (Estee) | 1 T. (.5 oz.) | 10 | 0.0 | | | 0 |
| Herb & spice (Featherweight) | 1 T. | 5 | 0.0 | | | |
| Italian: | | | | | | |
| (USDA) | 1 T. | 118 | .7 | .2 | .6 | |
| (Estee) creamy | 1 T. | 30 | 0.0 | | | 5 |
| (Featherweight) | 1 T. | 127 | 0.0 | | | |
| (Henri's): | | | | | | |
| Authentic | 1 T. | 260 | 1.0 | | | |
| Creamy | 1 T. | 200 | 1.0 | | | |
| (Walden Farms): | | | | | | |
| *Classico* | 1 T. | 300 | Tr. | | | 0 |
| Sodium free | 1 T. | 5 | Tr. | | | 0 |
| (Wish-Bone) creamy | 1 T. (.5 oz.) | 200 | 3.0 | | | 0 |
| Onion & chive (Wish-Bone) | 1 T. | 160 | 3.0 | | | 0 |
| Ranch (Pritikin) | 1 T. | 0 | 0.0 | | | 0 |
| Russian: | | | | | | |
| (Pritikin) | 1 T. | 20 | 0.0 | | | 0 |
| (Wish-Bone) | 1 T. (.5 oz.) | 140 | Tr. | | | 0 |
| Thousand island: | | | | | | |
| (Henri's) | 1 T. | 160 | 2.0 | | | |
| (Wish-Bone) | 1 T. | 110 | 3.0 | | | 10 |
| Tomato (Pritikin) | 1 T. | 0 | 0.0 | | | 0 |
| Vinaigrette (Pritikin) | 1 T. | 0 | 0.0 | | | 0 |

(USDA): United States Department of Agriculture
*Prepared as Package Directs

| Food and Description | Measure or Quantity | Sodium (mg.) | Total | — Fats in grams — Satu- rated | Unsatu- rated | Choles- terol (mg.) |
|---|---|---|---|---|---|---|
| *Yogonaise* (Henri's) | 1 T. | 120 | 5.0 | | | |
| *Yogowhip* (Henri's) | 1 T. | 125 | 4.0 | | | |
| **\*SALAD DRESSING MIX** | | | | | | |
| (Good Seasons): | | | | | | |
| Regular: | | | | | | |
| Bleu cheese | 1 T. | 216 | <6.0 | | | <1 |
| Classic herb | 1 T. | 147 | | | | 0 |
| French, old fashioned | 1 T. | 185 | | | | 0 |
| Garlic, cheese | 1 T. | 173 | <10 | | | <1 |
| Italian: | | | | | | |
| Regular | 1 T. | 172 | <10 | | | 0 |
| Mild | 1 T. | 192 | <10 | | | 0 |
| Zesty | 1 T. | 122 | <10 | | | 0 |
| Dietetic, Italian: | | | | | | |
| Regular | 1 T. | 161 | | | | 0 |
| Lite, cheese | 1 T. | 181 | | | | <1 |
| **SALAD HERBS** (Spice Islands) | 1 tsp. | <1 | | | | (0) |
| **SALAD SEASONING,** (Durkee) | | | | | | |
| Regular | 1 tsp. (4 grams) | 1151 | .5 | | | |
| With cheese | 1 tsp. (3 grams) | 786 | .7 | | | |
| **SALAMI:** | | | | | | |
| (USDA): | | | | | | |
| Dry | 1 oz. | | 10.8 | | | |
| Cooked | 1 oz. | | 7.3 | | | |
| (Eckrich): | | | | | | |
| For beer | 1 oz. | 350 | 6.0 | | | |
| Cooked, chub | 1 oz. | 360 | 6.0 | | | |
| Cotto, beef | .7-oz. slice | 240 | 4.0 | | | |
| Cotto, meat | 1-oz. slice | 340 | 5.0 | | | |
| Hard | 1 oz. | 600 | 12.0 | | | |
| (Hormel): | | | | | | |
| Beef | 1 slice | 110 | 2.5 | | | |
| Cotto, chub | 1 oz. | 385 | 9.0 | | | |
| Genoa: | | | | | | |
| *Di Lusso* | 1 oz. | 443 | 8.0 | | | |
| *San Remo Brand* | 1 oz. | 544 | 10.0 | | | |
| Hard: | | | | | | |
| Packaged, sliced | 1 slice | 169 | 3.5 | | | |
| Whole, regular | 1 oz. | 468 | 10.0 | | | |
| (Ohse) cooked | 1 oz. | 330 | 5.0 | | | |

(USDA): United States Department of Agriculture
\*Prepared as Package Directs

| Food and Description | Measure or Quantity | Sodium (mg.) | Fats in grams — Total | Satu- rated | Unsatu- rated | Choles- terol (mg.) |
|---|---|---|---|---|---|---|
| (Oscar Mayer): | | | | | | |
| For beer, regular | .8-oz. slice | 282 | 4.4 | | | 16 |
| Cotto, beef | .8-oz. slice | 294 | 3.4 | | | 18 |
| Genoa | .3-oz. slice | 155 | 3.0 | | | 8 |
| Hard | .3-oz. slice | 167 | 2.8 | | | 7 |
| | | | | | | |
| **SALISBURY STEAK** frozen: | | | | | | |
| (Armour): | | | | | | |
| *Classic Lite* | 10-oz. meal | 870 | 13.0 | | | 75 |
| *Dinner Classics* | 11-oz. meal | 1,400 | 27.0 | | | 110 |
| (Banquet): | | | | | | |
| Dinner: | | | | | | |
| *American Favorites* | 11-oz. dinner | 1,333 | 26.0 | | | |
| *Extra Helping* | 19-oz. dinner | 2,175 | 65.0 | | | |
| Entree for one | 5-oz. pkg. | 766 | 18.0 | | | 35 |
| *Family Entree* | 2-lb. pkg. | 5,100 | 75.0 | | | |
| (Blue Star) *Dining Lite* | 9½-oz. meal | 1,460 | 9.3 | | | |
| (Stouffer's): | | | | | | |
| Regular, with onion gravy | 6 oz. | 1,150 | 15.0 | | | |
| *Lean Cuisine,* with Italian style sauce & vegetables | 9½-oz. meal | 820 | 13.0 | | | 95 |
| (Swanson): | | | | | | |
| Dinner, *Hungry-Man* | 16½-oz. dinner | 1,630 | 40.0 | | | |
| Entree: | | | | | | |
| Regular | 5½-oz. meal | 650 | 21.0 | | | |
| Main course | 10-oz. meal | 1,400 | 21.0 | | | |
| (Weight Watchers) beef | 8¾-oz. meal | 990 | 12.0 | | | |
| | | | | | | |
| **SALMON:** | | | | | | |
| Atlantic (USDA): | | | | | | |
| Raw, whole | 1 lb. (weighed whole) | | 39.5 | | | |
| Raw, meat only | 4 oz. | | 15.2 | | | |
| Canned, solids & liq., including bones | 4 oz. | | 13.8 | | | |
| Chinook or King (USDA): | | | | | | |
| Raw, steak | 1 lb. (weighed with bones) | 180 | 62.3 | 19. | 43. | |
| Raw, meat only | 4 oz. | 51 | 17.7 | 6. | 12. | |
| Canned, solids & liq., including bones, no salt added | 4 oz. | 51 | 15.9 | 4. | 11. | |

(USDA): United States Department of Agriculture
*Prepared as Package Directs

| Food and Description | Measure or Quantity | Sodium (mg.) | Fats in grams — Total | Satu- rated | Unsatu- rated | Choles- terol (mg.) |
|---|---|---|---|---|---|---|
| **Chum, (USDA):** | | | | | | |
| Raw, meat only | 4 oz. | 60 | | | | |
| Canned, solids & liq., including bones, no salt added | 4 oz. | 60 | 5.9 | | | |
| **Coho, (USDA):** | | | | | | |
| Raw, meat only | 4 oz. | 54 | | | | |
| Raw, meat only, dipped in brine | 4 oz. | 244 | | | | |
| Canned, solids & liq., no salt added | 4 oz. | 54 | 8.1 | | | |
| Canned, solids & liq., salt added | 4 oz. | 398 | 8.1 | | | |
| **Pink or Humpback (USDA):** | | | | | | |
| Raw, steak | 1 lb. (weighed with bones) | 255 | 14.8 | 4. | 11. | |
| Raw, meat only | 4 oz. | 73 | 4.2 | 1. | 3. | |
| Raw, meat only, dipped in brine | 4 oz. | 536 | 4.2 | 1. | 3. | |
| Canned, solids & liq.: | | | | | | |
| No salt added (USDA) | 4 oz. | 73 | 6.7 | 2. | 4. | |
| Salt added (USDA) | 4 oz. | 439 | 6.7 | 2. | 4. | |
| (Del Monte) | 7¾-oz. can | 1,371 | 9.2 | | | |
| (Del Monte) | 1 cup (8 oz.) | 1,414 | 9.5 | | | |
| **Sockeye or Red or Blueback:** | | | | | | |
| Raw, meat only (USDA) | 4 oz. | 54 | | | | 40 |
| Raw, steak (USDA) | 1 lb. | 192 | | | | 141 |
| Canned, solids & liq.: | | | | | | |
| Including bones, no salt added (USDA) | 4 oz. | 54 | 10.5 | | | 40 |
| Including bones, salt added (USDA) | 4 oz. | 592 | 10.5 | | | 40 |
| (Del Monte) | 7¾-oz. can | 1,217 | 16.7 | | | |
| (Del Monte) | 1 cup (8 oz.) | 1,255 | 17.2 | | | |
| **Unspecified kind of salmon, baked or broiled with vegetable shortening:** | | | | | | |
| (USDA) | 4-oz. steak (approx. 4″ × 3″ × ½″, 4.2 oz.) | 139 | 8.9 | | | 53 |
| (USDA) | 6¾″ × 2½″ × 1″ (5.1 oz.) | 168 | 10.7 | | | 68 |

(USDA): United States Department of Agriculture
*Prepared as Package Directs

| Food and Description | Measure or Quantity | Sodium (mg.) | — Fats in grams — | | | Choles- terol (mg.) |
|---|---|---|---|---|---|---|
| | | | Total | Satu- rated | Unsatu- rated | |
| **SALMON RICE LOAF,** home recipe (USDA) | 4 oz. | | 5.1 | | | |
| **SALMON, SMOKED:** | | | | | | |
| (USDA) | 4 oz. | | 10.5 | | | |
| Lox, drained (Vita) | 4-oz. jar | | 6.7 | | | |
| Nova, drained (Vita) | 4-oz. can | | 14.6 | | | |
| **SALSIFY** (USDA): | | | | | | |
| Raw, without tops, freshly harvested | 1 lb. (weighed untrimmed) | | 2.4 | | | 0 |
| Raw, without tops, after storage | 1 lb. (weighed untrimmed) | | 2.4 | | | 0 |
| Boiled, drained, freshly harvested | 4 oz. | | .7 | | | 0 |
| Boiled, drained, after storage | 4 oz. | | .7 | | | 0 |
| **SALT:** | | | | | | |
| Butter-flavored, imitation: | | | | | | |
| (Durkee) | 1 tsp. (5 grams) | 1,362 | .3 | | | |
| (French's) | 1 tsp. (4 grams) | 1,090 | .9 | | | |
| Garlic (French's) | 1 tsp. (6 grams) | 1,850 | .1 | | | |
| Garlic, parslied (French's) | 1 tsp. (4 grams) | 1,050 | .1 | | | |
| Garlic (Lawry's) | 2.9-oz. pkg. | | .3 | | | |
| Garlic (Lawry's) | 1 tsp. (4 grams) | | Tr. | | | |
| Hickory smoke (French's) | 1 tsp. (4 grams) | 1,170 | Tr. | | | |
| Lite Salt (Morton) | 1 tsp. (6 grams) | 1,188 | 0.0 | | | |
| Onion (French's) | 1 tsp. (5 grams) | 1,620 | .1 | | | |
| Onion (Lawry's) | 3-oz. pkg. | | 1.0 | | | |
| Onion (Lawry's) | 1 tsp. (3 grams) | | <.1 | | | |
| Seasoning (French's) | 1 tsp. (5 grams) | 1,620 | .1 | | | |
| Seasoned (Lawry's) | 3-oz. pkg. | | .5 | | | |
| Seasoned (Lawry's) | 1 tsp. (5 grams) | | <.1 | | | |
| Substitute: | | | | | | |
| (Adolph's) | 1 tsp. (4 grams) | <1 | 0.0 | | | 0 |
| (Morton) | 1 tsp. (6 grams) | <1 | 0.0 | | | |
| Substitute, seasoned: | | | | | | |
| (Adolph's) | 1 tsp. (4 grams) | <1 | <.1 | Tr. | Tr. | 0 |
| (Morton) | 1 tsp. (6 grams) | <1 | 0.0 | | | |
| Table: | | | | | | |
| (USDA) | 1 tsp. (6 grams) | 2,325 | 0.0 | | | 0 |
| (Morton) | 1 tsp. (6 grams) | 2,544 | 0.0 | | | (0) |

(USDA): United States Department of Agriculture
*Prepared as Package Directs

| Food and Description | Measure or Quantity | Sodium (mg.) | — Fats in grams — | | | Choles- terol (mg.) |
|---|---|---|---|---|---|---|
| | | | Total | Satu- rated | Unsatu- rated | |
| **SALT PORK,** raw (USDA): | | | | | | |
| With skin | 1 lb. (weighed with skin) | 5,278 | 370.0 | 141. | 229. | |
| Without skin | 1 oz. | 344 | 24.1 | 9. | 15. | |
| **SALT STICK** (See **BREAD STICK**) | | | | | | |
| **SAND DAB,** raw (USDA): | | | | | | |
| Whole | 1 lb. (weighed whole) | 117 | 1.2 | | | |
| Meat only | 4 oz. | 88 | .9 | | | |
| **SANDWICH SPREAD:** | | | | | | |
| (USDA) | 1 cup (8.7 oz.) | 1,540 | 89.1 | | | |
| (USDA) | 1 T. (.5 oz.) | 94 | 5.4 | | | |
| (USDA) low calorie | 1 T. (.5 oz.) | 94 | 1.4 | | | |
| (Hellmann's)[1] | 1 T. (.5 oz.) | 191 | 6.2 | | | 27 |
| (Oscar Mayer) | 1 oz. | 261 | 4.9 | | | 10 |
| **SAPODILLA,** fresh (USDA): | | | | | | |
| Whole | 1 lb. (weighed with skin & seeds) | 44 | 4.0 | | | 0 |
| Flesh only | 4 oz. | 14 | 1.2 | | | 0 |
| **SAPOTE OR MARMALADE PLUM,** fresh (USDA): | | | | | | |
| Whole | 1 lb. (weighed with skin & seeds) | | 2.1 | | | 0 |
| Flesh only | 4 oz. | | .7 | | | 0 |
| **SARDINE:** | | | | | | |
| Atlantic, canned in oil (USDA): | | | | | | |
| Solids & liq. | 3¾-oz. can | 541 | 25.9 | | | 127 |
| Drained solids | 3¾-oz. can | 757 | 10.2 | | | 129 |
| Atlantic, canned in tomato sauce, solids & liq. (Del Monte) | 1½ large sardines | 321 | 6.8 | | | |
| Norwegian, canned: | | | | | | |
| (Snow's) | 1 oz. | | 6.3 | | | |

(USDA): United States Department of Agriculture
*Prepared as Package Directs
[1]Principal source of fat: oil.

| Food and Description | Measure or Quantity | Sodium (mg.) | —Fats in grams— | | | Choles- terol (mg.) |
|---|---|---|---|---|---|---|
| | | | Total | Satu- rated | Unsatu- rated | |
| In mustard sauce (Underwood) | 3¾-oz. can | 837 | 14.2 | | | |
| In oil, drained (Underwood) | 3¾-oz. can | 182 | 16.0 | | | |
| In tomato sauce (Underwood) | 3¾-oz. can | 422 | 9.8 | | | |
| Pacific (USDA): | | | | | | |
| Raw | 4 oz. | | 9.8 | | | |
| Canned, in brine or mustard, solids & liq. | 4 oz. | 862 | 13.6 | | | |
| Canned in tomato sauce, solids & liq. | 4 oz. | 454 | 13.8 | | | |
| **SAUCE:** | | | | | | |
| Regular: | | | | | | |
| *A-1* | 1 T. | 275 | Tr. | | | |
| Barbecue: | | | | | | |
| *Chris' & Pitt's* | 1 T. | 141 | .1 | | | |
| (French's) smoky | 1 T. | 280 | 0.0 | | | |
| (Hunt's) | 1 T. | 190 | 0.0 | | | |
| *Open Pit* (General Foods) original | 1 T. | 236 | Tr. | | | 0 |
| Burrito (Del Monte) | ¼ cup | 355 | 0.0 | | | |
| Chili (See **CHILI SAUCE**) | | | | | | |
| *Escoffier* Sauce Diable | 1 T. | 160 | Tr. | | | |
| *Escoffier* Sauce Robert | 1 T. | 70 | Tr. | | | |
| *Famous Sauce* | 1 T. | 67 | 7.0 | | | |
| Hot, *Frank's* | 1 tsp. | 131 | 0.0 | | | |
| Italian (See also **SPAGHETTI SAUCE or TOMATO SAUCE**): | | | | | | |
| (Contadina) | 4-oz. serving | 601 | 2.4 | | | |
| (Ragú) red cooking | 3½-oz. serving | | 2.0 | | | |
| Salsa Mexicana (Contadina) | 4 fl. oz. | 570 | .4 | | | |
| Salsa Picante (Del Monte) regular | ¼ cup | 385 | 0.0 | | | |
| Salsa Roja (Del Monte) | ¼ cup | 510 | 0.0 | | | |
| Seafood cocktail (Del Monte) | 1 T. | 228 | Tr. | | | |
| Soy: | | | | | | |
| (Kikkoman) | 1 T. | 921 | Tr. | | | Tr. |
| (La Choy) | 1 T. | 974 | .1 | | | Tr. |
| *Steak Supreme* | 1 T. | 125 | Tr. | | | |
| Sweet & sour: | | | | | | |
| (Chun King) | 1.8 oz. | 234 | .1 | | | 0 |

(USDA): United States Department of Agriculture
*Prepared as Package Directs

| Food and Description | Measure or Quantity | Sodium (mg.) | —Fats in grams— | | | Choles-terol (mg.) |
|---|---|---|---|---|---|---|
| | | | Total | Satu-rated | Unsatu-rated | |
| (Contadina) | 4 fl. oz. | 500 | 3.0 | | | 0 |
| (La Choy) | 1-oz. serving | | | | | |
| *Tabasco* | ¼ tsp. | 9 | Tr. | | | |
| Taco: | | | | | | |
| *Old El Paso,* hot or mild | 1 T. | 66 | Tr. | | | |
| (Ortega) hot | 1 oz. | 207 | .1 | | | 0 |
| Tartar (Hellmann's) | 1 T. | 182 | 7.9 | | | 5 |
| Teriyaki (Kikkoman) | 1 T. | 612 | Tr. | | | Tr. |
| *V8* | 1-oz. serving | 270 | 1.0 | | | |
| White, medium (USDA) | ¼ cup | 241 | 7.9 | 4.4 | 3.5 | 9 |
| Worcestershire (French's) | | | | | | |
| regular or smoky | 1 T. | 200 | 0.0 | | | |
| Dietetic (Estee): | | | | | | |
| Barbecue | 1 T. | 3 | 0.0 | | | 0 |
| Cocktail | 1 T. | 35 | 0.0 | | | 0 |
| Taco | 1 oz. | 25 | 0.0 | | | 0 |
| | | | | | | |
| **SAUCE MIX:** | | | | | | |
| Regular: | | | | | | |
| A la King (Durkee) | 1-oz. pkg. | 1,384 | 8.0 | | | |
| *Cheese: | | | | | | |
| (Durkee) | ½ cup | 446 | 10.5 | | | |
| (French's) | ½ cup | 425 | 4.0 | | | |
| Hollandaise: | | | | | | |
| (Durkee) | 1-oz. pkg. | 548 | 14.0 | | | |
| *(French's) | 1 T. | 97 | 1.3 | | | |
| *Sour cream (French's) | ⅔ cup | 727 | 7.0 | | | |
| *Sweet & sour (Kikkoman) | 1 T. | 63 | 0.0 | | | 0 |
| Teriyaki (Kikkoman) | 1.5-oz. pkg. | 400 | .4 | | | 0 |
| Dietetic (Weight Watchers) | | | | | | |
| lemon butter | 1 pkg. | 1,895 | 0.0 | | | |
| | | | | | | |
| **SAUERKRAUT,** canned: | | | | | | |
| Solids & liq. (USDA) 1.9% salt | 1 cup (8.3 oz.) | 1,755 | .5 | | | 0 |
| Drained solids (USDA) | 1 cup (5 oz.) | | .4 | | | 0 |
| Solids & liq. (Del Monte) | 1 cup (8 oz.) | 1,550 | .4 | | | 0 |
| Solids & liq. (Stokely-Van Camp's) | 1 cup (7.8 oz.) | | .4 | | | |
| | | | | | | |
| **SAUERKRAUT JUICE,** canned | | | | | | |
| (USDA) 2% salt | ½ cup (4.3 oz.) | 952 | Tr. | | | 0 |

(USDA): United States Department of Agriculture
*Prepared as Package Directs

| Food and Description | Measure or Quantity | Sodium (mg.) | —Fats in grams— | | | Cholesterol (mg.) |
|---|---|---|---|---|---|---|
| | | | Total | Saturated | Unsaturated | |
| **SAUGER,** raw (USDA): | | | | | | |
| Whole | 1 lb. (weighed whole) | | 13.2 | | | |
| Meat only | 4 oz. | | .9 | | | |
| **SAUSAGE:** | | | | | | |
| Brown & serve: | | | | | | |
| (USDA) | 1 oz. | | 10.2 | | | |
| *(USDA) | 1 oz. | | 10.7 | | | |
| *(Hormel) | 1 sausage | 215 | 6.5 | | | |
| Country-style, smoked links | | | | | | |
| (USDA) | 1 oz. | | 8.8 | 3.1 | 5.7 | |
| Links, hot (Ohse) | 1 oz. | 310 | 3.0 | | | |
| Patty (Hormel): | | | | | | |
| Hot | 1 patty | 549 | 13.0 | | | |
| Mild | 1 patty | 541 | 13.0 | | | |
| Polish-style: | | | | | | |
| (Eckrich) meat: | | | | | | |
| Regular | 1 oz. | 260 | 9.0 | | | |
| Skinless | 1 oz. | 250 | 8.0 | | | |
| (Hormel): | | | | | | |
| Regular | 1 sausage | 287 | 7.0 | | | |
| Kielbasa | ½ link | 826 | 14.0 | | | |
| Kolbase | 3 oz. | 904 | 19.0 | | | |
| (Ohse): | | | | | | |
| Regular | 1 oz. | 290 | 7.0 | | | |
| Hot | 1 oz. | 270 | 5.0 | | | |
| Pork: | | | | | | |
| (USDA) links or bulk: | | | | | | |
| Uncooked | 1 oz. | 210 | 14.4 | 5.1 | 9.3 | |
| Cooked | 1 oz. | 272 | 12.5 | 5.0 | 8. | |
| Cooked, 16 links per lb. | | | | | | |
| raw | 1 link | 125 | 5.7 | 2.1 | 3.7 | |
| (Eckrich): | | | | | | |
| Links | 1-oz. link | | 10.0 | | | |
| Patty | 2-oz. patty | | 26.0 | | | |
| *(Hormel): | | | | | | |
| *Little Sizzlers* | 1 sausage | 96 | 4.5 | | | |
| Midget links | 1 sausage | 163 | 6.5 | | | |
| Smoked | 1 oz. | | 9.0 | | | |
| (Jimmy Dean) | 2 oz. | 338 | | | | 48 |
| *(Oscar Mayer): | | | | | | |
| *Little Friers* | 1-oz. link | 218 | 7.5 | | | 17 |
| Patty, southern brand | 1.5-oz. patty | 282 | 11.3 | | | 27 |

(USDA): United States Department of Agriculture
*Prepared as Package Directs

| Food and Description | Measure or Quantity | Sodium (mg.) | Total | Satu-rated | Unsatu-rated | Choles-terol (mg.) |
|---|---|---|---|---|---|---|
| | | | —Fats in grams— | | | |
| Smoked: | | | | | | |
| (Eckrich): | | | | | | |
| Beef | 2 oz. | 520 | 17.0 | | | |
| Cheese | 2 oz. | 500 | 15.0 | | | |
| Ham, *Smok-Y-Links* | .8-oz. link | 280 | 6.5 | | | |
| Meat | 2 oz. | 530 | 17.0 | | | |
| Meat, hot | 2.7-oz. link | 640 | 21.0 | | | |
| (Hormel) Smokies: | | | | | | |
| Regular | 1 sausage | 298 | 7.0 | | | |
| Cheese | 1 sausage | 311 | 7.5 | | | |
| (Ohse) | 1 oz. | 320 | 7.0 | | | |
| (Oscar Mayer): | | | | | | |
| Regular | 1.5-oz. link | 432 | 11.2 | | | 27 |
| Regular | 4-oz. link | 1,135 | 29.4 | | | 71 |
| Beef | 1.5-oz. link | 430 | 11.0 | | | 27 |
| Cheese | 1.5-oz. link | 453 | 11.2 | | | 28 |
| Pork, Little Smokies | .3-oz. link | 91 | 2.5 | | | 6 |
| Turkey: | | | | | | |
| *(Louis Rich) | 1 oz. | | 3.0 | | | |
| (Ohse) breakfast | 1 oz. | 180 | 5.3 | | | |
| Vienna, canned: | | | | | | |
| (Hormel) no broth: | | | | | | |
| Regular | 1 sausage | 120 | 4.5 | | | |
| Chicken | 1 sausage | NA | 4.0 | | | |
| (Libby's): | | | | | | |
| In barbecue sauce | ½ of 5-oz. can | | 15.0 | | | |
| In beef broth | 1 link (5-oz. can) | 94 | 4.3 | | | |
| In beef broth | 1 link (9-oz. can) | 86 | 4.0 | | | |
| **SAUTERNES:** | | | | | | |
| (Barton & Guestier) French white Bordeaux, 13% alcohol | 3 fl. oz. | 3 | 0.0 | | | (0) |
| (Gold Seal) dry, 12% alcohol | 3 fl. oz. | 3 | 0.0 | | | (0) |
| (Gold Seal) semi-soft, 12% alcohol | 3 fl. oz. (3.2 oz.) | 3 | 0.0 | | | (0) |
| (Great Western) Aurora, 12.5% alcohol | 3 fl. oz. | 34 | 0.0 | | | 0 |
| **SAVORY** (Spice Islands) | 1 tsp. | <1 | | | | (0) |

**SCALLION** (See **ONION, GREEN**)

(USDA): United States Department of Agriculture
*Prepared as Package Directs

319

| Food and Description | Measure or Quantity | Sodium (mg.) | — Fats in grams — | | | Cholesterol (mg.) |
|---|---|---|---|---|---|---|
| | | | Total | Saturated | Unsaturated | |
| **SCALLOP:** | | | | | | |
| Raw, muscle only[1] (USDA) | 4 oz. | 289 | .2 | | | 40 |
| Steamed (USDA) | 4 oz. | 301 | 1.6 | | | 60 |
| Frozen: | | | | | | |
| Breaded, fried, reheated (USDA) | 4 oz. | | 9.5 | | | |
| (Mrs. Paul's): | | | | | | |
| Breaded & french fried | 1/2 of 7-oz. pkg. | 545 | 7.0 | | | |
| Mediterranean | 11-oz. pkg. | 775 | 5.0 | | | |
| (Stouffer's) *Lean Cuisine,* oriental, & vegetable with rice | 11-oz. pkg. | 1,325 | 2.0 | | | 20 |
| **SCALLOP & SHRIMP MARINER,** frozen (Stouffer's) with rice | 10 1/4-oz. pkg | 1,120 | 16.0 | | | |
| *SCOTCH-COMFORT* | 1 fl. oz. | Tr. | 0.0 | | | (0) |
| **SCOTCH WHISKY** (See **DISTILLED LIQUOR**) | | | | | | |
| **SCRAPPLE** (USDA) | 4 oz. | | 15.4 | | | |
| **SCREWDRIVER COCKTAIL,** (Mr. Boston) 12 1/2% alcohol | 3 fl. oz. | 104 | 0.0 | | | |
| **SCUP** (See **PORGY**) | | | | | | |
| **SEABASS, WHITE,** raw, meat only (USDA) | 4 oz. | | .6 | | | |
| **SEAFOOD DINNER OR ENTREE,** frozen: | | | | | | |
| (Armour) *Classic Lite* natural herbs | 11 1/2-oz. pkg. | 1,240 | 6.0 | | | 20 |
| (Mrs. Paul's): | | | | | | |
| Combination, breaded & fried | 9-oz. serving | 1,340 | 25.0 | | | |
| Newberg | 8 1/2-oz. serving | 610 | 13.0 | | | |

(USDA): United States Department of Agriculture
*Prepared as Package Directs
[1]Frozen scallops, possibly brined.

| Food and Description | Measure or Quantity | Sodium (mg.) | — Fats in grams — | | | Choles- terol (mg.) |
|---|---|---|---|---|---|---|
| | | | Total | Satu- rated | Unsatu- rated | |
| *SEGO* **DIET FOOD,** canned: | | | | | | |
| Regular: | | | | | | |
| Very chocolate, very chocolate malt or very dutch chocolate | 10-fl.-oz. can | 445 | 1.0 | | | |
| Very strawberry or very vanilla | 10-fl.-oz. can | 360 | 5.0 | | | |
| Lite: | | | | | | |
| Chocolate, chocolate jamocha almond, chocolate malt, double chocolate or dutch chocolate | 10-fl.-oz. can | 475 | 3.0 | | | |
| French vanilla, strawberry or vanilla | 10-fl.-oz. can | 390 | 4.0 | | | |
| **SESAME SEED:** | | | | | | |
| Dry, whole (USDA) | 1 oz. | 17 | 13.9 | 2. | 12. | 0 |
| Dry, hulled (USDA) | 1 oz. | | 15.1 | 2. | 13. | 0 |
| Hulled (Spice Islands) | 1 tsp. | 2 | | | | (0) |
| Liquid, Tahini (Sahadi) | 1 T. (8 grams) | | 5.1 | | | |
| **7 WHOLE GRAIN,** cereal (Loma Linda): | | | | | | |
| Crunchy | 1 oz. | 90 | 2.0 | | | |
| No sugar | 1 oz. | 75 | 1.0 | | | |
| **SHAD** (USDA): | | | | | | |
| Raw, whole | 1 lb. (weighed whole) | 118 | 21.8 | | | |
| Raw, meat only | 4 oz. | 61 | 11.3 | | | |
| Cooked, home recipe: | | | | | | |
| Baked with butter or margarine & bacon slices | 4 oz. | 90 | 12.8 | | | |
| Creole, made with tomatoes, onion, green pepper, butter & flour | 4 oz. | 83 | 9.9 | | | |
| Canned, solids & liq. | 4 oz. | | 10.0 | | | |
| **SHAD, GIZZARD,** raw (USDA): | | | | | | |
| Whole | 1 lb. (weighed whole) | | 21.0 | | | |
| Meat only | 4 oz. | | 15.9 | | | |

(USDA): United States Department of Agriculture
*Prepared as Package Directs

| Food and Description | Measure or Quantity | Sodium (mg.) | —Fats in grams— | | | Cholesterol (mg.) |
|---|---|---|---|---|---|---|
| | | | Total | Satu-rated | Unsatu-rated | |

**SHAKE 'N BAKE,** seasoned
  mixes:
  Chicken:

| | | | | | | |
|---|---|---|---|---|---|---|
| Original | 2.4-oz. envelope | 2,363 | 10.2 | | | Tr. |
| Barbecue | 3.5-oz. envelope | 3,280 | 7.6 | | | Tr. |
| Crispy country mild | 2.4-oz. envelope | 2,041 | 14.9 | | | Tr. |
| Fish | 2-oz. envelope | 1,049 | 7.9 | | | Tr. |
| Italian | 2.4-oz. envelope | 2,098 | 10.3 | | | 1 |
| Pork, original | 2.4-oz. envelope | 2,541 | 4.2 | | | 0 |
| Pork & ribs, barbecue | 2.9-oz. envelope | 2,644 | 6.5 | | | Tr. |

**SHAKEY'S:**
  Chicken, fried, & potatoes:

| | | | | | | |
|---|---|---|---|---|---|---|
| 3-piece | 1 order | 2,293 | 56.0 | | | |
| 5-piece | 1 order | 5,327 | 90.0 | | | |
| Ham & cheese sandwich, hot | 1 sandwich | 2,135 | 21.0 | | | |

  Pizza:
  Cheese:

| | | | | | | |
|---|---|---|---|---|---|---|
| Thin | 13″ pizza | 3,160 | 45.0 | | | |
| Thick | 13″ pizza | 5,740 | 43.0 | | | |

  Onion, green pepper, olive &
    mushroom:

| | | | | | | |
|---|---|---|---|---|---|---|
| Thin | 13″ pizza | 3,950 | 54.0 | | | |
| Thick | 13″ pizza | 4,340 | 52.0 | | | |

  Pepperoni:

| | | | | | | |
|---|---|---|---|---|---|---|
| Thin | 13″ pizza | 4,550 | 83.0 | | | |
| Thick | 13″ pizza | 4,940 | 81.0 | | | |

  Sausage & mushroom:

| | | | | | | |
|---|---|---|---|---|---|---|
| Thin | 13″ pizza | 4,160 | 58.0 | | | |
| Thick | 13″ pizza | 4,450 | 56.0 | | | |

  Sausage & pepperoni:

| | | | | | | |
|---|---|---|---|---|---|---|
| Thin | 13″ pizza | 5,870 | 102.0 | | | |
| Thick | 13″ pizza | 6,260 | 100.0 | | | |

  Special:

| | | | | | | |
|---|---|---|---|---|---|---|
| Thin | 13″ pizza | 5,760 | 98.0 | | | |
| Thick | 13″ pizza | 6,060 | 96.0 | | | |
| Potatoes | 15-piece order | 3,703 | 36.0 | | | |

  Spaghetti with meat sauce &
    garlic bread

| | | | | | | |
|---|---|---|---|---|---|---|
| garlic bread | 1 order | 1,904 | 33.0 | | | |
| Super hot hero | 1 sandwich | 2,688 | 44.0 | | | |

**SHALLOT,** raw (USDA):

| | | | | | | |
|---|---|---|---|---|---|---|
| With skin | 1 oz. | 3 | <.1 | | | 0 |
| With skin removed | 1 oz. | 3 | <.1 | | | 0 |

(USDA): United States Department of Agriculture
*Prepared as Package Directs

| Food and Description | Measure or Quantity | Sodium (mg.) | — Fats in grams — | | | Choles- terol (mg.) |
|---|---|---|---|---|---|---|
| | | | Total | Satu- rated | Unsatu- rated | |

**SHEEFISH** (See **INCONNU**)

**SHEEPSHEAD,** Atlantic, raw (USDA):

| | | | | | | |
|---|---|---|---|---|---|---|
| Whole | 1 lb. (weighed whole) | 142 | 3.9 | | | |
| Meat only | 4 oz. | 115 | 3.2 | | | |

**SHELLS, PASTA, STUFFED,** frozen:
(Celentano):

| | | | | | | |
|---|---|---|---|---|---|---|
| Broccoli & cheese stuffed | 11¼-oz. pkg. (4 shells) | 480 | 17.0 | | | 130 |
| Cheese stuffed: | | | | | | |
| without sauce | ½ of 12½-oz. pkg. | 265 | 15.0 | | | |
| with sauce | ½ of 16-oz. box | 425 | 14.0 | | | 75 |
| (Stouffer's): | | | | | | |
| Beef & spinach stuffed with tomato sauce | 9-oz. pkg. | 1,315 | 11.0 | | | |
| Cheese stuffed with meat sauce | 9-oz. pkg. | 1,310 | 14.0 | | | |
| Chicken stuffed with cheese sauce | 9-oz. pkg. | 1,060 | 22.0 | | | |

**\*SHELLS AND SAUCE**
(Lipton):

| | | | | | | |
|---|---|---|---|---|---|---|
| Creamy garlic | ½ cup | 535 | 9.0 | | | |
| Herb tomato | ½ cup | 435 | 6.0 | | | |

**SHERBET OR SORBET:**

| | | | | | | |
|---|---|---|---|---|---|---|
| Cassis (Häagen-Dazs) | 4 fl. oz. | 11 | Tr. | | | |
| Daiquiri ice (Baskin-Robbins) | 4 fl. oz. | 18 | 0.0 | | | |
| Lemon (Häagen-Dazs) | 4 fl. oz. | 22 | Tr. | | | |
| Orange: | | | | | | |
| (USDA) | ¼ pt. (3.4 oz.) | 10 | 1.2 | | | 0 |
| (Baskin-Robbins) | 4 fl. oz. | 46 | 2.4 | | | |
| (Borden) | ½ cup | 40 | 1.0 | | | |
| (Häagen-Dazs) | 4 fl. oz. | 22 | Tr. | | | |
| (Howard Johnson's) | ½ cup | | 1.5 | | | |
| Raspberry: | | | | | | |
| (Baskin-Robbins) | 4 fl. oz. | 42 | 0 | | | |
| (Häagen-Dazs) | 4 fl. oz. | 17 | Tr. | | | |
| (Sealtest) | ½ cup | 20 | | | | |

(USDA): United States Department of Agriculture
\*Prepared as Package Directs

| Food and Description | Measure or Quantity | Sodium (mg.) | — Fats in grams — | | | Choles- terol (mg.) |
|---|---|---|---|---|---|---|
| | | | Total | Satu- rated | Unsatu- rated | |
| **SHERRY:** | | | | | | |
| (Great Western) Solera, 18% alcohol | 3 fl. oz. | 34 | 0.0 | | | 0 |
| Cocktail (Gold Seal) 19% alcohol | 3 fl. oz. (3.1 oz.) | 3 | 0.0 | | | (0) |
| Cooking (Great Western) 18% alcohol | 3 fl. oz. | 31 | 0.0 | | | 0 |
| Cream (Gold Seal) 19% alcohol | 3 fl. oz. (3.3 oz.) | 3 | 0.0 | | | (0) |
| Cream (Great Western) 18% alcohol | 3 fl. oz. | 32 | 0.0 | | | 0 |
| Dry (Great Western) Solera, 18% alcohol | 3 fl. oz. | 34 | 0.0 | | | 0 |
| **SHORTENING** (See **FATS**) | | | | | | |
| **SHREDDED OATS,** cereal (USDA)[1] | 1 oz. | 173 | .6 | Tr. | < 1. | 0 |
| **SHREDDED WHEAT,** cereal: | | | | | | |
| (USDA) plain, without salt | 1 cup (1.2 oz.) | 1 | .7 | Tr. | < 1. | 0 |
| (USDA) with malt, salt & sugar | 1 cup (2.1 oz.) | 418 | 1.7 | Tr. | 2. | 0 |
| (Kellogg's) cinnamon or sugar-frosted, *Mini-Wheats* | 4 biscuits (1 oz.) | 4 | .3 | | | (0) |
| (Nabisco) | 1 biscuit (.9 oz.) | < 1 | 1.0 | | | (0) |
| (Nabisco) *Spoon Size* | 2/3 cup (1 oz.) | < 1 | 1.0 | | | (0) |
| (Quaker) | 2 biscuits (1 1/3 oz.) | < 1 | .4 | | | (0) |
| **SHRIMP:** | | | | | | |
| Raw (USDA): | | | | | | |
| Whole | 1 lb. (weighed in shell) | 438 | 2.5 | | | 470 |
| Meat only | 4 oz. | 159 | 9 | | | 170 |
| Canned, dry pack or drained (USDA) | 1 cup (22 large or 76 small, 4.5 oz.) | | 1.4 | | | 192 |
| Cooked, french-fried[2] (USDA) | 4 oz. | 211 | 12.2 | | | |

(USDA): United States Department of Agriculture
*Prepared as Package Directs
[1]Includes protein & other added nutrients.
[2]Dipped in egg, bread crumbs & flour or in batter.

| Food and Description | Measure or Quantity | Sodium (mg.) | Fats in grams Total | Satu- rated | Unsatu- rated | Choles- terol (mg.) |
|---|---|---|---|---|---|---|
| Frozen: | | | | | | |
| Raw: | | | | | | |
| Breaded, not more than 50% breading (USDA) | 4 oz. | | .8 | | | |
| Breaded (Gorton's) | ¼ of 1-lb. pkg. | 80 | .8 | | | |
| Cooked (Sau-Sea) | 5 oz. | 330 | 2.0 | | | 173 |
| **SHRIMP COCKTAIL,** (Sau-Sea) | 4-oz. jar | 1,020 | 1.0 | | | 102 |
| **SHRIMP DINNER OR ENTREE,** frozen: | | | | | | |
| (Armour) *Classic Lite,* in sherried cream sauce | 10½-oz. pkg. | 1,220 | 8.0 | | | 110 |
| (Blue Star) *Dining Lite,* creole, with rice | 10 oz. | 820 | 1.9 | | | |
| (Conagra) *Light & Elegant* creole | 10-oz. entree | 1,050 | 2.0 | | | 120 |
| (Gorton's) *Light Recipe:* | | | | | | |
| Oriental | 1 pkg. | 740 | 2.0 | | | |
| & pasta | 1 pkg. | 550 | 19.0 | | | |
| Scampi | 1 pkg. | 420 | 24.0 | | | |
| Stuffed | 1 pkg. | 950 | 15.0 | | | |
| (Mrs. Paul's): | | | | | | |
| Breaded & fried | 3 oz. | 525 | 10.0 | | | |
| Oriental | 11 oz. | 940 | 2.0 | | | |
| Parmesan | 11 oz. | 1,185 | 9.0 | | | |
| (Stouffer's) newberg | 6½ oz. | 555 | 23.0 | | | |
| **SHRIMP PASTE,** canned (USDA) | 1 oz. | | 2.7 | | | |
| **SHRIMP PUFF,** frozen (Durkee) | 1 piece (.5 oz.) | | 4.3 | | | |
| **SKATE,** raw, meat only (USDA) | 4 oz. | | .8 | | | |
| **SLENDER** (Carnation): | | | | | | |
| Bar: | | | | | | |
| Chocolate | 1 bar | 142 | 7.0 | | | < 1 |
| Chocolate peanut butter | 1 bar | 142 | 7.5 | | | < 1 |
| Vanilla | 1 bar | 160 | 7.5 | | | < 1 |
| Dry: | | | | | | |
| Chocolate[1] | 1 pkg. (1 oz.) | 110 | 1.0 | Tr. | Tr. | 3 |

(USDA): United States Department of Agriculture
*Prepared as Package Directs
[1]Principal sources of fat: milk, cocoa & lecithin.

| Food and Description | Measure or Quantity | Sodium (mg.) | — Fats in grams — | | | Cholesterol (mg.) |
|---|---|---|---|---|---|---|
| | | | Total | Saturated | Unsaturated | |
| Dutch chocolate [1] | 1 pkg. (1 oz.) | 110 | .9 | < 1. | Tr. | 2 |
| Vanilla, French | 1 pkg. (1 oz.) | 110 | .2 | Tr. | Tr. | 3 |
| Liquid: | | | | | | |
| Chocolate [2] | 10-fl.-oz. can | 515 | 4.0 | | | 4 |
| Chocolate fudge [2] | 10-fl.-oz. can | 550 | 4.0 | | | 4 |
| Chocolate malt [3] | 10-fl.-oz. can | 530 | 4.0 | | | 4 |
| Milk chocolate [2] | 10-fl.-oz. can | 520 | 4.0 | | | 4 |
| Vanilla [4] | 10-fl.-oz. can | 550 | 4.0 | | | 5 |

**SLOPPY JOE:**
Canned:

| | | | | | | |
|---|---|---|---|---|---|---|
| (Hormel) *Short Orders* | 7½-oz. can | | 23.0 | | | |
| (Libby's) beef | ⅓ cup (2.5 oz.) | 190 | 7.0 | | | |
| Frozen (Morton) | 5-oz. pkg. | 730 | 13.0 | | | 33 |

**SLOPPY JOE SAUCE** (Ragú)

| | | | | | | |
|---|---|---|---|---|---|---|
| *Joe Sauce* | ¼ of 14-oz. jar | 645 | 0.0 | | | 0.0 |

**SLOPPY JOE SEASONING MIX:**
*(Durkee):

| | | | | | | |
|---|---|---|---|---|---|---|
| Regular | 1¼ cups | 1,788 | 48.5 | | | |
| Pizza flavor | 1¼ cups | 1,515 | 51.0 | | | |
| (French's) | 1 pkg. | 3,040 | 0.0 | | | |
| *(Hunt's) *Manwich* | 5.9-oz. serving | 590 | 13.0 | | | |

**SMELT,** Atlantic, jack & bay (USDA):

| | | | | | | |
|---|---|---|---|---|---|---|
| Raw, whole | 1 lb. (weighed whole) | | | | | |
| Raw, meat only | 4 oz. | | 2.4 | | | |
| Canned, solids & liq. | 4 oz. | | 15.3 | | | |

**SMURF-BERRY CRUNCH,**

| | | | | | | |
|---|---|---|---|---|---|---|
| cereal (Post) | 1 cup (1 oz.) | 65 | .9 | | | |

**SNACK** (See **CRACKER, POPCORN, POTATO CHIPS,** etc.)

(USDA): United States Department of Agriculture
*Prepared as Package Directs
[1]Principal sources of fat: milk, cocoa & lecithin.
[2]Principal sources of fat: milk, cocoa & corn oil.
[3]Principal sources of fat: wort solids, milk, cocoa & corn oil.
[4]Principal sources of fat: milk & corn oil.

| Food and Description | Measure or Quantity | Sodium (mg.) | Total | Fats in grams — Satu-rated | Unsatu-rated | Choles-terol (mg.) |
|---|---|---|---|---|---|---|
| **SNACK BAR** (Pepperidge Farm): | | | | | | |
| Apple nut | 1.7-oz. piece | 90 | 5.0 | | | |
| Blueberry | 1.7-oz. piece | 90 | 3.0 | | | |
| Brownie nut | 1.5-oz. piece | 100 | 7.0 | | | |
| Date nut | 1.5-oz. piece | 90 | 7.0 | | | |
| Raisin spice | 1.5-oz. piece | 80 | 6.0 | | | |
| **SNAIL,** raw: | | | | | | |
| (USDA) | 4 oz. | | 1.6 | | | |
| Giant African (USDA) | 4 oz. | | 1.6 | | | |
| **SNAPPER** (See **RED SNAPPER**) | | | | | | |
| **SNO-BALLS** (Hostess) 2 to pkg. | 1 cake (1.5 oz.) | 170 | 3.8 | | | 2 |
| **SOFT DRINK:** | | | | | | |
| Sweetened: | | | | | | |
| Apple (Slice) | 6 fl. oz. | 2 | 0.0 | | | 0 |
| Birch beer (Canada Dry) | 6 fl. oz. | 14 | 0.0 | | | 0 |
| Bitter lemon (Schweppes) | 6 fl. oz. | 13 | 0.0 | | | 0 |
| *Bubble Up* | 6 fl. oz. | 16 | 0.0 | | | 0 |
| *Cactus Cooler* (Canada Dry) | 6 fl. oz. | 16 | 0.0 | | | 0 |
| Cherry: | | | | | | |
| (Canada Dry) | 6 fl. oz. | 16 | 0.0 | | | 0 |
| (Shasta) black | 6 fl. oz. | 13 | 0.0 | | | 0 |
| Cherry-lime (Spree) | 6 fl. oz. | 1 | 0.0 | | | 0 |
| Chocolate (Yoo-Hoo) | 6 fl. oz. | 87 | .7 | | | 0 |
| Citrus mist (Shasta) | 6 fl. oz. | 9 | 0.0 | | | 0 |
| Club: | | | | | | |
| (Shasta) | 6 fl. oz. | 23 | 0.0 | | | 0 |
| (Schweppes) | 6 fl. oz. | 25 | 0.0 | | | 0 |
| Cola: | | | | | | |
| (Canada Dry) *Jamaica* | 6 fl. oz. | Tr. | 0.0 | | | 0 |
| *Coca-Cola:* | | | | | | |
| Regular or caffeine free | 6 fl. oz. | 3 | 0.0 | | | 0 |
| Cherry or classic | 6 fl. oz. | 7 | 0.0 | | | 0 |
| *Pepsi-Cola* | 6 fl. oz. | 1 | 0.0 | | | 0 |
| *RC 100* | 6 fl. oz. | <1 | 0.0 | | | 0 |
| (Royal Crown) | 6 fl. oz. | Tr. | 0.0 | | | 0 |

(USDA): United States Department of Agriculture
*Prepared as Package Directs

| Food and Description | Measure or Quantity | Sodium (mg.) | — Fats in grams — | | | Cholesterol (mg.) |
|---|---|---|---|---|---|---|
| | | | Total | Saturated | Unsaturated | |
| (Shasta): | | | | | | |
| Regular or caffeine free | 6 fl. oz. | Tr. | 0.0 | | | 0 |
| Cherry | 6 fl. oz. | 11 | 0.0 | | | 0 |
| (Slice) cherry | 6 fl. oz. | 2 | 0.0 | | | 0 |
| (Spree) | 6 fl. oz. | Tr. | 0.0 | | | 0 |
| Collins or Tom Collins mix: | | | | | | |
| (Canada Dry) | 6 fl. oz. | 13 | 0.0 | | | 0 |
| (Schweppes) | 6 fl. oz. | 51 | 0.0 | | | 0 |
| (Shasta) | 6 fl. oz. | 11 | 0.0 | | | 0 |
| Cream (Shasta) | 6 fl. oz. | 12 | 0.0 | | | 0 |
| Dr. Diablo (Shasta) | 6 fl. oz. | 7 | 0.0 | | | 0 |
| Dr. Nehi (Royal Crown) | 6 fl. oz. | 13 | 0.0 | | | 0 |
| Dr Pepper | 6 fl. oz. | 9 | 0.0 | | | 0 |
| Fruit Punch: | | | | | | |
| (Nehi) | 6 fl. oz. | 8 | 0.0 | | | 0 |
| (Shasta) | 6 fl. oz. | 16 | 0.0 | | | 0 |
| Ginger Ale: | | | | | | |
| (Canada Dry): | | | | | | |
| Regular | 6 fl. oz. | 5 | 0.0 | | | 0 |
| Golden | 6 fl. oz. | 18 | 0.0 | | | 0 |
| (Fanta) | 6 fl. oz. | 13 | 0.0 | | | 0 |
| (Schweppes) | 6 fl. oz. | 10 | 0.0 | | | 0 |
| (Spree) | 6 fl. oz. | Tr. | 0.0 | | | 0 |
| Ginger beer (Schweppes) | 6 fl. oz. | 30 | 0.0 | | | 0 |
| Grape: | | | | | | |
| (Canada Dry) | 6 fl. oz. | 16 | 0.0 | | | 0 |
| (Fanta) | 6 fl. oz. | 7 | 0.0 | | | 0 |
| (Hi-C) | 6 fl. oz. | 6 | 0.0 | | | 0 |
| (Nehi) | 6 fl. oz. | 8 | 0.0 | | | 0 |
| (Shasta) | 6 fl. oz. | 17 | 0.0 | | | 0 |
| Grapefruit: | | | | | | |
| (Schweppes) | 6 fl. oz. | 28 | 0.0 | | | 0 |
| (Spree) | 6 fl. oz. | Tr. | 0.0 | | | 0 |
| Half & Half (Canada Dry) | 6 fl. oz. | 13 | 0.0 | | | 0 |
| Hi-Spot (Canada Dry) | 6 fl. oz. | 19 | 0.0 | | | 0 |
| Island Lime (Canada Dry) | 6 fl. oz. | 14 | 0.0 | | | 0 |
| Kick (Royal Crown) | 6 fl. oz. | 25 | 0.0 | | | 0 |
| Lemon (Hi-C) | 6 fl. oz. | 6 | 0.0 | | | 0 |
| Lemon-lime (Shasta) | 6 fl. oz. | 9 | 0.0 | | | 0 |
| Lemon-tangerine (Spree) | 6 fl. oz. | Tr. | 0.0 | | | 0 |
| Mandarin Lime (Spree) | 6 fl. oz. | Tr. | 0.0 | | | 0 |
| Mello Yello | 6 fl. oz. | 13 | 0.0 | | | 0 |
| Mr. PiBB | 6 fl. oz. | 11 | 0.0 | | | 0 |

(USDA): United States Department of Agriculture
*Prepared as Package Directs

| Food and Description | Measure or Quantity | Sodium (mg.) | — Fats in grams — | | | Choles- terol (mg.) |
|---|---|---|---|---|---|---|
| | | | Total | Satu- rated | Unsatu- rated | |
| *Mountain Dew* | 6 fl. oz. | 16 | 0.0 | | | 0 |
| Orange: | | | | | | |
| (Canada Dry) | 6 fl. oz. | 16 | 0.0 | | | 0 |
| (Fanta) | 6 fl. oz. | 7 | 0.0 | | | 0 |
| (Hi-C) | 6 fl. oz. | 7 | 0.0 | | | 0 |
| (Nehi) | 6 fl. oz. | 11 | 0.0 | | | 0 |
| (Schweppes) | 6 fl. oz. | 17 | 0.0 | | | 0 |
| (Shasta) | 6 fl. oz. | 14 | 0.0 | | | 0 |
| (Slice) | 6 fl. oz. | 11 | 0.0 | | | 0 |
| Peach (Nehi) | 6 fl. oz. | 16 | 0.0 | | | 0 |
| Pineapple (Canada Dry) | 6 fl. oz. | 16 | 0.0 | | | 0 |
| Purple Passion (Canada Dry) | 6 fl. oz. | 14 | 0.0 | | | 0 |
| Quinine or tonic water: | | | | | | |
| (Canada Dry) | 6 fl. oz. | 5 | 0.0 | | | 0 |
| (Schweppes) | 6 fl. oz. | 8 | 0.0 | | | 0 |
| Red berry (Shasta) | 6 fl. oz. | 10 | 0.0 | | | 0 |
| *Red Pop* (Shasta) | 6 fl. oz. | 10 | 0.0 | | | 0 |
| Root beer: | | | | | | |
| *Barrelhead* | 6 fl. oz. | 13 | 0.0 | | | 0 |
| (Dad's) | 6 fl. oz. | 14 | 0.0 | | | 0 |
| (Fanta) | 6 fl. oz. | 9 | 0.0 | | | 0 |
| *On Tap* | 6 fl. oz. | 9 | 0.0 | | | 0 |
| (Ramblin) | 6 fl. oz. | 10 | 0.0 | | | 0 |
| *Rooti* | 6 fl. oz. | 13 | 0.0 | | | 0 |
| (Shasta) | 6 fl. oz. | 15 | 0.0 | | | 0 |
| (Spree) | 6 fl. oz. | 1 | 0.0 | | | 0 |
| Seltzer (Schweppes) | 6 fl. oz. | 3 | 0.0 | | | 0 |
| *7 UP* | 6 fl. oz. | 10 | 0.0 | | | 0 |
| *Slice* | 6 fl. oz. | 5 | 0.0 | | | 0 |
| *Sprite* | 6 fl. oz. | 22 | 0.0 | | | 0 |
| Strawberry (Shasta) | 6 fl. oz. | 18 | 0.0 | | | 0 |
| Whiskey sour (Canada Dry) | 6 fl. oz. | 13 | 0.0 | | | 0 |
| *Wink* (Canada Dry) | 6 fl. oz. | 14 | 0.0 | | | 0 |
| Dietetic: | | | | | | |
| Apple (Slice) | 6 fl. oz. | 2 | 0.0 | | | 0 |
| Birch beer (Shasta) | 6 fl. oz. | 17 | 0.0 | | | 0 |
| Cherry, black: | | | | | | |
| (No-Cal) | 6 fl. oz. | 44 | 0.0 | | | 0 |
| (Shasta) | 6 fl. oz. | 20 | 0.0 | | | 0 |
| Chocolate: | | | | | | |
| (No-Cal) | 6 fl. oz. | 33 | 0.0 | | | 0 |
| (Shasta) | 6 fl. oz. | 18 | 0.0 | | | 0 |
| Coffee (No-Cal) | 6 fl. oz. | 45 | 0.0 | | | 0 |

(USDA): United States Department of Agriculture
*Prepared as Package Directs

| Food and Description | Measure or Quantity | Sodium (mg.) | —Fats in grams— | | | Choles-terol (mg.) |
|---|---|---|---|---|---|---|
| | | | Total | Satu-rated | Unsatu-rated | |
| Cola: | | | | | | |
| (Canada Dry) | 6 fl. oz. | 20 | 0.0 | | | 0 |
| *Coca-Cola* | 6 fl. oz. | 4 | 0.0 | | | 0 |
| *Pepsi-Cola* | 6 fl. oz. | 2 | 0.0 | | | 0 |
| Cream: | | | | | | |
| (No-Cal) | 6 fl. oz. | 33 | 0.0 | | | 0 |
| (Shasta) | 6 fl. oz. | 21 | 0.0 | | | 0 |
| *Dr Pepper* | 6 fl. oz. | Tr. | 0.0 | | | 0 |
| *Fresca* | 6 fl. oz. | Tr. | 0.0 | | | 0 |
| Ginger ale: | | | | | | |
| (Canada Dry) | 6 fl. oz. | 22 | 0.0 | | | 0 |
| (Schweppes) | 6 fl. oz. | 39 | 0.0 | | | 0 |
| (Shasta) | 6 fl. oz. | 20 | 0.0 | | | 0 |
| Grape (Shasta) | 6 fl. oz. | 18 | 0.0 | | | 0 |
| Grapefruit (Shasta) | 6 fl. oz. | 18 | 0.0 | | | 0 |
| Lemon-lime: | | | | | | |
| (No-Cal) | 6 fl. oz. | 29 | 0.0 | | | 0 |
| (Shasta) | 6 fl. oz. | 23 | 0.0 | | | 0 |
| *Mr. PiBB* | 6 fl. oz. | 19 | 0.0 | | | 0 |
| Orange: | | | | | | |
| (Canada Dry) | 6 fl. oz. | 19 | 0.0 | | | 0 |
| (Fanta) | 6 fl. oz. | 24 | 0.0 | | | 0 |
| (No-Cal) | 6 fl. oz. | 19 | 0.0 | | | 0 |
| (Shasta) | 6 fl. oz. | 19 | 0.0 | | | 0 |
| (Slice) | 6 fl. oz. | 11 | 0.0 | | | 0 |
| Quinine or tonic: | | | | | | |
| (Canada Dry) | 6 fl. oz. | 18 | 0.0 | | | 0 |
| (No-Cal) | 6 fl. oz. | 15 | 0.0 | | | 0 |
| Root beer: | | | | | | |
| *Barrelhead* | 6 fl. oz. | 19 | 0.0 | | | 0 |
| (Dad's): | | | | | | |
| Diet | 6 fl. oz. | 14 | 0.0 | | | 0 |
| Sugar free | 6 fl. oz. | 41 | 0.0 | | | 0 |
| (No-Cal) | 6 fl. oz. | 30 | 0.0 | | | 0 |
| (Shasta) | 6 fl. oz. | 18 | 0.0 | | | 0 |
| *7 Up* | 6 fl. oz. | 16 | 0.0 | | | 0 |
| *Slice* | 6 fl. oz. | 5 | 0.0 | | | 0 |
| *Sprite* | 6 fl. oz. | Tr. | 0.0 | | | 0 |
| **SOLE:** | | | | | | |
| Raw, whole (USDA) | 1 lb. (weighed whole) | 117 | 1.2 | | | |
| Raw, meat only (USDA) | 4 oz. | 88 | .9 | | | |

(USDA): United States Department of Agriculture
*Prepared as Package Directs

| Food and Description | Measure or Quantity | Sodium (mg.) | — Fats in grams — | | | Cholesterol (mg.) |
|---|---|---|---|---|---|---|
| | | | Total | Saturated | Unsaturated | |

| Food and Description | Measure or Quantity | Sodium (mg.) | Total | Satu-rated | Unsatu-rated | Choles-terol (mg.) |
|---|---|---|---|---|---|---|
| **Frozen:** | | | | | | |
| (Frionor) *Norway Gourmet* | 4-oz. fillet | 350 | 0.0 | | | 0 |
| (Gorton's): | | | | | | |
|   *Fishmarket Fresh* | 4 oz. | 110 | 1.0 | | | |
|   Light recipe, fillet, with | | | | | | |
|     lemon butter | 1 pkg. | 730 | 13.0 | | | |
| (Mrs. Paul's) breaded & | | | | | | |
|   fried, light & natural | 6-oz. fillet | 700 | 13.0 | | | |
| (Van de Kamps): | | | | | | |
|   Regular, batter dipped, | | | | | | |
|     french fried | 2-oz. piece | 289 | 7.6 | | | |
|   *Today's Catch* | 4 oz. | 220 | 0.0 | | | |
| (Weight Watchers) in lemon | | | | | | |
|   sauce | 9 1/8-oz. serving | 810 | 5.0 | | | |
| **SORGHUM** (USDA), grain | 1 oz. | | .9 | Tr. | < 1. | 0 |
| **SORREL** (See **DOCK**) | | | | | | |
| **SOUFFLE:** | | | | | | |
| Cheese: | | | | | | |
|   Home recipe (USDA) | 4 oz. | 413 | 19.4 | 10. | 9.2 | 189 |
|   Frozen (Stouffer's) | 1/2 of 12-oz. pkg. | 1,260 | 26.0 | | | |
| Corn, frozen (Stouffer's) | 4 oz. | 510 | 7.0 | | | |
| **SOUP:** | | | | | | |
| Canned, regular pack: | | | | | | |
|   *Asparagus (Campbell), | | | | | | |
|     condensed: | | | | | | |
|     Cream of | 8-oz. serving | 900 | 4.0 | | | |
|     *Creamy Natural* | 8-oz. serving | 840 | 14.0 | | | |
|   Bean: | | | | | | |
|     (Campbell's): | | | | | | |
|       *Chunky,* with ham, old | | | | | | |
|        fashioned: | | | | | | |
|       Small | 11-oz. can | 1,150 | 9.0 | | | |
|       Large | 19 1/4-oz. can | 2,020 | 16.0 | | | |
|       *Condensed, with bacon | 8-oz. serving | 860 | 5.0 | | | |
|       Semi-condensed, *Soup* | | | | | | |
|       *For One,* with ham | 11-oz. serving | 1,400 | 7.0 | | | |
|     (Grandma Brown's) | 8-oz. serving | | 3.4 | | | |
|   Bean, black: | | | | | | |
|     *(Campbell's) condensed | 8-oz. serving | 980 | 2.0 | | | |

(USDA): United States Department of Agriculture
*Prepared as Package Directs

331

| Food and Description | Measure or Quantity | Sodium (mg.) | — Fats in grams — | | | Cholesterol (mg.) |
|---|---|---|---|---|---|---|
| | | | Total | Saturated | Unsaturated | |
| (Crosse & Blackwell) with sherry | 6½-oz. serving | 757 | 1.0 | | | |
| Beef: | | | | | | |
| (Campbell's): | | | | | | |
| *Chunky:* | | | | | | |
| Regular: | | | | | | |
| Small | 10¾-oz. can | 1,110 | 5.0 | | | |
| Large | 19-oz. can | 1,940 | 8.0 | | | |
| Stroganoff style | 10¾-oz. can | 1,290 | 15.0 | | | |
| *Condensed: | | | | | | |
| Regular | 8-oz. serving | 850 | 2.0 | | | |
| Broth | 8-oz. serving | 860 | 0.0 | | | |
| Consommé | 8-oz. serving | 780 | 0.0 | | | |
| Mushroom | 8-oz. serving | 960 | 3.0 | | | |
| Noodle: | | | | | | |
| Regular | 8-oz. serving | 870 | 3.0 | | | |
| Homestyle | 8-oz. serving | 810 | 4.0 | | | |
| (Swanson) | 7¼-oz. can | 750 | 1.0 | | | |
| Borscht (See **BORSCHT**) | | | | | | |
| *Broccoli (Campbell's) condensed, *Creamy Natural* | 8-oz. serving | 860 | 8.0 | | | |
| *Cauliflower (Campbell's) condensed, *Creamy Natural* | 8-oz. serving | 850 | 13.0 | | | |
| Celery: | | | | | | |
| *(Campbell's) condensed, cream of | 8-oz. serving | 860 | 7.0 | | | |
| *(Rokeach): | | | | | | |
| Prepared with milk | 10-oz. serving | 1,020 | 9.0 | | | |
| Prepared with water | 10-oz. serving | 950 | 4.0 | | | |
| *Cheddar cheese (Campbell's) | 8-oz. serving | 800 | 8.0 | | | |
| Chicken: | | | | | | |
| (Campbell's): | | | | | | |
| *Chunky:* | | | | | | |
| Noodle, with mushrooms | 10¾-oz. can | 1,190 | 7.0 | | | |
| Old fashioned: | | | | | | |
| Small | 10¾-oz. can | 1,340 | 5.0 | | | |
| Large | 19-oz. can | 2,360 | 8.0 | | | |
| With rice | 19-oz. can | 2,160 | 8.0 | | | |
| Vegetable | 19-oz. can | 2,200 | 12.0 | | | |

(USDA): United States Department of Agriculture
*Prepared as Package Directs

| Food and Description | Measure or Quantity | Sodium (mg.) | — Fats in grams — | | | Choles- terol (mg.) |
|---|---|---|---|---|---|---|
| | | | Total | Satu- rated | Unsatu- rated | |
| *Condensed: | | | | | | |
| Alphabet | 8-oz. serving | 870 | 3.0 | | | |
| Broth: | | | | | | |
| Plain | 8-oz. serving | 790 | 2.0 | | | |
| Noodles | 8-oz. serving | 870 | 2.0 | | | |
| & rice | 8-oz. serving | 880 | 1.0 | | | |
| Cream of | 8-oz. serving | 850 | 7.0 | | | |
| & dumplings | 8-oz. serving | 980 | 3.0 | | | |
| Gumbo | 8-oz. serving | 910 | 2.0 | | | |
| Mushroom, creamy | 8-oz. serving | 940 | 8.0 | | | |
| Noodle | 8-oz. serving | 920 | 3.0 | | | |
| NoodleO's | 8-oz. serving | 840 | 2.0 | | | |
| & rice | 8-oz. serving | 840 | 2.0 | | | |
| & stars | 8-oz. serving | 920 | 2.0 | | | |
| Vegetable | 8-oz. serving | 870 | 3.0 | | | |
| *Semi-condensed, Soup For One: | | | | | | |
| & noodles, golden | 11-oz. serving | 1,450 | 4.0 | | | |
| Vegetable, full flavored | 11-oz. serving | 1,500 | 6.0 | | | |
| (Swanson) broth | 7 1/4-oz. can | 910 | 2.0 | | | |
| Chili beef (Campbell's): | | | | | | |
| Chunky: | | | | | | |
| Small | 11-oz. can | 1,150 | 7.0 | | | |
| Large | 19 1/2-oz. can | 1,240 | 12.0 | | | |
| *Condensed | 8-oz. serving | 900 | 5.0 | | | |
| Chowder: | | | | | | |
| Beef'n vegetable (Hormel) | | | | | | |
| Short Orders | 7 1/2-oz. can | | 5.0 | | | |
| Clam: | | | | | | |
| Manhattan style: | | | | | | |
| (Campbell's): | | | | | | |
| Chunky: | | | | | | |
| Small | 10 3/4-oz. can | 1,230 | 5.0 | | | |
| Large | 19-oz. can | 2,260 | 8.0 | | | |
| *Condensed | 8-oz. serving | 860 | 2.0 | | | |
| (Crosse & Blackwell) | 6 1/2-oz. serving | 803 | 1.0 | | | |
| New England Style: | | | | | | |
| *(Campbell's): | | | | | | |
| Chunky: | | | | | | |
| Small | 10 3/4-oz. can | 1,180 | 17.0 | | | |
| Large | 19-oz. can | 2,080 | 30.0 | | | |

(USDA): United States Department of Agriculture
*Prepared as Package Directs

333

| Food and Description | Measure or Quantity | Sodium (mg.) | Fats in grams — Total | Satu- rated | Unsatu- rated | Choles- terol (mg.) |
|---|---|---|---|---|---|---|
| Condensed: | | | | | | |
| Made with milk | 8-oz. serving | 930 | 7.0 | | | |
| Made with water | 8-oz. serving | 880 | 3.0 | | | |
| Semi-condensed, *Soup For One:* | | | | | | |
| Made with milk | 11-oz. serving | 1,410 | 8.0 | | | |
| Made with water | 11-oz. serving | 1,360 | 4.0 | | | |
| (Crosse & Blackwell) | 6½-oz. serving | 637 | 3.0 | | | |
| *(Gorton's) | 1 can | | | | | |
| Ham'n potato (Hormel) *Short Orders* | 7½-oz. can | | 6.0 | | | |
| Consommé madrilene (Crosse & Blackwell) | 6½-oz. serving | 609 | 2.0 | | | |
| Crab (Crosse & Blackwell) | 6½-oz. serving | 933 | 1.0 | | | |
| Gazpacho: | | | | | | |
| *(Campbell's) condensed | 8-oz. serving | 590 | 0.0 | | | |
| (Crosse & Blackwell) | 6½-oz. serving | 1,653 | 2.0 | | | |
| Ham'n butter bean (Campbell's) *Chunky* | 10¾-oz. can | 1,180 | 10.0 | | | |
| Lentil (Crosse & Blackwell) with ham | 6½-oz. serving | 979 | 2.0 | | | |
| *Meatball alphabet (Campbell's) condensed | 8-oz. serving | 970 | 4.0 | | | |
| Minestrone: | | | | | | |
| (Campbell's): | | | | | | |
| *Chunky* | 19-oz. can | 1,880 | 10.0 | | | |
| *Condensed | 8-oz. serving | 930 | 2.0 | | | |
| (Crosse & Blackwell) | 6½-oz. serving | 720 | 2.0 | | | |
| Mushroom: | | | | | | |
| *(Campbell's) condensed: | | | | | | |
| Cream of | 8-oz. serving | 820 | 7.0 | | | |
| Golden | 8-oz. serving | 900 | 3.0 | | | |
| (Crosse & Blackwell) cream of, bisque, | 6½-oz. serving | 923 | 5.0 | | | |
| *(Rokeach) cream of, prepared with water | 10-oz. serving | 1,050 | 10.0 | | | |
| *Noodle (Campbell's): | | | | | | |
| Curly, & chicken | 8-oz. serving | 960 | 3.0 | | | |
| & ground beef | 8-oz. serving | 840 | 4.0 | | | |
| *Onion (Campbell's): | | | | | | |
| Regular | 8-oz. serving | 950 | 2.0 | | | |
| Cream of: | | | | | | |
| Made with water | 8-oz. serving | 830 | 5.0 | | | |
| Made with water & milk | 8-oz. serving | 860 | 7.0 | | | |

(USDA): United States Department of Agriculture
*Prepared as Package Directs

| Food and Description | Measure or Quantity | Sodium (mg.) | Total | Fats in grams — Satu- rated | Unsatu- rated | Choles- terol (mg.) |
|---|---|---|---|---|---|---|
| *Oyster stew (Campbell's): | | | | | | |
| Made with milk | 8-oz. serving | 900 | 9.0 | | | |
| Made with water | 8-oz. serving | 850 | 5.0 | | | |
| *Pea, green (Campbell's): | | | | | | |
| condensed | 8-oz. serving | 840 | 3.0 | | | |
| Pea, split: | | | | | | |
| (Campbell's): | | | | | | |
| Chunky, with ham: | | | | | | |
| Small | 10¾-oz. can | 1,070 | 6.0 | | | |
| Large | 19-oz. can | 1,900 | 10.0 | | | |
| *Condensed, with ham | | | | | | |
| & bacon | 8-oz. serving | 800 | 4.0 | | | |
| (Grandma Brown's) | 8-oz. serving | | 3.0 | | | |
| *Pepper pot (Campbell's) | 8-oz. serving | 960 | 4.0 | | | |
| *Potato (Campbell's): | | | | | | |
| cream of, made with water | 8-oz. serving | 930 | 3.0 | | | |
| cream of, made with water | | | | | | |
| & milk | 8-oz. serving | 960 | 4.0 | | | |
| Creamy Natural | 8-oz. serving | 860 | 15.0 | | | |
| *Scotch broth (Campbell's) | | | | | | |
| condensed | 8-oz. serving | 890 | 3.0 | | | |
| Shrimp: | | | | | | |
| *(Campbell's) condensed, cream of: | | | | | | |
| Made with milk | 8-oz. serving | 850 | 10.0 | | | |
| Made with water | 8-oz. serving | 790 | 6.0 | | | |
| (Crosse & Blackwell) | 6½-oz. serving | 1,459 | 4.0 | | | |
| Sirloin burger (Campbell's) Chunky: | | | | | | |
| Small | 10¾-oz. can | 1,280 | 9.0 | | | |
| Large | 19-oz. can | 2,260 | 16.0 | | | |
| *Spinach (Campbell's) condensed, Creamy Natural | 8-oz. serving | 700 | 10.0 | | | |
| Steak & potato (Campbell's) Chunky: | | | | | | |
| Small | 10¾-oz. can | 1,250 | 5.0 | | | |
| Large | 19-oz. can | 2,230 | 8.0 | | | |
| Tomato: | | | | | | |
| (Campbell's): | | | | | | |
| Condensed: | | | | | | |
| Regular: | | | | | | |
| Made with milk | 8-oz. serving | 770 | 6.0 | | | |
| Made with water | 8-oz. serving | 720 | 2.0 | | | |

(USDA): United States Department of Agriculture
*Prepared as Package Directs

| Food and Description | Measure or Quantity | Sodium (mg.) | Total | —Fats in grams— Satu- rated | Unsatu- rated | Choles- terol (mg.) |
|---|---|---|---|---|---|---|
| Bisque | 8-oz. serving | 830 | 3.0 | | | |
| *Creamy Natural* | 8-oz. serving | 750 | 7.0 | | | |
| & rice, old fashioned | 8-oz. serving | 760 | 2.0 | | | |
| Semi-condensed, *Soup for One,* Royale | 11-oz. serving | 1,080 | 3.0 | | | |
| *(Rokeach): | | | | | | |
| Plain, made with water | 10-oz. serving | 980 | 1.0 | | | |
| & rice | 10-oz. serving | 815 | 5.0 | | | |
| Turkey (Campbell's): | | | | | | |
| *Chunky* | 18¾-oz. can | 2,160 | 12.0 | | | |
| *Condensed: | | | | | | |
| Noodle | 8-oz. serving | 910 | 2.0 | | | |
| Vegetable | 8-oz. serving | 820 | 3.0 | | | |
| Vegetable: | | | | | | |
| (Campbell's): | | | | | | |
| *Chunky:* | | | | | | |
| Regular: | | | | | | |
| Small | 10¾-oz. can | 1,100 | 4.0 | | | |
| Large | 19-oz. can | 1,940 | 8.0 | | | |
| Beef, old fashioned: | | | | | | |
| Small | 10¾-oz. can | 1,210 | 5.0 | | | |
| Large | 19-oz. can | 2,140 | 8.0 | | | |
| Mediterranean | 19-oz. can | 2,040 | 10.0 | | | |
| *Condensed: | | | | | | |
| Regular | 8-oz. serving | 770 | 2.0 | | | |
| Beef | 8-oz. serving | 820 | 2.0 | | | |
| Old fashioned | 8-oz. serving | 910 | 2.0 | | | |
| Vegetarian | 8-oz. serving | 770 | 2.0 | | | |
| *Semi-condensed, *Soup For One:* | | | | | | |
| Barley, with beef & bacon | 11-oz. serving | 1,480 | 5.0 | | | |
| Old world | 11-oz. serving | 1,470 | 4.0 | | | |
| *(Rokeach) vegetarian | 10-oz. serving | 1,055 | 3.0 | | | |
| Vichyssoise (Crosse & Blackwell) cream of | 6½-oz. serving | 702 | 4.0 | | | |
| *Won ton (Campbell's) | 8-oz. serving | 870 | 1.0 | | | |
| Canned, dietetic pack: | | | | | | |
| Beef (Campbell's) *Chunky,* & mushroom, low sodium | 10¾-oz. can | 65 | 7.0 | | | |
| Chicken: | | | | | | |
| (Campbell's) low sodium Vegetable | 10¾-oz. can | 95 | 11.0 | | | |
| (Estee) & vegetable | 7½-oz. serving | 60 | 6.0 | | | |

(USDA): United States Department of Agriculture
*Prepared as Package Directs

| Food and Description | Measure or Quantity | Sodium (mg.) | —Fats in grams—<br>Total | Satu-rated | Unsatu-rated | Choles-terol (mg.) |
|---|---|---|---|---|---|---|
| Minestrone (Estee) | 7½-oz. serving | 30 | 5.0 | | | |
| Mushroom: | | | | | | |
| (Campbell's) cream of, low sodium | 10½-oz. can | 55 | 14.0 | | | |
| Onion (Campbell's) French, low sodium | 10½-oz. can | 50 | 4.0 | | | |
| Pea, split (Campbell's) low sodium | 10¾-oz. can | 25 | 5.0 | | | |
| Tomato (Campbell's) low sodium, with tomato pieces | 10½-oz. can | 40 | 5.0 | | | |
| Vegetable: | | | | | | |
| (Campbell's) low sodium, *Chunky* | 10¾-oz. can | 60 | 5.0 | | | |
| (Estee) & beef | 7½-oz. serving | 130 | 7.0 | | | |
| Frozen: | | | | | | |
| *Barley & mushroom (Mother's Own) | 8-oz. serving | 490 | Tr. | | | |
| Chowder, clam, New England style (Stouffer's) | 8-oz. serving | 510 | 10.0 | | | |
| Pea, split: | | | | | | |
| *(Mother's Own) | 8-oz. serving | 575 | 2.0 | | | |
| (Stouffer's) with ham | 8¼-oz. serving | 695 | 3.0 | | | |
| Spinach (Stouffer's) cream of | 8-oz. serving | 885 | 15.0 | | | |
| *Vegetable (Mother's Own) | 8-oz. serving | 560 | 1.0 | | | |
| *Won ton (La Choy) | ½ of 15-oz. pkg. | 1,050 | 1.0 | | | |
| Mix, regular: | | | | | | |
| Beef: | | | | | | |
| *Carmel Kosher | 6 fl. oz. | | .1 | | | |
| *(Lipton) Cup-A-Soup: | | | | | | |
| Regular: | | | | | | |
| Noodle | 6 fl. oz. | 830 | Tr. | | | |
| Vegetable | 6 fl. oz. | 820 | Tr. | | | |
| Lots-A-Noodles | 7 fl. oz. | 780 | 2.0 | | | |
| *Chicken: | | | | | | |
| Carmel Kosher | 6 fl. oz. | | .1 | | | |
| (Lipton): | | | | | | |
| Regular, noodle | 8 fl. oz. | 900 | Tr. | | | |
| Cup-A-Broth | 6 fl. oz. | 780 | Tr. | | | |
| Cup-A-Soup: | | | | | | |
| Regular: | | | | | | |
| Cream of | 6 fl. oz. | 840 | 4.0 | | | |
| & noodles with meat | 6 fl. oz. | 770 | 1.0 | | | |

(USDA): United States Department of Agriculture
*Prepared as Package Directs

| Food and Description | Measure or Quantity | Sodium (mg.) | — Fats in grams — Total | Satu- rated | Unsatu- rated | Choles- terol (mg.) |
|---|---|---|---|---|---|---|
| & rice | 6 fl. oz. | 750 | Tr. | | | |
| & vegetable | 6 fl. oz. | 800 | Tr. | | | |
| Country style: | | | | | | |
|   Hearty | 6 fl. oz. | 970 | 1.0 | | | |
|   Supreme | 6 fl. oz. | 870 | 5.0 | | | |
| *Lots-A-Noodles:* | | | | | | |
|   Regular | 7 fl. oz. | 855 | 1.0 | | | |
|   Cream of | 7 fl. oz. | 755 | 5.0 | | | |
| *Minestrone (Manischewitz) | 6 fl. oz. | 160 | Tr. | | | |
| *Mushroom: | | | | | | |
| *Carmel Kosher* | 6 fl. oz. | | .1 | | | |
| (Lipton): | | | | | | |
|   Regular: | | | | | | |
|     Beef | 8 fl. oz. | 995 | Tr. | | | |
|     Onion | 8 fl. oz. | 995 | 1.0 | | | |
|   *Cup-A-Soup,* cream of | 6 fl. oz. | 830 | 4.0 | | | |
| *Noodle (Lipton): | | | | | | |
|   With chicken broth | 8 fl. oz. | 785 | 2.0 | | | |
|   *Giggle Noodle* | 8 fl. oz. | 925 | 2.0 | | | |
|   *Ring-O-Noodle* | 8 fl. oz. | 855 | 1.0 | | | |
| *Onion: | | | | | | |
| *Carmel Kosher* | 6 fl. oz. | | .1 | | | |
| (Lipton): | | | | | | |
|   Regular: | | | | | | |
|     Plain | 8 fl. oz. | 640 | Tr. | | | |
|     Beefy | 8 fl. oz. | 950 | 1.0 | | | |
|   *Cup-A-Soup* | 6 fl. oz. | 870 | 1.0 | | | |
| *Pea, green (Lipton) | | | | | | |
| *Cup-A-Soup:* | | | | | | |
|   Regular, green | 6 fl. oz. | 710 | 4.0 | | | |
|   Country style, Virginia | 6 fl. oz. | 870 | 5.0 | | | |
| *Pea, split (Manischewitz) | 6 fl. oz. | 320 | Tr. | | | |
| *Tomato (Lipton): | | | | | | |
| *Cup-A-Soup:* | | | | | | |
|   Regular | 6 fl. oz. | 650 | 1.0 | | | |
|   Lots-A-Noodles, | | | | | | |
|     vegetable | 7 fl. oz. | 885 | 1.0 | | | |
|   Hearty, vegetable noodle | 8 fl. oz. | 930 | 1.0 | | | |
| *Vegetable: | | | | | | |
| (Lipton): | | | | | | |
|   Regular: | | | | | | |
|     Beef stock | 8 fl. oz. | 995 | Tr. | | | |

(USDA): United States Department of Agriculture
*Prepared as Package Directs

| Food and Description | Measure or Quantity | Sodium (mg.) | — Fats in grams — | | | Cholesterol (mg.) |
|---|---|---|---|---|---|---|
| | | | Total | Saturated | Unsaturated | |
| Country | 8 fl. oz. | 995 | 1.0 | | | |
| For dip | 8 fl. oz. | 995 | 1.0 | | | |
| *Cup-A-Soup:* | | | | | | |
| Regular: | | | | | | |
| Beef | 6 fl. oz. | 820 | Tr. | | | |
| Spring | 6 fl. oz. | 865 | 1.0 | | | |
| Country Style, harvest | 6 fl. oz. | 625 | Tr. | | | |
| *Lots-A-Noodles,* | | | | | | |
| garden | 7 fl. oz. | 745 | 2.0 | | | |
| (Manischewitz) | 6 fl. oz. | 25 | Tr. | | | |
| *Mix, dietetic: | | | | | | |
| Beef (Lipton) *Cup-A-Soup,* | | | | | | |
| trim | 6 fl. oz. | 695 | 0.0 | | | |
| Beef noodle (Estee) | 6 fl. oz. | 140 | Tr. | | | 1 |
| Beefy tomato (Lipton) | | | | | | |
| *Cup-A-Soup,* trim | 6 fl. oz. | 440 | 0.0 | | | |
| Chicken (Lipton) | | | | | | |
| *Cup-A-Soup,* trim | 6 fl. oz. | 560 | 0.0 | | | |
| Chicken noodle (Estee) | 6 fl. oz. | 135 | Tr. | | | 4 |
| Herb vegetable (Lipton) | | | | | | |
| *Cup-A-Soup,* trim | 6 fl. oz. | 560 | 0.0 | | | |
| Mushroom, cream of (Estee) | 6 fl. oz. | 115 | <2.0 | | | 1 |
| Onion (Estee) | 6 fl. oz. | 140 | <1.0 | | | 1 |
| Tomato (Estee) | 6 fl. oz. | 95 | <1.0 | | | 0 |
| **SOURSOP,** raw (USDA): | | | | | | |
| Whole | 1 lb. (weighed with skin & seeds) | 43 | .9 | | | 0 |
| Flesh only | 4 oz. | 16 | .3 | | | 0 |
| **SOUSE** (USDA)[1] | 1 oz. | | 3.8 | 1. | 2. | |
| ***SOUTHERN COMFORT*** | 1 fl. oz. | Tr. | 0.0 | | | (0) |
| **SOYBEAN** (USDA): | | | | | | |
| Young seeds: | | | | | | |
| Raw | 1 lb. (weighed in pods) | | 12.3 | 2. | 10. | 0 |
| Cooked without salt, drained | 4 oz. | | 5.8 | 1. | 5. | 0 |
| Canned, solids & liq. | 4 oz. | 268 | 3.6 | 1. | 2. | 0 |
| Canned, drained solids | 4 oz. | 268 | 5.7 | 1. | 5. | 0 |

(USDA): United States Department of Agriculture
*Prepared as Package Directs
[1]Principal source of fat: pork.

| Food and Description | Measure or Quantity | Sodium (mg.) | — Fats in grams — | | | Choles- terol (mg.) |
|---|---|---|---|---|---|---|
| | | | Total | Satu- rated | Unsatu- rated | |
| **Mature seeds, dry:** | | | | | | |
| Raw | 1 lb. | 23 | 80.3 | 12. | 68. | 0 |
| Raw | 1 cup (7.4 oz.) | 10 | 37.2 | 6. | 31. | 0 |
| Cooked without salt | 4 oz. | 2 | 6.5 | 1. | 5. | 0 |
| Roasted: | | | | | | |
| Unsalted, *Soy Town* | 1 oz. | 6 | 10.5 | 1. | 9. | 0 |
| Sea-salted, *Soy Town* | 1 oz. | 249 | 10.5 | 1. | 9. | 0 |
| **SOYBEAN CURD OR TOFU** | | | | | | |
| (USDA) | 4.2-oz. cake (2¾" × 2½" × 1") | 8 | 5.0 | 1. | 4. | 0 |
| **SOYBEAN FLOUR** (See **FLOUR**) | | | | | | |
| **SOYBEAN GRITS,** high fat | | | | | | |
| (USDA) | 1 cup (4.9 oz.) | 1 | 16.7 | 3. | 14. | 0 |
| **SOYBEAN MILK** (USDA): | | | | | | |
| Fluid | 4 oz. | | 1.7 | | | 0 |
| Powder | 1 oz. | | 5.8 | <1. | 5. | 0 |
| Sweetened: | | | | | | |
| Liquid concentrate [1] | 4 oz. (by wt.) | 49 | 8.0 | 1. | 7. | 0 |
| Dry powder [2] | 1 oz. | <1 | 6.6 | 3. | 4. | 0 |
| **SOYBEAN PROTEIN** (USDA) | 1 oz. | 60 | <.1 | | | 0 |
| **SOYBEAN PROTEINATE** | | | | | | |
| (USDA) | 1 oz. | 340 | <.1 | | | 0 |
| **SOYBEAN SPROUT** (See **BEAN SPROUT**) | | | | | | |
| **SOYNUT,** unsalted, *Soy Ahoy* | 1 oz. | 6 | 10.2 | 1. | 9. | 0 |
| **SOY SAUCE** (See **SAUCE**) | | | | | | |
| **SPAGHETTI:** | | | | | | |
| Dry: | | | | | | |
| (USDA) | 1 oz. | Tr. | .3 | | | 0 |
| (Pritikin) whole wheat | 1 oz. | 20 | 1.0 | | | 0 |

(USDA): United States Department of Agriculture
*Prepared as Package Directs
[1]Principal source of fat: soybean.
[2]Principal sources of fat: soybean, coconut oil & olive oil.

| Food and Description | Measure or Quantity | Sodium (mg.) | Fats in grams — Total | Satu- rated | Unsatu- rated | Choles- terol (mg.) |
|---|---|---|---|---|---|---|
| Cooked (USDA): | | | | | | |
| 8-10 minutes | 1 cup (5.1 oz.) | 1 | .7 | | | 0 |
| 14-20 minutes | 1 cup (4.9 oz.) | 1 | .6 | | | 0 |
| Canned: | | | | | | |
| Regular: | | | | | | |
| (Franco-American): | | | | | | |
| Regular: | | | | | | |
| With meatballs in | | | | | | |
| tomato sauce | 7³⁄₈-oz. can | 820 | 8.0 | | | |
| In meat sauce | 7¹⁄₂-oz. can | 1,110 | 8.0 | | | |
| SpaghettiOs: | | | | | | |
| With meatballs in | | | | | | |
| tomato sauce | 7³⁄₈-oz. can | 910 | 8.0 | | | |
| With sliced franks | 7³⁄₈-oz. can | 990 | 9.0 | | | |
| (Hormel) & beef | 7¹⁄₂-oz. can | 1,091 | 14.0 | | | |
| Dietetic, with meatballs: | | | | | | |
| (Estee) | 7¹⁄₂-oz. can | 130 | 15.0 | | | |
| (Featherweight) | 7¹⁄₂-oz. serving | 95 | 5.0 | | | |
| Frozen: | | | | | | |
| (Armour) Dinner Classics | 11-oz. meal | 1,130 | 21.0 | | | 95 |
| (Banquet): | | | | | | |
| Casserole | 8-oz. casserole | 1,242 | 8.0 | | | |
| Dinner | 9¹⁄₂-oz. dinner | 1,317 | 14.0 | | | |
| (Blue Star) Dining Lite, with | | | | | | |
| beef & mushrooms | 11-oz. dinner | 1,550 | 8.3 | | | |
| (Conagra) Light & Elegant | 10¹⁄₄-oz. entree | 700 | 8.0 | | | 35 |
| (Morton) dinner | 11¹⁄₂-oz. dinner | 1,300 | 11.4 | | | |
| (Stouffer's) Lean Cuisine | 11¹⁄₂-oz. dinner | 1,455 | 7.0 | | | 20 |
| (Weight Watchers) with meat | | | | | | |
| sauce | 10¹⁄₂-oz. meal | 1,100 | 6.0 | | | |
| **SPAGHETTI SAUCE,** canned: | | | | | | |
| Regular pack: | | | | | | |
| Beef (Prego Plus) ground | | | | | | |
| sirloin | 4 oz. | 420 | 7.0 | | | |
| Gardenstyle (Ragú): | | | | | | |
| Green pepper & | | | | | | |
| mushroom | ¹⁄₄ of 15¹⁄₂-oz. can | 400 | 2.0 | | | 0 |
| Mushroom & onion | ¹⁄₄ of 15¹⁄₂-oz. can | 400 | 3.0 | | | |
| Homestyle (Ragú): | | | | | | |
| Plain | 4 oz. | 400 | 2.0 | | | |
| Meat flavor | 4 oz. | 400 | 2.0 | | | |

(USDA): United States Department of Agriculture
*Prepared as Package Directs

| Food and Description | Measure or Quantity | Sodium (mg.) | —Fats in grams— | | | Cholesterol (mg.) |
|---|---|---|---|---|---|---|
| | | | Total | Saturated | Unsaturated | |
| Marinara (Ragú) | 4 oz. | 740 | 4.0 | | | 0 |
| Meat or meat flavored: | | | | | | |
| (Hunt's) | 4 oz. | 520 | 2.0 | | | |
| (Prego) | 4 oz. | 680 | 6.0 | | | |
| (Ragú) Extra thick & zesty | 4 oz. | 740 | 4.0 | | | 2 |
| Meatless or plain: | | | | | | |
| (Hain) | 4 oz. | | .8 | | | 0 |
| (Prego) | 4 oz. | 670 | 6.0 | | | |
| (Ragú) | 4 oz. | 740 | 3.0 | | | 0 |
| Mushroom: | | | | | | |
| (Hain) | 4 oz. | | 1.7 | | | 0 |
| (Hunt's) | 4 oz. | 520 | 2.0 | | | |
| (Prego) | 4 oz. | 640 | 5.0 | | | |
| (Ragú) | 4 oz. | 740 | 4.0 | | | 0 |
| Sausage & green pepper (Prego Plus) | 4 oz. | 480 | 9.0 | | | |
| Veal (Prego Plus) & sliced mushroom | 4 oz. | 380 | 5.0 | | | |
| Dietetic: | | | | | | |
| (Featherweight) | 2/3 cup | <10 | 3.0 | | | |
| (Furman's) | 1/2 cup | <10 | | | | |
| (Prego) | 4 oz. | 25 | 6.0 | | | |
| (Pritikin) plain or mushroom | 4 oz. | 35 | 0.0 | | | 0 |
| Mushroom with meat (Heinz) | 1/2 cup | 822 | 3.9 | | | |
| **\*SPAGHETTI SAUCE MIX:** | | | | | | |
| (Durkee): | | | | | | |
| Plain | 1/2 cup | 747 | .2 | | | |
| With mushroom | 1 1/3 cups | 1,553 | .4 | | | |
| (French's): | | | | | | |
| Italian style | 5/8 cup | 900 | 4.0 | | | |
| Mushroom | 5/8 cup | 1,045 | 4.0 | | | |
| Thick homemade style | 7/8 cup | 1,455 | 7.0 | | | |
| (Spatini) | 1/2 cup | 546 | 0.0 | | | |
| ***SPAM** (Hormel), canned: | | | | | | |
| Regular | 3 oz. | 1,296 | 24.0 | | | |
| & cheese | 3 oz. | 1,215 | 24.0 | | | |
| **SPANISH MACKEREL,** raw (USDA): | | | | | | |
| Whole | 1 lb. (weighed whole) | 188 | 28.8 | | | |
| Meat only | 4 oz. | 77 | 11.8 | | | |

(USDA): United States Department of Agriculture
\*Prepared as Package Directs

| Food and Description | Measure or Quantity | Sodium (mg.) | —Fats in grams— | | | Choles-terol (mg.) |
|---|---|---|---|---|---|---|
| | | | Total | Satu-rated | Unsatu-rated | |
| **SPARKLING COOLER CITRUS** (La Croix) 3½% alcohol | 12 fl. oz. | 10 | 0.0 | | | 0 |
| **SPECIAL K,** cereal (Kellogg's) | 1 cup (1 oz.) | 220 | 0.0 | | | |
| **SPINACH:** | | | | | | |
| Raw (USDA): | | | | | | |
| Untrimmed | 1 lb. (weighed with large stems & roots) | 232 | 1.0 | | | 0 |
| Trimmed or packaged | 1 lb. | 322 | 1.4 | | | 0 |
| Trimmed, whole leaves | 1 cup (1.2 oz.) | 23 | <.1 | | | 0 |
| Trimmed, chopped | 1 cup (1.8 oz.) | 37 | .2 | | | 0 |
| Boiled without salt, whole leaves, drained (USDA) | 1 cup (5.5 oz.) | 78 | .5 | | | 0 |
| Canned, regular pack: | | | | | | |
| Solids & liq. (USDA) | ½ cup (4.1 oz.) | 274 | .5 | | | 0 |
| Drained solids (USDA) | ½ cup (4 oz.) | 264 | .7 | | | 0 |
| Drained liq. (USDA) | 4 oz. | 268 | 0.0 | | | 0 |
| Drained solids (Del Monte) | ½ cup (4 oz.) | 389 | .6 | | | 0 |
| Solids & liq. (Stokely-Van Camp's) | ½ cup (3.9 oz.) | | .5 | | | (0) |
| Canned, dietetic pack, low-sodium: | | | | | | |
| Solids & liq. (USDA) | 4 oz. | 39 | .5 | | | 0 |
| Drained solids (USDA) | 4 oz. | 36 | .6 | | | 0 |
| Drained liq. (USDA) | 4 oz. | 36 | 0.0 | | | 0 |
| Solids & liq. (Blue Boy) | 4 oz. | 39 | .4 | | | (0) |
| Frozen: | | | | | | |
| Chopped: | | | | | | |
| Not thawed (USDA) | 4 oz. | 65 | .3 | | | 0 |
| Boiled, drained (USDA) | 4 oz. | 59 | .3 | | | 0 |
| (Birds Eye) | ⅓ of 10. oz. pkg. | 82 | .3 | | | 0 |
| Deviled, with cheddar cheese, casserole (Green Giant) | ⅓ of 10-oz. pkg. | 387 | 3.3 | | | |
| In cream sauce (Green Giant) | ⅓ of 10-oz. pkg. | 359 | 2.8 | | | |
| Leaf: | | | | | | |
| Not thawed (USDA) | 4 oz. | 60 | .3 | | | 0 |
| Boiled, drained (USDA) | 4 oz. | 56 | .3 | | | 0 |
| (Birds Eye) | ⅓ of 10-oz. pkg. | 82 | .3 | | | 0 |

(USDA): United States Department of Agriculture
*Prepared as Package Directs

| Food and Description | Measure or Quantity | Sodium (mg.) | — Fats in grams — | | | Cholesterol (mg.) |
|---|---|---|---|---|---|---|
| | | | Total | Saturated | Unsaturated | |
| Creamed (Birds Eye) | ⅓ of 10-oz. pkg. | 277 | 3.8 | | | Tr. |
| In butter sauce (Green Giant) | ⅓ of 10-oz. pkg. | 340 | 2.6 | | | |

**SPINACH, NEW ZEALAND (See NEW ZEALAND SPINACH)**

**SPINY LOBSTER** (See **CRAYFISH**)

**SPLEEN,** raw (USDA):

| | | | | | | |
|---|---|---|---|---|---|---|
| Beef & calf | 4 oz. | | 3.4 | | | |
| Hog | 4 oz. | | 4.3 | | | |
| Lamb | 4 oz. | | 4.4 | | | |

**SPOT,** fillets (USDA):

| | | | | | | |
|---|---|---|---|---|---|---|
| Raw[1] | 1 lb. | 277 | 72.1 | | | |
| Baked, salt added | 4 oz. | 354 | 24.8 | | | |

**SQUAB,** pigeon, raw (USDA):

| | | | | | | |
|---|---|---|---|---|---|---|
| Dressed | 1 lb. (weighed with feet, inedible viscera & bones) | | 45.1 | | | |
| Meat & skin | 4 oz. | | 27.0 | | | |
| Meat only | 4 oz. | | 8.5 | | | |
| Light meat only, without skin | 4 oz. | | 4.8 | | | |
| Giblets | 1 oz. | | 2.0 | | | |

**SQUASH SEEDS,** dry (USDA):

| | | | | | | |
|---|---|---|---|---|---|---|
| In hull | 4 oz. | | 39.2 | 7. | 32. | 0 |
| Hulled | 1 oz. | | 13.2 | 2. | 11. | 0 |

**SQUASH, SUMMER:**
Fresh (USDA):
Crookneck & Straightneck, yellow:

| | | | | | | |
|---|---|---|---|---|---|---|
| Whole | 1 lb. (weighed untrimmed) | 4 | .9 | | | 0 |
| Boiled, drained, diced | ½ cup (3.6 oz.) | 1 | .2 | | | 0 |
| Boiled, drained, slices | ½ cup (3.1 oz.) | <1 | .2 | | | 0 |

(USDA): United States Department of Agriculture
*Prepared as Package Directs
[1]Based on samples caught in October. Fat content may vary greatly in samples caught at other seasons of year.

| Food and Description | Measure or Quantity | Sodium (mg.) | Total | Satu- rated | Unsatu- rated | Choles- terol (mg.) |
|---|---|---|---|---|---|---|
| | | | — Fats in grams — | | | |
| Scallop, white & pale green: | | | | | | |
| Whole | 1 lb. (weighed untrimmed) | 4 | .4 | | | 0 |
| Boiled, drained, mashed | ½ cup (4.2 oz.) | 1 | .1 | | | 0 |
| Zucchini & Cocozelle, green: | | | | | | |
| Whole | 1 lb. (weighed untrimmed) | 4 | .4 | | | 0 |
| Boiled, drained slices | ½ cup (2.7 oz.) | < 1 | 2.1 | | | 0 |
| Canned, zucchini in tomato sauce (Del Monte) | ½ cup (4.1 oz.) | 485 | .1 | | | |
| Frozen: | | | | | | |
| Not thawed (USDA) | 4 oz. | 3 | .1 | | | 0 |
| Boiled, drained (USDA) | 4 oz. | 3 | .1 | | | 0 |
| Fried, breaded, zucchini (Mrs. Paul's) | 9-oz. pkg. | | 30.1 | | | |
| Parmesan, zucchini (Mrs. Paul's) | 12-oz. pkg. | | 13.5 | | | |
| Summer squash, slices (Birds Eye) | ½ cup (3.3 oz.) | 3 | .1 | | | 0 |
| Zucchini (Birds Eye) | ⅓ of 10-oz. pkg. | 3 | .1 | | | 0 |
| **SQUASH, WINTER:** | | | | | | |
| Fresh (USDA): | | | | | | |
| Acorn: | | | | | | |
| Whole | 1 lb. (weighed with skin & seeds) | 3 | .3 | | | 0 |
| Baked, flesh only, mashed | ½ cup (3.6 oz.) | 1 | .1 | | | 0 |
| Boiled, mashed | ½ cup (4.1 oz.) | 1 | .1 | | | 0 |
| Butternut: | | | | | | |
| Whole | 1 lb. (weighed with skin & seeds) | 3 | .3 | | | 0 |
| Baked, flesh only | 4 oz. | 1 | .1 | | | 0 |
| Boiled, flesh only | 4 oz. | 1 | .1 | | | 0 |
| Hubbard: | | | | | | |
| Whole | 1 lb. (weighed with skin & seeds) | 3 | .9 | | | 0 |
| Baked, flesh only | 4 oz. | 1 | .5 | | | 0 |
| Baked, flesh only, mashed | ½ cup (3.6 oz.) | 1 | .4 | | | 0 |
| Boiled, flesh only, diced | ½ cup (4.2 oz.) | 1 | .4 | | | 0 |
| Boiled, flesh only, mashed | ½ cup (4.3 oz.) | 1 | .3 | | | 0 |

(USDA): United States Department of Agriculture
*Prepared as Package Directs

| Food and Description | Measure or Quantity | Sodium (mg.) | Total | Fats in grams — Satu- rated | Unsatu- rated | Choles- terol (mg.) |
|---|---|---|---|---|---|---|
| Frozen: | | | | | | |
| Not thawed (USDA) | 4 oz. | 1 | .3 | | | 0 |
| Heated (USDA) | ½ cup (4.2 oz.) | 1 | .4 | | | 0 |
| (Birds Eye) | ⅓ of 12-oz. pkg. | 1 | .3 | | | 0 |
| **SQUID,** raw, meat only (USDA) | 4 oz. | | 10.2 | | | |
| **STARCH** (See **CORNSTARCH**) | | | | | | |
| **STOMACH, PORK,** scalded (USDA) | 4 oz. | | 10.2 | | | |
| **STRAINED FOOD** (See **BABY FOOD**) | | | | | | |
| **STRAWBERRY:** | | | | | | |
| Fresh, whole (USDA) | 1 lb. (weighed with caps & stems) | 4 | 2.2 | | | 0 |
| Fresh, whole, capped | 1 cup (5.1 oz.) | 1 | .7 | | | 0 |
| Canned, unsweetened or low calorie water pack, solids & liq. | 4 oz. | 1 | .1 | | | 0 |
| Frozen: | | | | | | |
| Sweetened, whole, not thawed: | | | | | | |
| (USDA) | 16-oz. can | 5 | .9 | | | 0 |
| (USDA) | ½ cup (4.5 oz.) | 1 | .3 | | | 0 |
| Sweetened, sliced, not thawed (USDA) | 10-oz. pkg. | 3 | .6 | | | 0 |
| Sweetened, sliced, not thawed (USDA) | ½ cup (4.5 oz.) | 1 | .3 | | | 0 |
| Whole (Birds Eye) | ¼ of 1 lb. pkg. | 1 | .2 | | | 0 |
| **STRAWBERRY FRUIT JUICE,** canned (Smucker's) | 8 fl. oz. | 5 | 0.0 | | | |
| **STRAWBERRY JELLY:** | | | | | | |
| Sweetened (Home Brand) | 1 T. | 7 | 0.0 | | | |
| Dietetic (Diet Delight) | 1 T. | 30 | 0.0 | | | |
| **STRAWBERRY KRISPIES,** cereal (Kellogg's) | ¾ cup (1 oz.) | 200 | 0.0 | | | |

(USDA): United States Department of Agriculture
*Prepared as Package Directs

| Food and Description | Measure or Quantity | Sodium (mg.) | —Fats in grams— | | | Cholesterol (mg.) |
|---|---|---|---|---|---|---|
| | | | Total | Satu-rated | Unsatu-rated | |
| **STRAWBERRY NECTAR,** | | | | | | |
| canned (Libby's) | 6 fl. oz. | 5 | 0.0 | | | |
| **STRAWBERRY PRESERVE OR JAM:** | | | | | | |
| Sweetened (Bama) | 1 T. (.7 oz.) | 7 | 0.0 | | | 0 |
| Dietetic or low calorie: | | | | | | |
| (Estee) | 1 T. | <3 | 0.0 | | | 0 |
| (Featherweight) | 1 T. | 40–50 | 0.0 | | | (0) |
| (Louis Sherry) | 1 T. | <3 | 0.0 | | | 0 |
| **STRAWBERRY SHORTCAKE,** | | | | | | |
| cereal (General Mills) | 1 cup (1 oz.) | 190 | 1.0 | | | |
| **STUFFING MIX:** | | | | | | |
| *Beef (Stove Top) | ½ cup | 582 | 8.7 | | | 21 |
| *Chicken: | | | | | | |
| (Bell's) | ½ cup | 536 | 8.0 | | | |
| (Stove Top) | ½ cup | 640 | 8.0 | | | 21 |
| Cornbread: | | | | | | |
| (Pepperidge Farm) | ⅛ of 8-oz. pkg. | 320 | 1.0 | | | |
| *(Stove Top) | ½ cup | 666 | 8.6 | | | 21 |
| Cube (Pepperidge Farm) | 1 oz. | 430 | 1.0 | | | |
| *Pork (Stove Top) | ½ cup | 621 | 8.9 | | | 21 |
| *Premium Blend (Bell's) | ½ cup | 420 | 6.0 | | | |
| *Turkey (Stove Top) | ½ cup | 634 | 8.8 | | | 21 |
| **STURGEON** (USDA): | | | | | | |
| Raw, section | 1 lb. (weighed with skin & bones) | | 7.3 | | | |
| Raw, meat only | 4 oz. | | 2.2 | | | |
| Smoked | 4 oz. | | 2.0 | | | |
| Steamed | 4 oz. | 122 | 6.5 | | | |
| **SUCCOTASH,** frozen: | | | | | | |
| Not thawed (USDA) | 4 oz. | 51 | .5 | | | 0 |
| Boiled, drained (USDA) | ½ cup (3.4 oz.) | 36 | .4 | | | 0 |
| (Birds Eye) | ½ cup (3.3 oz.) | 33 | .5 | | | 0 |
| **SUCKER, CARP,** raw (USDA): | | | | | | |
| Whole | 1 lb. (weighed whole) | | 5.7 | | | |
| Meat only | 4 oz. | | 3.6 | | | |

(USDA): United States Department of Agriculture
*Prepared as Package Directs

| Food and Description | Measure or Quantity | Sodium (mg.) | — Fats in grams — | | | Cholesterol (mg.) |
|---|---|---|---|---|---|---|
| | | | Total | Saturated | Unsaturated | |
| **SUCKER,** including **WHITE and MULLET,** raw (USDA): | | | | | | |
| Whole | 1 lb. (weighed whole) | 109 | 3.5 | | | |
| Meat only | 4 oz. | 64 | 2.0 | | | |
| **SUET,** raw (USDA) | 1 oz. | | 26.6 | | | |
| **SUGAR,** beet or cane (There is no difference in values among brands): | | | | | | |
| Brown: | | | | | | |
| (USDA) | 1 lb. | 136 | 0.0 | | | 0 |
| Brownulated (USDA) | 1 cup (5.4 oz.) | 46 | 0.0 | | | 0 |
| Firm-packed (USDA) | 1 cup (7.5 oz.) | 64 | 0.0 | | | 0 |
| Firm-packed (USDA) | 1 T. (.5 oz.) | 4 | 0.0 | | | 0 |
| Confectioners': | | | | | | |
| (USDA) | 1 lb. | 5 | 0.0 | | | 0 |
| Unsifted (USDA) | 1 cup (4.3 oz.) | 1 | 0.0 | | | 0 |
| Unsifted (USDA) | 1 T. (8 grams) | <1 | 0.0 | | | 0 |
| Sifted (USDA) | 1 cup (3.4 oz.) | <1 | 0.0 | | | 0 |
| Sifted (USDA) | 1 T. (6 grams) | <1 | 0.0 | | | 0 |
| Stirred (USDA) | 1 cup (4.2 oz.) | 1 | 0.0 | | | 0 |
| Stirred (USDA) | 1 T. (8 grams) | <1 | 0.0 | | | 0 |
| Granulated: | | | | | | |
| (USDA) | 1 lb. | 5 | 0.0 | | | 0 |
| (USDA) | 1 cup (6.9 oz.) | 2 | 0.0 | | | 0 |
| (USDA) | 1 T. (.4 oz.) | <1 | 0.0 | | | 0 |
| (USDA) | 1 lump (1⅛" × ¾" × ⅜", 6 grams | <1 | 0.0 | | | 0 |
| Maple (USDA) | 1 lb. | 64 | 0.0 | | | 0 |
| Maple (USDA) | 1¾" × 1¼" × ½" piece (1.2 oz.) | 4 | 0.0 | | | 0 |
| **SUGAR APPLE,** raw (USDA): | | | | | | |
| Whole | 1 lb. (weighed with skin & seeds) | 22 | .6 | | | 0 |
| Flesh only | 4 oz. | 12 | .3 | | | 0 |
| **SUGAR *CHEX*,** cereal, dry | ⅞ cup (1 oz.) | 220 | 2.2 | | | (0) |

(USDA): United States Department of Agriculture
*Prepared as Package Directs

| Food and Description | Measure or Quantity | Sodium (mg.) | —Fats in grams— | | | Choles- terol (mg.) |
|---|---|---|---|---|---|---|
| | | | Total | Satu- rated | Unsatu- rated | |
| **SUGAR FROSTED FLAKES,** cereal (Kellogg's) | ¾ cup (1 oz.) | 170 | 0.0 | | | (0) |
| **SUGAR JETS,** cereal (General Mills) | 1 cup (1 oz.) | 218 | 1.1 | | | (0) |
| **SUGAR POPS,** cereal (Kellogg's) | 1 cup (1 oz.) | 68 | .1 | | | (0) |
| **SUGAR PUFFS,** cereal (Malt-O-Meal) | ⅞ cup (1 oz.) | 26 | 0.0 | | | |
| **SUGAR SMACKS,** cereal (Kellogg's) | 1 cup (1 oz.) | 22 | .5 | | | (0) |
| **SUGAR SUBSTITUTE:** | | | | | | |
| (Estee) fructose | 1 tsp. | 0 | 0.0 | | | 0 |
| Sprinkle Sweet (Pillsbury) | 1 tsp. | 1 | 0.0 | | | 0 |
| Spoon-For-Spoon | 1 tsp. | 0 | 0.0 | | | 0 |
| Sweet 'N Low: | | | | | | |
| Brown | 1 tsp. | 19 | 0.0 | | | 0 |
| Granulated | 1-gram packet | 3 | 0.0 | | | 0 |
| Liquid | 1 drop | 0 | 0.0 | | | 0 |
| Sweet *10 (Pillsbury) | ⅛ tsp. | 2 | 0.0 | | | 0 |
| **SUKI-YAKI DINNER,** canned: | | | | | | |
| *(Chun King) stir fry | 6 oz. | 405 | 16.7 | | | 52 |
| *(La Choy) | ¾ cup | 990 | 9.0 | | | |
| **SUKI-YAKI MIX:** | | | | | | |
| (Durkee) | 1.7-oz. pkg. | 6,271 | .9 | | | |
| *With meat & vegetables (Durkee) | 6 cups (1.7-oz. pkg.) | 7,226 | 122.7 | | | |
| **SUNFLOWER SEED** (USDA): | | | | | | |
| In hulls | 4 oz. (weighed in hull) | 18 | 29.0 | 4. | 25. | 0 |
| Hulled | 1 oz. | 9 | 13.4 | 2. | 12. | 0 |
| **SUNSHINE PUNCH DRINK,** canned, Ssips (Johanna Farms) | 8.45-fl.-oz. cont. | 10 | 0.0 | | | |

(USDA): United States Department of Agriculture
*Prepared as Package Directs

| Food and Description | Measure or Quantity | Sodium (mg.) | Total | Satu-rated | Unsatu-rated | Choles-terol (mg.) |
|---|---|---|---|---|---|---|
| | | | | —Fats in grams— | | |
| **SURIMI,** *Crab Delights* (Louis Kemp), chunks, flakes or legs | 2 oz. | 550 | < 1.0 | | | 10 |
| **SUNFLOWER SEED FLOUR** (See **FLOUR**) | | | | | | |
| **SURINAM CHERRY** (See **PITANGA**) | | | | | | |
| **SUZY QS** (Hostess): | | | | | | |
| Banana | 2¼-oz. piece | 195 | 8.9 | | | 22 |
| Chocolate | 2¼-oz. piece | 303 | 9.6 | | | 16 |
| **SWAMP CABBAGE** (USDA): | | | | | | |
| Raw, whole | 1 lb. (weighed untrimmed) | | 1.1 | | | 0 |
| Boiled, trimmed, drained | 4 oz. | | .2 | | | 0 |
| **SWEETBREADS** (USDA): | | | | | | |
| Beef, raw | 1 lb. | 435 | 72.6 | | | 1134 |
| Beef, braised | 4 oz. | 132 | 26.3 | | | 528 |
| Calf, raw | 1 lb. | | 9.1 | | | |
| Calf, braised | 4 oz. | | 3.6 | | | |
| Hog (See **PANCREAS**) | | | | | | |
| Lamb, raw | 1 lb. | | 17.2 | | | |
| Lamb, braised | 4 oz. | | 6.9 | | | |
| **SWEET POTATO:** | | | | | | |
| Raw (USDA): | | | | | | |
| All kinds, unpared | 1 lb. (weighed whole) | 37 | 1.5 | | | 0 |
| All kinds, pared | 4 oz. | 11 | .5 | | | 0 |
| Firm-fleshed, Jersey types, pared | 4 oz. | 11 | .8 | | | 0 |
| Soft-fleshed, Puerto Rico variety, pared | 4 oz. | 11 | .3 | | | 0 |
| Baked, peeled after baking (USDA) | 3.9-oz. sweet potato (5″ × 2″) | 13 | .6 | | | 0 |
| Boiled, peeled after boiling (USDA) | 5-oz. sweet potato (5″ × 2″) | 15 | .6 | | | 0 |

(USDA): United States Department of Agriculture
*Prepared as Package Directs

| Food and Description | Measure or Quantity | Sodium (mg.) | —Fats in grams— | | | Cholesterol (mg.) |
|---|---|---|---|---|---|---|
| | | | Total | Saturated | Unsaturated | |
| Candied, home recipe (USDA)[1] | 6.2-oz. sweet potato (3½" × 2¼") | 74 | 5.8 | 4. | 2. | 0 |
| Canned (Trappey's): | | | | | | |
| Cut, in light syrup | ½ cup (4.3 oz.) | 25 | 0 | | | 0 |
| Mashed | ½ cup | 80 | 0 | | | 0 |
| Whole, in heavy syrup | ½ cup | 35 | 0 | | | 0 |
| Canned, dietetic pack, without added sugar & salt (USDA) | 4 oz. | 14 | .1 | | | 0 |
| Dehydrated flakes, dry (USDA) | ½ cup (2 oz.) | 105 | .3 | | | 0 |
| *Dehydrated flakes, prepared with water (USDA) | ½ cup (4.4 oz.) | 57 | .1 | | | 0 |
| Frozen: | | | | | | |
| Candied (Mrs. Paul's) | ⅓ of 12-oz. pkg. | 105 | Tr. | | | |
| Sweets & Apples, candied (Mrs. Paul's) | ⅓ of 12-oz. pkg. | 50 | 1.0 | | | |
| **SWEET POTATO PIE:** | | | | | | |
| Home recipe, made with lard (USDA)[2] | ⅙ of 9" pie (5.4 oz.) | 331 | 17.2 | 6. | 11. | |
| Home recipe, made with vegetable shortening (USDA)[3] | ⅙ of 9" pie (5.4 oz.) | 331 | 17.2 | 5. | 13. | |
| (Tastykake) | 4-oz. pie | | 15.0 | | | |
| **SWEETSOP** (See **SUGAR APPLE**) | | | | | | |
| **SWEET & SOUR CHICKEN** (La Choy): | | | | | | |
| *Canned, bi-pack | ¾ cup | 440 | 2.0 | | | |
| Frozen | 12-oz. entree | 2,010 | 1.0 | | | |
| ***SWEET & SOUR ORIENTAL,** canned (La Choy): | | | | | | |
| Chicken | ¾ cup | 1,420 | 2.0 | | | |
| Pork | ¾ cup | 1,540 | 4.0 | | | |

(USDA): United States Department of Agriculture
*Prepared as Package Directs
[1]Principal source of fat: butter.
[2]Principal sources of fat: lard & butter.
[3]Principal sources of fat: vegetable shortening & butter.

| Food and Description | Measure or Quantity | Sodium (mg.) | —Fats in grams— | | | Choles-terol (mg.) |
|---|---|---|---|---|---|---|
| | | | Total | Satu-rated | Unsatu-rated | |

**SWEET & SOUR PORK,**
frozen:

| Food and Description | Measure or Quantity | Sodium (mg.) | Total | Satu-rated | Unsatu-rated | Choles-terol (mg.) |
|---|---|---|---|---|---|---|
| (La Choy) | 12-oz. entree | 2,200 | 6.0 | | | |
| (Van de Kamp's) & rice | 11-oz. serving | 590 | 17.0 | | | |
| **SWISS STEAK,** frozen: | | | | | | |
| (Green Giant) baked, in gravy, with stuffed potato | 1 meal | 1,235 | 13.0 | | | |
| (Swanson) | 10-oz. dinner | 830 | 14.0 | | | |
| **SWORDFISH** (USDA): | | | | | | |
| Raw, meat only | 1 lb. | | 18.1 | | | |
| Broiled, with butter or margarine | 3″ × 3″ × ½″ steak (4.4 oz.) | | 7.5 | | | |
| Canned, solids & liq. | 4 oz. | | 3.4 | | | |
| **SYRUP:** | | | | | | |
| Regular: | | | | | | |
| Apricot (Smucker's) | 1 T. | <5 | Tr. | | | |
| Chocolate: | | | | | | |
| (USDA): | | | | | | |
| Fudge type[1] | 1 T. (.7 oz.) | 17 | 2.6 | 1.3 | 1.3 | |
| Thin type | 1 T. (.7 oz.) | 10 | .4 | .2 | .2 | |
| Bosco | 1 T. | 25 | .1 | | | |
| (Hershey's) | 1 T. (.5 oz.) | 15 | .5 | | | |
| (Nestlé) Quik | 1 oz. | 35 | 0.0 | | | |
| Corn: | | | | | | |
| (USDA) | 1 T. | 14 | 0.0 | | | 0 |
| Karo: | | | | | | |
| Dark | 1 T. | 37 | 0.0 | | | (0) |
| Light | 1 T. | 29 | 0.0 | | | (0) |
| Cane (USDA) | 1 T. | | 0.0 | | | 0 |
| Maple: | | | | | | |
| (USDA) | 1 T. | 2 | 0.0 | | | 0 |
| (Home Brand) | 1 oz. | 25 | 0.0 | | | (0) |
| Karo, imitation | 1 T. | 32 | 0.0 | | | (0) |
| Pancake or waffle: | | | | | | |
| (Aunt Jemima) | 1 T. | 15 | 0.0 | | | (0) |
| Karo | 1 T. | 32 | 0.0 | | | 11 |
| Log Cabin: | | | | | | |
| Regular | 1 T. | 6 | 0.0 | | | 0 |
| Buttered | 1 T. | 38 | .3 | | | 11 |

(USDA): United States Department of Agriculture
*Prepared as Package Directs
[1]Principal sources of fat: chocolate, animal & vegetable shortening & milk.

| Food and Description | Measure or Quantity | Sodium (mg.) | Total | Satu-rated | Unsatu-rated | Choles-terol (mg.) |
|---|---|---|---|---|---|---|
| *Mrs. Butterworth's* | 1 T. | 24 | .2 | | | 1 |
| Strawberry (Smucker's) | 1 T. | 2 | Tr. | | | |
| Dietetic: | | | | | | |
| Blueberry: | | | | | | |
| (Dia-Mel) | 1 T. | 15 | 0.0 | | | 0 |
| (Estee) | 1 T. | 0 | 0.0 | | | 0 |
| (Featherweight) | 1 T. | <25 | 0.0 | | | 0 |
| Chocolate: | | | | | | |
| (Diet Delight) | 1 T. | 10 | 0.0 | | | |
| (Estee) *Choco-Syp* | 1 T. | 3 | 0.0 | | | 0 |
| Pancake or waffle: | | | | | | |
| (Aunt Jemima) | 1 T. | 29 | 0.0 | | | (0) |
| (Dia-Mel) | 1 T. | 10 | 0.0 | | | 0 |
| (Diet Delight) | 1 T. | 30 | 0.0 | | | (0) |
| (Estee) | 1 T. | 0 | 0.0 | | | (0) |

# T

**TACO:**

| | | | | | | |
|---|---|---|---|---|---|---|
| *Canned (Ortega) | 1 oz. | 104 | 3.6 | | | 18 |
| Mix: | | | | | | |
| *(Durkee) | 1 cup | 1,115 | 48.6 | | | |
| (French's) | ⅙ of 1¼-oz. pkg. | 365 | 0.0 | | | |
| (Old El Paso) | 1 pkg. | 3,569 | 1.4 | | | |
| Shell: | | | | | | |
| (Gebhardt) | .4-oz. shell | 0 | 2.0 | | | |
| (Old El Paso) | .4-oz. shell | 47 | 3.0 | | | |
| (Ortega) | .4-oz. shell | 55 | 2.0 | | | |
| (Rosarita) | .4-oz. shell | 0 | 2.0 | | | |

**TACO BELL:**

| | | | | | | |
|---|---|---|---|---|---|---|
| *Bellbeefer:* | | | | | | |
| Regular | 5-oz. serving | 710 | 8.8 | | | 23 |
| With cheese | 5½-oz. serving | 670 | 11.5 | | | 27 |
| Burrito: | | | | | | |
| Bean | 7.2-oz. serving | 935 | 14.6 | | | 19 |
| Beef | 6.7-oz. serving | 989 | 19.0 | | | 54 |
| Combination | 8.4-oz. serving | 777 | 13.2 | | | 29 |
| Supreme | 5.6-oz. serving | 855 | 18.5 | | | 28 |
| Crispas, cinnamon | 2.2-oz. serving | 158 | 21.8 | | | 2 |

(USDA): United States Department of Agriculture
*Prepared as Package Directs

| Food and Description | Measure or Quantity | Sodium (mg.) | Fats in grams — Total | Satu- rated | Unsatu- rated | Choles- terol (mg.) |
|---|---|---|---|---|---|---|
| Enchirito | 6½-oz. serving | 1,030 | 10.7 | | | 40 |
| Nachos: | | | | | | |
| Regular | 3.3-oz. serving | 319 | 19.1 | | | 11 |
| *Bellgrande* | 10.6-oz. serving | 1,140 | 38.4 | | | 44 |
| Pintos & cheese | 5.1-oz. serving | 732 | 9.6 | | | 7 |
| Taco: | | | | | | |
| Regular | 3.1-oz. serving | 279 | 12.3 | | | 34 |
| *Bellgrande* | 5.2-oz. serving | 353 | 18.5 | | | 36 |
| Light | 5.0-oz. serving | 426 | 22.3 | | | 39 |
| Taco salad | 18.3-oz. serving | 1,455 | 56.6 | | | 69 |
| Tostada: | | | | | | |
| Regular | 5.7-oz. serving | 534 | 12.5 | | | 9 |
| Beefy | 7.4-oz. serving | 714 | 19.3 | | | 49 |

**TAMALE:**

Canned:

(Hormel) beef:

| | | | | | | |
|---|---|---|---|---|---|---|
| Regular | 1 tamale | 275 | 5.0 | | | |
| Hot & spicy | 1 tamale | 306 | 5.0 | | | |
| *Short Orders* | 7½-oz. can | 1,140 | 19.0 | | | |
| (Old El Paso) with chili gravy | 1 tamale | 189 | 6.0 | | | |
| (Pride of Mexico) beef | 1 tamale (2 oz.) | 310 | 8.5 | | | |
| Frozen (Hormel) beef | 1 tamale | 555 | 7.0 | | | |

**TAMARIND,** fresh (USDA):

| | | | | | | |
|---|---|---|---|---|---|---|
| Whole | 1 lb. (weighed with pods & seeds) | 111 | 1.3 | | | 0 |
| Flesh only | 4 oz. | 58 | .7 | | | 0 |

**\*TANG,** instant breakfast drink:

| | | | | | | |
|---|---|---|---|---|---|---|
| Grape | 6 fl. oz. | 5 | Tr. | | | 0 |
| Orange | 6 fl. oz. | 1 | .1 | | | 0 |

**TANGELO,** fresh (USDA):

| | | | | | | |
|---|---|---|---|---|---|---|
| Juice from whole fruit | 1 lb. (weighed with peel, membrane & seeds) | | .3 | | | 0 |
| Juice | ½ cup (4.4 oz.) | | .1 | | | 0 |

(USDA): United States Department of Agriculture
*Prepared as Package Directs

| Food and Description | Measure or Quantity | Sodium (mg.) | Total | Satu-rated | Unsatu-rated | Choles-terol (mg.) |
|---|---|---|---|---|---|---|
| | | | —Fats in grams— | | | |

**TANGERINE OR MANDARIN ORANGE,** fresh:

| Food and Description | Measure or Quantity | Sodium (mg.) | Total | Satu-rated | Unsatu-rated | Choles-terol (mg.) |
|---|---|---|---|---|---|---|
| Whole (USDA) | 1 lb. (weighed with peel, membrane & seeds) | 7 | .7 | | | 0 |
| Whole (USDA) | 4.1-oz. tangerine (2⅜″ dia.) | 2 | .2 | | | 0 |
| Peeled (Sunkist) | 1 large tangerine (4.1 oz.) | 2 | Tr. | | | 0 |
| Sections, without membranes (USDA) | 1 cup (6.8 oz.) | 4 | .4 | | | 0 |

**TANGERINE JUICE:**

| | | | | | | |
|---|---|---|---|---|---|---|
| Fresh (USDA) | ½ cup (4.4 oz.) | 1 | .2 | | | 0 |
| Canned, unsweetened (USDA) | ½ cup (4.4 oz.) | 1 | .2 | | | 0 |
| Canned, sweetened (USDA) | ½ cup (4.4 oz.) | 1 | .2 | | | 0 |
| Frozen concentrate, unsweetened: | | | | | | |
| Undiluted (USDA) | 6-oz. can | 4 | 1.5 | | | 0 |
| *Prepared with 3 parts water by volume (USDA) | ½ cup (4.4 oz.) | 1 | .2 | | | 0 |
| Frozen concentrate, sweetened: | | | | | | |
| *(Minute Maid) | ½ cup (4.2 oz.) | 1 | <.1 | | | 0 |
| *(Snow Crop) | ½ cup (4.2 oz.) | 1 | <.1 | | | 0 |

**TAPIOCA,** dry, quick cooking, granulated:

| | | | | | | |
|---|---|---|---|---|---|---|
| (USDA) | 1 cup (5.4 oz.) | 5 | .3 | | | 0 |
| (USDA) | 1 T. (10 grams) | <1 | <.1 | | | 0 |
| (Minute Tapioca) | 1 T. | 2 | Tr. | | | |

**TAQUITO,** frozen (Van de Kamp's) beef, shredded

| | | | | | | |
|---|---|---|---|---|---|---|
| | 8-oz. serving | 990 | 25.0 | | | |

**TARO,** raw (USDA):

| | | | | | | |
|---|---|---|---|---|---|---|
| Tubers, whole | 1 lb. (weighed with skin) | 27 | .8 | | | 0 |
| Tubers, skin removed | 4 oz. | 8 | .2 | | | 0 |
| Leaves & stems | 1 lb. | | 3.6 | | | 0 |

**TARRAGON** (Spice Islands)

| | | | | | | |
|---|---|---|---|---|---|---|
| | 1 tsp. | <1 | | | | (0) |

(USDA): United States Department of Agriculture
*Prepared as Package Directs

| Food and Description | Measure or Quantity | Sodium (mg.) | —Fats in grams— | | | Choles- terol (mg.) |
|---|---|---|---|---|---|---|
| | | | Total | Satu- rated | Unsatu- rated | |
| **_TASTEEOS_**, cereal (Ralston Purina) | 1¼ cups (1 oz.) | 210 | .7 | | | |
| **TAUTOG OR BLACKFISH,** raw (USDA): | | | | | | |
| Whole | 1 lb. (weighed whole) | | 1.8 | | | |
| Meat only | 4 oz. | | 1.2 | | | |
| **TEA:** | | | | | | |
| Bag: | | | | | | |
| *(Celestial Seasonings): | | | | | | |
| After dinner: | | | | | | |
| _Amaretto Nights, Cinnamon Vienna_ or _Swiss Mint_ | 1 cup | < 1 | Tr. | | | |
| _Bavarian Chocolate Orange_ | 1 cup | 5 | Tr. | | | |
| _Irish Cream Mist_ | 1 cup | 1 | Tr. | | | |
| Caffeine-free | 1 cup | 5 | Tr. | | | |
| Fruit & tea | 1 cup | < 1 | Tr. | | | |
| Herb: | | | | | | |
| _Almond Sunset, Emperor's Choice_ or _Red Zinger_ | 1 cup | 2 | Tr. | | | |
| _Cranberry Cove_ | 1 cup | 6 | Tr. | | | |
| _Mellow Mint_ or _Mo's 24 Herb_ | 1 cup | 8 | Tr. | | | |
| Peppermint | 1 cup | 8 | Tr. | | | |
| *(Lipton) regular, herbal or decaf | 1 cup | 0 | 0.0 | | | |
| Canned (Lipton) | 12 fl. oz. | 12 | | | | (0) |
| Instant: | | | | | | |
| Dry powder, slightly sweetened (USDA) | 1 tsp. (< 1 gram) | | Tr. | | | 0 |
| *Beverage, slightly sweetened (USDA) | 1 cup (8.4 oz.) | | Tr. | | | 0 |
| *(Lipton) | 1 cup | 0 | 0.0 | | | (0) |
| _Nestea_ | 1 tsp. (< 1 gram) | 7 | 0.0 | | | (0) |
| (Tender Leaf) | 1 rounded tsp. | Tr. | Tr. | | | 0 |
| **_TEAM,_** cereal | 1 cup (1 oz.) | 190 | 1.0 | | | (0) |

(USDA): United States Department of Agriculture
*Prepared as Package Directs

| Food and Description | Measure or Quantity | Sodium (mg.) | Total | Fats in grams Satu- rated | Unsatu- rated | Choles- terol (mg.) |
|---|---|---|---|---|---|---|
| **TEA MIX,** iced: | | | | | | |
| *All flavors (Salada) | 1 cup (.5 oz. dry) | 6 | <.1 | | | (0) |
| *(Tender Leaf) | 1 cup | 80 | | | | 0 |
| Lemon-flavored: | | | | | | |
| *Low calorie (Lipton) | 1 cup | 0 | <.1 | | | (0) |
| *Low calorie (Tender Leaf) | 1 cup | 50 | Tr. | | | 0 |
| **TENDERGREEN** (See **MUSTARD SPINACH**) | | | | | | |
| **TEQUILA** (See **DISTILLED LIQUOR**) | | | | | | |
| **TEQUILA SUNRISE COCKTAIL** (Mr. Boston) 12½% alcohol | 3 fl. oz. | 130 | 0.0 | | | |
| **TERIYAKI:** | | | | | | |
| *Canned (La Choy) chicken, bi-pack | ¾ cup | 850 | 2.0 | | | |
| Frozen: | | | | | | |
| (Armour) *Dinner Classics:* | | | | | | |
| Chicken | 10½-oz. meal | 1,520 | 15.0 | | | |
| Steak | 10-oz. meal | 1,550 | 16.0 | | | |
| (Conagra) *Light & Elegant,* beef | 8-oz. entree | 625 | 3.0 | | | |
| **TERIYAKI BASTE & GLAZE OR SAUCE:** | | | | | | |
| (Kikkoman) | 1 T. (.8 oz.) | 487 | Tr. | | | 0 |
| (La Choy) | 1 oz. | 1,640 | 0.0 | | | |
| **TERRAPIN, DIAMOND BACK,** raw (USDA): | | | | | | |
| In shell | 1 lb. (weighed in shell) | | 3.3 | | | |
| Meat only | 4 oz. | | 4.0 | | | |
| **TEXTURED VEGETABLE PROTEIN:** | | | | | | |
| Breakfast links, *Morningstar Farms* | 1 link (.8 oz.) | 225 | 5.7 | | | 0 |

(USDA): United States Department of Agriculture
*Prepared as Package Directs

| Food and Description | Measure or Quantity | Sodium (mg.) | Total | Satu-rated | Unsatu-rated | Choles-terol (mg.) |
|---|---|---|---|---|---|---|
| | | | | —Fats in grams— | | |
| Breakfast patties, *Morningstar Farms* | 1 pattie (1.3 oz.) | 470 | 7.2 | | | 0 |
| Breakfast slices, *Morningstar Farms* | 1 slice (1 oz.) | 468 | 3.1 | 1. | 2. | 0 |
| **THURINGER,** sausage: | | | | | | |
| (USDA) | 1 oz. | | 6.9 | | | |
| (Eckrich): | | | | | | |
| Sliced | 1-oz. slice | 380 | 7.0 | | | |
| *Smoky Tang* | 1 oz. | 350 | 7.0 | | | |
| (Hormel): | | | | | | |
| Packaged, sliced | 1 slice | 353 | 5.5 | | | |
| Whole: | | | | | | |
| Regular | 1 oz. | 332 | 9.0 | | | |
| Beefy | 1 oz. | 313 | 9.0 | | | |
| *Old Smokehouse* | 1 oz. | 328 | 8.0 | | | |
| (Ohse): | | | | | | |
| Regular | 1 oz. | 340 | 5.0 | | | |
| Beef | 1 oz. | 330 | 6.0 | | | |
| (Oscar Mayer): | | | | | | |
| Beef | .8-oz. slice | 316 | 6.3 | | | 17 |
| Meat | 1-oz. slice | 327 | 8.1 | | | 21 |
| Summer sausage, pure beef (Oscar Mayer) | .8-oz. slice | 278 | 5.8 | | | (0) |
| **THYME** (Spice Islands) | 1 tsp. | <1 | | | | (0) |
| **TIGER TAIL** (Hostess) | 2¼-oz. piece | 249 | 7.0 | | | 27 |
| **TILEFISH** (USDA): | | | | | | |
| Raw, whole | 1 lb. (weighed whole) | | 1.2 | | | |
| Baked, meat only | 4 oz. | | 4.2 | | | |
| **TOASTED WHEAT AND RAISINS,** cereal (Nabisco) | 1 oz. | 0 | 1.0 | | | |
| **TOASTER CAKE OR PASTRY:** | | | | | | |
| *Pop-Tarts* (Kellogg's): | | | | | | |
| Regular: | | | | | | |
| Blueberry | 1.8-oz. piece | 220 | 6.0 | | | |
| Brown sugar cinnamon | 1¾-oz. piece | 215 | 8.0 | | | |

(USDA): United States Department of Agriculture
*Prepared as Package Directs

| Food and Description | Measure or Quantity | Sodium (mg.) | Total | —Fats in grams— Satu- rated | Unsatu- rated | Choles- terol (mg.) |
|---|---|---|---|---|---|---|
| Cherry | 1.8-oz. piece | 230 | 6.0 | | | |
| Strawberry | 1.8-oz. piece | 225 | 4.0 | | | |
| Frosted: | | | | | | |
| Blueberry | 1.8-oz. piece | 220 | 5.0 | | | |
| Cherry | 1.8-oz. piece | 230 | 5.0 | | | |
| Concord grape, dutch apple, raspberry or strawberry | 1.8-oz. piece | 215 | 6.0 | | | |
| Toaster Strudel (Pillsbury): | | | | | | |
| Blueberry, raspberry or strawberry | 1 piece | 205 | 8.0 | | | |
| Cinnamon | 1 piece | 200 | 8.0 | | | |
| Toastettes (Nabisco): | | | | | | |
| Regular: | | | | | | |
| Apple | 1 piece | 170 | 5.0 | | | |
| Blueberry, cherry or strawberry | 1 piece | 200 | 5.0 | | | |
| Frosted: | | | | | | |
| Fudge | 1 piece | 210 | 6.0 | | | |
| Strawberry | 1 piece | 200 | 5.0 | | | |
| Toast-R-Cakes (Thomas'): | | | | | | |
| Blueberry | 1.2-oz. piece | 158 | 3.3 | | | |
| Bran | 1.2-oz. piece | 163 | 2.9 | | | |
| Corn | 1.2-oz. piece | 142 | 4.0 | | | |
| **TOASTIES,** cereal (Post) | 1¼ cups (1 oz.) | 298 | .1 | | | |
| **TOASTY O'S,** cereal (Malt-O-Meal) | 1¼ cups (1 oz.) | 281 | 2.0 | | | |
| **TODDLER FOOD** (See **BABY FOOD**) | | | | | | |
| **TOFU** (See **SOYBEAN CURD**) | | | | | | |
| **TOFUTTI:** | | | | | | |
| Frozen: | | | | | | |
| Chocolate supreme | 4 fl. oz. | 130 | 13.0 | | | 0 |
| Maple walnut | 4 fl. oz. | 95 | 14.0 | | | 0 |
| Vanilla | 4 fl. oz. | 90 | 11.0 | | | 0 |
| Wildberry supreme | 4 fl. oz. | 100 | 12.0 | | | 0 |
| Cuties: | | | | | | |
| Chocolate | 1 piece | 130 | 5.0 | | | 0 |
| Vanilla | 1 piece | 110 | 5.0 | | | 0 |

(USDA): United States Department of Agriculture
*Prepared as Package Directs

| Food and Description | Measure or Quantity | Sodium (mg.) | Total | —Fats in grams— Satu- rated | Unsatu- rated | Choles- terol (mg.) |
|---|---|---|---|---|---|---|
| *Love Drops:* | | | | | | |
| Cappuccino | 4 fl. oz. | 120 | 12.0 | | | 0 |
| Chocolate or vanilla | 4 fl. oz. | 100 | 12.0 | | | 0 |
| Soft serve: | | | | | | |
| Banana pecan, chocolate, maple walnut, peanut butter, strawberry, vanilla or wildberry | 4 fl. oz. | 65 | 8.0 | | | 0 |
| Hi-Lite | 4 fl. oz. | 75 | 1.0 | | | 0 |

## TOMATO:

| Food and Description | Measure or Quantity | Sodium (mg.) | Total | —Fats in grams— Satu- rated | Unsatu- rated | Choles- terol (mg.) |
|---|---|---|---|---|---|---|
| Fresh, green, whole, untrimmed (USDA) | 1 lb. (weighed with core & stem end) | 12 | .8 | | | 0 |
| Fresh, green, trimmed, unpeeled (USDA) | 4 oz. | 3 | .2 | | | 0 |
| Fresh, ripe (USDA): | | | | | | |
| Whole, eaten with skin | 1 lb. | 14 | .9 | | | 0 |
| Whole, peeled | 1 lb. (weighed with skin, stem ends & hard core) | 12 | .8 | | | 0 |
| Whole, peeled | 1 med. (2" × 2½", 5.3 oz.) | 4 | .3 | | | 0 |
| Whole, peeled | 1 small (1¾" × 2¼", 3.9 oz.) | 3 | .2 | | | 0 |
| Sliced, peeled | ½ cup (3.2 oz.) | 3 | .2 | | | 0 |
| Cooked without salt | ½ cup (4.3 oz.) | 5 | .2 | | | 0 |
| Canned, regular pack: | | | | | | |
| Whole, solids & liq. (USDA) | ½ cup (4.2 oz.) | 155 | .2 | | | 0 |
| (Contadina) | ½ cup (4 oz.) | 225 | Tr. | | | |
| Solids & liq. (Del Monte) | ½ cup (4.2 oz.) | 159 | 1.0 | | | 0 |
| Diced, in puree (Contadina) | ½ cup (4 oz.) | 232 | Tr. | | | (0) |
| Sliced (Contadina) | ½ cup (4 oz.) | 352 | Tr. | | | (0) |
| Stewed (Contadina) | ½ cup (4 oz.) | 216 | Tr. | | | (0) |
| Stewed (Del Monte) | ½ cup (4.2 oz.) | 342 | .2 | | | 0 |
| Wedges, solids & liq. (Del Monte) | ½ cup (4.1 oz.) | 336 | .2 | | | 0 |
| Whole, peeled (Hunt's) | ½ cup (4.2 oz.) | 415 | 0.0 | | | (0) |
| Whole, solids & liq. (Stokely-Van Camp's) | ½ cup (4.1 oz.) | | .2 | | | (0) |

(USDA): United States Department of Agriculture
*Prepared as Package Directs

| Food and Description | Measure or Quantity | Sodium (mg.) | — Fats in grams — | | Choles-terol (mg.) |
|---|---|---|---|---|---|
| | | | Total | Satu-rated | Unsatu-rated | |

| Food and Description | Measure or Quantity | Sodium (mg.) | Total | Saturated | Unsaturated | Cholesterol (mg.) |
|---|---|---|---|---|---|---|
| Canned, dietetic pack, low sodium: | | | | | | |
| Solids & liq. (USDA) | 4 oz. | 3 | .2 | | | 0 |
| Solids & liq. (Tillie Lewis) | ½ cup (4.3 oz.) | 15 | .2 | | | 0 |
| Whole, peeled (Diet Delight) | ½ cup (4.3 oz.) | 9 | .1 | | | 0 |
| Whole, unseasoned (S&W) | | | | | | |
| *Nutradiet* | 4 oz. | 10 | .1 | | | 0 |
| **TOMATO JUICE:** | | | | | | |
| Canned, regular pack: | | | | | | |
| (USDA) | 6 fl. oz. (6.4 oz.) | 364 | .2 | | | 0 |
| (USDA) | ½ cup (4.3 oz.) | 244 | .1 | | | 0 |
| (Campbell's) | 6 fl. oz. | 570 | 0.0 | | | (0) |
| (Libby's) | 6 fl. oz. | 455 | 0.0 | | | (0) |
| (Welch's) | 6 fl. oz. | 550 | 0.0 | | | (0) |
| Canned, dietetic pack, low sodium: | | | | | | |
| (USDA) | 4 oz. (by wt.) | 3 | .1 | | | 0 |
| (Diet Delight) | 6 fl. oz. | 20 | 0.0 | | | (0) |
| Unseasoned (S&W) | | | | | | |
| *Nutradiet* | 6 fl. oz. | 20 | 0.0 | | | (0) |
| Concentrate, canned (USDA) | 4 oz. (by wt.) | 896 | .5 | | | 0 |
| *Concentrate, canned, diluted with 3 parts water by volume | | | | | | |
| (USDA) | 4 oz. (by wt.) | 237 | .1 | | | 0 |
| Dehydrated (USDA) | 1 oz. | 1,115 | .6 | | | 0 |
| *Dehydrated (USDA) | ½ cup (4.3 oz.) | 312 | .1 | | | 0 |
| **TOMATO JUICE COCKTAIL:** | | | | | | |
| (USDA) | 4 oz. (by wt.) | 227 | .1 | | | 0 |
| *Snap-E-Tom* | 6 fl. oz. | 980 | 0.0 | | | |
| **TOMATO PASTE,** canned: | | | | | | |
| (USDA) regular, no salt added | 6-oz. can | 65 | .7 | | | 0 |
| (USDA) regular, no salt added | ½ cup (4.6 oz.) | 49 | .5 | | | 0 |
| (USDA) regular, no salt added | 1 T. (.6 oz.) | 61 | .6 | | | 0 |
| (USDA) salt added | 6-oz. can | 1,343 | .7 | | | 0 |
| (USDA) salt added | ½ cup (4.6 oz.) | 1,019 | .5 | | | 0 |
| (USDA) salt added | 1 T. (.6 oz.) | 126 | .6 | | | 0 |
| (Contadina) regular | 6 oz. | 135 | 0.0 | | | 0 |
| (Del Monte) | ¾ cup (6 oz.) | 110 | 1.0 | | | |
| (Hunt's): | | | | | | |
| Regular | 6 oz. | 450 | 0.0 | | | |

(USDA): United States Department of Agriculture
*Prepared as Package Directs

| Food and Description | Measure or Quantity | Sodium (mg.) | — Fats in grams — | | | Choles- terol (mg.) |
|---|---|---|---|---|---|---|
| | | | Total | Satu- rated | Unsatu- rated | |
| Italian style | 6 oz. | 1,575 | 0.0 | | | |
| Dietetic | 6 oz. | 75 | 0.0 | | | |
| **TOMATO, PICKLED,** canned | | | | | | |
| (Claussen) | 1 oz. | 326 | Tr. | | | |
| **TOMATO PUREE:** | | | | | | |
| Canned, regular pack: | | | | | | |
| (USDA) | 1 cup (8.8 oz.) | 998 | .5 | | | 0 |
| (Contadina) | 1 cup | 180 | 0.0 | | | (0) |
| (Hunt's) | 1 cup (8.8 oz.) | 370 | 0.0 | | | (0) |
| Canned, dietetic pack (USDA) | 8 oz. | 14 | .5 | | | 0 |
| **TOMATO SALAD,** jellied | | | | | | |
| (Contadina) | 1/2 cup | 592 | Tr. | | | (0) |
| **TOMATO SAUCE,** canned: | | | | | | |
| (Contadina) regular | 1 cup | 1,020 | 0.0 | | | (0) |
| (Del Monte) plain | 1 cup (8.8 oz.) | 1,330 | 1.0 | | | (0) |
| (Del Monte) with onions | 1 cup (8.8 oz.) | 1,180 | 1.0 | | | |
| (Hunt's) plain | 1 cup (8.7 oz.) | 1,330 | 0.0 | | | (0) |
| (Hunt's) herb[1] | 1 cup (8.8 oz.) | 990 | 8.5 | | | |
| (Hunt's) with cheese[2] | 1 cup (8.8 oz.) | 1,590 | 2.0 | | | |
| (Hunt's) with mushrooms | 1 cup (8.8 oz.) | 1,420 | 0.0 | | | |
| (Hunt's) with onions | 1 cup (8.8 oz.) | 1,340 | 0.0 | | | |
| **TOMCOD, ATLANTIC,** raw (USDA): | | | | | | |
| Whole | 1 lb. (weighed whole) | | .7 | | | |
| Meat only | 4 oz. | | .5 | | | |
| **TOM COLLINS:** | | | | | | |
| Cocktail (Mr. Boston) 12 1/2% alcohol | 3 fl. oz. | 39 | 0.0 | | | (0) |
| *Mix (Bar-Tender's Brand) | 6 fl. oz. | 32 | 0.0 | | | 0 |
| **TONGUE** (USDA): | | | | | | |
| Beef, medium fat, raw, untrimmed | 1 lb. | | 52.0 | | | |
| Beef, medium fat, braised | 4 oz. | 69 | 18.9 | | | |
| Beef, smoked | 4 oz. | | 32.7 | | | |

(USDA): United States Department of Agriculture
*Prepared as Package Directs
[1]Principal source of fat: cottonseed oil.
[2]Principal source of fat: cheese.

| Food and Description | Measure or Quantity | Sodium (mg.) | Total | Saturated | Unsaturated | Cholesterol (mg.) |
|---|---|---|---|---|---|---|
| | | | | — Fats in grams — | | |
| Calf, raw, untrimmed | 1 lb. | | 18.5 | | | |
| Calf, braised | 4 oz. | | 6.8 | | | |
| Hog, raw, untrimmed | 1 lb. | | 53.8 | | | |
| Hog, braised | 4 oz. | | 19.7 | | | |
| Lamb, raw, untrimmed | 1 lb. | | 50.7 | | | |
| Lamb, braised | 4 oz. | | 20.6 | | | |
| Sheep, raw, untrimmed | 1 lb. | | 72.2 | | | |
| Sheep, braised | 4 oz. | | 28.7 | | | |

**TONGUE, CANNED:**

| Food and Description | Measure or Quantity | Sodium (mg.) | Total | Saturated | Unsaturated | Cholesterol (mg.) |
|---|---|---|---|---|---|---|
| Pickled (USDA) | 1 oz. | | 5.8 | | | |
| Potted or deviled (USDA) | 1 oz. | | 6.5 | | | |
| (Hormel) pork, cured | 3 oz. (12-oz. can) | 966 | 13.0 | | | |

**TOPPING** (See also
**CHOCOLATE SYRUP**):
Sweetened:

| Food and Description | Measure or Quantity | Sodium (mg.) | Total | Saturated | Unsaturated | Cholesterol (mg.) |
|---|---|---|---|---|---|---|
| Butterscotch (Smucker's) | 1 T. | 37 | .5 | | | Tr. |
| Caramel (Smucker's): | | | | | | |
|   Regular | 1 T. | 55 | .5 | | | |
|   Hot | 1 T. | 37 | 2.0 | | | |
| Chocolate: | | | | | | |
|   (Hershey's) fudge | 1 T. | 15 | Tr. | | | |
|   (Smucker's): | | | | | | |
|     Regular | 1 T. | 17 | 0.0 | | | |
|     Fudge | 1 T. | 22 | .5 | | | |
|     Fudge, hot | 1 T. | 27 | 2.0 | | | |
| Nut (Planters) | 1 T. | 0 | 8.0 | | | 0 |
| Pecans, in syrup (Smucker's) | 1 T. | 0 | .5 | | | |
| Pineapple (Smucker's) | 1 T. | 0 | 0.0 | | | |
| Peanut butter caramel | | | | | | |
|   (Smucker's) | 1 T. | 52 | 1.0 | | | |
| Strawberry (Smucker's) | 1 T. | 0 | 0.0 | | | |
| Walnuts in syrup (Smucker's) | 1 T. | 0 | .5 | | | |
| Dietetic, chocolate (Diet | | | | | | |
|   Delight) | 1 T. (.6 oz.) | 9 | Tr. | | | |

**TOPPING, WHIPPED:**

| Food and Description | Measure or Quantity | Sodium (mg.) | Total | Saturated | Unsaturated | Cholesterol (mg.) |
|---|---|---|---|---|---|---|
| (USDA) pressurized | 1 cup (2.5 oz.) | | 17.0 | 15. | 2. | |
| (USDA) pressurized | 1 T. (4 grams) | | 1.0 | <1. | Tr. | |
| (Birds Eye) *Cool Whip* | 1 T. (4 grams) | 2 | 1.2 | | | Tr. |
| *Dover Farms* | 1 T. | 3 | Tr. | | | Tr. |
| (Johanna) | 1 T. | 2 | .7 | | | 4 |

(USDA): United States Department of Agriculture
*Prepared as Package Directs

| Food and Description | Measure or Quantity | Sodium (mg.) | Total | Fats in grams — Satu-rated | Unsatu-rated | Choles-terol (mg.) |
|---|---|---|---|---|---|---|
| **TOPPING, WHIPPED, MIX:** | | | | | | |
| *(D-Zerta) | 1 T. | 6 | .6 | | | Tr. |
| *(Dream Whip) | 1 T. (.2 oz.) | 4 | .8 | | | Tr. |
| *(Lucky Whip) | 1 T. (4 grams) | 3 | .6 | Tr. | <1. | 0 |
| | | | | | | |
| **TORTILLA** (USDA) | 7-oz. tortilla (5″) | | .6 | | | |
| | | | | | | |
| **TOSTADA,** frozen (Van de Kamp's) beef | 8½-oz. pkg. | 720 | 30.0 | | | |
| | | | | | | |
| **TOSTADA SHELL:** | | | | | | |
| (Old El Paso) | .4-oz. shell | 66 | 3.2 | | | |
| (Ortega) | .4-oz. shell | | 2.0 | | | |
| | | | | | | |
| ***TOTAL,*** cereal (General Mills): | | | | | | |
| Regular | 1 cup (1 oz.) | 375 | 1.0 | | | |
| Corn | 1 cup (1 oz.) | 310 | 1.0 | | | |
| | | | | | | |
| **TOWEL GOURD,** raw (USDA): | | | | | | |
| Unpared | 1 lb. (weighed with skin) | | .8 | | | 0 |
| Pared | 4 oz. | | .2 | | | 0 |
| | | | | | | |
| **TRIPE,** beef (USDA): | | | | | | |
| Commercial | 4 oz. | 82 | 2.3 | | | |
| Pickled | 4 oz. | 52 | 1.5 | | | |
| | | | | | | |
| ***TRIX,*** cereal (General Mills) | 1 cup (1 oz.) | 170 | 1.0 | | | |
| | | | | | | |
| **TROUT:** | | | | | | |
| Brook, fresh, whole (USDA) | 1 lb. (weighed whole) | | 4.7 | | | |
| Brook, fresh, meat only (USDA) | 4 oz. | | 2.4 | | | |
| Lake (See **LAKE TROUT**) | | | | | | |
| Rainbow (USDA): | | | | | | |
| Fresh, meat with skin | 4 oz. | | 12.9 | 3. | 10. | 62 |
| Canned | 4 oz. | | 15.2 | 5. | 11. | |
| Frozen (1000 Springs): | | | | | | |
| Boned | 5-oz. trout | 29 | 4.2 | | | |
| Dressed | 5-oz. trout | 35 | 5.1 | | | |

(USDA): United States Department of Agriculture
*Prepared as Package Directs

| Food and Description | Measure or Quantity | Sodium (mg.) | — Fats in grams — | | | Choles- terol (mg.) |
|---|---|---|---|---|---|---|
| | | | Total | Satu- rated | Unsatu- rated | |
| **TUNA:** | | | | | | |
| Raw, bluefin, meat only (USDA) | 4 oz. | | 4.6 | 1. | 4. | |
| Raw, yellowfin, meat only (USDA) | 4 oz. | 42 | 3.4 | 1. | 2. | |
| Raw, yellowfin, meat only, brined (USDA) | 4 oz. | 498 | 3.4 | 1. | 2. | |
| Canned in oil: | | | | | | |
| Solids & liq.: | | | | | | |
| (USDA)[1] | 6½-oz. can | 1,472 | 37.7 | 9. | 29. | 100 |
| (Breast O' Chicken) | 6½-oz. can | | 36.8 | | | |
| Chunk, light (Chicken of the Sea) | 6-oz. can | 1,196 | 25.6 | 3. | 22. | 74 |
| Chunk, light (Del Monte) | 6½-oz. can | 1,150 | 32.8 | | | |
| Chunk, light (Del Monte) | 1 cup (4.7 oz.) | 831 | 23.7 | | | |
| White albacore (Del Monte) | 6½-oz. can | 1,019 | 37.7 | | | |
| White albacore (Del Monte) | 1 cup (4.7 oz.) | 528 | 27.3 | | | |
| Drained solids: | | | | | | |
| (USDA)[1] | 6½-oz. can | | 12.9 | 5. | 8. | 102 |
| Albacore (Del Monte) | 1 cup (5.6 oz.) | 858 | 13.1 | | | |
| Chunk, light (Chicken of the Sea) | 6½-oz. can | 1,072 | 12.5 | 2. | 11. | 36 |
| Canned in water: | | | | | | |
| Solids & liq., no salt added: (USDA) | 6½-oz. can | 75 | 1.5 | | | 116 |
| Solids & liq., salt added: (USDA) | 6½-oz. can | 1,610 | 1.5 | | | 116 |
| (Breast O' Chicken) | 6½-oz. can | | 1.8 | | | |
| Drained, solid, light (Chicken of the Sea) | 6½-oz. can | 1,105 | 3.4 | | | |
| Drained, solid, white (Chicken of the Sea) | 6½-oz. can | 1,105 | 1.7 | | | |
| Canned, dietetic, drained, chunk, white (Chicken of the Sea) | 6½-oz. can | 74 | 2.6 | | | |
| | | | | | | |
| **TUNA PIE,** frozen: | | | | | | |
| (Banquet) | 8-oz. pie | 565 | 18.0 | | | |
| (Morton) | 8-oz. pie | 1,120 | 18.0 | | | |

(USDA): United States Department of Agriculture
*Prepared as Package Directs
[1]Principal sources of fat: cottonseed oil & tuna.

| Food and Description | Measure or Quantity | Sodium (mg.) | Fats in grams — Total | Satu- rated | Unsatu- rated | Choles- terol (mg.) |
|---|---|---|---|---|---|---|
| **TUNA SALAD,** home recipe [1,2] (USDA) | 4 oz. | | 11.9 | 3. | 9. | |
| **TURBOT, GREENLAND:** | | | | | | |
| Raw, whole (USDA) | 1 lb. (weighed whole) | | 19.8 | | | |
| Raw, meat only (USDA) | 4 oz. | 64 | 9.5 | 2. | 8. | |
| Frozen (Weight Watchers) | 18-oz. dinner | | 25.1 | | | |
| Frozen, with apple (Weight Watchers) | 9½-oz. luncheon | | 16.4 | | | |
| **TURF & SURF DINNER,** frozen (Armour) *Classic Lite* | 10-oz. meal | 890 | 7.0 | | | 80 |
| **TURKEY:** | | | | | | |
| Raw, ready-to-cook (USDA) | 1 lb. (weighed with bones) | | 48.7 | 14. | 35. | 272 |
| Raw, meat & skin only (USDA) | 4 oz. | | | | | 84 |
| Raw, dark meat (USDA) | 4 oz. | 92 | 4.9 | | | 85 |
| Raw, light meat (USDA) | 4 oz. | 58 | 1.4 | | | 68 |
| Raw, skin only (USDA) | 4 oz. | | 44.5 | | | 125 |
| Roasted (USDA): | | | | | | |
| Flesh, skin & giblets | From 13½-lb. raw, ready-to-cook turkey | | 603.5 | | | 3864 |
| Flesh & skin | From 13½-lb. raw, ready-to-cook turkey | | 338.9 | 106. | 233. | 3283 |
| Flesh & skin | 4 oz. | | 10.9 | 3. | 7. | 105 |
| Meat only: | | | | | | |
| Chopped | 1 cup (5 oz.) | 183 | 8.6 | 3. | 6. | |
| Dark | 4 oz. | 112 | 9.4 | 2. | 7. | 115 |
| Dark | 1 slice (2½" × 1⅝" × ¼", .7 oz.) | 21 | 1.8 | Tr. | 1. | 21 |
| Diced | 1 cup (4.8 oz.) | 176 | 8.2 | 3. | 6. | |
| Light | 4 oz. | 93 | 4.4 | 1. | 3. | 87 |
| Light | 1 slice (4" × 2" × ¼", 3 oz.) | 35 | 1.7 | Tr. | 1. | 32 |
| Skin only | 1 oz. | | 11.9 | 3. | 9. | 36 |

(USDA): United States Department of Agriculture
*Prepared as Package Directs
[1]Prepared with tuna, celery, mayonnaise, pickle, onion & egg.
[2]Principal sources of fat: cottonseed oil, soybean oil, corn oil, tuna & egg.

| Food and Description | Measure or Quantity | Sodium (mg.) | Total | Satu-rated | Unsatu-rated | Choles-terol (mg.) |
|---|---|---|---|---|---|---|
| | | | | — Fats in grams — | | |
| Giblets, simmered (USDA) | 2 oz. | | 8.7 | | | |
| Smoked, cooked, pressed (Oscar Mayer) | .8-oz. slice | 266 | .4 | | | |
| Canned, boned: | | | | | | |
| (USDA) | 4 oz. | | 14.2 | 5. | 10. | |
| Solids & liq. (Lynden Farms) | 5-oz. jar | 527 | 10.5 | 4. | 6. | |
| (Swanson) with broth | 5-oz. can | 760 | 14.0 | | | |
| Packaged: | | | | | | |
| (Carl Buddig) smoked, sliced: | | | | | | |
| Regular | 1 oz. | 400 | 3.0 | 1.0 | 2.0 | 6 |
| Ham | 1 oz. | 435 | .7 | .7 | | 19 |
| Salami | 1 oz. | 400 | .7 | .7 | | 19 |
| (Hormel) breast: | | | | | | |
| Regular | 1 slice | 242 | 1.0 | | | |
| Smoked | 1 slice | 270 | 1.0 | | | |
| (Ohse): | | | | | | |
| Oven cooked | 1 oz. | 190 | 1.0 | | | |
| Turkey bologna | 1 oz. | 300 | 6.0 | | | |
| Turkey salami | 1 oz. | 260 | 3.0 | | | |
| (Oscar Mayer) breast, sliced | ¾-oz. slice | 294 | .3 | .1 | .2 | 7 |
| **TURKEY DINNER OR ENTREE,** frozen: | | | | | | |
| (Armour) *Classic Lite,* parmesan | 11-oz. dinner | 480 | 8.0 | | | 70 |
| (Banquet) American Favorites | 11-oz. dinner | 1,416 | 9.0 | | | |
| (Conagra) *Light & Elegant* sliced | 8-oz. entree | 1,020 | 5.0 | | | 55 |
| (Le Menu) | 11¼-oz. dinner | 1,140 | 24.0 | | | |
| (Morton) regular | 11¼-oz. dinner | 1,100 | 4.9 | | | |
| (Stouffer's) casserole with gravy & dressing | 9¾-oz. pkg. | 1,125 | 18.0 | | | |
| (Swanson): | | | | | | |
| Dinner, *Hungry-Man* | 18½-oz. dinner | 2,150 | 18.0 | | | |
| Entree, main course, with gravy | 9¼-oz. meal | 1,120 | 10.0 | | | |
| (Weight Watchers) stuffed breast | 8½-oz. meal | 1,070 | 10.0 | | | |
| **TURKEY GIZZARD** (USDA): | | | | | | |
| Raw | 4 oz. | 66 | 8.3 | | | 164 |
| Simmered | 4 oz. | 58 | 9.8 | | | 260 |

(USDA): United States Department of Agriculture
*Prepared as Package Directs

| Food and Description | Measure or Quantity | Sodium (mg.) | Fats in grams Total | Saturated | Unsaturated | Cholesterol (mg.) |
|---|---|---|---|---|---|---|
| **TURKEY PIE:** | | | | | | |
| Home recipe, baked (USDA)[1] | 1/3 of 9″ pie (8.2 oz.) | 633 | 31.3 | 9. | 22. | 72 |
| Frozen: | | | | | | |
| Commercial, unheated (USDA)[1] | 8 oz. | 837 | 23.6 | 7. | 17. | 20 |
| (Banquet) | 8-oz. pie | 1,111 | 41.0 | | | |
| (Swanson) | 8-oz. pie | 800 | 25.0 | | | |
| (Swanson) *Chunky* | 10-oz. pie | 950 | 31.0 | | | |
| **TURKEY, POTTED** (USDA) | 1 oz. | | 5.4 | | | |
| **TURKEY SALAD,** canned | | | | | | |
| (Carnation) *Spreadable* | 1/4 of 7 1/2-oz. can | 245 | 7.5 | | | 16 |
| **TURKEY TETRAZZINI,** frozen | | | | | | |
| (Stouffer's) | 12-oz. pkg. | 1,240 | 28.0 | | | |
| **TURMERIC** (Spice Islands) | 1 tsp. | 1 | | | | (0) |
| **TURNIP** (USDA): | | | | | | |
| Fresh, without tops | 1 lb. (weighed with skins) | 191 | .8 | | | 0 |
| Fresh, pared, diced | 1/2 cup (2.4 oz.) | 33 | .1 | | | 0 |
| Fresh, pared, slices | 1/2 cup (2.3 oz.) | 31 | .1 | | | 0 |
| Boiled without salt, drained, diced | 1/2 cup (2.8 oz.) | 27 | .2 | | | 0 |
| Boiled without salt, drained, mashed | 1/2 cup (4 oz.) | 39 | .2 | | | 0 |
| **TURNIP GREENS,** leaves & stems: | | | | | | |
| Fresh (USDA) | 1 lb. (weighed untrimmed) | | 1.1 | | | 0 |
| Boiled, in small amount water, short time, drained (USDA) | 1/2 cup (2.5 oz.) | | .1 | | | 0 |
| Boiled, in large amount of water, long time, drained (USDA) | 1/2 cup (2.5 oz.) | | .1 | | | 0 |

(USDA): United States Department of Agriculture
*Prepared as Package Directs
[1]Principal sources of fat: vegetable shortening, cream, turkey & butter.

| Food and Description | Measure or Quantity | Sodium (mg.) | Total | Fats in grams — Satu- rated | Unsatu- rated | Choles- terol (mg.) |
|---|---|---|---|---|---|---|
| Canned, solids & liq.: | | | | | | |
| (USDA) | ½ cup (4.1 oz.) | 274 | .4 | | | 0 |
| (Stokely-Van Camp's) | ½ cup (3.9 oz.) | | .4 | | | (0) |
| Frozen: | | | | | | |
| Not thawed (USDA) | 4 oz. | 26 | .3 | | | 0 |
| Boiled, drained (USDA) | ½ cup (2.9 oz.) | 14 | .2 | | | 0 |
| Chopped (Birds Eye) | ½ cup (3.3 oz.) | 22 | .3 | | | 0 |
| **TURNOVER:** | | | | | | |
| Frozen (Pepperidge Farm): | | | | | | |
| Apple | 3.1-oz. piece | 220 | 17.0 | | | |
| Blueberry | 3.1-oz. piece | 240 | 19.0 | | | |
| Cherry | 3.1-oz. piece | 290 | 19.0 | | | |
| Refrigerated (Pillsbury): | | | | | | |
| Apple | 1 piece | 320 | 8.0 | | | |
| Blueberry or cherry | 1 piece | 310 | 8.0 | | | |
| **TURTLE, GREEN** (USDA): | | | | | | |
| Raw, in shell | 1 lb. (weighed in shell) | | .5 | | | |
| Raw, meat only | 4 oz. | | .6 | | | |
| Canned | 4 oz. | | .8 | | | |
| ***TWINKIES*** (Hostess): | | | | | | |
| Regular | 1 cake (1.5 oz.) | 149 | 5.1 | | | 21 |
| Devil's Food | 1 cake (1.5 oz.) | 213 | 5.1 | | | 10 |

# U

| Food and Description | Measure or Quantity | Sodium (mg.) | Total | | | Choles- terol (mg.) |
|---|---|---|---|---|---|---|
| ***UFOS,*** canned (Franco-American): | | | | | | |
| Regular | 7½-oz. serving | 780 | 3.0 | | | |
| With meatballs | 7½-oz. serving | 790 | 9.0 | | | |

# V

| Food and Description | Measure or Quantity | Sodium (mg.) | Total | Satu- rated | Unsatu- rated | Choles- terol (mg.) |
|---|---|---|---|---|---|---|
| **VANILLA,** bean (Spice Islands) | 2″ piece | <1 | | | | (0) |
| **VEAL,** medium fat (USDA): | | | | | | |
| Chuck, raw | 1 lb. (weighed with bone) | 327 | 36.0 | 17. | 19. | 258 |

(USDA): United States Department of Agriculture
*Prepared as Package Directs

VEAL (Continued)

| Food and Description | Measure or Quantity | Sodium (mg.) | Fats in grams Total | Saturated | Unsaturated | Cholesterol (mg.) |
|---|---|---|---|---|---|---|
| Chuck, braised, lean & fat | 4 oz. | 91 | 14.5 | 7. | 8. | 115 |
| Flank, raw | 1 lb. (weighed with bone) | 404 | 121.0 | 60. | 61. | 319 |
| Flank, stewed, lean & fat | 4 oz. | 91 | 36.6 | 18. | 18. | 115 |
| Foreshank, raw | 1 lb. (weighed with bone) | 212 | 19.0 | 10. | 9. | 168 |
| Foreshank, stewed, lean & fat | 4 oz. | 91 | 11.8 | 6. | 6. | 115 |
| Loin, raw | 1 lb. (weighed with bone) | 338 | 41.0 | 20. | 21. | 267 |
| Loin, broiled, medium done, chop, lean & fat | 4 oz. | 91 | 15.2 | 8. | 7. | 115 |
| Plate, raw | 1 lb. (weighed with bone) | 322 | 61.0 | 30. | 31. | 254 |
| Plate, stewed, lean & fat | 4 oz. | 91 | 24.0 | 12. | 12. | 115 |
| Rib, raw, lean & fat | 1 lb. (weighed with bone) | 314 | 49.0 | 23. | 26. | 248 |
| Rib, roasted, medium done, lean & fat | 4 oz. | 91 | 19.2 | 9. | 10. | 115 |
| Round & rump, raw | 1 lb. (weighed with bone) | 314 | 31.0 | 16. | 15. | 248 |
| Round & rump, broiled, steak or cutlet, lean & fat | 4 oz. (weighed without bone) | 91 | 12.6 | 7. | 6. | 115 |
| **VEAL DINNER,** frozen: | | | | | | |
| (Armour) *Dinner Classics* parmigiana | 10¾-oz. meal | 1,430 | 22.0 | | | 75 |
| (Banquet) parmigiana: | | | | | | |
| Dinner | 11-oz. dinner | 1,310 | 21.0 | | | |
| Entree for one | 5-oz. entree | 842 | 11.0 | | | 35 |
| (Morton): | | | | | | |
| Regular | 12-oz. dinner | 1,300 | 8.2 | | | |
| Light | 11-oz. dinner | 1,300 | 7.0 | | | |
| (Swanson) parmigiana: | | | | | | |
| Regular | 12¾-oz. dinner | 1,120 | 21.0 | | | |
| *Hungry-Man* | 20-oz. dinner | 2,010 | 28.0 | | | |
| (Weight Watchers) parmigiana | 8 1/16-oz. meal | 1,040 | 9.0 | | | |
| **VEAL STEAK,** frozen (Hormel): | | | | | | |
| Regular | 4 oz. | | 4.0 | | | |
| Breaded | 4 oz. | | 13.0 | | | |

(USDA): United States Department of Agriculture
*Prepared as Package Directs

| Food and Description | Measure or Quantity | Sodium (mg.) | —Fats in grams— | | | Cholesterol (mg.) |
|---|---|---|---|---|---|---|
| | | | Total | Satu-rated | Unsatu-rated | |

## VEGETABLE BOUILLON
### CUBE:
| | | | | | | |
|---|---|---|---|---|---|---|
| (Herb-Ox) | 1 cube (4 grams) | 920 | .1 | | | |
| (Wyler's) | 1 tsp. | 910 | < 1.0 | | | |

## VEGETABLE FAT (See FAT)

## VEGETABLE JUICE
### COCKTAIL, canned:
| | | | | | | |
|---|---|---|---|---|---|---|
| (USDA) | 4 oz. (by wt.) | 227 | .1 | | | 0 |
| Unseasoned (S & W) *Nutradiet* | 4 oz. (by wt.) | 25 | 0.0 | | | (0) |
| *V8* (Campbell's) | 6 fl. oz. | 625 | 0.0 | | | (0) |

## VEGETABLES, MIXED:
Canned, solids & liq.:
Regular pack:

| | | | | | | |
|---|---|---|---|---|---|---|
| (Del Monte) | ½ cup | 355 | Tr. | | | |
| (La Choy) Chinese | ½ cup | 35 | Tr. | | | Tr. |

Dietetic:

| | | | | | | |
|---|---|---|---|---|---|---|
| (Featherweight) | ½ cup | 25 | 0.0 | | | |
| (Larsen) *Fresh-Lite* | ½ cup | 25 | 0.0 | | | |

Frozen:
(Birds Eye):
Regular:

| | | | | | | |
|---|---|---|---|---|---|---|
| Broccoli, cauliflower & carrots in butter sauce | 3.3 oz. | 308 | 2.4 | | | |
| Medley in butter sauce | 3.3 oz. | 188 | 1.8 | | | |
| Mixed | 3.3 oz. | 43 | .4 | | | 0 |
| With onion sauce | ⅓ of 8-oz. pkg. | 357 | 5.3 | | | Tr. |

*Farm Fresh:*

| | | | | | | |
|---|---|---|---|---|---|---|
| Broccoli, corn & red pepper | ⅕ of 16-oz. pkg. | 11 | Tr. | | | 0 |
| Pea, carrot & pearl onion | ⅕ of 16-oz. pkg. | 85 | Tr. | | | 0 |

(Frosty Acres):

| | | | | | | |
|---|---|---|---|---|---|---|
| Regular | 3.3 oz. | 50 | 0.0 | | | |
| Italian style | 3.2 oz. | 20 | 0.0 | | | |
| Soup mix | 3 oz. | 35 | 0.0 | | | |
| Stew mix | 3 oz. | 21 | 0.0 | | | |
| (Le Sueur) pea, onion & carrot in butter sauce | ½ cup | 100 | 3.0 | | | |

(Larsen):

| | | | | | | |
|---|---|---|---|---|---|---|
| Regular | 3.3 oz. | 45 | 0.0 | | | |

(USDA): United States Department of Agriculture
*Prepared as Package Directs

| Food and Description | Measure or Quantity | Sodium (mg.) | — Fats in grams — | | | Cholesterol (mg.) |
|---|---|---|---|---|---|---|
| | | | Total | Saturated | Unsaturated | |
| California blend | 3.3 oz. | 20 | 0.0 | | | |
| Italian blend | 3.3 oz. | 20 | 0.0 | | | |
| Oriental blend | 3.3 oz. | 10 | 0.0 | | | |

**VEGETABLE OYSTER** (See **SALSIFY**)

**VEGETABLES IN PASTRY,**
frozen (Pepperidge Farm):

| Food and Description | Measure or Quantity | Sodium (mg.) | Total | Saturated | Unsaturated | Cholesterol (mg.) |
|---|---|---|---|---|---|---|
| Asparagus with mornay sauce | ½ of 7½-oz. pkg. | 245 | 17.0 | | | |
| Broccoli with cheese | ½ of 7½-oz. pkg. | 455 | 17.0 | | | |
| Mushrooms dijon | ½ of 7½-oz. pkg. | 415 | 16.0 | | | |
| Spinach almondine | ½ of 7½-oz. pkg. | 325 | 18.0 | | | |

**VEGETABLE STEW,** canned
(Hormel) *Dinty Moore* — 8 oz. — 1,047 — 8.0

**"VEGETARIAN FOODS":**
Canned or dry:

| Food and Description | Measure or Quantity | Sodium (mg.) | Total | Saturated | Unsaturated | Cholesterol (mg.) |
|---|---|---|---|---|---|---|
| Chicken, fried (Loma Linda) with gravy | 1½-oz. piece | 170 | 5.0 | | | |
| Chili (Worthington) | ½ cup | 626 | 7.2 | | | |
| Dinner cut (Loma Linda) | 2.1-oz. piece | 330 | <1.0 | | | |
| Dinner loaf (Loma Linda) | ¼ cup | 380 | 1.0 | | | 0 |
| Franks (Loma Linda) big | 1.8-oz. piece | 220 | 5.0 | | | 0 |
| Frichick (Worthington) | 1.6-oz. piece | 273 | 4.5 | | | |
| Gran Burger (Worthington) | 1 oz. | 622 | .4 | | | 0 |
| Linketts (Loma Linda) | 1.3-oz. piece | 170 | 4.0 | | | |
| Numete (Worthington) | ½" slice | 370 | 9.3 | | | |
| Nuteena (Loma Linda) | ½" slice | 120 | 12.0 | | | |
| Proteena (Loma Linda) | ½" slice | 460 | 6.0 | | | |
| Protose (Worthington) | ½" slice | 476 | 7.5 | | | |
| Redi-burger (Loma Linda) | ½" slice | 270 | 6.0 | | | |
| Stew Pac (Loma Linda) | 2 oz. | 220 | 2.0 | | | |
| Tender Bits (Loma Linda) | .5-oz. piece | 85 | .5 | | | |
| Vege-Burger (Loma Linda) no salt added | ½ cup | 55 | 2.0 | | | |
| Veg-scallops (Loma Linda) | 1 piece | 30 | .2 | | | 0 |

(USDA): United States Department of Agriculture
*Prepared as Package Directs

| Food and Description | Measure or Quantity | Sodium (mg.) | — Fats in grams — | | | Choles- terol (mg.) |
|---|---|---|---|---|---|---|
| | | | Total | Satu- rated | Unsatu- rated | |
| **Frozen:** | | | | | | |
| Bologna (Loma Linda) | 1-oz. slice | 245 | 4.5 | | | |
| Chicken, fried (Loma Linda) | 2-oz. piece | 510 | 14.0 | | | 0 |
| Chicken-like slices (Worthington) | 1-oz. slice | 288 | 2.8 | | | |
| *Chik-Nuggets* (Loma Linda) | .6-oz. piece | 126 | 2.2 | | | |
| Corn dogs (Loma Linda) | 2½-oz. piece | 300 | 19.0 | | | 0 |
| Meatballs (Loma Linda) | 1 piece | 53 | 1.0 | | | |
| Meatless salami (Worthington) | ¾-oz. slice | 300 | 2.2 | | | |
| Olive loaf (Loma Linda) | 1 slice | 261 | 2.8 | | | |
| *Stripples* (Worthington) | .3-oz. slice | 123 | 1.3 | | | |
| **VENISON,** raw, lean meat only (USDA) | 4 oz. | | 4.5 | 3. | 1. | |
| **VERMOUTH,** dry or sweet (Great Western) 16% alcohol | 3 fl. oz. | 20 | | | | |
| **VINEGAR:** | | | | | | |
| Cider: | | | | | | |
| (USDA) | ½ cup (4.2 oz.) | 1 | 0.0 | | | 0 |
| (USDA) | 1 T. (.5 oz.) | <1 | 0.0 | | | 0 |
| Distilled: | | | | | | |
| (USDA) | ½ cup (4.2 oz.) | 1 | | | | 0 |
| (USDA) | 1 T. (.5 oz.) | <1 | | | | 0 |
| Red or white wine (Regina) | 1 T. (.5 oz.) | <1 | Tr. | | | (0) |
| Red wine: | | | | | | |
| Plain (Spice Islands) | 2 T. | 6 | | | | (0) |
| Eschalot (Spice Islands) | 2 T. | 10 | | | | (0) |
| Garlic (Spice Islands) | 2 T. | 9 | | | | (0) |
| Rose (Spice Islands) | 2 T. | 10 | | | | (0) |
| White wine: | | | | | | |
| Plain (Spice Islands) | 2 T. | 11 | | | | (0) |
| Tarragon (Spice Islands) | 2 T. | 10 | | | | (0) |
| **VINESPINACH OR BASELLA,** raw (USDA) | 4 oz. | | .3 | | | 0 |

**VIN ROSE** (See **ROSE WINE**)

**VODKA,** unflavored (See **DISTILLED LIQUOR**)

(USDA): United States Department of Agriculture
*Prepared as Package Directs

373

| Food and Description | Measure or Quantity | Sodium (mg.) | —Fats in grams— | | | Choles-terol (mg.) |
|---|---|---|---|---|---|---|
| | | | Total | Satu-rated | Unsatu-rated | |

# W

**WAFER** (See **COOKIE** or **CRACKER**)

**WAFFLE:**

| Food and Description | Measure or Quantity | Sodium | Total | Satu-rated | Unsatu-rated | Chol. |
|---|---|---|---|---|---|---|
| Home recipe (USDA)[1] | 2.6-oz. waffle (7" dia.) | 356 | 7.4 | 2. | 5. | |
| Frozen: | | | | | | |
| (USDA)[2] | 1.6-oz. waffle (8 in 13-oz. pkg.) | 296 | 2.9 | <.1 | 2. | |
| (USDA)[2] | .8-oz. waffle (6 in 5-oz. pkg.) | 155 | 1.5 | Tr. | 1. | |
| (Aunt Jemima) buttermilk | 1 section (¾ oz.) | 170 | 2.3 | | | |
| Jumbo: | | | | | | |
| Plain | 1¼-oz. piece | 261 | 2.1 | | | |
| Blueberry | 1¼-oz. piece | 243 | 2.1 | | | |
| Buttermilk | 1¼-oz. piece | 267 | 2.1 | | | |
| Original | 1 section (¾ oz.) | 160 | 2.4 | | | |
| (Eggo): | | | | | | |
| Plain | 1.4-oz. piece | 265 | 5.0 | | | |
| Blueberry | 1.4-oz. piece | 260 | 5.0 | | | |
| Buttermilk | 1.4-oz. piece | | 5.0 | | | |
| Strawberry | 1.4-oz. piece | 265 | 5.0 | | | |
| **WAFFLE MIX** (USDA) (See also **PANCAKE & WAFFLE MIX**): | | | | | | |
| Dry, complete mix[2] | 1 oz. | 291 | 5.4 | 1. | 4. | |
| *Prepared with water[2] | 2.6-oz. waffle (½" × 4½" × 5½", 7" dia.) | 420 | 10.5 | 2. | 8. | |
| Dry, incomplete mix | 1 oz. | 406 | .5 | | | |
| *Prepared with egg & milk[1] | 2.6-oz. waffle (7" dia.) | 514 | 8.0 | 3. | 5. | 45 |
| *Prepared with egg & milk[1] | 7.1-oz. waffle (9" × 9" × ⅝", 1⅛ cup batter) | 1,372 | 21.2 | 8. | 13. | 120 |
| **WAFFLEOS,** cereal (Ralston Purina) | 1 cup (1 oz.) | 116 | 1.2 | | | |

(USDA): United States Department of Agriculture
*Prepared as Package Directs
[1]Principal sources of fat: vegetable shortening, egg & milk.
[2]Principal sources of fat: vegetable shortening & egg.

| Food and Description | Measure or Quantity | Sodium (mg.) | —Fats in grams— | | | Choles-terol (mg.) |
|---|---|---|---|---|---|---|
| | | | Total | Satu-rated | Unsatu-rated | |

**WAFFLE SYRUP** (See **SYRUP**)

**WALNUT:**
Black:

| | | | | | | |
|---|---|---|---|---|---|---|
| In shell, whole (USDA) | 1 lb. (weighed in shell) | 3 | 59.2 | 4. | 55. | 0 |
| Shelled, whole (USDA) | 4 oz. | 3 | 67.2 | 5. | 63. | 0 |
| Chopped (USDA) | ½ cup (2.1 oz.) | 2 | 35.6 | 2. | 33. | 0 |
| Kernels (Hammons) | 4 oz. | | 63.8 | | | 0 |

English or Persian:

| | | | | | | |
|---|---|---|---|---|---|---|
| In shell, whole (USDA) | 1 lb. (weighed in shell) | 4 | 130.6 | 9. | 122. | 0 |
| Shelled, whole (USDA) | 4 oz. | 2 | 72.6 | 4.5 | 68. | 0 |
| Chopped (USDA) | ½ cup (2.1 oz.) | 1 | 38.4 | 2. | 36. | 0 |
| Chopped (USDA) | 1 T. (8 grams) | <1 | 4.8 | Tr. | 4. | 0 |
| Halves (USDA) | ½ cup (1.8 oz.) | 1 | 32.0 | 2. | 30. | 0 |
| (Diamond) | 3-oz. bag (¾ cup) | 2 | 54.7 | 5. | 50. | (0) |
| (Diamond) | 15 halves (.5 oz.) | <1 | 9.7 | <1. | 9. | (0) |

**WATER** (See page 386)

**WATER CHESTNUT, CHINESE,** raw (USDA):

| | | | | | | |
|---|---|---|---|---|---|---|
| Whole | 1 lb. (weighed unpeeled) | 70 | .7 | | | 0 |
| Peeled | 4 oz. | 23 | .2 | | | 0 |

**WATERCRESS,** raw (USDA):

| | | | | | | |
|---|---|---|---|---|---|---|
| Untrimmed | ½ lb. (weighed untrimmed) | 108 | .6 | | | 0 |
| Trimmed | ½ cup (.6 oz.) | 8 | <.1 | | | 0 |

**WATERMELON,** fresh (USDA):

| | | | | | | |
|---|---|---|---|---|---|---|
| Whole | 1 lb. (weighed with rind) | 2 | .4 | | | 0 |
| Wedge | 2-lb. wedge (4″ × 8″, measured with rind) | 4 | .9 | | | 0 |
| Slice | ½ slice (12.2 oz., ¾″ × 10″) | 2 | .3 | | | 0 |
| Diced | 1 cup (5.6 oz.) | 2 | .3 | | | 0 |

(USDA): United States Department of Agriculture
*Prepared as Package Directs

| Food and Description | Measure or Quantity | Sodium (mg.) | Total | —Fats in grams— Satu- rated | Unsatu- rated | Choles- terol (mg.) |
|---|---|---|---|---|---|---|
| **WATERMELON RIND** (Crosse & Blackwell) | 1 T. (.6 oz.) | 210 | 0.0 | | | (0) |
| **WAX GOURD,** raw (USDA): | | | | | | |
| Whole | 1 lb. (weighed with skin & cavity contents) | 19 | .6 | | | 0 |
| Flesh only | 4 oz. | 7 | .2 | | | 0 |
| **WEAKFISH** (USDA): | | | | | | |
| Raw, whole | 1 lb. (weighed whole) | 163 | 12.2 | | | |
| Broiled, meat only, salt added | 4 oz. | 635 | 12.9 | | | |
| **WELSH RAREBIT:** | | | | | | |
| Home recipe (USDA)[1] | 1 cup (8.2 oz.) | 770 | 31.6 | 16. | 15. | 72 |
| Canned (Snow's) | 4 oz. | | 11.4 | | | |
| Frozen (Stouffer's) | 5 oz. | 660 | 29.0 | | | |
| **WENDY'S:** | | | | | | |
| Bacon, breakfast | 1 strip | 223 | 5.0 | | | 7 |
| Bacon cheeseburger | 5.2-oz. serving | 860 | 28.0 | | | 65 |
| Breakfast sandwich | 4.5-oz. sandwich | 770 | 19.0 | | | 200 |
| Buns: | | | | | | |
| Wheat, multi-grain | 1.7-oz. piece | 220 | 3.0 | | | 2 |
| White | 1.8-oz. piece | 266 | 3.0 | | | Tr. |
| Chicken sandwich on wheat bun | 4½-oz. sandwich | 500 | 10.0 | | | 59 |
| Chili | 8-oz. serving | 1,070 | 8.0 | | | 30 |
| Condiments: | | | | | | |
| Bacon | ½ strip | 112 | 2.7 | | | 3 |
| Cheese, American | .6-oz. slice | 260 | 6.0 | | | 15 |
| Ketchup | 1 tsp. | 65 | Tr. | | | 0 |
| Lettuce | 1 piece | 0 | Tr. | | | 0 |
| Mayonnaise | 1 T. | 80 | 11.0 | | | 10 |
| Mustard | 1 tsp. | 50 | Tr. | | | 0 |
| Onions | .3-oz. piece | 0 | Tr. | | | 0 |
| Pickles, dill | 4 slices | 125 | Tr. | | | 0 |
| Relish | .3-oz. serving | 70 | Tr. | | | 0 |
| Tomatoes | 1 slice | 0 | Tr. | | | 0 |
| Danish | 3-oz. piece | 340 | 18.0 | | | |

(USDA): United States Department of Agriculture
*Prepared as Package Directs
[1]Principal sources of fat: cheese, butter & milk.

| Food and Description | Measure or Quantity | Sodium (mg.) | —Fats in grams— | | | Choles- terol (mg.) |
|---|---|---|---|---|---|---|
| | | | Total | Satu- rated | Unsatu- rated | |
| **Drinks:** | | | | | | |
| Coffee, black | 6 fl. oz. | 0 | Tr. | | | 0 |
| Cola: | | | | | | |
| Regular | 12 fl. oz. | 15 | Tr. | | | 0 |
| Dietetic | 12 fl. oz. | 20 | Tr. | | | 0 |
| Fruit flavored | 12 fl. oz. | 10 | Tr. | | | 0 |
| Hot chocolate | 6 fl. oz. | 145 | 3.0 | | | |
| Milk: | | | | | | |
| Regular | 8 fl. oz. | 120 | 8.0 | | | 35 |
| Chocolate | 8 fl. oz. | 150 | 8.0 | | | 30 |
| Orange juice | 6 fl. oz. | 0 | Tr. | | | 0 |
| Tea: | | | | | | |
| Hot | 6 fl. oz. | 15 | Tr. | | | 0 |
| Iced | 12 fl. oz. | 20 | Tr. | | | 0 |
| **Eggs, scrambled** | 3.2-oz. serving | 160 | 12.0 | | | 450 |
| **Hamburgers:** | | | | | | |
| Double, on white bun | 7-oz. serving | 575 | 34.0 | | | 125 |
| Kids meal | 2.6-oz. serving | 265 | 8.0 | | | 20 |
| Single: | | | | | | |
| On wheat bun | 4.2-oz. serving | 290 | 17.0 | | | 67 |
| On white bun | 4.2-oz. serving | 410 | 18.0 | | | 65 |
| **Omelets:** | | | | | | |
| Ham & cheese | 1 omelet | 405 | 17.0 | | | 450 |
| Ham, cheese, onion & green pepper | 1 omelet | 485 | 19.0 | | | 525 |
| Mushroom, onion & green pepper | 1 omelet | 200 | 15.0 | | | 460 |
| **Potatoes:** | | | | | | |
| Baked, hot stuffed: | | | | | | |
| Plain | 8.8-oz. potato | 60 | 2.0 | | | Tr. |
| Broccoli & cheese | 12.9-oz. potato | 430 | 25.0 | | | 22 |
| Chili & cheese | 14.1-oz. potato | 610 | 20.0 | | | 22 |
| Sour cream & chives | 10.9-oz. potato | 230 | 24.0 | | | 15 |
| French fries | 3½-oz. serving | 95 | 14.0 | | | 15 |
| Home fries | 2.6-oz. serving | 745 | 22.0 | | | 20 |
| **Salad bar:** | | | | | | |
| Alfalfa sprouts | 2 oz. | | Tr. | | | 0 |
| Bacon bits | ⅛ oz. | 95 | Tr. | | | 5 |
| Blueberries | 1 T. | 0 | Tr. | | | |
| Breadsticks | 1 piece | | 1.0 | | | 0 |
| Broccoli | ½ cup (1.6 oz.) | 10 | Tr. | | | 0 |
| Cantaloupe | 2 pieces (2 oz.) | 35 | 0.0 | | | 0 |
| Carrots | ¼ cup (1 oz.) | 15 | Tr. | | | 0 |

(USDA): United States Department of Agriculture
*Prepared as Package Directs

| Food and Description | Measure or Quantity | Sodium (mg.) | Fats in grams — Total | Satu- rated | Unsatu- rated | Choles- terol (mg.) |
|---|---|---|---|---|---|---|
| Cauliflower | ½ cup (1.8 oz.) | 5 | Tr. | | | 0 |
| Cheese: | | | | | | |
| American | 1 oz. | | 5.0 | | | |
| Cottage | ½ cup | 425 | 6.0 | | | 0 |
| Mozzarella | 1 oz. | 320 | 7.0 | | | 1 |
| Swiss | 1 oz. | 450 | 6.0 | | | 1 |
| Chow mein noodles | ¼ cup | 80 | 3.0 | | | 0 |
| Cole slaw | ½ cup | 70 | 8.0 | | | |
| Crackers, saltine | 1 piece | 37 | .5 | | | 1 |
| Croutons | 1 piece | 5 | .1 | | | |
| Cucumber | ¼ cup | 0 | Tr. | | | 0 |
| Mushrooms | ¼ cup (.6 oz.) | 5 | Tr. | | | 0 |
| Onions, red | 1 T. | 0 | Tr. | | | |
| Pasta salad | ½ cup (3.5 oz.) | 400 | 6.0 | | | |
| Peas, green | ½ cup (2.8 oz.) | 90 | Tr. | | | 0 |
| Pineapple chunks in juice | ½ cup | 0 | Tr. | | | 0 |
| Watermelon | 1 piece (1 oz.) | 0 | Tr. | | | 0 |
| Salad dressing: | | | | | | |
| Regular: | | | | | | |
| Blue cheese | 1 T. | 85 | 7.0 | | | 12 |
| French, red | 1 T. | 130 | 5.0 | | | 0 |
| Italian, golden | 1 T. | 260 | 4.0 | | | 0 |
| Ranch | 1 T. | 155 | 9.0 | | | 0 |
| Dietetic: | | | | | | |
| Bacon & tomato | 1 T. | 160 | 4.0 | | | 0 |
| Italian | 1 T. | 180 | 2.0 | | | 0 |
| Thousand island | 1 T. | 125 | 4.0 | | | 5 |
| Wine vinegar | 1 T. | 5 | Tr. | | | 0 |
| Sausage patty | 1.6-oz. patty | 410 | 18.0 | | | 30 |
| Toast: | | | | | | |
| Regular, with margarine | 1.2-oz. slice | 205 | 4.5 | | | 0 |
| French | 2.4-oz. slice | 425 | 9.5 | | | 57 |

**WEST INDIAN CHERRY** (See **ACEROLA**)

**WHALE MEAT,** raw (USDA)

| | | | | | | |
|---|---|---|---|---|---|---|
| | 4 oz. | 88 | 8.5 | 1. | 7. | |

**WHEAT FLAKES,** cereal, crushed (USDA)

| | | | | | | |
|---|---|---|---|---|---|---|
| | 1 cup (2.5 oz.) | 722 | 1.1 | | | 0 |

**WHEAT GERM,** crude, commercial, milled (USDA)

| | | | | | | |
|---|---|---|---|---|---|---|
| | 1 oz. | <1 | 3.1 | <1. | 3. | 0 |

(USDA): United States Department of Agriculture
*Prepared as Package Directs

| Food and Description | Measure or Quantity | Sodium (mg.) | Total | Fats in grams — Satu- rated | Unsatu- rated | Choles- terol (mg.) |
|---|---|---|---|---|---|---|
| **WHEAT GERM, CEREAL:** | | | | | | |
| (USDA) | ¼ cup (1 oz.) | <1 | 3.2 | <1. | 3. | 0 |
| (Kretschmer) | ¼ cup (1 oz.) | 1 | 3.1 | | | (0) |
| With sugar & honey (Kretschmer) | ¼ cup (1 oz.) | | 2.3 | | | (0) |
| **WHEATIES,** cereal (General Mills) | 1 cup (1 oz.) | 370 | 1.0 | | | (0) |
| **WHEAT, PUFFED,** cereal: | | | | | | |
| Added nutrients, without salt (USDA) | 1 cup (.4 oz.) | <1 | 2.0 | | | 0 |
| Frosted with sugar and honey (USDA) | 1 cup (.4 oz.) | 19 | 3.0 | | | 0 |
| (Checker) | ½ oz. | 3 | 3.0 | | | (0) |
| (Quaker) | ⅓ cups (½ oz.) | <1 | 2.0 | | | (0) |
| (Sunland) | ½ oz. | 3 | 3.0 | | | (0) |
| (Whiffs) | ½ oz. | 3 | 3.0 | | | (0) |
| **WHEAT, ROLLED** (USDA): | | | | | | |
| Uncooked | 1 cup (3.1 oz.) | 2 | 1.7 | | | 0 |
| Cooked, salt added | 1 cup (7.7 oz.) | 640 | .9 | | | 0 |
| **WHEAT, SHREDDED,** cereal (See **SHREDDED WHEAT**) | | | | | | |
| **WHEY,** fluid (USDA) | 1 cup (8.6 oz.) | | .7 | | | |
| **WHISKEY OR WHISKY** (See **DISTILLED LIQUOR**) | | | | | | |
| **WHITE CASTLE:** | | | | | | |
| Bun | .89-oz. bun | 131 | .9 | | | |
| Cheese | .3-oz. piece | 154 | 1.6 | | | |
| Cheeseburger | 2.3-oz. serving | 361 | 11.2 | | | |
| Chicken sandwich | 2¼-oz. serving | 497 | 7.4 | | | |
| Fish sandwich, without tartar sauce | 2.1-oz. sandwich | 201 | 5.0 | | | |
| French fries | 1 order | 193 | 14.7 | | | |
| Hamburger | 2.1-oz. burger | 266 | 7.9 | | | |
| Onion chips | 3.3-oz. order | 823 | 16.5 | | | |
| Onion rings | 1 order | 566 | 13.4 | | | |

(USDA): United States Department of Agriculture
*Prepared as Package Directs

| Food and Description | Measure or Quantity | Sodium (mg.) | Fats in grams — Total | Saturated | Unsaturated | Cholesterol (mg.) |
|---|---|---|---|---|---|---|
| Sausage & egg sandwich | 3.4-oz. sandwich | 698 | 22.0 | | | |
| Sausage sandwich | 1.7-oz. sandwich | 488 | 12.3 | | | |
| **WHITEFISH, LAKE** (USDA): | | | | | | |
| Raw, whole | 1 lb. (weighed whole) | 111 | 17.5 | | | |
| Raw, meat only | 4 oz. | 59 | 9.3 | | | |
| Baked, stuffed, home recipe[1] | 4 oz. | 221 | 15.9 | | | |
| Smoked | 4 oz. | | 8.3 | | | |
| **WHITEFISH & PIKE** (See **GEFILTE FISH**) | | | | | | |
| **WIENER** (See **FRANKFURTER**) | | | | | | |
| **WILD RICE,** raw (USDA) | ½ cup (2.9 oz.) | 6 | .6 | | | 0 |
| **WINE** (Most wines are listed by kind, brand, vineyard, region or grape name): | | | | | | |
| Cooking, Sauterne or Burgundy (Regina) | ½ cup (3.9 oz.) | 657 | 0.0 | | | (0) |
| Cooking, Sherry (Regina) | ½ cup (3.9 oz.) | 657 | 0.0 | | | (0) |
| Dessert (USDA) 18.8% alcohol | 3 fl. oz. (3.1 oz.) | 4 | 0.0 | | | 0 |
| Table (USDA) 12.2% alcohol | 3 fl. oz. (3.1 oz.) | 4 | 0.0 | | | 0 |
| **WORCESTERSHIRE SAUCE** (See **SAUCE,** Worcestershire) | | | | | | |
| **WRECKFISH,** raw, meat only (USDA) | 4 oz. | | 4.4 | | | |

# Y

| Food and Description | Measure or Quantity | Sodium (mg.) | Fats in grams — Total | Saturated | Unsaturated | Cholesterol (mg.) |
|---|---|---|---|---|---|---|
| **YAM** (USDA): | | | | | | |
| Raw, whole | 1 lb. (weighed with skin) | | .8 | | | 0 |
| Raw, flesh only | 4 oz. | | .2 | | | 0 |
| Canned & frozen (See **SWEET POTATO**) | | | | | | |

(USDA): United States Department of Agriculture
*Prepared as Package Directs
[1]Prepared with bacon, butter, onion, celery & bread crumbs.

| Food and Description | Measure or Quantity | Sodium (mg.) | — Fats in grams — | | | Choles- terol (mg.) |
|---|---|---|---|---|---|---|
| | | | Total | Satu- rated | Unsatu- rated | |

**YAM BEAN,** raw (USDA):

| Food and Description | Measure or Quantity | Sodium (mg.) | Total | Satu- rated | Unsatu- rated | Choles- terol (mg.) |
|---|---|---|---|---|---|---|
| Unpared tuber | 1 lb. (weighed unpared) | | .8 | | | 0 |
| Pared tuber | 4 oz. | | .2 | | | 0 |

**YEAST:**
Baker's:

| | | | | | | |
|---|---|---|---|---|---|---|
| Compressed (USDA) | 1 oz. | 5 | .1 | | | 0 |
| Compressed (Fleischmann's) | 3/5-oz. cake | 3 | .1 | | | |
| Dry (USDA) | 1 oz. | 15 | .5 | | | 0 |
| Dry (USDA) | 1 pkg. (7 grams) | 4 | .1 | | | 0 |
| Dry (Fleischmann's) | 1/4 oz. (pkg. or jar) | 5 | .1 | | | 0 |
| Brewer's dry, debittered (USDA) | 1 oz. | 34 | .3 | | | 0 |
| Brewer's dry, debittered (USDA) | 1 T. (8 grams) | 10 | <.1 | | | 0 |

**YELLOWTAIL,** raw, meat only (USDA):

| | | | | | | |
|---|---|---|---|---|---|---|
| (USDA) | 4 oz. | | 6.1 | | | |

**YOGURT:**

| | | | | | | |
|---|---|---|---|---|---|---|
| Made from whole milk (USDA) | 1/2 cup (4.3 oz.) | 57 | 4.1 | 2. | 2. | |
| Made from partially skimmed milk, plain or vanilla: | | | | | | |
| (USDA) | 1/2 cup (4.3 oz.) | 62 | 2.1 | 1. | <1. | 10 |
| (USDA) | 8-oz. container | 116 | 3.9 | 2. | 2. | 18 |
| Made from partially skimmed milk, fruit-flavored (USDA) | 8-oz. container | | 2.7 | | | 15 |
| Regular: | | | | | | |
| Plain: | | | | | | |
| (Colombo): | | | | | | |
| Regular | 8-oz. container | 160 | 7.0 | | | 34 |
| *Natural Lite* | 8-oz. container | 182 | 0.0 | | | 4 |
| (Johanna) | 8-oz. container | 140 | 4.0 | | | 14 |
| (La Yogurt) | 6-oz. container | 140 | 6.0 | | | |
| *Lite-Line* (Borden's) | 8-oz. container | 150 | 2.0 | | | |
| (Meadow Gold) | 8-oz. container | 160 | 5.0 | | | |
| (Mountain High) | 8-oz. container | 140 | 9.0 | | | |
| (Whitney's) | 6-oz. container | 140 | 7.0 | | | |
| *Yoplait* | 6-oz. container | 135 | 5.0 | | | |
| Apple: | | | | | | |
| (Colombo) | 8-oz. container | | 6.0 | | | |

(USDA): United States Department of Agriculture
*Prepared as Package Directs

| Food and Description | Measure or Quantity | Sodium (mg.) | Fats in grams — Total | Satu- rated | Unsatu- rated | Choles- terol (mg.) |
|---|---|---|---|---|---|---|
| (Dannon) Dutch, | | | | | | |
| Fruit-on-the-bottom | 8-oz. container | 120 | 3.0 | | | 10 |
| (New Country) | 8-oz. container | | 3.0 | | | |
| (Sweet 'n Low) | 8-oz. container | 170 | 0.0 | | | |
| Apple cinnamon, *Yoplait* | 6-oz. container | 95 | 5.0 | | | |
| Apple & raisins (Whitney's) | 6-oz. container | 95 | 5.0 | | | |
| Banana (Dannon) | | | | | | |
| Fruit-on-the-bottom | 8-oz. container | 120 | 3.0 | | | 10 |
| Blueberry: | | | | | | |
| (Breyers) | 8-oz. container | 125 | | | | |
| (Colombo) | 8-oz. container | | 7.0 | | | |
| (Dannon): | | | | | | |
| *Fresh Flavors* | 8-oz. container | 160 | 4.0 | | | 10 |
| Fruit-on-the-bottom | 8-oz. container | 120 | 3.0 | | | 10 |
| (Mountain High) | 8-oz. container | 140 | 6.0 | | | |
| (Sweet'n Low) | 8-oz. container | 170 | 0.0 | | | |
| (Whitney's) | 6-oz. container | 95 | 5.0 | | | |
| Boysenberry: | | | | | | |
| (Dannon) | | | | | | |
| Fruit-on-the-bottom | 8-oz. container | 120 | 3.0 | | | 10 |
| (Sweet'n Low) | 8-oz. container | 170 | 0.0 | | | |
| (Whitney's) | 6-oz. container | 95 | 5.0 | | | |
| Cherry: | | | | | | |
| (Breyers) black | 8-oz. container | 124 | | | | |
| (Dannon) | | | | | | |
| Fruit-on-the-bottom | 8-oz. container | 120 | 3.0 | | | 10 |
| (Sweet'n Low) | 8-oz. container | 170 | 0.0 | | | |
| (Whitney's) | 6-oz. container | 95 | 5.0 | | | |
| Cherry-vanilla, *Lite-Line* | | | | | | |
| (Borden's) | 8-oz. container | 150 | 2.0 | | | |
| Coffee: | | | | | | |
| (Dannon) *Fresh Flavors* | 8-oz. container | 140 | 3.0 | | | 10 |
| (Johanna) | 8-oz. container | 140 | 4.0 | | | |
| (Whitney's) | 6-oz. container | 125 | 6.0 | | | |
| Exotic fruit (Dannon) | | | | | | |
| Fruit-on-the-bottom | 8-oz. container | 120 | 3.0 | | | 10 |
| Lemon: | | | | | | |
| (Dannon) | 8-oz. container | 140 | 3.0 | | | 10 |
| (Johanna) | 8-oz. container | 140 | 4.0 | | | |
| (Sweet'n Low) | 8-oz. container | 170 | 0.0 | | | |
| (Whitney's) | 6-oz. container | 125 | 6.0 | | | |
| Mixed berries (Dannon): | | | | | | |
| Extra smooth | 4.4-oz. serving | 80 | 2.0 | | | 10 |

(USDA): United States Department of Agriculture
*Prepared as Package Directs

| Food and Description | Measure or Quantity | Sodium (mg.) | Fats in grams — Total | Saturated | Unsaturated | Cholesterol (mg.) |
|---|---|---|---|---|---|---|
| Fruit-on-the-bottom | 8-oz. container | 120 | 3.0 | | | 10 |
| *Hearty Nuts and Raisins* | 8-oz. container | 120 | 3.0 | | | 10 |
| Peach: | | | | | | |
| (Dannon) | | | | | | |
| Fruit-on-the-Bottom | 8-oz. container | 120 | 3.0 | | | 10 |
| *Lite-Line* (Borden's) | 8-oz. container | 150 | 2.0 | | | |
| (Sweet'n Low) | 8-oz. container | 170 | 0.0 | | | |
| (Whitney's) | 6-oz. container | 95 | 5. | | | |
| Pina colada (Dannon) | | | | | | |
| Fruit-on-the-bottom | 8-oz. container | 120 | 3.0 | | | 10 |
| Pineapple: | | | | | | |
| (Breyers) | 8-oz. container | 125 | | | | |
| (Light N' Lively) | 8-oz. container | 120 | | | | |
| Raspberry: | | | | | | |
| (Dannon): | | | | | | |
| Extra smooth | 4.4-oz. container | 80 | 2.0 | | | 10 |
| *Fresh Flavors* | 8-oz. container | 160 | 4.0 | | | 10 |
| Fruit-on-the-bottom | 8-oz. container | 120 | 3.0 | | | 10 |
| (Meadow Gold) | 8-oz. container | 160 | 4.0 | | | |
| (Sweet'n Low) | 8-oz. container | 170 | 0.0 | | | |
| (Whitney's) | 6-oz. container | 95 | 5.0 | | | |
| Strawberry: | | | | | | |
| (Dannon): | | | | | | |
| Extra smooth | 4.4-oz. container | 80 | 2.0 | | | 10 |
| *Fresh Flavors* | 8-oz. container | 160 | 4.0 | | | 10 |
| Fruit-on-the-bottom | 8-oz. container | 120 | 3.0 | | | 10 |
| *Lite-Line* (Borden's) | 8-oz. container | 150 | 2.0 | | | |
| (Sweet'n Low) | 8-oz. container | 170 | 0.0 | | | |
| (Whitney's) | 6-oz. container | 95 | | | | |
| Strawberry-banana: | | | | | | |
| (Dannon) | | | | | | |
| Fruit-on-the-bottom | 8-oz. container | 120 | 3.0 | | | 10 |
| (Sweet'n Low) | 8-oz. container | 170 | 0.0 | | | |
| (Whitney's) | 6-oz. container | 95 | 5.0 | | | |
| Tropical fruit (Sweet'n Low) | 8-oz. container | 170 | 0.0 | | | |
| Vanilla: | | | | | | |
| (Dannon) | 8-oz. container | 140 | 3.0 | | | 10 |
| (La Yogurt) | 6-oz. container | 100 | 4.0 | | | |
| (Whitney's) | 6-oz. container | 125 | 6.0 | | | |
| Frozen: | | | | | | |
| Hard: | | | | | | |
| Banana (Danny) | | | | | | |
| *Danny-in-a-Cup* | 8 fl. oz. | | 2.0 | | | 8 |

(USDA): United States Department of Agriculture
*Prepared as Package Directs

383

| Food and Description | Measure or Quantity | Sodium (mg.) | Total | Fats in grams — Saturated | Unsaturated | Cholesterol (mg.) |
|---|---|---|---|---|---|---|
| Boysenberry (Dannon) *Danny-on-a-Stick,* carob coated | 2½-fl.-oz. pop | 15 | 8.0 | | | 5 |
| Chocolate: | | | | | | |
| (Colombo) bar, chocolate covered | 1 bar | | 8. | | | |
| (Dannon): | | | | | | |
| *Danny-in-a-Cup* | 8 fl. oz. | | 3.0 | | | < 10 |
| *Danny-on-a-Stick:* | | | | | | |
| Uncoated | 2½-fl.-oz. bar | 15 | 1.0 | | | 5 |
| Chocolate coated | 2½-fl.-oz. bar | 15 | 8.0 | | | 5 |
| Soft-serve: | | | | | | |
| (Colombo) | 6 fl. oz. | | 2.0 | | | |
| (Dannon) *Danny-Yo* | 3½-fl.-oz. serving | | 1.0 | | | 5 |
| **YOGURT DRINK** (Dannon) *Dan'Up* | 8 oz. | 110 | 4.0 | | | 10 |
| **YOUNGBERRY,** fresh (See **BLACKBERRY,** fresh) | | | | | | |

# Z

| Food and Description | Measure or Quantity | Sodium (mg.) | Total | Saturated | Unsaturated | Cholesterol (mg.) |
|---|---|---|---|---|---|---|
| ***ZING,*** cereal beverage, 0.4% alcohol | 12 fl. oz. (12 oz.) | 41 | | | | 0 |
| **ZITI,** frozen: | | | | | | |
| (Morton) light | 11-oz. dinner | 790 | 6.0 | | | |
| (Weight Watchers) | 11¼-oz. meal | 1,387 | 9.0 | | | |
| **ZITI,** baked, with sauce, frozen (Buitoni) | 4 oz. | | 1.6 | | | |
| **ZUCCHINI** (See **SQUASH, SUMMER**) | | | | | | |
| **ZWIEBACK:** | | | | | | |
| (USDA)[1] | 1 oz. | 71 | 2.5 | < 1. | 2. | |
| (Nabisco) | 1 piece (7 grams) | 10 | .5 | | | |

(USDA): United States Department of Agriculture
*Prepared as Package Directs
[1]Principal sources of fat: vegetable shortening & egg.

# BIBLIOGRAPHY

Dawson, Elsie H., Gilpin, Gladys L., and Fulton, Lois H., *Average weight of a measured cup of various foods.* U.S.D.A. ARS 61-6, February 1969, 19 pp.

Durfor, C. N., and Becker, E., *Geological Survey Water Supply Paper* 1812, Washington, U. S. Government Printing Office, 1964, pp. 1–364.

Feeley, R. M., Criner, P. E., and Watt, B. K., "Cholesterol Content of Food," *Journal of the American Dietetic Association,* 61, August 2, 1972, pp. 134–149.

Kraus, Barbara, *The Barbara Kraus Cholesterol Counter,* Perigee Books, 1985, 128 pp.

Merrill, A. L. and Watt, B. K., *Energy value of foods—basis and derivation.* U.S.D.A. Handb. 74, 1955, 105 pp.

Pecot, Rebecca K., Jaeger, Carol M., and Watt, Bernice K., *Proximate composition of beef from carcass to cooked meat: Method of derivation and tables of values.* U.S.D.A. Home Economics Research Report 31, 1965, 32 pp.

Pecot, Rebecca K. and Watt, Bernice K., *Food yields: Summarized by different stages of preparation.* U.S.D.A. Handb. 102, 1956, 93 pp.

U.S.D.A. *Nutritive value of foods.* Home and Garden Bul. 72, 1964, 36 pp., and revised edition, 1970, 41 pp.

U.S.D.A. Unpubl. Data 1969.

Watt, Bernice K., Merrill, Annabel L., *et al., Composition of foods: Raw, processed, prepared.* U.S.D.A. Agriculture Handb. 8, 1963, 190 pp.

# APPENDIXES

## Sodium Content of Local Water Supplies

This chart covers the largest cities in the United States and their principal sources of water supplies. The two types of resources are ground water (wells and infiltration galleries) and surface water (streams, lakes and reservoirs). Most cities use but one source; a second group always uses more than one source; a third group uses different sources only part of the year. Therefore, the column headed "% of water supply" includes both primary and auxiliary sources wherever used.

| State, city & plant, reservoir or lake | % of water supply | Finished water or raw water | Sodium (mg.) 1 cup |
|---|---|---|---|
| **ALABAMA:** | | | |
| Birmingham: | | | |
| Inland Lake | 10% | R | .5 |
| Putnam Station filtration plant | 10% | F | .4 |
| Cahaba River | 90% | R | 2.4 |
| Shades Mountain filtration plant | 90% | F | 2.3 |
| Mobile: | | | |
| Big Creek | 100% | R | .5 |
| Treatment plant | 100% | F | .6 |
| Montgomery: | | | |
| Court Street plant, 18 wells | 39% | R | 12.1 |
| Court Street treatment plant | 39% | F | 13.0 |
| Day Street plant, 31 wells | 61% | R | 12.1 |
| Day Street treatment plant | 61% | F | 12.6 |
| **ARIZONA:** | | | |
| Phoenix: | | | |
| Verde River | 12% | R | 31.0 |
| Verde River filtration plant | 12% | F | 31.0 |
| Squaw Peak filtration plant | 30% | F | 32.7 |
| Verde well field | 17% | F | 9.7 |
| Scottsdale well 36 | 15% | F | 22.8 |
| Tucson: | | | |
| Composite of southside wells | 33% | F | 15.9 |
| Composite of northside wells | 33% | F | 8.1 |
| Composite of Upper Santa Cruz wells | 33% | F | 7.8 |

| State, city & plant, reservoir or lake | % of water supply | Finished water or raw water | Sodium (mg.) 1 cup |
|---|---|---|---|
| **CALIFORNIA:** | | | |
| Fresno: | | | |
| Composite of wells | 100% | R | 4.0 |
| Long Beach: | | | |
| Long Beach well water | | R | 16.8 |
| Long Beach treatment plant | 60% | F | 17.5 |
| La Verne treatment plant | 40% | F | 46.9 |
| Los Angeles: | | | |
| Colorado River | 20% | R | 21.8 |
| San Fernando Reservoir | 60% | F | 7.6 |
| Weymouth treatment plant | 20% | F | 35.8 |
| Oakland: | | | |
| Orinda filtration plant | 99% | F | .6 |
| San Pablo filtration plant | | F | .2 |
| Upper San Leandro filtration plant | | F | 1.6 |
| Chabot filtration plant | | F | 5.5 |
| Sacramento: | | | |
| Sacramento River | 85% | R | 2.4 |
| Filtration plant | 85% | F | 2.8 |
| San Diego: | | | |
| Lake Hodges Reservoir | 10% | R | 23.5 |
| Alvarado treatment plant | 47% | F | 23.5 |
| Torrey Pines treatment plant | 10% | F | 25.4 |
| Lower Otay Reservoir | 4% | R | 21.3 |
| San Francisco: | | | |
| Calaveres Reservoir | 18% | F | 2.8 |
| Crystal Springs Reservoir | 8% | F | .8 |
| San Andreas Reservoir | 2% | F | 1.2 |
| Hetch Hetchy Reservoir | 72% | R | .3 |
| Hetch Hetchy treatment plant | 72% | F | .7 |
| San Jose: | | | |
| Wells | 80% | F | 6.9 |
| **COLORADO:** | | | |
| Denver: | | | |
| Frazer River & Williams Fork | 47% | R | .5 |
| Moffat filtration plant | 46% | F | .6 |
| South Platte River & Bear Creek | 38% | R | 5.7 |
| Marston Lake, northside filtration plant | 31% | F | 5.7 |
| South Platte River | 15% | R | 8.1 |
| Kassler filtration plant | 15% | F | 7.3 |
| Marston Lake, southside filtration plant | 8% | F | 6.4 |
| **CONNECTICUT:** | | | |
| Bridgeport: | | | |
| Easton Reservoir | 21% | R | .9 |
| Easton treatment plant | 21% | F | .9 |
| Hemlocks Reservoir | 51% | R | .9 |

## SODIUM CONTENT OF LOCAL WATER SUPPLIES

| State, city & plant, reservoir or lake | % of water supply | Finished water or raw water | Sodium (mg.) 1 cup |
|---|---|---|---|
| Hemlocks treatment plant | 51% | F | .9 |
| Trap Falls Reservoir | 26% | R | .9 |
| Trap Falls treatment plant | 26% | F | 1.0 |
| Hartford: | | | |
| West Hartford filtration plant | 97% | F | .7 |
| New Haven: | | | |
| Whitney filtration plant | 13% | F | 1.4 |
| Lake Gaillard | 41% | F | .7 |
| Lake Saltonstall | 12% | F | 1.5 |
| Woodbridge system | 12% | F | .9 |
| Lake Wintergreen | 9% | F | .6 |
| Lake Bethany | 4% | F | .8 |
| Beaver Brook Lake | 4% | F | 2.6 |
| Maltby Lakes | 2% | F | 1.3 |
| **WASHINGTON, D.C.:** | | | |
| Potomac River | 100% | R | 1.8 |
| Dalecarlia filtration plant | 45% | F | 1.9 |
| McMillan filtration plant | 55% | F | 2.4 |
| **FLORIDA:** | | | |
| Jacksonville: | | | |
| Well | 100% | R | 3.3 |
| Chlorination plant | 100% | F | 3.3 |
| Miami: | | | |
| Hialeah well fields | 40% | R | 5.2 |
| Hialeah treatment plant | 40% | F | 5.5 |
| Orr well field | 60% | R | 2.8 |
| Orr treatment plant | 60% | F | 3.1 |
| St. Petersburg: | | | |
| Cosme well field | 100% | R | 1.4 |
| Treatment plant | 100% | F | 1.4 |
| Tampa: | | | |
| Hillsborough River | 97% | R | 1.9 |
| Tampa waterworks | 97% | F | 1.9 |
| **GEORGIA:** | | | |
| Atlanta: | | | |
| Chattahoochee River | 100% | R | .5 |
| Hemphill filtration plant | 100% | F | .5 |
| Savannah: | | | |
| Abercorn Creek | 100% | R | .8 |
| Cherokee Hill plant | 100% | F | 1.0 |
| Well 2 | 100% | R | 2.1 |
| **HAWAII:** | | | |
| Honolulu: | | | |
| Kaimuki pumping station | 13% | R | 15.2 |
| Beretania pumping station | 23% | R | 8.3 |
| Kalihi underground station | 21% | R | 8.1 |

## SODIUM CONTENT OF LOCAL WATER SUPPLIES

| State, city & plant, reservoir or lake | % of water supply | Finished water or raw water | Sodium (mg.) 1 cup |
|---|---|---|---|
| **ILLINOIS:** | | | |
| Chicago: | | | |
| Lake Michigan | 100% | R | .9 |
| Chicago Avenue station | 46% | F | .9 |
| Lake View station | 20% | F | .9 |
| South District filtration plant | 34% | F | 1.0 |
| Rockford: | | | |
| Unit well 15 | 92% | F | .8 |
| Composite of 6 group wells | 8% | F | 1.8 |
| **INDIANA:** | | | |
| Evansville: | | | |
| Filtration plant | 100% | F | 3.1 |
| Fort Wayne: | | | |
| St. Joseph River (impounded) | 100% | R | 2.3 |
| Three Rivers filtration plant | 100% | F | 3.6 |
| Gary: | | | |
| Gary-Hobart filtration plant | 100% | F | 1.1 |
| Indianapolis: | | | |
| Fall Creek purification plant | 45% | F | 1.9 |
| White River purification plant | 55% | F | 3.3 |
| South Bend: | | | |
| Coquillard Station well 3 | 18% | F | 1.8 |
| Pinhook Station well 3 | 18% | F | 1.3 |
| North Station wells 5 & 7 | 18% | F | 2.0 |
| Oliver Station well 4 | 20% | F | 2.8 |
| **IOWA:** | | | |
| Des Moines: | | | |
| Infiltration gallery | 75% | R | 3.1 |
| Des Moines waterworks | 77% | F | 7.8 |
| **KANSAS:** | | | |
| Kansas City: | | | |
| Missouri River | 100% | R | 6.2 |
| Quindaro treatment plant | 100% | F | 5.9 |
| Topeka: | | | |
| Kansas River | 100% | R | 1.7 |
| Treatment plant | 100% | F | 26.3 |
| Well 2 | 1% | R | 15.6 |
| Well 3 | 1% | R | 16.6 |
| Wichita: | | | |
| Wells in Equus Beds | 100% | R | 14.2 |
| Treatment plant | 100% | F | 14.5 |
| Well 4 near Bentley | | R | 35.1 |
| **KENTUCKY:** | | | |
| Louisville: | | | |
| Ohio River | 100% | R | 3.8 |
| Filtration plant | 100% | F | 6.2 |

| State, city & plant, reservoir or lake | % of water supply | Finished water or raw water | Sodium (mg.) 1 cup |
|---|---|---|---|
| **LOUISIANA:** | | | |
| Baton Rouge: | | | |
| Lula Street plant, 7 wells | 26% | F | 17.1 |
| Lafayette Street plant, 3 wells | 10% | F | 23.0 |
| Government Street plant, 5 wells | 37% | F | 18.5 |
| Bankston Street plant, 5 wells | 27% | F | 15.9 |
| New Orleans: | | | |
| Mississippi River | 100% | R | 4.0 |
| Algiers purification plant | 3% | F | 4.3 |
| Carrollton purification plant | 97% | F | 4.3 |
| Shreveport: | | | |
| Cross Lake | 100% | R | 5.7 |
| Cross Lake treatment plant | 74% | F | 5.7 |
| McNeill Street treatment plant | 26% | F | 5.7 |
| **MARYLAND:** | | | |
| Baltimore: | | | |
| Loch Raven Reservoir | 55% | R | 9 |
| Montebello filtration plant | 55% | F | .7 |
| Liberty Reservoir | 45% | R | .9 |
| Ashburton filtration plant | 45% | F | .9 |
| **MASSACHUSETTS:** | | | |
| Boston: | | | |
| Quabbin Reservoir | 100% | R | .4 |
| Norumbega Reservoir | 100% | F | .6 |
| Springfield: | | | |
| Little River (Cobble Mountain Reservoir) | 91% | F | .7 |
| Ludlow Reservoir | 9% | F | .7 |
| Worcester: | | | |
| Holden Reservoir | 35% | F | .5 |
| Lynde Brook & Holden Reservoir | 65% | F | .8 |
| **MICHIGAN:** | | | |
| Detroit: | | | |
| Detroit River | 100% | R | 1.0 |
| Water Works Park Station | 100% | F | .9 |
| Flint: | | | |
| Flint River (impounded) | 100% | R | 3.6 |
| Filtration plant | 100% | F | 6.6 |
| Grand Rapids: | | | |
| Lake Michigan | 100% | R | 1.0 |
| Filtration plant | 100% | F | 1.2 |
| **MINNESOTA:** | | | |
| Minneapolis: | | | |
| Mississippi River | 100% | R | 1.7 |
| Fridley filtration plant | 51% | F | 1.6 |
| Columbia Heights filtration plant | 49% | F | 1.5 |

| State, city & plant, reservoir or lake | % of water supply | Finished water or raw water | Sodium (mg.) 1 cup |
|---|---|---|---|
| **St. Paul:** | | | |
| Mississippi River | 90% | R | 1.6 |
| McCarron purification plant | 90% | F | 1.4 |
| **MISSISSIPPI:** | | | |
| Jackson: | | | |
| Treatment plant | 100% | F | .8 |
| **MISSOURI:** | | | |
| Kansas City: | | | |
| Missouri River | 100% | R | 8.3 |
| Treatment plant | 100% | F | 9.0 |
| St. Louis: | | | |
| Missouri River | 34% | R | 4.0 |
| Howard Bend purification plant | 34% | F | 5.2 |
| Mississippi River | 66% | R | 4.0 |
| Chain of Rocks purification plant | 66% | F | 5.2 |
| **NEBRASKA:** | | | |
| Lincoln: | | | |
| Composite of Ashland wells, 6, 9, 54-1, -4, -7, -9, -11 | 96% | R | 5.9 |
| Lincoln wells | 4% | R | 5.9 |
| Ashland purification plant | 100% | F | 5.9 |
| Omaha: | | | |
| Missouri River | 100% | R | 15.4 |
| Minne Lusa treatment plant | 100% | F | 15.4 |
| **NEW JERSEY:** | | | |
| Jersey City: | | | |
| Boonton Reservoir | 100% | F | 1.1 |
| Newark: | | | |
| Wanaque River | 45% | R | .9 |
| Wanaque Reservoir | | F | .8 |
| Cedar Grove treatment plant | 55% | F | 1.0 |
| Paterson: | | | |
| Passaic River | 47% | R | .5 |
| Little Falls treatment plant | 47% | F | 1.1 |
| Wanaque River | 53% | R | .9 |
| Wanaque Reservoir | | F | .8 |
| **NEW MEXICO:** | | | |
| Albuquerque: | | | |
| West Mesa Station, 40 wells | 4% | F | 25.4 |
| Santa Barbara Station | 34% | F | 12.3 |
| Eubank Station, 44 wells | 50% | F | 7.8 |
| Thomas Station, 8 wells | 6% | F | 11.1 |
| **NEW YORK:** | | | |
| Albany: | | | |
| Alcove Reservoir | 92% | R | .4 |
| Feura Bush filtration plant | 92% | F | .4 |

## SODIUM CONTENT OF LOCAL WATER SUPPLIES

| State, city & plant, reservoir or lake | % of water supply | Finished water or raw water | Sodium (mg.) 1 cup |
|---|---|---|---|
| **Buffalo:** | | | |
| Lake Erie | 100% | R | 2.3 |
| Filtration plant | 100% | F | 2.2 |
| **New York City:** | | | |
| Catskill & Delaware supplies | 79% | F | .4 |
| Croton supply | 18% | F | 1.0 |
| Jamaica wells (8, 8A, 17A & 31) | 3% | F | 4.0 |
| **Rochester:** | | | |
| Lake Ontario | 21% | R | |
| Lake Ontario filtration plant | 21% | F | 2.4 |
| Hemlock Lake | 79% | R | 1.2 |
| Upland supply | 79% | F | 1.1 |
| Candice Lake | | R | .7 |
| **Syracuse:** | | | |
| Skaneateles Lake | 100% | R | 3.8 |
| Treatment plant | 100% | F | 4.0 |
| **Yonkers:** | | | |
| Saw Mill Reservoir | 18% | F | 4.7 |
| Grassy Sprain Reservoir | 17% | F | 4.5 |
| Catskill Aqueduct | 65% | F | .4 |
| **NORTH CAROLINA:** | | | |
| Charlotte: | | | |
| Catawba River | 100% | R | .9 |
| Hoskins treatment plant | 100% | F | 1.0 |
| Greensboro: | | | |
| Lake Brandt | 100% | R | .7 |
| Filtration plant | 100% | F | .6 |
| **OHIO:** | | | |
| Akron: | | | |
| Treatment plant | 100% | F | 1.5 |
| Cincinnati: | | | |
| Ohio River | 100% | R | |
| Treatment plant | 100% | F | 4.3 |
| Cleveland: | | | |
| Nottingham filtration plant | 100% | F | 2.6 |
| Columbus: | | | |
| Big Walnut Creek | | R | |
| Morse Road treatment plant | 55% | F | 13.7 |
| Scioto River | | R | |
| Dublin Road treatment plant | 45% | F | 8.1 |
| Dayton: | | | |
| Well water | 100% | R | 2.6 |
| Ottawa Street treatment plant | 100% | F | 4.0 |
| Toledo: | | | |
| Lake Erie | 100% | R | 2.8 |
| Collins Park treatment plant | 100% | F | 2.8 |

| State, city & plant, reservoir or lake | % of water supply | Finished water or raw water | Sodium (mg.) 1 cup |
|---|---|---|---|
| Youngstown: | | | |
| Meander Creek treatment plant | 100% | F | 6.2 |
| **OKLAHOMA:** | | | |
| Oklahoma City: | | | |
| Lake Hefner | 100% | R | 21.3 |
| Lake Hefner treatment plant | 100% | F | 19.9 |
| Tulsa: | | | |
| Sapvinaw Creek | | R | |
| Treatment plant | 100% | F | 1.0 |
| **OREGON:** | | | |
| Portland: | | | |
| Bull Run Headworks | 100% | F | .3 |
| **PENNSYLVANIA:** | | | |
| Erie: | | | |
| Lake Erie | 100% | F | 1.9 |
| Chestnut Street filtration plant | 100% | F | 2.8 |
| Philadelphia: | | | |
| Delaware River | | R | |
| Torresdale filtration plant | 50% | F | 1.1 |
| Schuykill River | | R | |
| Belmont filteration plant | 50% | F | 1.7 |
| Pittsburgh: | | | |
| Allegheny River | | F | |
| Aspinwall filtration plant | 60% | F | 1.6 |
| Aldrich filtration plant | 40% | F | 4.0 |
| **RHODE ISLAND:** | | | |
| Providence: | | | |
| Scituate Reservoir | 92% | R | .7 |
| Filtration plant | 92% | F | .8 |
| **TENNESSEE:** | | | |
| Chattanooga: | | | |
| Tennessee River | 100% | R | 1.9 |
| Treatment plant | 100% | F | 2.0 |
| Memphis: | | | |
| Allen well field | 28% | R | 1.8 |
| Allen filtration plant | 28% | F | 1.8 |
| Sheadan well field | 28% | R | 2.8 |
| Sheadan filtration plant | 28% | F | 2.8 |
| McCord well field | 16% | R | 1.5 |
| McCord filtration plant | 16% | F | 1.5 |
| Parkway well field | 28% | R | 4.0 |
| Parkway filtration plant | 28% | F | 4.0 |
| Nashville: | | | |
| Cumberland River | 100% | R | .7 |
| Treatment plant | 100% | F | .8 |

## SODIUM CONTENT OF LOCAL WATER SUPPLIES

| State, city & plant, reservoir or lake | % of water supply | Finished water or raw water | Sodium (mg.) 1 cup |
|---|---|---|---|
| **TEXAS:** | | | |
| Amarillo: | | | |
| Composite of wells southwest of city | 55% | F | 5.9 |
| Palo Duro well field | | R | 4.5 |
| McDonald well 2 | | R | 4.0 |
| Bush well 4 | | R | 6.9 |
| Westex well 3 | | R | 6.4 |
| Well 6, section 49 | | R | 8.3 |
| Composite of 25 wells in Carson County | 45% | F | 5.0 |
| Austin: | | | |
| Colorado River | 100% | R | 8.1 |
| Filteration plant 1 | 53% | F | 7.8 |
| Filteration plant 2 | 47% | F | 7.8 |
| Tap at 807 Brazos Street | 100% | F | 7.8 |
| Corpus Christi: | | | |
| Nueces River | 100% | R | 14.7 |
| Cunningham treatment plant | 100% | F | 14.7 |
| Dallas: | | | |
| Garza-Little Elm Reservoir | 67% | R | 9.2 |
| Elm Fork treatment plant | 67% | F | 9.7 |
| Grapevine & Garza-Little Elm Reservoir | 26% | R | 8.1 |
| Bachman plant | 26% | F | 9.7 |
| Lake Lavon | 7% | F | 3.6 |
| El Paso: | | | |
| Rio Grande | 14% | R | 39.1 |
| Rio Grande treatment plant | 14% | F | 43.6 |
| Wells at Mesa Station | 16% | F | 22.0 |
| Canutillo Station, 6 wells | 25% | F | 20.9 |
| Airport Station, 3 wells | 13% | F | 28.2 |
| Nevins Station 7 wells | 14% | F | 20.1 |
| Well V-70 in lower valley | 15% | F | 40.8 |
| Fort Worth: | | | |
| Lake Worth | 99% | R | 4.7 |
| North Holly treatment plant | 99% | F | 4.7 |
| Lake Benbrook | | R | 3.6 |
| Houston: | | | |
| Heights well field | 14% | F | 26.3 |
| East End well field | 5% | F | 41.9 |
| South Park well field | 3% | F | 38.2 |
| South End well field | 6% | F | 23.7 |
| Meyerland well | 1% | F | 20.6 |
| Northeast well field | 9% | F | 25.1 |
| Southwest well field | 18% | F | 20.4 |
| Central well field | 3% | F | 33.9 |
| San Jacinto River | 24% | R | 2.6 |
| San Jacinto purification plant | 24% | F | 2.6 |

| State, city & plant, reservoir or lake | % of water supply | Finished water or raw water | Sodium (mg.) 1 cup |
|---|---|---|---|
| Lubbock: | | | |
| City well 62 at Northwest well field | 7% | R | 30.6 |
| Composite of wells in South part Lubbock | 4% | F | 26.3 |
| Northeast well field | 13% | F | 25.1 |
| Composite of wells in Sand Hills well field | 65% | F | 6.4 |
| Well 102 in Shallowater well field | 10% | R | 24.2 |
| San Antonio: | | | |
| Market Street Station, 4 wells | | F | 1.9 |
| Wells of Bexar Metropolitan | | | |
| Water District | | R | 2.1 |
| Artesia Station, 5 wells | | F | 1.8 |
| Mission Station, 5 wells | | F | 2.4 |
| Basin Station, 4 wells | | F | 1.7 |
| 34th Street Station, 3 wells | | F | 1.6 |
| **UTAH:** | | | |
| Salt Lake City: | | | |
| Deer Creek Reservoir | 24% | R | 1.0 |
| Little Cottonwood treatment plant | 11% | F | 2.8 |
| Big Cottonwood Creek | 33% | R | 1.0 |
| Big Cottonwood treatment plant | 30% | F | 1.3 |
| Mountain Dell treatment plant | 14% | F | 5.2 |
| City Creek treatment plant | 9% | F | 1.0 |
| Artesian wells, 3rd East Station | 4% | F | 6.6 |
| **VIRGINIA:** | | | |
| Norfolk: | | | |
| Lake Wright | 62% | R | 3.3 |
| Moores Bridges treatment plant | 62% | F | 2.6 |
| Lake Prince | 38% | R | 1.1 |
| 37th Street treatment plant | 38% | F | 1.4 |
| Lake Burnt Mills | | R | 1.0 |
| Richmond: | | | |
| James River | 100% | R | .7 |
| Douglasdale Road filtration plant | 100% | F | .9 |
| **WASHINGTON:** | | | |
| Seattle: | | | |
| Cedar River | 100% | R | .5 |
| Lake Youngs purification plant | 100% | F | .4 |
| Spokane: | | | |
| Parkway well 5 | 32% | F | .7 |
| Electric well 2 | 45% | F | .7 |
| Tacoma: | | | |
| Treatment plant | 94% | F | .6 |
| Treatment plant | | F | .5 |
| **WISCONSIN:** | | | |
| Madison: | | | |
| Main Station wells | 25% | F | .9 |

395

## SODIUM CONTENT OF LOCAL WATER SUPPLIES

| State, city & plant, reservoir or lake | % of water supply | Finished water or raw water | Sodium (mg.) 1 cup |
|---|---|---|---|
| Unit well 6 | 25% | F | .7 |
| Unit well 11 | 25% | F | .7 |
| Unit well 12 | 25% | F | .5 |
| Milwaukee: | | | |
| Lake Michigan | 100% | R | 1.0 |
| Linnwood Avenue purification plant | 100% | F | 1.0 |

# Visual Meat Portions and Their Sodium, Fat, and Cholesterol Content

*(Source: USDA)*

This Thick

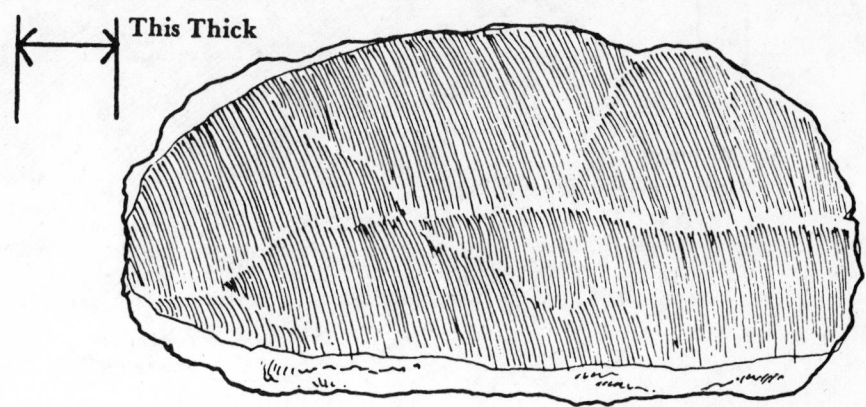

One piece of *round steak* (lean only) of this size (3 oz., cooked medium) has approximately 5 gr. total fat, of which 2 gr. are saturated and 3 gr. are unsaturated; 77 mg. of cholesterol; and 51 mg. of sodium (See also p. 50).

**This Thick**

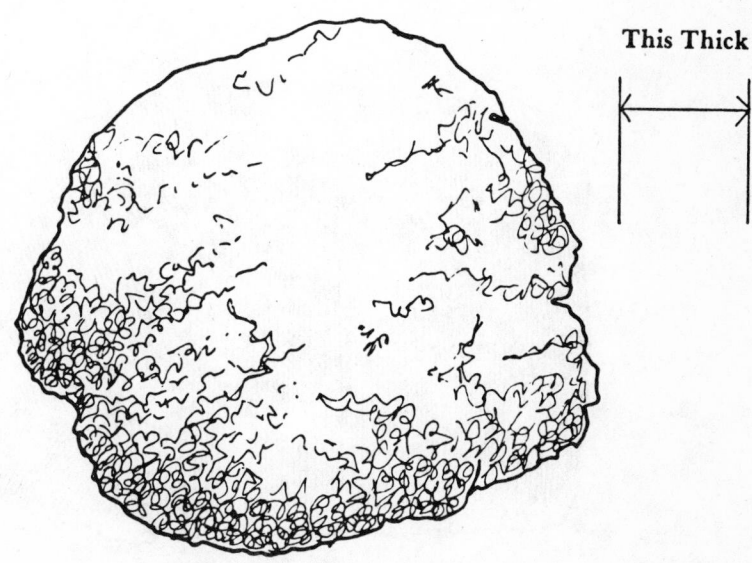

One *hamburger* (lean only) of this size (3 oz., cooked medium) has approximately 10 gr. total fat, of which 5 gr. are saturated and 5 gr. are unsaturated; 77 mg. of cholesterol; and 41 mg. of sodium (See also p. 49).

**This Thick**

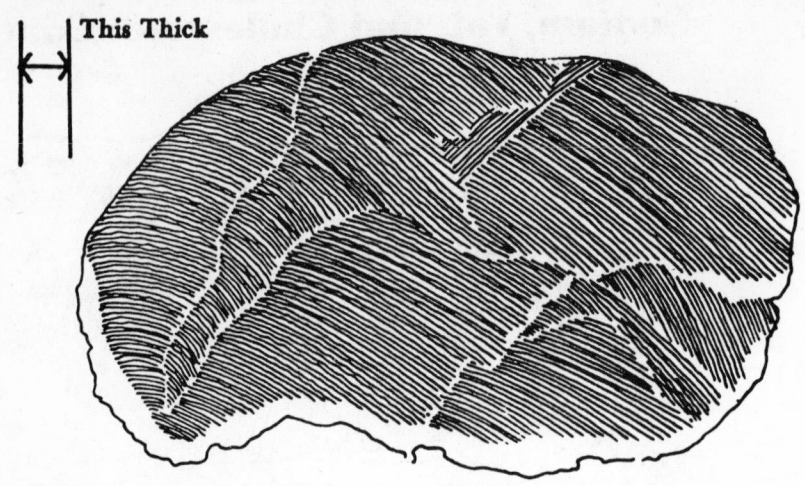

Two slices of *roast beef round* (lean only) of this size (3 oz., cooked medium) have approximately 5 gr. total fat, of which 2 gr. are saturated and 3 gr. are unsaturated; 77 mg. of cholesterol; and 51 mg. of sodium (See also p. 50).

**This Thick**

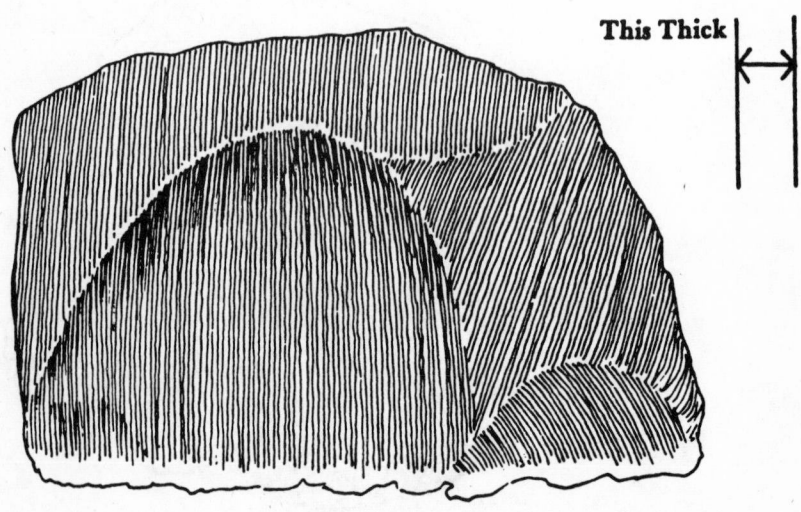

Two slices of *cured ham* (lean only) of this size (3 oz., cooked) have approximately 8 gr. total fat, of which 3 gr. are saturated and 5 gr. are unsaturated; 75 mg. of cholesterol; and 790 mg. of sodium (See also p. 282).

**This Thick**

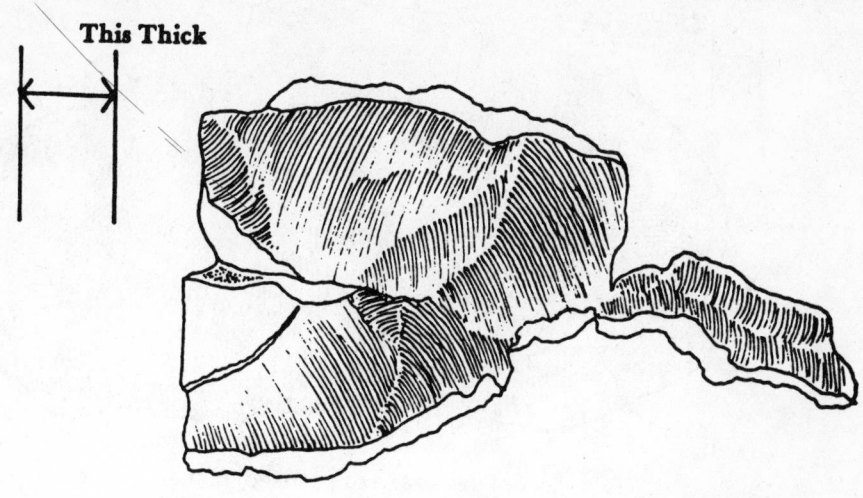

Two *lamb chops* (lean only) of this size (3 oz., cooked medium) have approximately 7 gr. total fat, of which 4 gr. are saturated and 3 gr. are unsaturated; 85 mg. of cholesterol; and 60 mg. of sodium (See also p. 210).

**This Thick**

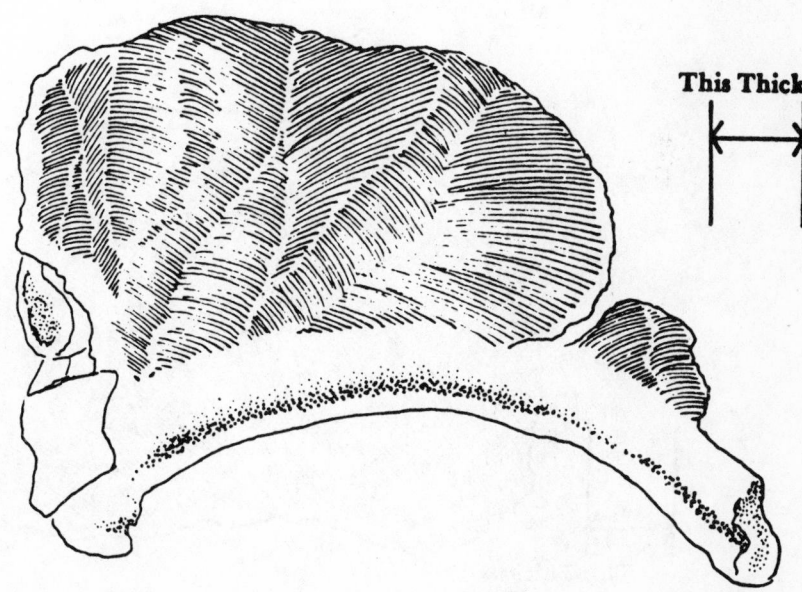

Two *pork chops* (lean only) of this size (3 oz., cooked) have approximately 13 gr. total fat, of which 5 gr. are saturated and 8 gr. are unsaturated; 75 mg. of cholesterol; and 55 mg. of sodium (See also p. 281).

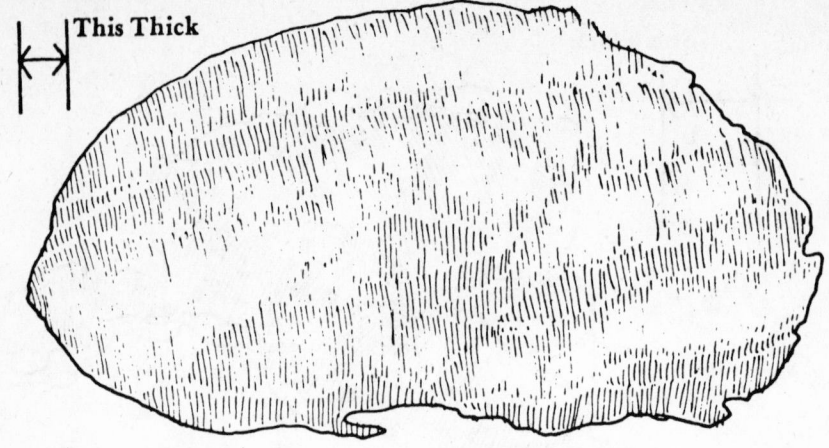

**This Thick**

Two slices of this size (3 oz., cooked) of the light meat of a *roast turkey* have approximately 3 gr. total fat, of which 1 gr. is saturated and 2 gr. are unsaturated; 55 mg. of cholesterol; and 70 mg. of sodium. Two slices of this size (3 oz., cooked) of the dark meat of a *roast turkey* have approximately 7 gr. total fat, of which 2 gr. are saturated and 5 gr. are unsaturated; 73 mg. of cholesterol; and 84 mg. of sodium (See also p. 366).

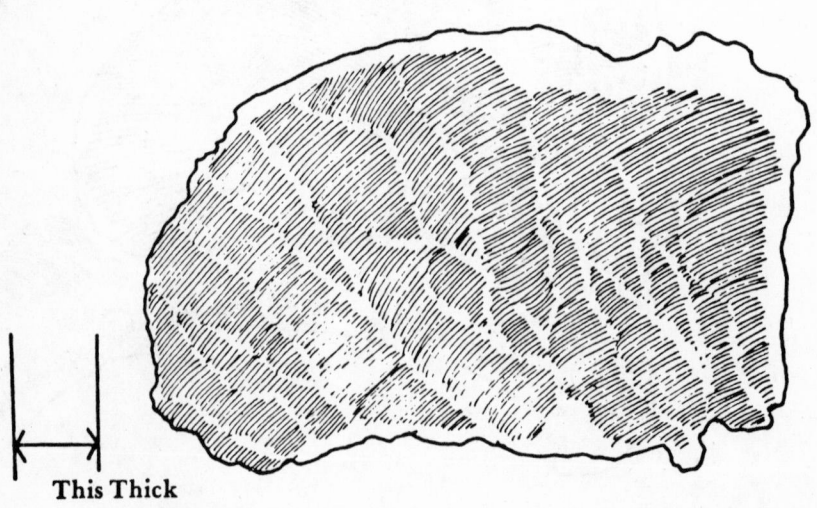

**This Thick**

One *veal cutlet* (trimmed) of this size (3 oz., cooked medium) has approximately 10 gr. total fat, of which 5 gr. are saturated and 5 gr. are unsaturated; 84 mg. of cholesterol; and 68 mg. of sodium (See also p. 370).